D1278828

The Psychosurgery Debate

A Series of Books in Psychology

Editors:

Richard C. Atkinson
Jonathan Freedman
Gardner Lindzey
Richard F. Thompson

The Psychosurgery Debate

Scientific, Legal, and Ethical Perspectives

Edited by
Elliot S. Valenstein
University of Michigan

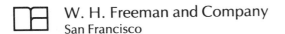

W. H. Freeman and Company
San Francisco

Sponsoring Editor: *W. Hayward Rogers*
Project Editor: *Pearl C. Vapnek*
Manuscript Editor: *Joan Westcott*
Designer: *Sharon Helen Smith*
Production Coordinator: *Fran Mitchell*
Illustration Coordinator: *Cheryl Nufer*
Compositor: *Graphic Typesetting Service*
Printer and Binder: *The Maple-Vail Book Manufacturing Group*

Library of Congress Cataloging in Publication Data
Main entry under title:

The Psychosurgery debate.

(Series of books in psychology)
Bibliography: p.
Includes index.
1.   Psychosurgery.   2.   Psychosurgery—Law
and legislation.   3.   Psychosurgery—Moral and
religious aspects.   I.   Valenstein, Elliot S.
[DNLM: 1.   Psychosurgery.   WL370 P9755]
RD594.P73   615.8'52   80-11187
ISBN 0-7167-1156-7
ISBN 0-7167-1157-5 pbk.

Printed in the United States of America

9   8   7   6   5   4   3   2   1

Contents

v

Preface

A scientist at the end of a long and distinguished career suddenly finds himself the target of a public protest and is accused of using public funds to mutilate cats in senseless research. A neurosurgeon who believes that he is offering very disturbed mental patients a chance for a more normal life is charged with using people as guinea pigs in Nazi-like experiments. Similar confrontations have become commonplace as increasing numbers of people feel that it is not only their right, but also their responsibility to monitor the social and ethical implications of new developments in science, technology, and medicine. Scientists and physicians, who had formerly never thought about these issues, have been forced to consider the social implications of their work and the limits of their responsibilities. Legislators, judges, and various public officials have had to wrestle with the problem of making decisions in complex fields.where even the experts disagree about the possible dangers and the potential benefits of different courses of action. In the process, it became obvious that our educational system had been turning out specialists who were seldom required to consider questions of ethics or social responsibility.

Traditionally, the teaching of ethics had been left to philosophers searching for those abstract principles that could distinguish ethical from unethical behavior. As honorable as that search might be, it seemed evident that there was no readily available set of principles that could resolve any of the current controversies. In fact, many of the controversies did not seem to involve differences in ethical values, as people on all sides of disputes frequently argued passionately that their position was consistent with the most noble of ethical goals. What seemed to be in dispute in most controversies were disagreements over the correct estimates of potential risks and benefits, how to resolve these disagreements, and what kinds of controls should be imposed.

In response to the deficiencies in our educational system, universities started offering many more courses designed to help people make "ethical" decisions. It is now estimated that there are at least 12,000 courses in ethics being taught in the United States, 1,000 of which are undergraduate courses in medical or bioethics. Almost all medical and law schools have introduced courses in ethics, many of which devote significant time to considering the issues that arise out of controversies about practices in the mental health field.

Because it seemed to me that there was an inadequate amount of source material available for courses in biomedical ethics, I decided to take one intensely disputed controversy, the psychosurgery debate, and to explore in depth the scientific, legal, ethical, and social issues raised by this dispute. While no single controversy can serve as a perfect model for all current concerns in the biomedical field, psychosurgery appeared to be a particularly instructive topic for several reasons. First, because the current controversy over this practice has been raging for about a decade, a great range of opinions have been expressed on all aspects of the problem. Many of these opinions raised arguments that applied equally well to almost all controversial interventions in the mental health field. Second, a commission (National Commission for the Protection of Human Subjects of Biomedical and Behavioral Research) had been mandated to study the problem and make recommendations to the government. It seemed most important to examine the procedures employed, particularly because of the possibility that a permanent commission to deal with all such issues in the future might be established. Third, a number of legislative solutions have been proposed to control or prohibit psychosurgery, and two states have had "psychosurgery laws" in existence for several years. Much could be learned by studying the effect of these legislative interventions into medicine. Fourth, lawyers have been involved in the malpractice suits that have to a great extent been generated by the controversy. Most important is the fact that several legal scholars have used the psychosurgery debate as a vehicle to discuss the special problems of mental patients either in prison or in institutions, having been committed against their will, and also to consider broad constitutional questions such as the implications of "mind-altering interventions" for civil liberties. Fifth, it was clear that the controversy did not involve only physicians and the general public. The basic research of scientists has contributed significantly to the development of psychosurgery, so that scientists are also involved in the evaluation of psychosurgery. Finally, several aspects of the psychosurgery debate made made it clear that we need to scrutinize not only the practices under discussion, but also the recommendations offered to resolve the disputes. Hastily adopted recommendations can produce consequences that are more undesirable than the problems to which they are addressed. It has become clear that no society can remain static and survive, that attempts to eliminate all risks may prove to be very costly.

Hopefully, the present volume presents a readable account of the scientific and social issues raised by the psychosurgery debate. Perhaps more significant is the fact that all the authors broadened their perspectives in an attempt to contribute to similar controversies that have already arisen or that will surely arise in the future. This volume is offered, therefore, in the hope that it will be useful not only to students in many fields, but also to scientists, lawyers, physicians, policymakers, and all those who are, or should be, concerned with the process of resolving controversies at the interface of science and society.

The organization of this book, a substantial amount of the research, and some of the writing of my contributions were accomplished while I was a Fellow at the Center for Advanced Study in the Behavioral Sciences. I am greatly indebted to the Center for providing such a congenial and supportive environment. In truth, the atmosphere at the Center was so free of any pressure that had I not produced anything under such idyllic circumstances, my feelings of guilt would have been unbearable. A sabbatical leave granted by the University of Michigan made it possible for me to work on this book. I am also pleased to acknowledge the very significant role of my secretary, Judy Baughn, who not only patiently accepted the work necessitated by many revisions but somehow managed to maintain order in the face of chaos. Judith Lehman provided very valuable assistance during the final stages of transition from manuscript to completed book. By no means last in importance is my feeling of gratitude for the valuable contribution made by the staff of W. H. Freeman and Company. W. Hayward Rogers provided constant encouragement without harassment, while Pearl C. Vapnek was most efficient in supervising the production of the volume. Joan Westcott edited all the manuscripts with awesome attention not only to small details but also to many conceptual issues, immensely improving the final version of the book.

June 1980   Elliot S. Valenstein

Contributors

George J. Annas, J.D., P.M.H.
Associate Professor of Law and Medicine
Boston University Schools of Medicine
  and Public Health
Boston, Massachusetts

H. Thomas Ballantine, Jr., M.D.
Clinical Professor of Surgery (Neurosurgery)
Harvard Medical School
  and Massachusetts General Hospital
Boston, Massachusetts

Peter R. Breggin, M.D.
Executive Director
Center for the Study of Psychiatry, Inc.
Washington, D.C.

M. Hunter Brown, M.D.
Senior Neurosurgeon
St. John's Hospital and Health Center
Santa Monica, California

William A. Carnahan, LL.M.
Partner
LeBoeuf, Leiby & MacRae
Washington, D.C.

Stephan L. Chorover, Ph.D.
Professor, Department of Psychology
Massachusetts Institute of Technology
Cambridge, Massachusetts

Suzanne Corkin, Ph.D.
Principal Research Scientist
Department of Psychology
and
Senior Investigator
Clinical Research Center
Massachusetts Institute of Technology
Cambridge, Massachusetts

Richard Delgado, J.D.
Professor of Law
University of California Law School
Los Angeles, California

Robert J. Grimm, M.D.
Neurological Sciences Institute
Portland, Oregon

Gabe Kaimowitz
Senior Staff Attorney
Michigan Legal Services
Detroit, Michigan

Alan E. Kazdin, Ph.D.
Professor, Department of Psychology
Pennsylvania State University
University Park, Pennsylvania

Vernon H. Mark, M.D., M.S., F.A.C.S.
Director, Neurosurgical Service
Boston City Hospital
and
Associate Professor of Surgery
Harvard Medical School
Boston, Massachusetts

Allan F. Mirsky, Ph.D.
Professor of Psychiatry (Neuropsychology)
  and Neurology
Division of Psychiatry
  and Department of Neurology
Boston University Medical Center
Boston, Massachusetts

Stephen J. Morse, J.D., Ph.D.
Professor of Law and Psychiatry
University of Southern California Law Center
and
Professor of Psychiatry and Behavioral Sciences
University of Southern California School of Medicine
Los Angeles, California

Maressa Hecht Orzack, M.D.
Associate Professor of Psychiatry (Psychology)
Division of Psychiatry and Department of Neurology
Boston University Medical Center
Boston, Massachusetts

Gerald T. Perkoff, M.D.
Curators Professor and Associate Chairman
Department of Family and Community Medicine
and
Professor of Medicine
University of Missouri-Columbia
Columbia, Missouri

Francis C. Pizzulli, J.D.
Weissburg and Aronson, Inc.
Los Angeles, California

Stanley Rachman, Ph.D.
Professor of Abnormal Psychology
Institute of Psychiatry
London, England

Michael H. Shapiro, M.A., J.D.
Professor of Law
University of Southern California Law Center
Los Angeles, California

Samuel I. Shuman, Ph.D., S.J.D.
Professor, Wayne State University School of Law
and
Professor, Department of Psychiatry
Wayne State University School of Medicine
Detroit, Michigan

Elliot S. Valenstein, Ph.D.
Professor and Chairman, Psychobiology Area
Department of Psychology and Neuroscience Laboratory
University of Michigan
Ann Arbor, Michigan

Introduction

Anyone who has followed the psychosurgery controversy during the past ten years is well aware of the extent of polarization of views on the subject. Opinions have been so extreme and emotions so strong that meaningful discussion of the issues has been practically impossible. The participants in this controversy assumed the position of moral crusaders. Those opposed to psychosurgery have accused their opponents of using "brain-control techniques" in "Nazi-like experiments"; those practicing psychosurgery have considered their opponents to be irresponsible "demagogues" who have prevented doctors from helping patients and have used every trick of distorting the truth to support their own political philosophy.

Recently, however, there were indications that the emotions had run their course and that most people recognized the futility of repeating the same accusations and counteraccusations. It seemed that those most actively involved in the debate might now be willing to start working toward solutions. At the very least, the time seemed right to present a logical analysis of the issues, rather than simply adding more fuel to the controversy. Therefore, I asked the principals in the debate and also others who had thought about the problem to consider the ethical, social, and legal issues that are raised by psychosurgery and other controversial therapeutic interventions in the mental health field. The great majority of the people contacted agreed to try to offer comments that would be constructive in tone, although it became obvious that strongly held positions influenced (as perhaps they should) both the form and the content of many of the contributions.

A few potential contributors, however, felt that psychosurgery could not be used as a vehicle to discuss more general ethical, social, and legal issues in the mental health field. They expressed the view that it was not possible to generalize from psychosurgery, either because the subject was too controversial or because the scientific rationale for these operations was inherently untestable. Quite commonly, it was also asserted that because psychosurgery involved destruction of healthy brain tissue it raised unique problems, and therefore it could not be used to discuss more general concerns.

After weighing these objections carefully, I decided that they were not well founded. In the first place, the very controversy surrounding psychosurgery was what made this an especially valuable topic to discuss. A great range of opinions on almost all aspects of the controversy had been expressed. Most important was the fact that in contrast to the questions raised by other controversial medical procedures, many of which could be resolved by a well-controlled study, the issues raised by psychosurgery are more varied and complex. Although any discussion of psychosurgery could benefit from reliable, valid, and current information on the outcome of these operations, many of the issues raised seem to go beyond questions of effectiveness, as usually defined. Psychosurgery might be effective in reducing or eliminating symptoms troublesome to the patient and to others, but might accomplish this (as some people claim and others deny) at a risk of reduced capacity for emotional experience and potential for creativity. Assuming for the moment that these gains and losses are real, there is no way of balancing them that can be divorced from one's personal value system. The subjective weights given to such gains and losses would be quite different when assigned, for example, by a person responsible for maintaining order in an institution than they would be when assigned by someone who regards individual expression as one of mankind's most valued characteristics.

In addition, there had been a number of legislative proposals for controlling or prohibiting psychosurgery, and two states (Oregon and California) now have "psychosurgery laws." Clearly we need to examine very carefully the effects of such legislative interventions into the practice of medicine (see Part V). Psychosurgery has also been the subject of three studies sponsored by a commission (National Commission for the Protection of Human Subjects of Biomedical and Behavioral Research) charged by the federal government with the task of holding hearings and obtaining the information necessary to make recommendations. While perhaps not without precedent, it is clear that this procedure has been used only rarely in the past. In view of the suggestion that the National Commission should become a permanent body, the information-gathering procedures used and the process of generating recommendations to Congress need to be closely scrutinized.

The argument that psychosurgery is unrepresentative of most controversial medical practices, in that it is an irreversible procedure involving destruction of healthy tissue, has to be answered. Furthermore, because it is brain cells that are destroyed, it is argued that memories, emotions, values, and all other attributes that together comprise an individual's personality are necessarily impaired. The destruction of healthy tissue is clearly a very important consideration, but not a unique one that should automatically close all debate. There are, for example, several less controversial therapeutic interventions that also involve destruction of healthy tissue and irreversible procedures, such as the removal of normal endocrine glands to arrest the growth of cancer. Although it clearly increases the seriousness of a medical procedure, the production of irreversible damage to healthy tissue is not, by itself, a sufficient reason to rule out a therapeutic practice.

Moreover, while it is certainly true that the brain is the organ most responsible for our individuality, it does not follow that all brain damage, whether it be from a tumor, stroke, accident, or psychosurgery, must have a dramatic impact on personality or even that any of its effects will be detectable under ordinary conditions. Obviously, any changes in personality or emotional or intellectual functioning will depend upon many variables, but particularly on the amount and the location of the brain damage. With respect to the irreversibility argument as applied to psychosurgery, it is certainly true that the destruction of a nerve cell is irreversible. (It might be noted in passing that the capacity of remaining cells to make new connections and to utilize other compensatory mechanisms is now known to be greater than was previously thought.) More meaningful to the patient, however, are questions about whether there are also irreversible losses in intellectual, emotional, or behavioral capacities.

Arguments about the inviolability of the brain and the irreversibility of the operations serve the very important function of counteracting any attempt to minimize the seriousness of a surgical intervention. We should never forget that the complex interrelations among the elements of the brain evolved over millions of years. The possible consequences of destroying one part of the brain should never be underestimated. Nor should we be so arrogant as to overestimate our knowledge of the way the brain functions. None of these arguments should, however, substitute for data describing the actual changes produced by specific psychosurgical operations. This is not meant to imply that the problem can be easily resolved. What needs to be thoroughly discussed is the adequacy of our test instruments and the other sources of data used to evaluate the outcome of psychosurgery or for that matter any intervention intended to change the mental status of patients (see Part III).

Another important issue raised by psychosurgery that has implications for all of psychiatry is the way mental illnesses are conceptualized. Explanatory models of psychiatric disorders vary widely, and a strong bias toward any particular model will greatly influence attitudes toward different therapeutic interventions. Many models have been proposed. Perhaps at one extreme are those theories that emphasize the importance of culturally determined values in assigning "disease labels" to socially unacceptable behavior (Kittrie, 1971; Laing, 1971; Szasz, 1972; Torrey, 1974). According to these theories, psychiatry should be considered a social science rather than a branch of biology or medicine. Szasz (1974), for example, rejects the "disease model." Describing mental illness as a "myth" perpetuated by the "mental health industry," he contends that "what people call mental illness are for the most part communications expressing unacceptable ideas." Most of the theorists in this group consider psychoses and neuroses to be merely deviant behaviors reflecting unconventional beliefs and values. Particularly subjected to criticism is the modern tendency to constantly expand the range of psychiatric diseases requiring medical treatment by including, for example, not only excessive eating, smoking, and gambling, but also criminal behavior and unconventional political ideas. It should not be surprising, therefore, that those opposed to the "disease model" have charged that many therapeutic interventions violate basic democratic freedoms in the name of therapy. This is an extreme view, and there are relatively few people who believe that most psychiatric disorders are nothing more than a society's way of labeling deviant behavior. Nevertheless, the supporters of this position have been very prolific writers and have had a significant impact in making people aware of the coercive aspects of psychiatric treatment and mental institutions.

Still others argue against the "disease model" and reject a biological or medical orientation because of a conviction that most psychiatric disorders are learned and maladaptive patterns of thinking and behaving. Behaviorally oriented therapists are primarily, but not exclusively, nonmedically trained psychologists who emphasize "principles of behavior" and learning theories in both explanations and treatment of psychological problems (see Kazdin and also Rachman in this volume).

In recent years, the number of people who believe in the appropriateness of a "disease model" for most psychiatric disorders has been growing. It is argued by those holding this view that there is increasingly good evidence that at least the more serious psychiatric disorders are caused by some biological dysfunction (Snyder, 1974; Usdin et al., 1977). They point to several disorders that in the past were considered to have a "psychogenic" origin but are now known to have biological causes ranging from viral infections to inborn metabolic abnormalities that produce biochemical imbalances in the brain. Also pointed to as supporting the "disease model" are the evidence of a significant genetic component in the susceptibility to certain psychiatric disorders and the relative effectiveness of certain classes of pharmacological agents in alleviating some psychiatric symptoms.

There is no logical reason that one should be forced to choose between the different models of psychiatric disorders, as depending on the circumstances and the particular psychiatric problem in question one or another model may be more appropriate. Nevertheless, most people tend to subscribe primarily to one model (there are many more than the examples provided), and this has a significant influence on their attitude, not only toward psychosurgery, but toward other therapeutic interventions as well. Although it is certainly possible to argue that a psychiatric disorder may be learned but best treated by a biological intervention, or the converse, most people tend to more readily accept therapeutic interventions that are consistent with their assumptions about the probable cause of the disorder.

Other issues raised by psychosurgery apply not only to the broader field of mental health but to almost all medical controversies. Psychosurgery is clearly a medical procedure about which physicians (as well as laymen) disagree. How does one decide when a medical procedure is an "experimental," "innovative," or "standard" procedure, and how should these terms be defined? In the courtroom, psychosurgery has often been called "experimental," as a means of influencing jurors by conveying the simultaneous impressions that humans were treated as "guinea pigs," that the techniques used were untested, or at least controversial, and that the main purpose of the intervention was research rather than therapy. But for the sake of clarity it is essential to distinguish these different meanings by using different terminology. It has been suggested that the term "innovative" be used for therapeutic interventions that are either relatively new or significantly changed, and that the label "experimental" be reserved for studies involving the systematic collection of research data, irrespective of the general acceptance of the therapeutic procedures employed. It should be noted that according to these suggested definitions a therapeutic intervention can be "controversial" without being "innovative" or "experimental." That is, if a technique has been used for a number of years it is not "innovative," and if the purpose is solely therapeutic it is not "experimental." It may, however, be "controversial" if there is serious disagreement about the appropriateness of using the technique at all, or for the purpose intended. A problem that has to be faced, however, is that it is not clear how much disagreement, and from whom, is sufficient to justify the label "controversial." Obviously, this question transcends the psychosurgery controversy.

In the case of a new drug, there are regulated procedures that govern its use through various stages of animal and human testing before it is released for more general use. There are no such specific regulations of "innovative" or "controversial" surgical procedures. Moreover, the problem is much more complicated in the case of psychosurgery because of obvious differences in experience and skill between surgeons. A procedure that may be highly successful after a surgeon gains some experience may have been very risky at an earlier time. When does a surgical procedure change from being "innovative" to being a "standard" procedure? One neurosurgeon argued that the fact that psychosurgical procedures are covered by medical insurance plans indicates that they are "standard" operations. Obviously, not everyone would accept the validity of this argument. How should differences in opinions be resolved, and who should be considered an expert in presenting arguments and testimony for resolving these issues? Here, too, it is obvious that some guidelines are needed, and they would have applications beyond the field of psychosurgery.

The majority of the so-called "ethical issues" that have been discussed as part of the psychosurgery controversy primarily reflect concerns about patient protection and are not exclusively psychosurgery issues. Questions about informed consent, possible conflicts between research goals and patient protection (including the morality of randomly assigning patients to different treatment groups), socioeconomic or ethnic biases in the selection of subjects used for testing new procedures, and rules that should protect incompetent or committed patients and prisoner-patients could be asked about any controversial medical procedure.

Nor are the many legal and legislative issues that have been discussed in the context of psychosurgery applicable only to this field. State legislators in Oregon and California have passed laws specifying the procedures that must be followed prior to the performance of any psychosurgery. Some people believe these laws have introduced so many hurdles that they have achieved a *de facto* prohibition and argue that medical controversies should not be resolved by state legislatures responding to political pressure. Others would disagree. In any case, it is clear that the advisability of a legislation solution needs to be examined closely, as this route has already been proposed for resolving debates over electroconvulsive shock, antipsychotic (neuroleptic) drugs, and other medical controversies. It is most important, therefore, to study the factors leading up to the passage of psychosurgical legislation and the experience with these laws since they have been enacted for what can be learned that may be applicable to similar proposals in the future.

Lastly, the psychosurgery controversy has raised the issue of using medical procedures for accomplishing social goals. It may be true that no one who performs psychosurgery believes it should be used for anything but individual therapy. On closer examination, however, it is clear that neurosurgeons and others disagree about how much criminal and particularly violent behavior is attributable to brain disease, whether psychosurgery is effective in reducing violent behavior, and whether these operations should be performed on prisoners. The interest expressed in psychosurgery by some members of the criminal justice community has aroused fears that "troublesome" people in or out of prison may be considered "sick" and subjected to procedures designed primarily to make them more manageable. The great amount of discussion of psychosurgery as a means of treating violent and sexually deviant behavior has increased these fears. Questions about the "fuzzy border" between individual therapy and social control do not apply only to psychosurgery. Most people believe that the use of drugs, for example, constitutes a greater danger of wide-scale application to social problems.

These are typical of the issues discussed by the contributors to this volume. While these complex issues are certainly not resolved, the contributors have all given a great amount of thought to some aspect of the problem. Of course, the editor could not possibly agree with all the opinions expressed, as the contributors were selected to represent different views. What is most important is that all the views need to be aired and discussed in the process of seeking solutions most consistent with the need to protect patients and to facilitate research—or, to put it more broadly, the needs of the individual and society.

PART I

Overview

CHAPTER 1

Historical Perspective

Elliot S. Valenstein

Judgments about any medical practice cannot be made in a vacuum. What may be reasonable treatment at one time may be completely indefensible in a new scientific, social, and intellectual context. Although it is not always clear whether progress is involved, medical knowledge, like other knowledge, is always evolving. It is generally acknowledged, therefore, that the "state of the art" must be considered in any fair evaluation.

Progress in medicine often results from the activities of physicians who are willing and able to explore new methods when conventional treatments seem fruitless. Until recently, however, the risks involved in these explorations have generally been assumed by the patient and not the physician; the physician could only gain if the innovations proved successful. There are obvious dangers in such an arrangement—and it is presently undergoing reevaluation as a result of malpractice lawsuits, public pressure, and a general heightened awareness of ethical issues in the practice of medicine. We are currently in a period of searching for the proper measure of restraint to assure maximum protection of patients without unduly interfering with scientific progress and freedom to test new therapeutic procedures. In essence, this is what this book is all about. Using psychosurgery as a model, the contributors have all addressed themselves to various scientific, legal, social, or ethical issues that should be considered in seeking the proper balance between restraint and freedom in medical practice.

The Definition of Psychosurgery

Among those involved in its practice, *psychosurgery* is defined as a destruction of some region of the brain in order to alleviate severe, and otherwise intractable, psychiatric disorders. In order to distinguish present surgical techniques from the earlier and cruder "lobotomy" operations, the term *psychiatric surgery* has been adopted by many of the advocates of psychosurgery. Those most opposed to these operations are likely to define them as mutilations of the brain aimed at making psychiatric patients more manageable by stunting their emotions and intellect. The question of which definition is more appropriate is best addressed by the data on the results of psychosurgery and the related discussion presented by a number of the contributors to this book.

In any case, regardless of differences in attitudes toward psychosurgery, it is necessary to focus its definition more sharply. Psychosurgery involves the destruction of apparently normal brain tissue —or at least tissue that has not been demonstrated to be diseased, injured, or pathological in any way. Therefore, brain surgery directed toward repairing damage or alleviating symptoms resulting from tumors, strokes, traumatic accidents, infections, or from other causes where evidence of brain impairment is clear, is not considered psychosurgery, even if the patient has serious behavioral and emotional symptoms (see the discussion by Mark and Carnahan in Chapter 7 of this volume).

Brain operations performed to alleviate nonpsychiatric medical problems such as movement disorders (Parkinson's disease, spastic conditions, and tremors) are not considered psychosurgical procedures, even though in most of these cases it would not have been possible to prove that the specific neural area destroyed was pathological. Similarly, brain surgery for epilepsy has frequently involved destruction or removal of portions of the brain that were not demonstrated to be the specific focal origin of the seizures. However, because the surgery is done to alleviate intractable seizures, which are

generally considered a neurological rather than a psychiatric problem, it is not viewed as psychosurgery. In some cases, epileptic
patients may also have serious psychiatric problems, and consequently it is not always clear (even in the mind of the surgeon)
whether the operation was performed primarily to alleviate the seizures or the psychiatric problem (see Valenstein, 1973, pp. 197–208,
for a discussion of these "borderline" cases).

Brain surgery to alleviate intractable pain has usually been considered a special subtopic under psychosurgery. This is not only because serious emotional disturbances frequently accompany chronic
pain, but also because the total preoccupation with the symptoms
can be quite similar to that seen in phobic, obsessive-compulsive,
depressed, and very anxious patients. Moreover, quite commonly
the same brain operations are performed (primarily cingulotomies
today, although frontal lobe and thalamic targets have been used)[1]
on patients suffering from either pain or emotional problems (see,
for example, the contribution by Corkin in this volume). The brain
targets in these cases of operations for intractable pain also cannot
by any presently available techniques be demonstrated to be pathological. Operations on the spinal cord or the peripheral nervous system to relieve intractable pain are directed toward sensory pathways
known to be conveying pain information to the brain and are not
considered to be psychosurgery.

It is necessary to make some additional comments on the question of the normality of the brain tissue destroyed in psychosurgery.
Among neurosurgeons performing these operations, there appear to
be some significant differences in viewpoint. Some of these neurosurgeons do not dispute the assertion that psychosurgery destroys
normal brain tissue, but justify the operations by their ability to
relieve otherwise intractable psychiatric conditions (see Chapter 2
on the rationale for psychosurgery). Other neurosurgeons, however,
appear to believe that ultimately it will be possible to demonstrate
that the brain areas destroyed are pathological in some sense.
Although the distinction between normal and pathological brain
tissue may seem to be a very clear issue, in reality it is not always
that clear, and the distinction may become increasingly blurred in
the future. Many neuroscientists as well as neurosurgeons believe
that we may soon be able to find evidence of brain pathology underlying some of the more serious psychiatric disorders. For them,

---

[1] See Chapter 2 for a description of psychosurgical procedures.

however, pathology is not restricted to gross brain damage; it may include also functional abnormalities resulting from chemical imbalances or differences in the responsiveness of nerve cells to the chemical transmitters of information between nerve cells.

At present, our techniques for obtaining such evidence from patients are clearly limited. Obviously, it is not feasible to remove sections of a patient's brain in order to examine them under the electron microscope or to subject them to various biochemical tests. Evidence of brain pathology is often inferred from such "soft neurological signs" as abnormal behavior and "suspicious" electroencephalographic recordings. In the future, however, it is likely that relatively noninvasive diagnostic techniques such as X-ray scanning techniques combined with injections of radioactive substances will be able to reveal biochemical deficiencies and excesses in different parts of the brain. It will be a long time, however, before sufficient data will be available to establish firmly the nature of the relationships between biochemical and other biological data and psychiatric disorders. In the interim, there is a danger that such data may be prematurely used as evidence of the *cause* of a psychiatric illness when they might actually be an *effect*.

Precursors of Psychosurgery

The belief that mental aberrations could be the result of disturbances in brain function undoubtedly goes back to primitive people's first observations that severe head injuries could produce radical changes in behavior. The practice of trepanning skulls may have begun as a means of treating head injuries. It must have been discovered quite early that the elevation of the part of a skull that was depressed after an injury could produce a very dramatic elimination of symptoms. It would be surprising if these observations did not lead to speculation that disturbances of the brain were the cause of mental aberrations even in the absence of traumatic injury. There is much evidence that trepanning for magical-medical purposes in the absence of any skull damage was performed extensively over wide areas of the world (Lisowski, 1967).

The practice of trepanning skulls to rid the brain of the offending "spirits," bad "humours," and even "insect larvae" has in fact continued up until very recent times in some areas of the world, such as certain South Pacific Islands, Algeria, and particularly Kenya. Thomas and Sandra McNett's film "Trepanation, East Africa 1968" shows the procedure as it is practiced by one tribe in Kenya as a therapeutic operation for post-traumatic headaches.[2] The young man shown being operated on in the film later wrote the McNetts that after a six-month period of recuperation and rest he had been headache-free for over three years.

While the earliest records of trepanation have been dated between 1500 and 2000 B.C., there are numerous references to its practice throughout the Middle Ages that indicate many medical authorities considered this procedure therapeutically useful (Lisowski, 1967). During the later Middle Ages and Renaissance, charlatans took advantage of earlier medical beliefs by performing "stone operations"—that is, pretending to remove stones from incisions they made in the heads of patients thought to be mad. "Stone operations" are depicted in paintings from the fifteenth to the seventeenth century by such artists as Hieronymus Bosch, Brueghel, and Jan de Bray (see Figure 1.1). The humorous nature of most of these paintings indicates the artists' awareness that these operations were performed by charlatans. Nevertheless, the fact that many people still sought out these charlatans indicates that, at least among the uneducated rural people, there were still many who believed in the "stone operations." (The expression "rocks in his head" probably dates from this time.)

The strange practice of "stone operations" could only have arisen following a period when the value of trepanation was widely accepted. Evidence for its acceptance in this earlier period can be seen in such passages as the following, translated from the Latin of Rogerius Frugardi, known as "Roger of Salerno," a leading twelfth-century surgeon.

> For mania and melancholy the skin at the top of the head should be incised in a cruciate fashion and the skull perforated to allow matter to escape [Rogerius Frugardi of Salerno].

Considering this advice and Frugardi's published descriptions of operations to repair damage to the skull, it is likely that trepanning was performed on mentally disturbed patients during the twelfth century.

Similarly, Robert Burton relates in his *Anatomy of Melancholy*, published in 1652 (cited by Sargant and Slater, 1963), that the observations that sword wounds penetrating the skull sometimes produced a cure for insanity led to operations to let out the "fuliginous humours" by boring the skull. Burton noted, however, that Alexan-

---

[2] This film, copyrighted by Michigan State University, 1970, is available through that university's Film Rental Department.

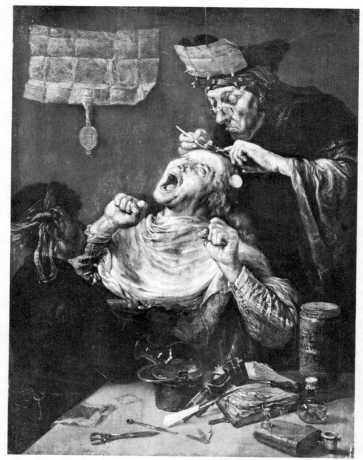

Figure 1.1 Jan de Bray, "The Cutting of the Stone," Museum Boymans–van Beuningen, Rotterdam (circa 1660). Copyright Frequin Photos.

der Messaria, a Professor of Padua, argued that these humours were too thick to be vented in that way. In one form or another, arguments and discussions about the characteristics of brain humours and their effect on mental state persisted until surprisingly modern times. Mental problems could result from the humours being too hot or cold, moist or dry, or thick or thin. Apparently, it was not always necessary to drill a hole in the skull. The sixteenth-century Dutch physician Levinus Lemnius recommended only shaving the head to allow the "grosse vapours" offending the brain to "have more scope to evaporate the fume out" (reprinted in Hunter and Macalpine, 1963).

During the seventeenth century, neurotic states were commonly called "vapours" by the English and "maladies vaporeuses" by the French, and these concepts continued to influence medical thinking in later periods. For example, the use of irritants ("counterirritants") on the shaven heads of mentally disturbed patients was common during the last century. Various animal, vegetable, and mineral substances were used to create pustules and other running sores that would allow the "black vapours" to escape. Such remedies were not proposed only by charlatans. Even the illustrious Edward Jenner, the discoverer of the smallpox vaccine, was convinced that counterirritants could cure insanity. A number of accounts published during the 1880s and even later mention the common use of counterirritation therapy in England and Scandinavia. A strange variation of the scalp irritant technique used in the late 1830s may have had historical links to the earlier stone operations. In a little book presenting medical and surgical reminiscences, Augustin Prichard recalled that:

> My father [James C. Prichard] originated the plan of making the long issue in the scalp in brain diseases; and although a strong remedy, it was sometimes undoubtedly the means of saving life. A cut was rapidly made with a sharp scalpel, through the thickness of the scalp from just above the occipital protuberance to the edge of the hair in front, and filled with a string of peas, which soon set up the needed suppuration as counter-irritation to the morbid process going on within the skull. We had, in addition, not unfrequently to insert setons [thread] or make an issue in the arm or elsewhere by incision or caustic [Prichard, 1896, pp. 19–20].

It should not be assumed that these ideas are so archaic as to have had no influence on more modern practices. The practice of placing a manic patient in warm water and cooling the head, for example, continued to be used in Scandinavian countries until the 1930s (Retterstol, 1975). Fever therapies were also used fairly extensively during the early part of this century. During this time, Wagner von Jauregg injected tuberculin, typhoid, and other vaccines into psychiatric patients, and later he infected patients suffering from dementia paralytica—also called general paralysis of the insane (GPI) and now believed to have mostly been neurosyphilis—with malaria. Jauregg received the Nobel Prize in 1927 "for his discovery of the therapeutic value of malaria innoculation in the treatment of dementia paralytica." Jauregg noted in his Nobel acceptance speech that the idea came to him after observing that "a febrile infection malady or a protracted suppuration often preceded the improvement in the state of the disease" (from Jauregg's Nobel Prize speech).

Although the terminology has changed and more contemporary physicians tend to speak of "energy" rather than "humours," it is not difficult to trace the continuity of ideas. Thus, Henry Monroe, the last of five generations of Monroes specializing in insanity, stated in 1850 (in *Remarks on Insanity*, published in London by Churchill) that mental illness could be attributed to a "depression of vitality, and a consequent morbid accumulation and suspension of nervous energy." In the 1920s, Arthur S. Loevenhart, who was on the faculty of the University of Wisconsin, tried in various ways to produce "cerebral stimulation" in psychiatric patients. In early experiments, Loevenhart injected sodium cyanide, local anesthetics, and antisyphilitic drugs into catatonic patients. Later, Loevenhart and his colleagues had patients suffering from "dementia praecox," "manic-depressive insanity," and "involutional melancholia" breathe a gas mixture containing a 10 to 15 percent concentration of carbon dioxide, a powerful respiratory stimulant (Loevenhart, Lorenz, and Waters, 1929). Very striking improvement was reported, particularly in catatonic and mute patients, and CO_2 therapy was used fairly extensively thereafter. In 1931, Walter Freeman, who not very long afterward became a leading figure in psychosurgery, experimented (using facilities at a navy yard) with the effects of high and low pressures on "cerebral stimulation." *Time* magazine ran a picture of Freeman with the caption "Give the nitwit oxygen" (Freeman, 1968, p. 28). In 1961, when the present author was visiting laboratories in the Soviet Union, he learned of a "new" experimental program that involved moving catatonic and mute patients to a station high on Mt. Elbris. It was said that when these patients returned to sea-level atmospheric pressure after spending weeks in rarefied air they frequently started talking coherently and displayed greater freedom of movement than they had for years.

Even this very sketchy account demonstrates the persistance of the idea that serious mental illnesses could be alleviated by physical manipulations, often directed at the brain. To trace the continuity of these ideas, however, is not to deny the very significant knowledge about the nervous system that has accumulated during the past 150 years. A great amount of anatomical and functional information about brain circuits has been acquired with the introduction of new techniques. The discovery of techniques for studying the effects of activating or destroying specific brain regions in experimental animals contributed important information about the function of different brain areas. The development of the cathode ray oscilloscope made it possible to study the electrical correlates of activity in different neural circuits. The electrical recording studies originating with Berger's 1929 description of the brain waves associated with different mental states started to contribute valuable information of theoretical and practical diagnostic importance by the mid-1930s. Equally important, however, was the acceptance of rules of evidence prescribed by the "experimental method." It became more difficult, but not impossible, to have colleagues accept claims that "humours" or even "cerebral energy" could be changed by one method or another unless it was possible to specify what exactly was changed and the operations used to measure these changes. In clinical medicine, however, where it was often impossible, for ethical as well as technical reasons, to obtain the measurements needed to give substance to hypotheses, styles of thinking characteristic of older periods often persisted. As will be seen later, speculations about how psychosurgery worked commonly made reference to implied processes that could neither be measured nor even adequately defined.

The Introduction of Psychosurgery

The first published record of both the procedure and rationale for the surgical destruction of a portion of the uninjured brain of a psychiatric patient was the report presented in 1891 by Gottlieb Burckhardt. Burckhardt, the director of the Insane Asylum in Prefargier, Switzerland, hoped to calm agitated and hallucinating patients by destroying the strip of cerebral cortex between the brain areas controlling sensory and motor functions (see Figure 1.2). The justification for the operation was based on a very tenuous extrapolation from the reports of changes in animal behavior following the experimental destruction of parts of the cerebral cortex. These operations were vigorously opposed by the local medical community, presumably on several grounds, but especially because one of Burckhardt's six patients died from the surgery and another developed epilepsy. Burckhardt, however, believed that one of the patients improved significantly after the surgery. Although he was forced to discontinue these operations, he expressed the "hope that my colleagues will nonetheless, while utilizing my experience, themselves tread the path of cortical extirpation with even better and more satisfying results." In 1910, Ludwig Puusepp, a well-known St. Petersburg

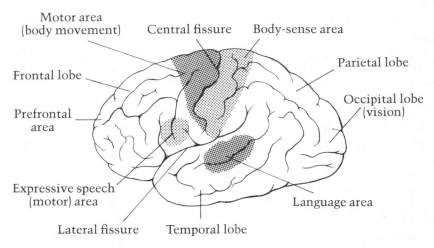

Motor area (body movement)   Central fissure   Body-sense area

Frontal lobe

Prefrontal area

Parietal lobe

Occipital lobe (vision)

Expressive speech (motor) area

Language area

Lateral fissure   Temporal lobe

Figure 1.2 Major subdivisions (lobes) of the brain and some functional areas mentioned in the text.

neurosurgeon who had been trained by the famous Russian neurologist Vladimir Bechterev, made knife cuts between the frontal and parietal brain lobes in three manic-depressive patients. Puusepp regarded the outcome as very poor and stated that he did not plan to "do any more operations of this kind." Nevertheless, in 1936 and 1937 Puusepp (1937), having moved to Italy, performed fourteen psychosurgical operations using a new procedure that had just been described by Moniz.

The Portuguese neurologist Egas Moniz is generally considered to have been responsible for triggering the widespread adoption of psychosurgery in 1935. Moniz, who was sixty-one at the time, had as a young man been made Director of the new Neurological Institute in Lisbon—as well as a member of the Portuguese parliament and later Foreign Minister—and had achieved wide recognition in neurology as the founder of cerebral angiography, a technique using X-rays and opaque dyes for visualizing blood vessels in the brain. Obviously a man in a position to have a great influence, Moniz started prefrontal psychosurgical procedures in 1935 just a few months after listening to Carlyle Jacobsen present his paper at the Second International Neurological Conference in London. Jacobsen reported that destruction of the prefrontal brain area of monkeys and chimpanzees produced a number of deficits in various problem-solving tasks, but what seemed to impress Moniz most was the observation that some of the more excitable animals became much calmer following the surgery.[3]

Initially, Moniz and his colleague Almeida Lima used alcohol injections to destroy a portion of the frontal lobes of psychiatric patients, but they soon switched to a technique of cutting nerve fibers with a surgical leucotome (leuco—white nerve fibers; tome—a cutting instrument). In a monograph published in French in 1936, not very long after he and Lima started to operate, Moniz reported very encouraging results from the initial 20 patients. The first operation was performed on November 12, 1935, on a sixty-three-year-old former prostitute with syphilis, who was diagnosed as an involutional melancholic. She had a history of being in and out of mental institutions and prisons and was considered psychotic. Two months after the lobotomy (a time clearly too short for an adequate judgment), Moniz reported that the patient was cured. In total, Moniz reported in his monograph that 7 patients were cured, 7 improved, and 6 unimproved. It is really not surprising that these results, reported by a highly respected neurologist at a time when psychiatry was offering so little help to the more seriously ill mental patients, encouraged neurosurgeons and neuropsychiatrists around the world to explore the usefulness of psychosurgery.

Although they were not the first to adopt prefrontal lobotomy after Moniz's report,[4] Walter Freeman and James Watts were destined to play the major part in popularizing these operations. Watts was the neurosurgeon of this team, but Freeman, who was a neuropsychiatrist, was clearly the major spokesman for psychosurgery in the United States, if not worldwide. Often described in disparaging terms by those opposed to psychosurgery, Freeman was in fact a complex personality—intelligent, extremely hard-working, dedicated to his work and patients, and prolific in his writing and lecturing, and at the same time ambitious, status-seeking, and flam-

---

[3]Moniz heatedly denied that it was Jacobsen's report on animal experiments that gave him the idea of trying psychosurgery; he claimed that he had been thinking along these lines for several years prior to 1935 (Moniz, 1956). Nevertheless, the fact that Moniz stood up after Jacobsen's presentation and asked "Why would it not be feasible to relieve anxiety states in man by surgical means?" and the fact that the first of the operations was performed only a few months after the conference suggested that at the very least the animal experiments served as a catalyst.

[4]Freeman and Watts (1950, p. xx) state that Lyerly, Grant, Love, Mixter, Davidoff, Myers, and Glaser were among the first to perform prefrontal lobotomies in the United States. They also mention Mattos Pimenta's four cases from Brazil in 1937 and Ramirez Corria's three cases from Cuba. Rizzatti and several other Italian neurosurgeons also performed these operations very soon after Moniz.

boyant.[5] A well-trained neuropsychiatrist, Freeman had a Ph.D. in neuroanatomy as well as a medical degree and had written a well-regarded book on neuropathology before becoming involved in psychosurgery. He was well organized in his work and could even be compulsive about details, but he also had a flair for the dramatic. Watts' earliest recollection of seeing the man who was to become his lifetime associate was at a neurology conference in Atlantic City, where Freeman "strolled down the boardwalk wearing a beard (when beards were not in fashion), a Texas sombrero, and carrying a cane."

Freeman loved performing under the spotlight. He carefully planned his presentations at meetings so that they would receive maximum coverage by the media. Dax [1977] recalled that Freeman learned Portuguese specially for the First International Congress on Psychosurgery held in Lisbon in 1948 and commented on his "tremendous energy," which "scattered the considerable opposition" to psychosurgery. In the exhibit halls at scientific meetings, he often behaved like a barker at a circus, using a "cricket" noisemaker to attract people to his booth. Nor was Freeman shy and retiring in his professional activities. He was eager to try most new physical therapies. Prior to turning to psychosurgery, Freeman had been the first physician in Washington, D.C., to use insulin, metrazol, and electroshock treatment. Also characteristic was Freeman's comment on Benjamin Rush's "gyrator." Rush, the eighteenth-century physician who has been called the "father of American psychiatry," had invented a whirling frame upon which a patient could be strapped and then rotated, with the head outward, in order to force more blood into the brain. Freeman commented: "To my knowledge, the human centrifuge has not been tried in mental disorders. Maybe it should be" [Freeman, 1968, p. 152]. He was clearly a man anxious to make a great impact and destined to do so. Freeman seemed to have been guided by the advice given by John Bunyan more than three centuries ago:

> Physicians get neither name nor fame by pricking of wheals or picking out thistles or by laying of plasters to the scratch of a pin; every old woman can do this. But if they would have a name and a fame, if they will have it quickly, they must do some great and desperate cures. Let

---

[5] An interesting description of Freeman was presented by Watts in a talk entitled "Psychosurgery: The Story of the 20 Year Follow-up of the Freeman and Watts Lobotomy Series," delivered on November 4, 1974, to the Instituto Nacional de Neurologia in Mexico City. I am indebted to Dr. Watts for providing me with a copy of this unpublished talk.

them fetch one to life that was dead; let them recover one that was born blind to see, or let them give ripe wits to a fool. These are notable cures and he that can do thus, if he doth thus first, shall have the name and fame he deserves [cited by Porteus and Kepner, 1944, p. 8].

It would be a gross distortion, however, to describe Freeman as merely a hard-working self-promoter. In spite of the callous way he sometimes described patients, Freeman seemed to have a genuine, if somewhat paternalistic, concern for them. He followed up his patients for years, sometimes making a great number of telephone calls to track them down when he had lost contact. He exchanged Christmas cards and letters with them and kept careful records of their current states. At the end of his life, when he was suffering from cancer, he collected additional postoperative information by traveling around the country in a small van visiting former patients. He kept records on some patients for over thirty-five years, and, as Watts observed, he did all this "without support of any grants and without charging for postoperative consultations."

Considering his personality and also the fact that his exhibit booth at the 1935 Neurology Conference in London was next to Moniz's, it was not surprising that Freeman was quick to adopt psychosurgery. Freeman also received one of the earliest copies of Moniz's 1936 monograph in the United States. In September 1936, Freeman and Watts performed their first psychosurgical operations at George Washington University. Moniz and Lima's surgical technique was soon modified and the Freeman-Watts "standard" lobotomy procedure was developed. Other U.S. surgeons were also performing various lobotomy procedures (see Chapter 2 and Valenstein, 1973, for details on the evolution of psychosurgical procedures).

The Growth and Decline of Psychosurgery

Numerous histories of psychosurgery have been written by neurosurgeons and psychiatrists actively engaged in its practice and by persons from many different professions and widely differing attitudes toward this practice (for example, Freeman and Watts, 1950; Breggin, 1972a; Valenstein, 1973; Robin and Macdonald, 1975; Vaughan, 1975; Dax, 1977). There is little point in repeating this same information in detail here. For our purpose—establishing the background of the present controversy—it is more appropriate to emphasize the social and intellectual factors that stimulated both the growth of psychosurgery and the opposition to its practice.

Over the years many factors have helped to shape attitudes towards psychosurgery, but three of these were particularly important in creating the initial climate of receptivity to psychosurgery. First, as was mentioned previously, the belief that disturbances of the brain could be the cause of mental illness was a very old and widely held idea. Moreover, belief that at least the more serious mental illnesses would eventually be traced to brain aberrations may well have been the prevailing opinion during the late 1930s, when psychosurgery was introduced. This is not to deny the fact that it had been recognized for a long time that experiences could be the cause of some mental illness. But modern psychiatry has its roots in neurology, and most psychiatrists during the nineteenth century and early part of this century were trained in neurology and tended to emphasize biological causes and physical therapies. Parenthetically, it might be noted that to this day the specialties of neurology and psychiatry are not separate in Germany. This intellectual climate certainly made it easier to accept the idea that a brain operation such as psychosurgery could alleviate either the cause of intractable mental illnesses or the basis for their persistence.

An equally important factor contributing to the acceptance of psychosurgery was the lack of effective alternative treatments for serious mental illnesses. Psychotherapy was very time-consuming and, more important, generally ineffective. The main alternatives were other new physical therapies such as insulin coma and electric shock treatments, and these were clearly not successful in many instances. It is important to recall that during the period between 1936 and 1953, when psychosurgery was experiencing its greatest growth, there were no pharmacological treatments available. Chlorpromazine, the first psychoactive drug produced commercially, was not introduced until 1952, and it was not used widely enough to have a significant influence until after 1954. Psychiatric institutions were becoming increasingly crowded as more patients were being admitted than were discharged. The large number of World War II veterans requiring psychiatric treatment exacerbated the problem. There was clearly a desperate need to do something to remedy the situation. An editorial in *Lancet* (1972) described this period:

> such was the enormous pool of psychotic patients vegetating as chronic sick in the closed wards of mental hospitals, without effective drug control and without hope, that when it became possible to help them in any way, this new method was taken up with more enthusiasm than caution and with more technical skill than psychiatric and neurophysiological understanding [Editorial, *Lancet*, 1972, p. 69].

A third factor that contributed to the acceptance and rapid growth of psychosurgery was the relative newness of neurosurgery as a separate field. In the 1930s, neurosurgery was still a young discipline with very few specialists. The Society of Neurological Surgeons was not organized until 1920, and then only with eleven members. The *Journal of Neurosurgery*, the first journal published in English that was exclusively devoted to neurosurgery, did not appear until 1944. A 1937 review of neurosurgery began with the statement: "Neurosurgery is still a youth among the medical and surgical specialties, and as such, its development continues to be rapid, its complexion to change almost from day to day" (Pilcher, 1937). In this state, the field of neurosurgery was particularly responsive to influence from a small number of its more prominent members, who persuaded their fellow neurosurgeons that psychosurgery produced desirable results and that there was a reasonably good scientific rationale to explain why these operations worked.

It is important to try to reconstruct the growth of psychosurgery as accurately as possible, not because the exact numbers are so important, but because the record tends to reveal some of the factors that influence the process of growth and decline in the use of a medical procedure. Psychosurgery was practiced to some degree in almost all countries where neurosurgery was relatively advanced. Although the first report of psychosurgery did not appear until 1941 in England, by that time there was evidence that psychosurgical operations had been performed in Italy, France, Romania, Brazil, and Cuba, as well as in several different locations in the United States (Hutton et al., 1941). It has been estimated that between 350 and 500 psychosurgical operations had been performed throughout the world by 1941, with the 185 cases reported by Rizzatti in Italy being the largest number done by a single surgeon (Hutton, Fleming, and Fox, 1941). The following year, Freeman and Watts' book *Psychosurgery* was published. This book presented an impressive amount of anatomical detail about the frontal lobes and their connections to other parts of the brain, and in the process it surely created the impression of a much more solid scientific basis for psychosurgery than actually existed. A number of people have commented that Freeman and Watts' *Psychosurgery* was responsible for a dramatic increase in the amount of psychosurgery performed throughout the world (Dax, 1977; Walsh, 1978). The Freeman-Watts standard lobotomy technique was adopted by many neurosurgeons, including the Japanese during World War II. In addition to the countries already noted, by the end of the 1940s psychosurgery had been performed in the Soviet Union, Canada, Australia, Japan, and in a number of European and South American countries.

As already noted, the widespread adoption of psychosurgery can be understood in part by the pressing need for psychiatric treatment and the few alternatives that existed at the time. World War II made it evident that psychotherapy was inadequate to deal with the large number of psychiatric patients crowding hospital facilities. The psychiatrist William Menninger wrote that of the 15 million men examined for admission to the armed forces of the United States during World War II, 12 percent (1,846,000) were rejected for psychiatric reasons and 632,000 were discharged because of "mental breaks" after admission. With no pharmacological treatments available, little could be done for them. Soldiers and veterans often seemed to be just deteriorating in army and VA psychiatric facilities, and their families began to clamor for some effective treatment. The urgent need for an "efficient" treatment to cope with the many psychiatrically disturbed soldiers and veterans of World War II, combined with the optimistic reports of the results of prefrontal lobotomy, resulted in a wide-scale adoption of psychosurgery. In 1943, the Veterans' Administration issued a communication encouraging staff neurosurgeons affiliated with their hospitals to obtain special training in prefrontal lobotomy operations. Once trained, most of these neurosurgeons began to perform lobotomies in other hospitals as well.

One factor that undoubtedly increased the number of operations performed in the United States was Freeman's popularization of the transorbital lobotomy operation in the late 1940s. An Italian surgeon, Fiamberti, had originated the technique but appeared to have lost interest in pursuing it after having performed about 100 operations by early 1948. After experimenting on cadavers, Freeman performed his first transorbital lobotomy in January 1946. The only instrument needed was a simple penetrating and cutting tool, which was forced through the bony orbit over the eye to enter the region of the frontal lobes (see Valenstein, 1973, and Chapter 2 for a description of this technique). Freeman designed this tool, and in his characteristically blunt manner he referred to its resemblance to an ice pick. Thereafter, opponents of the technique referred to the operation as "ice pick surgery." Because transorbital lobotomies were relatively easy to perform and electroconvulsive shock was frequently used in place of anesthesia, the surgery was commonly performed by psychiatrists without the involvement of neurosurgeons, anesthetists, and surgical amphitheaters. In some instances, the operation was performed as an office procedure and the patient was taken home by the family a few hours after the operation. In the 1950 edition of Freeman and Watts' Psychosurgery, it is noted that Freeman had already performed around 400 transorbital operations since his first in 1946. Although Watts admitted that mortality and morbidity were less following transorbital lobotomies than following the standard Freeman-Watts operation, he objected to Freeman's attitude that this new procedure was a "minor operation." Pointing out that "of the first ten cases he [Freeman] reported, four were not disabled and six had been disabled less than six months"—that is, prior to the operation—he expressed his concern that transorbital lobotomies might be used too casually (Freeman and Watts, 1950, pp. 57–61). According to figures compiled by the National Institute of Mental Health, one-third of all psychosurgery in the United States between 1949 and 1951 used the transorbital procedure (Kramer, 1954), and only three years after its introduction the number of transorbital operations exceeded all other psychosurgical operations in state hospitals (Limburg, 1951). Before his retirement, Freeman had performed (or supervised) almost 3,600 psychosurgical operations; 600 were the standard Freeman-Watts lobotomies and 3,000 were transorbital lobotomies.

It is impossible to obtain accurate figures on the total number of prefrontal lobotomies (of one type or another) performed around the world. In England and Wales, one survey summarized the results on 10,365 patients lobotomized between 1942 and 1954 (Tooth and Newton, 1961), but this study did not include all of the psychosurgery done in the United Kingdom. Sargant and Slater (1963) estimated that 15,000 operations had been performed in Great Britain by 1962. Individual neurosurgeons reported large numbers of operations. For example, by April 1946, McKissock in London had performed his 500th operation, and Poppen (1948) at the Lahey Clinic in Boston reported having done 470 prefrontal lobotomies between 1943 and 1948. Baretto of São Paulo reported the results of 412 operations at the First International Congress of Psychosurgery held in 1948. It is generally agreed that the rate of performing these operations significantly decreased around the world after 1955, and the decline probably started a year or two before that date. One indication of the growth and decline in interest in psychosurgery is the number of publications on the topic. Using the listings in the Library of the Royal Society of Medicine, Kelly (1975) found that between 1936 and 1941 there were less than 12 publications a year. This figure increased to 300 per year by 1951, but then gradually decreased to about 12 a year during the 1960s.

It is frequently stated that 50,000 operations were performed in the United States during the "first wave" of lobotomies (for example, Breggin, 1972a), but this figure has not been supported by any documentation and probably is on the high side. In 1942, when Freeman and Watts published the first edition of *Psychosurgery*, they reported the results of operations on 80 patients. The great influence of this book has been already noted. Other U.S. surgeons were also performing various lobotomy procedures, and, according to a report in *Time* (Nov. 30, 1942, p. 46), a total of 300 psychosurgical operations had been performed in the United States by 1942. The rate of performing lobotomies began to increase, and by 1946 *Time* (Dec. 23, 1946, p. 67) reported that a total of 2,000 lobotomies had been done in the United States with "sensational results"; 200 of these operations had been done at the Boston Psychiatric Hospital. A few months later, *Life* confirmed (or simply repeated) the figure of 2,000 operations in the United States, performed, according to this account, "only on 'hopeless' patients who had failed to respond to other methods of treatment, people who had little to lose and everything to gain." *Life* concluded:

> The results were spectacular: about 30% of the lobotomized patients were able to return to everyday productive lives. Another 30% benefited considerably, finding relief from the painful anxiety and profound depression that their psychoses inflicted on them. The rest were mostly unaffected [*Life*, March 3, 1947, p. 93].

There is evidence that the article in *Life* and others like it in the popular press had a significant influence in increasing the referrals from psychiatrists and the requests from patients for these operations (Mayer, 1947–48; Koskoff and Goldhurst, 1968).[6] By 1950, when the second edition of *Psychosurgery* was published, Freeman and Watts could report the results of 1,000 of their operations.

Limburg (1951) surveyed 855 U.S. institutions, "including all Federal, State, private, and other mental hospitals, general hospitals with psychiatric wards, and all medical schools," and estimated that 150 operations were performed in 1945; 496 operations in 1946; 1,171 in 1947; 2,281 in 1948; and 5,074 in 1949. In total, it was calculated that 10,706 psychosurgical operations had been performed from 1936 through August 15, 1949. According to Limburg's

---

[6] A recent article in the *Reader's Digest* entitled "Should We Halt the Brain Probers? Evidence Indicates that Psychosurgery Can Help Many Victims of Severe Psychiatric Disorders" (Methvin, 1979) took a very pro-psychosurgery position and has produced a very similar effect. The article was written by a layman, who obviously depended on one neurosurgeon for most of his evidence. Over thirty million copies (in fifteen languages) of the *Reader's Digest* are sold each month. Although not a physician, the present author (ESV) received three phone calls from persons who were now thinking about psychosurgery after reading the article. More significant is the fact that the neurosurgeon cited in the article, H. Thomas Ballantine, has been "flooded" by inquiries that were clearly the result of this article.

survey, 56 percent of the operations had been performed in state hospitals, 16 percent in medical schools, 12 percent in Veterans' Administration hospitals, and 6 percent in private hospitals. (The remaining 10 percent were performed in other "psychopathic," city, and federal hospitals.) Freeman and Watts must have performed about 10 percent of these operations themselves, because in 1950, when the second edition of their book *Psychosurgery* was published, they reported results of 1,000 of their own operations. By 1951, 286 hospitals reported that they were practicing psychosurgery, whereas only 49 hospitals were engaged in this practice in 1945 (Kramer, 1954). There were only five states (Idaho, Maine, New Mexico, North Dakota, and Utah) in which no psychosurgery was performed in public hospitals between January 1, 1949 and June 30, 1951. In the last of the three Research Conferences on Psychosurgery sponsored by the National Institutes of Health during the early 1950s, Kramer (1954) reported the results of his survey, which indicated that there were a total of 18,608 operations performed in the United States from 1936 to June 30, 1951. Although a few operations were probably not included in the survey, these figures were probably quite accurate, as 897 of the 951 hospitals surveyed (94 percent) responded to Kramer's questionnaire. The nonresponding hospitals generally had small numbers of patients and were not known to be institutions where psychosurgery was being performed.

In Limburg's survey, 58 percent of the 164 hospitals reporting the use of psychosurgery in 1949 indicated that they expected the number of operations to increase in the future. In spite of this expectation of an increase, Kramer concluded from his 1951 survey that the number of operations showed a slight decline from its peak in 1949. Kramer reported that in 1950 there were 4,861 operations, but he estimated (projected from data obtained for the first six months) that the number declined to 4,700 during 1951. Everyone seems to agree that the rate had started to decline before 1955 and that it dropped very significantly after 1955. There are no accurate figures for the years 1952–1955, but given the increasing opposition to psychosurgery and the availability of psychoactive drugs, the total number of operations for this period probably did not exceed 10,000. Considering the general disfavor into which psychosurgery had fallen after 1955, a figure of 500 operations per year is probably a reasonably accurate estimate for the average for the years 1956 through 1978 (see Valenstein, 1977, and Chapter 3 for summaries of more recent surveys). These estimates and figures obtained from surveys indicate that approximately 35,000 psychosurgical operations were performed in the United States from 1936 through 1978.

The Early Psychosurgery Controversy

Although many people placed great hope in psychosurgery as a means of helping psychiatric patients (as indicated by Moniz's receipt of the 1949 Nobel Prize "for his discovery of the therapeutic value of prefrontal leucotomy in certain psychoses"), there was much opposition to this practice from the outset. Two contrasting editorials capture some of the flavor of this controversy:

The Lobotomy Delusion

. . . Lobotomy for frontal lobe malignant tumor we can understand, but by this extended lobotomy, one is supposed to be able to "pluck from the brain a hidden sorrow." It is claimed it can ameliorate or cure people suffering from obsessional and compulsion neuroses, and even bring restitution to the more cyclical and obstinate disorder. . . . we recommend these aspirants for neurosurgical honors to read and digest Karl Menninger's remarks on poly surgical castration devices, not those of strictly phallic significance but those that maim and destroy the creative functions of a non-mutilated body.

In the name of Madame Rowland who cried aloud concerning the many crimes committed in the cause of "liberty" we would call the attention of these mutilating surgeons to the Hippocratic oath [Unsigned editorial, *Medical Record*, 1940, *151*, 335].

The 1949 Nobel Prize in Medicine

The Nobel Prize for 1949 in medicine has been awarded [to] . . . Dr. Egas Moniz, a former professor of neurology in the University of Lisbon [who] . . . devised the revolutionary brain operation of prefrontal leucotomy, later known as lobotomy, now widely used in the treatment of certain forms of mental disease. In the last thirteen years, since his report in 1936, thousands of such operations, now modified into various patterns, have been carried out in many parts of the world, greatly to the betterment of patients with the more serious and prolonged types of mental aberration. A new psychiatry may be said to have been born in 1935, when Moniz took his first bold step in the field of psychosurgery [Editorial by Dr. Henry P. Viets, *New England Journal of Medicine*, 1949, *1241*, 1025–1026].

Other early evidence of the controversy can be gleaned from the fact that in 1949 the *Stanford Law Review* considered the possibility of drafting a statute regulating the use of lobotomy but concluded that "the greater good will be achieved by avoiding legislative fetters and relying for protection on the high standards of the medical profession and the individuals who compose it." The Soviet Union reached a different conclusion and outlawed psychosurgery in 1951 (Khachaturyan, 1951; but see the evidence in Chapter 2 that electrical stimulation is currently being used).

Opinions on psychosurgery have been divided almost since the practice's inception, with some viewing psychosurgery as a mutilation of the brain designed to eliminate troublesome behavior by transforming humans into permanent emotional and intellectual "vegetables" and others consistently asserting that these operations make it possible for patients who were suffering from crippling and otherwise intractable mental illnesses to live normal (or close to normal) lives. It has been proven very easy to select data to support either position. There is no doubt that there were a number of instances during the early lobotomy era in which patients died or suffered serious neurological consequences as a result of the surgery. Fatalities varied between 1.5 percent and 6 percent in different samples. (A 1947 report from the Joint Committee of State Mental Hospitals in Connecticut indicated that their record of 6 deaths (4 percent) out of 125 operations was below the national average.) The more common physical sequelae included epileptic seizures, incontinence, partial paralysis, huge weight gain, impairment of motor coordination, and endocrine problems. After the operation, some patients became emotionally unresponsive ("zombies"), while others became happy in a very shallow and irresponsible way. Many lobotomized patients showed just the opposite reaction and were characterized as "affectively incontinent," lacking tact and restraint in social relationships. It was frequently observed that some lobotomized individuals were "disinhibited," displaying lowered personal standards of morality or social decorum (swearing, kleptomania, urinating in the streets, and the like), and exhibited immature, impulsive, or extravagant behavior. Sometimes increased irritability was observed postoperatively, but this seldom was expressed as increased aggressive behavior. Many of these adverse physical and behavioral consequences of the surgery were temporary or were attenuated over time, but sometimes they persisted. Still, even the highly respected neurologist Kurt Goldstein, who was a critic of psychosurgery, wrote in 1950 that "it is certainly an exaggeration to refer to all lobotomized patients as human vegetables." Goldstein did note, however, that his testing methods revealed a loss in capacity for abstract reasoning—a loss that he believed followed almost any damage to the brain. Others were not able to replicate Goldstein's results with more standardized tests. In any case, Goldstein admitted that the consequences of psychosurgery were often difficult to separate from the effects of the psychiatric disorder itself. This difficulty continues to plague attempts to evaluate psychosurgery.

Contributing to the early psychosurgery controversy was the confusion over responsibility for the patient. The relatively abrupt appearance of psychosurgery on the scene forced neurosurgeons and psychiatrists to form referral networks hastily, without a clear understanding of the delegation of responsibility for the patient. A statement by the neurosurgeon James Poppen, written after he had already performed 500 psychosurgical operations, is revealing in this context:

> I feel strongly that it is the neurosurgeon's duty to perform the operation as safely and accurately as possible but that the burden of deciding whether a mental patient should be subjected to the procedures falls on the shoulders of competent neuropsychiatrists who have had an opportunity to study many patients before and after operation.
>
> No neurosurgeon wishes to be a technician only. In most instances, however, the neurosurgeon has not had the proper training nor has he the time to devote the many weeks and perhaps months of intimate contact with the patient and his relatives to reach a just decision. Therefore, he is not in a position to weigh justly the merits for or against operative interference [Poppen, 1948].

Psychiatrists, however, did not always assume the responsibilities implied in Poppen's statement. In many instances, they referred patients on to neurosurgeons because they could not cope with them, and that was the last they saw of the patients. This was particularly true in state hospitals, where patients were often transferred to another institution with the necessary surgical facilities and expertise. The unclear delegation of responsibility for the patient also hindered recognition of serious impairments sometimes caused by the psychosurgical operations.

Early Evaluations of Psychosurgery

Very commonly, psychosurgery has been attacked or defended on the grounds of unrepresentative results of a few extreme cases. It should be obvious that selected case reports of dramatic successes or tragic failures of psychosurgery cannot substitute for more representative data based on large samples of patients. Individual case records that demonstrate serious impairment produced by psychosurgery have been countered by equally dramatic cases of postoperative improvement, such as Walter Freeman's description of a young lobotomized physician who later headed a hospital with a staff of ten doctors and Sadao Hirose's (1979) account of a psychosurgical patient who subsequently held a very high and responsible position in the Japanese government.

Although there was much to criticize about the way the more systematic studies of psychosurgery were conducted, it is a matter of record that almost all of them concluded that the majority of patients were at least moderately, if not markedly, improved (see Valenstein, 1973, for a review). Some of the studies that reached this conclusion involved relatively long-term follow-ups and some, such as those conducted by the Connecticut Lobotomy Committee and the British Board of Control Study, included large samples of patients. The Columbia-Greystone Project is frequently cited (even though the patient group was not large) because it used a battery of thirty-five psychological tests and employed over sixty clinical investigators, many of whom were very prominent in the field. Although less evidence of improvement was found in this study than in others, it was concluded that there was no evidence that topectomy (one type of prefrontal psychosurgical operation) produced any permanent loss in learning ability, memory, creativity, imagination, intellectual achievement, social or ethical attitudes, or even sense of humor (Landis, Zubin, and Mettler, 1950; Mettler, 1952). In all probability, the generally favorable reports emerging from most of the earlier studies contributed to the wide-scale adoption of psychosurgery. It should be obvious that if the results were typically as bad as the tragic cases reported by those most vehemently opposed to psychosurgery, these operations would not have continued as long as they did.

There is little doubt that most of the early studies had serious scientific shortcomings, including generally poor methodology and especially a lack of experimental controls (see particularly Robin and Macdonald, 1975). Postoperative improvement was always attributed to the beneficial effects of psychosurgery, even though it might have taken more than six months, and in some cases almost two years, before improvement was evident. Generally lacking was a comparable, nonsurgical group of patients that would have made it possible to estimate the incidence of "spontaneous" remissions. Several early studies cited by Robin and Macdonald (1975) concluded that close to 50 percent of patients diagnosed as psychotic showed a significant improvement even though they were given no treatment or a placebo treatment. More recently, Klein and Davis (1969) pooled the results of thirty-six studies using a "placebo control group" and concluded that 39 percent of depressed patients improved without any specific treatment. Also generally ignored is the fact that psychiatric ailments tend to fluctuate in intensity. Psychosurgery is commonly performed when a patient is most desperate and usually most impaired; therefore, the probability of some improvement after the operation (particularly when periods up to two years are considered) is high, as improvement would be likely even without the operation. The standard response to this criticism is that lobotomies were done as a last resort and patients had all been seriously ill for long periods of time without any relief. The fact, however, is that some patients (it would be impossible to estimate how many) were referred for operations after quite short periods of alternative treatment, and not all were in such a poor state as was commonly implied; see, for example, Watts' comment on Freeman's first transorbital lobotomized patients (Freeman and Watts, 1950, pp. 57–61) and Rachman's contribution to this book.

Another difficulty in deciding how much weight should be given to the older evaluation studies is that it is usually impossible to separate out the consequences of psychosurgery from the effects of special attention or changes in attitude usually given to the patients by staff and family. Robin and Macdonald describe a striking example of the importance of this factor.

> J.X. was a 35 year old patient with several admissions to mental hospitals and the diagnosis of paranoid schizophrenia. She was well preserved in personality and in touch with her environment. Whether this attitude arose from the patient's illness or not, is not clear, but her parents appeared ambivalent towards her. Ensuring the highest standard of treatment by constantly criticizing the activities of the hospital, its doctors and nurses, they carefully avoided any personal involvement and resisted the average family contribution to her care, e.g. weekends at home. A leucotomy operation was eventually proposed, and a very high chance of success presented to both the patient and her parents. The operation started, but because of excessive bleeding, attributed by the surgeon to the fact that the patient was menstruating, was abandoned after trephine holes had been cut, but before brain surgery. The patient made an uneventful recovery and nothing was said to her about the extent of the operation performed—or the lack of it. Clinical improvement was observed from the date of operation for several months. Her parents took a renewed interest in her, and the question of discharge had been discussed, when a final interview was arranged at which they were further reassured with the advice that should the patient relapse, then they need have no particular fear as the operation had not in fact been done and could still be performed in the future. At this first intimation of the true situation regarding the operation, the patient's mother remarked "But surely, if she has not had the operation she cannot be better, and we could not possibly risk having her at home." Discharge was impossible. The patient, in due course, began to relapse. A full leucotomy operation was performed and no clinical improvement followed. The patient remains in hospital 20 years later [Robin and Macdonald, 1975, p. 20].

As striking as this case may seem, it may not really be representative, as there are several accounts of "sham operations" that were not followed by any improvement (Livingston, 1953, p. 377). Nevertheless, it is clearly possible that attitudes of the patient, staff, and family toward the operation can have a very significant influence on the outcome, even though it may be unethical to test their influence in a rigorously scientific manner because to do so would involve deceiving the patient and others (see the discussion of this issue by Corkin in this volume). Moreover, many neurosurgeons have argued that it would be unethical and dangerous to withhold treatment for experimental purposes.

Another factor that has to be considered is that the test instruments may not be sensitive to important changes in behavior capacities. Gosta Rylander (1948) frequently asserted that the major deficits seen after the operations were not detected by psychological tests. He maintained that it was necessary to live with the patients (or at least observe them very thoroughly in everyday activities) to appreciate the extent to which they had become less stable emotionally and less effective intellectually. It was frequently noted that intelligence as measured by an intelligence test was not impaired following psychosurgery, but motivational and emotional deficits made it less likely that intelligence would be used in everyday decisions. Porteus and Kepner (1944) concluded from a study of lobotomized patients at the Territorial Hospital in Hawaii that the capacity to plan ahead was always diminished by the operation, but if this capacity was high enough preoperatively the individual would "retain enough to enable him to function satisfactorily in community life." It was not always clear, however, in how many instances of "successful operations" the patients were actually returned to "community life." Most lobotomized patients lived sheltered lives in institutions or with their families where they were seldom confronted with the challenges that would reveal any diminished capacities. Although a few older evaluation studies did include information about the ability to hold a job, the nature of the job was rarely specified except to illustrate instances of dramatic success.

A number of studies that emphasized the positive results of psychosurgery gave too much weight to the elimination of behavior that was most troublesome to the hospital staff and family and placed less emphasis on the present quality of life of the lobotomized patients. There is a recurrent and disquieting theme throughout the older psychosurgical literature suggesting that problems of management played too large a role, both in the selection of patients and in the evaluation of the results. Burckhardt, for example, selected agitated patients for the first psychosurgery operations at the end of the last century, while Moniz, according to Freeman and Watts (1950), "compared in his own mind the querulous, the deluded, the agitated, and the obsessed" with Fulton and Jacobsen's ape that was calmed following destruction of its frontal lobes. Porteus and Kepner (1944) studied lobotomized patients in Hawaii and noted that:

> Among the criminally insane operated upon were three individuals whose collective convictions included three killings and five stabbings. All were improved and one was discharged as being no longer a menace to the community. *Other extremely dangerous patients have become amenable and easily managed* [Porteus and Kepner, 1944, p. 113, italics added].

Not infrequently, Freeman and Watts included comments such as, "She is not noisy and is now easy to manage" in their psychosurgery evaluations (Freeman and Watts, 1942, p. 241). After quoting a mother of a six-year-old girl that "she has not had one temper tantrum since the operation . . . it is a pleasure to dress her now . . . she seems perfectly happy all the time," Freeman and Watts (1950) added, "improvement has continued . . . she can be more easily managed at home." Particularly revealing is Draper's (1947) description of the first patient operated on by the eminent neurosurgeon Walter Dandy. One year later, the patient was still institutionalized:

> she lacks initiative and spontaneity, although occasionally she is the first to say "Good Morning." Her attention is not maintained . . . her judgment is poor and insight is only partial. Except for transient smiles she seems rather flat emotionally. However, our patient, we think, has been definitely helped by her prefrontal lobotomy of one year ago . . . she is comfortable and happy and showed definite improvement from the standpoint of manageability [Draper, 1947, pp. 6–7].

It is probably already apparent that even if everyone had agreed on the outcome of the older lobotomy operations, there would still have been strongly opposed attitudes toward these operations. Perhaps the most dramatic way to illustrate this point is to quote extensively from Freeman and Watts' (1944) description of the consequences of their "standard" lobotomy operation:

> Following the initial period (two to five days) of lethargy and disorientation after lobotomy during which the patient has to be tended like a baby, fed, watered, and changed because of incontinence, there appears a stage of serene relaxation and indolence that may last for several days. During this time there is placid acceptance of the attentions of relatives varied with playful gestures and remarks and not infrequently persistent stereotyped overactivity in a vague semidazed condition. . . . A good deal depends upon the prepsychotic personality of the patient, the duration of the psychosis, and the stereotyped na-

ture of the complaints or the compulsions. In patients who have manifested chronic anxiety as the outstanding symptom, normality returns—very rapidly; in those who have suffered from hallucinations, delusions, obsessions, hypochondriacal complaints, compulsions, and other specific and durable mental symptoms, the patterns of the reactions continue even though the emotional component has evaporated. One speaks of echo symptoms.

Once the patient returns to his home, about two weeks after lobotomy, the newly emerging personality is fairly well developed and continues its evolution for a period of many months or even years. It is not a healthy personality at first; probably the word immature best describes it. Granting that the disease symptoms have been relieved by operation, the patient manifests two outstanding traits that could be described as laziness and tactlessness. In some people indolence is outstanding, in others hastiness, explosiveness, petulance, talkativeness, laughter, and other signs of lack of self-control. . . . They are often buoyant and exuberant, and many times they have been likened to children by their observant relatives. Their interest span is short, they are distractable, but their good humor is almost invincible. They cannot be serious. They do not dream.

Further maturation of the personality occurs with the lapse of weeks and months. The housewife complains of forgetfulness when she is really describing distractability and lack of correct timing of the various household maneuvers. The man makes up his mind to look for a job but he can't quite summon up the energy necessary to overcome his inertia, and the many facets of the problem of obtaining employment are too numerous for his still limited capacity for consecutive and constructive thought. If he has a job to go back to he is apt to lose it because of errors of judgment and foresight. . . . Capacity for constructive thinking increases with lapse of time, and initiative also improves. Some patients even become overly energetic, seeming to lose themselves in their work, even oblivious to the state of normal fatigue. . . . Naturally indolent persons, however, who previously drove themselves beyond their capacity, are apt to be satisfied with activities far short of their previous aims.

As in the case with indolence, so also tactlessness tends to disappear in the months and years following lobotomy. Patients regain more or less completely their capacity to conduct themselves in a dignified and considerate manner particularly with strangers, although they may revert to their more immature behavior in the family surroundings. It is not that they don't know better, for many of them will confess their lapses, but they either cannot foresee the effect of their hasty words or actions, or they just don't give a damn.

It is this emotional "set" that characterizes people who have been operated upon. The outstanding feature is lack of self-consciousness in the sense that they are childlike in the expression of their attitudes. They do not take themselves seriously. They cannot be insulted; no matter what one says to them they do not take offense. They laugh easily and flare up in anger on slight nagging or frustration, but seldom weep. They enjoy the pleasures and avoid the disagreeable facts of life as much as they are allowed to. Life is enormously simplified by the relatively complete obliteration of the need for introspection. Basic intelligence is intact, planning capacity is adequate, foresight is direct, decision is abrupt, acceptance of the results is realistic, and the emotional responses are vivid though evanescent and lacking in depth. On the whole, a patient who has satisfactorily recovered from a psychosis through psychosurgery gives the impression of a pleasant and enthusiastic if somewhat immature individual whose willingness to fall in with the "set" of the other person's attitude makes him an agreeable companion. People on whom this operation has been performed are generous, steady, fairly reliable workers, friendly, and unembarrassed at being interviewed by strangers. They take things as they come [Freeman and Watts, 1944, pp. 520–522].

Several years later, Robinson, Freeman, and Watts (1951) concluded:

If the incisions lie far anteriorly, the chief effects appear to be loss of fantasy, of creative drive, of sensitivity, of sympathetic understanding of others. If the operation is radical, patients are likely to be somewhat gross in their appetites for food and sex, careless and slovenly in appearance, and largely impervious to criticism. Between these extremes lies a wide range of individual differences.

Are generalizations nevertheless possible? We became convinced that they are. Patients after lobotomy always show some lack of personality depth. They are cheerful and complacent and are indifferent to the opinions and feelings of others. Rather objective about their faults, they seldom give voice to defense mechanisms. Their goals are immediate—not remote. They can recall the past as well as ever, but it has diminished interpretive value for them, and they are not more interested in their own past emotional crises than if they had happened to someone else. They seem incapable of feeling guilt now for past misdeeds [Robinson, Freeman, and Watts, 1951, p. 159].

Although these descriptions of the consequences of psychosurgery were written by strong advocates of this operation, they contain much that could be used by those opposed to this practice. It would be interesting to know how many patients or members of patients' families were given comparable descriptions of the consequences of psychosurgery prior to consenting to the operation.

There is probably much that we can still learn from the early lobotomy literature, but it is important to keep in mind that this literature is more than a quarter century old and that the surgical procedures and the brain targets used today have changed considerably. Many of the critics of psychosurgery have refused to consider the possibility that the record of the "lobotomy era" may not apply to present conditions and have drawn most of their incriminating evidence from a literature that advocates of these operations consider to be no longer applicable. In Part III more current data on the results of psychosurgery will be presented.

The Revived Interest in Psychosurgery

It is generally acknowledged that even after psychoactive drugs became available there were (and still are) a great number of psychiatric patients who were not helped by any available treatment. Some of these patients, albeit a relatively small number, continued to be referred to neurosurgeons practicing psychosurgery. There were several factors responsible for the continuation of psychosurgery after 1955. Perhaps most important was the fact that some neurosurgeons and psychiatrists became convinced that sufficient knowledge had accumulated to avoid the major complications of the earlier lobotomy operations. The results of several studies comparing the behavioral outcomes of operations on the more lateral versus the medial areas of the prefrontal brain, for example, suggested that only the destruction of the lateral areas produced intellectual deficits. Experiments on monkeys also indicated that the lateral prefrontal area was more essential to various types of problem-solving behavior. At the same time, evidence from electrical stimulation and destruction studies on the brains of animals pointed to the ventromedial area's role in emotional behavior and in those physiological responses, such as increased heart rate and respiration, associated with emotional expression (see Valenstein, 1977, pp. 316–326). Thus, psychosurgical procedures used in the 1960s tended to avoid the more lateral prefrontal areas and concentrate either on the ventromedial prefrontal area or on brain structures anatomically connected to this medial area. Moreover, it proved possible to destroy smaller targets and with more accuracy by the use of electrodes—to make electrolytic or radio frequency lesions—and stereotaxic instruments combined with on-line X-ray visualization of brain landmarks during the electrode insertion. There could be little questioning the advantage of these techniques over the relatively free-hand insertion of knives into the brain guided only by gross skull landmarks. These technical advances certainly helped reduce the incidence of serious neurological impairment.

Although psychosurgery did continue at a relatively low level throughout the 1960s, the topic received virtually no public attention at all. In the 1970s, several factors combined to produce the present controversy. First of all, the awareness that these operations were still being done tended to create the impression of a "resurgence of psychosurgery." Actually, the number of operations had not increased significantly during the last ten years, but there was certainly evidence of increasing professional interest in the topic. For example, the International Congress of Psychosurgery, which had not met since it was first convened in Lisbon in 1948, was reactivated in 1970 and held its second meeting in Copenhagen. A third meeting was held in Cambridge in 1972, a fourth in Madrid in 1975, and a fifth in Boston in 1978. During this time, a number of articles appeared stating that the current "psychiatric surgery" was a much more sophisticated and discrete operation and that criticisms based on results of the older prefrontal lobotomies were completely irrelevant. It was claimed in these articles that much more was now known about the brain and that the frontal lobes should be "revisited." Many people not only viewed such statements with skepticism but also suspected them to be a prelude to large-scale applications of psychosurgery.

Undoubtedly, what caused the greatest concern were the suggestions that psychosurgery and other physical manipulations of the brain might be used to change socially (and politically) undesirable behavior. These suggestions generated a very emotional response, not only because they seemed to portend an explosion in the amount of psychosurgery performed, but also because they raised fears that these operations might be used as a means of social control (see the contributions by Breggin and Kaimowitz in this volume). It is only possible to speculate what course psychosurgery would have taken if the issue had not become the subject of such a heated dispute. Many have argued that no significant increase in the number of operations would have occurred because the availability of numerous psychoactive drugs and new forms of psychotherapy would have limited psychosurgery to a small number of otherwise intractable cases. Others continue to argue, however, that the proposed applications of psychosurgical techniques to recalcitrant prisoners, persons considered violent, and other "troublesome" individuals who might be classified as "functionally brain damaged" would have resulted in a very significant increase in the number of operations performed.

Even those most opposed to psychosurgery seem to concede at least now (although they did not initially) that present psychosurgical techniques have reduced the amount of gross physical and intellectual impairment sometimes produced by the older lobotomy operations. Nevertheless, these critics argue that regardless of the technical advances, all psychosurgical procedures tend to dehumanize people by reducing their capacity to respond emotionally. In addition, there is now a concern that was only rarely voiced during the earlier debate over psychosurgery. Those now opposed to psychosurgery maintain that the selection of psychosurgery patients by certain elements of the society's power structure for the express purpose of changing social behavior presents clear dangers to our social and political life (Breggin, 1975a; Chorover, 1976b; Chorover, 1979; Scheflin and Opton, 1978; Kaimowitz, in this volume). Although there was at least one instance during the older "lobotomy era" when psychosurgery was performed on a "consenting" criminal (the circumstances are described by Koskoff and Goldhurst, 1968), there was no widespread discussion of the possible use of biological techniques to modify socially undesirable behavior, as there is today. Moreover, the recent charge that women, blacks and other ethnic minorities, and political activists are (or will soon be) the main targets of psychosurgery has certainly added fuel to the current controversy, as well as broadening the group of people who believe they have a stake in the issue. This concern was expressed in an article in *Ebony* magazine entitled "Psychosurgery: A New Threat to Blacks" (Mason, 1973); in a statement by members of the Congressional Black Caucus; and in the testimony of Congressman Louis Stokes during the June 11, 1976, hearing on psychosurgery conducted by the National Commission for the Protection of Human Subjects of Biomedical and Behavioral Research.

There are understandable reasons for the concern over the social and political consequences of new developments in "brain control" techniques. While many of the techniques discussed in this context are, strictly speaking, not psychosurgery, many people feel that this distinction is only academic. The use of psychoactive drugs is not psychosurgery, but these drugs do make patients more manageable, at least in part by sedating them, and many of the "neuroleptic" drugs have been known to produce permanent brain damage. Similarly, the use of stimulating brain electrodes is technically not psychosurgery, but electrical stimulation can be used to alter the moods of patients and it has often been used in conjunction with psychosurgery. In the public's mind, these are all "brain control" techniques, which have been used (or at least tested) by groups working within, or for, the federal government. Evidence that governmental agencies had tested mind-altering drugs on unsuspecting employees (Scheflin and Opton, 1978) and that security agencies were interested in possible applications of implanted brain electrodes (Valenstein, 1973, pp. 68–69; Lilly, 1978, p. 91),[7] among many other revelations, has heightened the distrust of governmental power.

---

[7] In a chapter entitled "Control of the Brain and the Covert Intelligence Service," Lilly has recently described the circumstances surrounding the request made of him by the combined intelligence services of the United States to present his "brain-electrode technique for stimulating motivations within the brain" (Lilly, 1978, p. 91).

Over the last ten years the public has been bombarded with stories of new developments in the brain sciences that are reputed to be powerful means of modifying and controlling behavior. Michael Crichton's *The Terminal Man* is only one of many novels that has portrayed the dangers of trying to use brain stimulation techniques and computers to control human behavior. Taking a different tack, an article in *Esquire* magazine described a future "electroligarchy" where everyone is controlled through implanted brain electrodes (Rorvik, 1969). A television program appearing on "prime time" (Sunday, June 26, 1977, at 8:00 P.M.) depicted a plot to implant electrodes in a nightclub entertainer who resembled an African leader, in order to control his speech to the United Nations. Variations on these themes have appeared just about everywhere, including magazine and newspaper articles, introductory textbooks, television programs, motion pictures, science fiction stories, and even serious essays purporting to describe life in the not-too-distant future. (See Valenstein, 1973, for more examples.)

Even the stories meant only as entertainment have gradually begun to influence people's perceptions of what will soon be possible. Exaggerated descriptions of the power of brain control techniques are not, however, restricted to fiction. A *New York Times* article by Boyce Rensberger described the scientists who:

> have been learning to tinker with the brains of animals and men and to manipulate their thoughts and behaviors. Though their methods are still crude and not always predictable, there can remain little doubt that the next few years will bring a frightening array of refined techniques for making human beings act according to the will of the psychotechnologist [*New York Times*, September 12, 1971].

With more drama and expressing less reservation, Perry London (1969), a professional psychologist, wrote in a widely used textbook:

> All the ancient dreams of mastery over man and all the tales of zombies, golems, and Frankensteins involved some magic formula, or ritual, or incantation that would magically yield the key to dominion. But no one could be sure, from the old Greeks down to Mrs. Shelley, either by speculation or vivisection, whether there was any door for which to find that key.... This has been changing gradually, as knowledge of the brain has grown and been compounded since the nineteenth century, until today a whole technology exists for physically penetrating and controlling the brain's own mechanisms of control. It is sometimes called "brain manipulation," which means placing electrical or chemical stimulating devices in strategic brain tissues.... These methods have been used experimentally on myriad aspects of animal behavior, and clinically on a growing number of people.... The number of activities connected to specific places and

processes in the brain and aroused, excited, augmented, inhibited, or suppressed at will by stimulation of the proper site is simply huge. Animals and men can be oriented toward each other with emotions ranging from stark terror or morbidity to passionate affection and sexual desire. . . . Eating, drinking, sleeping, moving of bowels or limbs or organs of sensation gracefully or in spastic comedy, can all be managed on electrical demand by puppeteers whose flawless strings are pulled from miles away by the unseen call of radio and whose puppets, made of flesh and blood, look "like electronic toys," so little self-direction do they seem to have [London, 1969, p. 37].

It is little wonder that the feeling of being controlled by surreptitiously implanted brain devices has become an increasingly common delusion among paranoid patients.

While many people emphasize the potential misuse of these new brain-manipulating techniques, some have stressed what they believe is their positive potential. They see in them a possible cure not only for intractable psychiatric disorders but for intractable social problems as well, particularly those related to violent crimes and wars. The potential of biological techniques to achieve desirable social ends was expressed by Kenneth Clark in his presidential address to the 1971 convention of the American Psychological Association. Clark suggested that:

we might be on the threshold of that type of scientific biochemical intervention which could stabilize and make dominant the moral and ethical propensities of man and subordinate, if not eliminate, his negative and primitive behavioral tendencies [Clark, 1971, p. 1055].

The fact that this suggestion came from a social psychologist (a member of a group that normally emphasizes environmental causes and solutions) indicates the extent of the influence of these ideas. Clark went on to suggest that all candidates for political office should:

accept and use the earliest perfected form of psychotechnological, biochemical intervention which would assure their positive use of power and reduce or block the possibility of using power destructively [Clark, 1971, p. 1056].

Suggestions that brain-manipulating techniques may be applicable to social problems began to appear with great frequency. Two criminologists wrote an article for a professional journal—not a popular magazine—entitled "The Use of Electronics in the Observation and Control of Human Behavior and Its Possible Use in Rehabilitation and Parole." The article described devices that might be surgically implanted in paroled prisoners' bodies and brains for the purpose of keeping track of them, monitoring their physiological responses, and activating specific circuits to prevent any return to criminal tendencies. Brain electrodes, it was asserted, could be used to block undesirable behavior "through the production of fear, anxiety, disorientation, loss of memory and purpose, and even, if need be, by loss of consciousness" and to condition behavior "by the manipulation of rewarding and aversive stimuli." They describe the following scenario:

> a parolee with a past record of burglaries is tracked to a downtown shopping district (in fact, is exactly placed in a store known to be locked up for the night) and the physiological data reveals an increased respiration rate, a tension in the musculature and an increased flow of adrenalin. It would be a safe guess, certainly, that he was up to no good. The computer in this case, *weighing the probabilities*, would come to a decision and alert the police or parole officer so that they could hasten to the scene; or, if the subject were equipped with an implanted radiotelemeter it could transmit an electrical signal which could block further action by the subject by causing him to forget or abandon his project [Ingraham and Smith, 1972, p. 42].

Most of these suggestions for applying brain-manipulating techniques to social problems originated with people having little direct knowledge of or experience with these methods. It was viewed as quite a bit more serious, however, when it was learned that several people who were directly involved in performing brain surgery also appeared to be suggesting applications to social problems. For example, in 1972 Dr. M. Hunter Brown, a neurosurgeon, characterized the treatment of violent prisoners as "well intentioned but timid efforts with inadequate tools" and was quoted widely in newspapers as stating that:

> When this current effort fails, as it will, the state will turn to professionals for well-designed comprehensive programs including chromosome classification, activated electroencephalography, psychological testing, trials of newer medications that show promise, and finally neurosurgical intervention to specific targets as indicated. Until then, humanity must mark time [Brown, 1972].

Psychosurgery and Violence

Undoubtedly, the publication of *Violence and The Brain* (1970) by Vernon Mark and Frank Ervin played a major role in arousing concern about possible applications of brain surgery to social problems and in focusing the psychosurgery controversy on the subject of violence control. Mark and Ervin, a neurosurgeon and neuropsychiatrist, respectively, stated in the Preface that they had "written this book to stimulate a new and biologically oriented approach to the problem of human violence" and noted that:

> Violence is, without question, both prominent and prevalent in American life. In 1968 more Americans were the victims of murder and aggravated assault in the United States than were killed or wounded in seven-and-one-half years of the Vietnam War; and altogether almost half a million of us were the victims of homicide, rape, and assault [Mark and Ervin, 1970, p. 3].

They were clearly interested in the social impact of their book, as indicated by the comment in the Preface that they decided not to write a monograph for physicians because this "would discourage many potential readers for whom the social implications of the book might be of value."

Mark and Ervin followed up their introductory comments with a review of that part of the experimental and clinical literature which supported their position that aggressive and violent behavior often is the result of brain damage, particularly to such temporal lobe structures as the amygdala. They also observed that, while most people consider brain disease to be a rare phenomenon, in reality it is likely "that more than ten million Americans suffer from an obvious brain disease, and the brains of another five million have been subtly damaged" (Mark and Ervin, 1970, p. 5; see Appendix for supporting material). Juxtaposing these statements about the prevalence of both violence and "brain disease," Mark and Ervin concluded that abnormal brain foci were responsible for much more of the violence in society than had been previously suspected. In brief, they argued that abnormal brain foci in the amygdala frequently trigger both epileptic seizures and violent behavior (it is implied the two are closely associated), and they described how implanted electrodes can be used to locate these "brain triggers." The electrodes can be used either to record the presence of abnormal electrical activity or to stimulate the brain and provoke violent behavior, thereby supposedly revealing the neural foci that trigger such behavior. The technique for eliminating violent behavior is portrayed as effective, precise, and involving relatively little brain destruction. Thus, the implanted electrodes are:

> used to destroy a very small number of cells in a precisely determined area. As a surgical technique it has three great advantages over lobectomy: it requires much less of an opening in the surfaces of the brain than lobectomy does; it destroys less than one-tenth as much brain tissue; and once the electrodes have been inserted in the brain, they can be left without harm to the patient until the surgeon is sure which

brain cells are firing abnormally and causing the symptoms of seizures and violence [Mark and Ervin, 1970, p. 70].

The apparent simplicity and effectiveness of this technique made it seem very attractive to many. It also seemed to many that Mark and Ervin were suggesting that if violence was to be significantly reduced, much of this type of surgery would be required.

Elsewhere the present author has argued that only a very small amount of violence could possibly be attributed to a "sick brain" and that the correlation between temporal lobe epilepsy and violence was not at all strong (Valenstein, 1976). In fact, in a study of human violence that Frank Ervin participated in, it was concluded that:

> Those patients who are known to have some form of epilepsy get the highest scores on the Monroe Dyscontrol Scale as well as life adjustment problems, but get fairly low scores on measures of violence and sex drive. It thus seems reasonable to conclude that temporal lobe or any other form of epilepsy is not generally associated with violent behavior (although exceptions may exist). . . . Individuals who show much overt violence therefore tend to have poor control. However, the converse is not true. Those individuals with high scores on episodic dyscontrol (e.g., epileptics) do not necessarily get high scores on the violence index [Plutchik, Climent, and Ervin, 1976, p. 92].

Moreover, Mark and Ervin's claim that they had developed a very successful technique for localizing and destroying "brain triggers" of violence seems to have been greatly exaggerated (see, for example, Valenstein, 1973 and 1976). Mark's testimony as a defendant in a recently completed malpractice suit, for example, revealed that the successful operations described in *Violence and the Brain* were not based on actual patients, but were really "composite histories" with details taken from a number of different patients (Dickson, 1979).

This is not the appropriate place to present scientific arguments for and against the views expressed in *Violence and the Brain*. For present purposes, the important point is that a great number of people became frightened and angered over what they viewed as an argument justifying the large-scale application of brain-manipulating techniques to problems that were really social in origin. Mark and Ervin's conclusion that "we need to develop an 'early warning test' of limbic brain function to detect those humans who have a low threshold for impulsive violence" (p. 160) sounded dangerously open-ended, as did Sweet's comment in the Foreword that "knowledge gained about emotional brain function in violent persons with brain disease can be applied to combat the violence-triggering mechanisms in the brains of the nondiseased."

Additional fear and anger were generated by the discovery that these same influential clinical researchers had commented in an earlier letter to the *Journal of the American Medical Association* (written shortly after the Detroit race riots) that:

> It is important to realize that only a small number of the millions of slum dwellers have taken part in the riots, and that only a sub-fraction of these rioters have indulged in arson, sniping, and assault. Yet, if slum conditions alone determined and initiated riots, why are the vast majority of slum dwellers able to resist the temptations of unrestrained violence? Is there something peculiar about the violent slum dweller that differentiates him from his peaceful neighbor?
>
> There is evidence from several sources, recently collated by the Neuro-Research Foundation, that brain dysfunction related to a focal lesion plays a significant role in the violent and assaultive behavior of thoroughly studied patients.
>
> . . . we need intensive research and clinical studies of the *individuals* committing the violence. The goal of such studies would be to pinpoint, diagnose and treat those people with low violence thresholds before they contribute to further tragedies [Mark, Sweet, and Ervin, 1967, p. 895].

In a number of more recent articles, both Mark and Ervin have explicitly stated that they always were opposed to any psychosurgery for violent patients unless there was clear evidence of brain pathology and, moreover, that under foreseeable conditions psychosurgery on prison inmates could not be justified (Mark, 1974; Mark and Neville, 1973; Mark and Carnahan, this volume; Ervin, 1976). If this has always been their view, they have not succeeded in making their position clear. For example, Ernst Rodin, a neurologist and coauthor of the research proposal to study the effectiveness of psychosurgery in the violent "criminally insane" that led to the Kaimowitz case (see the contribution by Kaimowitz in this volume) has stated that he was misled by *Violence and the Brain* into believing that the operations were being recommended for violent persons who did not present clear evidence of brain pathology (Rodin's presentation at the Michigan Society for Neuroscience symposium, Ann Arbor, May 12, 1973 and Memorandum submitted as Exhibit AC-4 in *Kaimowitz* v. *Department of Mental Health*, Civil No. 73-19434-AW, Cir. Ct., Wayne County, Michigan, July 10, 1973). It is not difficult to understand why *Violence and the Brain* might have misled many people. The book emphasized the behavioral symptoms of a "dyscontrol syndrome" without stating explicitly that clear evidence of brain pathology was essential before surgery should be considered. Moreover, it was known at the time that there were several neurosurgeons who were performing similar operations directed toward the same brain target (the amygdala) on patients with only behavioral disorders (Small et al., 1977; Narabayashi, 1969; Balasubramaniam et al., 1970).

It should be noted that this growing interest in biological causes and treatment of violent behavior was spurred by public and governmental concern over the increasing incidence of "senseless" violence. Assassinations of public figures by people with very unclear motives did more than any statistics of street violence to dramatize the seriousness of the problem. It was easy to attribute violent behavior to brain abnormalities. Hence it was not surprising that when an ex-Marine, Charles Whitman, poured down a deadly rain of bullets from the University of Texas tower in August of 1966, Governor John Connally called on the neurosurgeon William Sweet to be a member of the panel charged with studying the case. In their description of the events surrounding the shootings, Sweet, Ervin, and Mark emphasized that "Whitman kept voluminous personal diaries, similar in detail to those of President Kennedy's murderer, Oswald," that he killed his wife and mother before going up to the tower to kill fifteen others and wound twenty-four; and that the postmortem examination of his brain, which was not performed in the standard way because the brain was badly damaged by gunshot wounds, revealed a walnut-sized malignant tumor—a glioblastoma multiforme —located "probably in the medial part of one temporal lobe" (Sweet, Ervin, and Mark, 1969, p. 338). Their emphases seem distinctly influenced by their own theory of violence. The information that Whitman kept a diary, for example, is significant only in light of reports that the "keeping of extensive diaries" is characteristic of some temporal lobe epileptics (Bear and Fedio, 1977). The description of the killings themselves implies that Whitman killed his mother, wife, and the fifteen others all in quick succession, in the throes of a sudden, episodic attack of violence. Sudden and unprovoked (so-called episodic) violence is described in *Violence and the Brain* as one of the main distinguishing characteristics of violence triggered by brain pathology. Actually, however, Whitman killed his mother and wife the night before, and his diary contained detailed plans for the tower shootings, including the clothing he would wear, the defense of his position on the tower, and plans for an escape. It also appears that the "evidence" about the location of the brain tumor was shaped to conform to the bias of the authors. The shotgun damage to the brain and its subsequent mishandling by the pathologists made it impossible to locate the tumor with any certainty. It could not be clearly established that the tumor was in the temporal lobes, let alone the "medial part," where, not too coincidentally, the amygdala (Mark and Ervin's main brain target) resides. Equally revealing are the omissions from the account. There was much in Whitman's childhood background and marine experiences that could have suggested alternative explanations of his mental disturbance and propensity for violence that was omitted from this account. (Note, for example, that Whitman's brother was subsequently shot and killed in a barroom fight.) It seems clear that the description of the events was filtered by a particular bias.

One of the recommendations of Governor Connally's panel was that substantial support be given to research on the relation of brain function to violent and aggressive behavior. A direct result was the arrangement of a symposium on the "Neural Bases of Violence and Aggression" to be held at the University of Texas Health Science Center during March 1972. Circulation of the agenda of this meeting was disturbing to a number of individuals who were monitoring developments in this field. They feared that the meeting would support the growing belief that the major causes of violence were biological rather than social. Some of the reasons for this fear and the steps that were taken in opposition are presented in a "Prologue" to the volume summarizing the presentations at the meeting (Fields and Sweet, 1975). The symposium included wide-ranging talks by basic scientists, clinicians doing brain surgery, and researchers in various disciplines studying hormonal and genetic causes of violence in the population at large and among prison inmates. The nature of the concern over the effect of this conference is expressed in the title of Breggin's contribution to the volume. Breggin, who has been one of the most vehement critics of psychosurgery, insisted on being placed on the program (he had not been invited) and gave a presentation entitled "Psychosurgery for the Control of Violence: A Critical Review" (Breggin, 1975b).

Actually, the number of violent persons among the psychosurgical patient population was relatively small, but most of the renewed controversy over psychosurgery in this period (1971–1978) centered on the issue of controlling violent behavior. Several factors combined to focus the controversy on questions about violence. As already noted, the publication of *Violence and the Brain* was a significant factor. Also, the number of inquiries from the Law Enforcement Assistants Agency (LEAA), the legal arm of the Justice Department, and from heads of Departments of Corrections (prison administrators) about biological factors causing violent behavior certainly added fuel to the growing concern. It was also learned that several clinicians had received government funds to study brain abnormalities in prison populations. Moreoever, it was revealed that brain operations had been performed under somewhat veiled circumstances on three prison inmates of California's Vacaville Prison (see, for example, Aarons, 1972).

There were many more signs that studies of biological solutions to violent behavior were receiving increasing attention and financial support from governmental agencies. This information has been reviewed elsewhere and need not be repeated here (see, for example, Scheflin and Opton, 1978). Not all the reports were accurate, and some of the inquiries by governmental agencies undoubtedly represented routine efforts to keep informed about any new developments relevant to their concerns. There is no doubt also that violence in prisons is a serious problem and that there might be good reasons for considering the establishment of so-called Maximum Psychiatric Diagnostic Units within the prison system. In total, however, there was much going on that justified concern and close scrutiny. Furthermore, because blacks constitute such a high percentage of the prison population in this country, it was not surprising that those concerned with racial prejudice would be especially suspicious of some of the plans that seemed to be brewing.

Chorover has described some of the events that sparked concern:

> In 1970, Dr. M. Hunter Brown, a California psychosurgeon, urged his colleagues at the Second International Congress of Psychosurgery "to initiate pilot programs for the precise (psychosurgical) rehabilitation of the prisoner-patient who is often young and intelligent, yet incapable of controlling various forms of violence." He also advanced an economic argument to make his psychosurgical pacification proposal appealing to taxpayers and beleaguered prison officials alike, pointing out that "each violent young criminal incarcerated from 20 years to life costs taxpayers perhaps $100,000. For roughly $6,000, society can provide medical treatment which will transform him into a responsible, well-adjusted citizen."
>
> In September 1971 (at the time of the Attica and San Quentin massacres) the chief of the California Department of Corrections wrote a letter to his board of supervisors, the California Council on Criminal Justice, which began by noting that the problem of treating the "aggressive, destructive inmate" has become particularly acute in recent years, although so far no satisfactory method of treatment has been developed. The letter went on to describe a plan "involving a complex neurosurgical evaluation and treatment program for the violent inmate," similar to the electrode implantation, stimulation, and destruction procedures practiced by Drs. Mark and Ervin [Chorover, 1979, p. 195].

It is difficult to know what might have happened had there been no public outcry. To reconstruct motives at this time is impossible because in all probability even the participants in the correspondence about psychosurgery had no specific goals in mind. One of the factors that contributed to the mood of suspicion, however, was the fact that inquiries were typically addressed to advocates of psychosurgery, who consistently made recommendations for studies of violent prisoners and sometimes suggested the establishment of "special units" (or even separate institutions) devoted to this problem.

Much of what was said and published during the period between 1971 and 1978 consisted of polemical diatribes. Evidence was commonly taken out of context to support the position that all neurosurgeons who performed psychosurgery were, at best, callous and uncaring. Typically, the work of "psychosurgeons" was compared to medical experiments performed by Nazi physicians. False claims that blacks and other minorities constituted the major group of patients served to muster political allies. Several members of the Black Caucas in Congress, for example, were persuaded by this misinformation to sponsor anti-psychosurgery legislation (see Chapter 4 for a discussion of the representation of minorities among the psychosurgical patient population). On the other side of the controversy, most psychiatrists and neurosurgeons who were pro-psychosurgery initially tended to maintain low profiles. Some of them exerted their influence as advisors on television programs, and many testified against proposed legislation that would have interfered with their freedom to practice.

An opponent of psychosurgery, neurologist Robert Grimm, warned that sociopolitical changes could put brain control technology in the hands of the state (Grimm, 1976). Predicting that "hard times" would follow the present difficult transitional period of "Western technocracy," Grimm declared that "ours may be the last generation to inquire openly about brain control of individuals by the state." In an attempt to maintain order, an authoritarian state would inevitably ask neuroscientists "to provide and transcribe brain control techniques for the state and . . . they will deliver when asked." According to this scenario, "physicians—and in particular psychiatrists—will become the principal agents of control," and their "task will be to change minds, not society" (pp. 110–111).

In the atmosphere created by "Watergate" and subsequent revelations of intrigue and deception, many people feared any governmental interest in "brain control" techniques. A number of people concluded that a more realistic danger was the prospect of a subtle change in attitudes toward psychosurgery, such as that reflected in a 1973 editorial in *The Times* of London (see Figure 1.3). On the surface, the editorial seemed very moderate and sensible. But a number of thoughtful people have expressed great concern over the growing

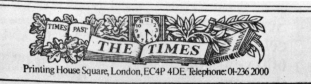

Printing House Square, London, EC4P 4DE. Telephone: 01-236 2000

THERAPY FOR CRIMINALS

Compared with other countries Britain has little experience of the medical and surgical treatment of sexual offenders and violent criminals. In Denmark, for example, castration is used in the treatment of repeated sexual offenders; in Germany and the United States brain surgery has been used for the same purpose and good results have been claimed for both procedures. A less draconic alternative is treatment with sex hormones, which induces a chemical castration, and the latest form of therapy is with drugs such as Benperidol which acts directly on the brain.

These treatments eliminate unwanted sexual impulses by eradication of any form of sexual desire but all have drawbacks particularly their side effects. Any brain operation intended to modify behaviour is likely to cause some flattening of personality so that drive and energy are reduced; sex hormone therapy has unpleasant physical effects including gain in weight and nausea; some powerful tranquillizers can cause permanent brain damage. Furthermore all such treatment is in a sense experimental since its long-term effects cannot be forecast with certainty and only time will show whether unexpected complications develop. There is of course the problem that patients of all kinds often cease to take drugs when side effects are unpleasant.

These are serious hazards but in practice they have been found acceptable by doctors with personal experience of the problem and by sexual offenders who have struggled for years with desires and impulses that they cannot suppress. For such men the risks and drawbacks of treatment seem preferable to a lifetime of anxiety that they may molest a child or commit some other violent assault.

Recently there has been growing criticism on ethical grounds of any treatment of offenders intended to remove their anti-social urges. Society has no right, it is argued, to set up standards of behaviour and then to assert that anyone who does not conform needs treatment—especially if he is already deprived of his liberty by being in prison. Discussion of this problem is, however, often too academic and concerned with concepts such as the integrity of the human personality and the choice between the welfare of society and individual freedom—it tends to ignore the needs and wishes of the offenders themselves.

Men who ask for treatment to modify their behaviour are not invariably convicted offenders; and even the critics of such treatment might acknowledge the liberty of an individual to choose it for himself in the absence of any specific pressures from society other than its disapproval of his sexual orientation. Consent by an adult is valid if he is capable of understanding the choices open to him and the risks and effects of the procedure have been fully explained. Consent is a much more difficult problem when a man is in prison or is on probation or parole.

The simple solution is to insist that in these circumstances treatment can never be offered as a condition of early release and that no form of irreversible treatment can be offered at all. In effect, this restricts its range to drug therapy for men whose term of imprisonment is fixed—though elegibility for parole qualifies even that conclusion. Unfortunately, many of the most severely disturbed offenders are those serving indeterminate sentences.

Often these men know that they will never be released until they are considered "safe". On any strict legal assessment their consent to treatment cannot be regarded as free—but is it equitable to say that these are the only men who cannot be offered treatment that might make them safe? That was the effect of a decision of an American court earlier this year which held that no one confined to an institution could give legal consent to an irreversible operation intended to remove his aggressive tendencies.

Too rigid an ethical stance could be to the disadvantage of offenders for there is likely to be further improvement in techniques of modification of personality by surgery and drugs, and these could play an important role in the rehabilitation of some types of offenders, provided satisfactory safeguards can be agreed. The proviso is all important. Outside prison the quality and nature of a man's consent to treatment is a matter between him and his doctor, but inside a prison the extra pressures justify an independent assessment. It is sometimes said that a committee simply spreads the responsibility for a decision and the guilt for failure; but a small group of independent experts could provide the necessary protection for the prisoner. Its role would be to establish that treatment was not being offered as a condition of parole or early release, that the prisoner fully understood the nature and risks of the procedure (including any likely modification of his condition due merely to the passage of time) and that the treatment had been adequately tested outside prison. With these safeguards society might in time have a better alternative for the repeated sexual offender than prolonged incarceration.

Figure 1.3 An editorial appearing in *The Times* of London, October 2, 1973, p. 17.

disillusionment with the possibility of rehabilitating criminals and the assumption that crime and rehabilitation require biological rather than social interventions. If opinion leaders and policy makers start to believe that crime is primarily a medical problem, they contended, the consequences could be far-reaching and dangerous.

In this atmosphere, it is not surprising that much of the debate about psychosurgery emphasized violent patients, prisoners, and the potential role of governmental agencies to use "brain control" techniques for their own purposes. There were very few serious discussions of whether the majority of the patients, who were not violent but were suffering from severe depression, obsessions and anxieties, were being helped (see Chapter 4 for a description of the patient population). The fate of the typical psychosurgical patient was usually not even a part of the dialogue. In fact, it gradually became clear in the early 1970s that there was no adequate outcome studies of the latest surgical procedures. Recognizing that it would be impossible to make recommendations without such information, the National Commission for the Protection of Human Subjects of Biomedical and Behavioral Research arranged in 1975 for one retrospective and one prospective study of patients to be conducted. The most recent results of these studies are reported by Mirsky and Orzack and Corkin in this volume.

It is also not surprising that the controversy was thrust into the political arena, where numerous proposals for protective legislation were made. Some of these were hastily conceived proposals aimed simply at prohibiting psychosurgery, with little thought given to the consequences of establishing a precedent of resolving disputes over medical practice by legislation motivated by political pressure. Some legislation defining the conditions under which psychosurgery may be performed has been passed in California and Oregon. It may be too soon to determine the full consequences of these laws, but the short-term effect appears to have been *de facto* prohibition of psychosurgery (see the chapter by Grimm for a description of the effect of the Oregon law and Valenstein's comments in Chapter 3 on the consequences of the California law). Legal issues are not restricted to laws passed by state legislatures. There are also legal precedents stemming from court decision, proposals of federal guidelines, issues related to constitutional guarantees, questions about responsibility as it relates to malpractice, and special legal problems that apply to children, prisoners, and committed patients. These and other issues are discussed in Part V of this volume.

Ethical issues were also raised frequently, but unfortunately these usually took the form of accusations. The charge and counter-charge atmosphere that was created was certainly not conducive to working out solutions to complex problems. Although it has been argued that operations on the brain present special ethical problems, the majority of "ethical" concerns expressed really dealt with patient protection and applied equally to all patients (at least to all psychiatric patients). It is not only psychosurgery that generates discussion about informed consent, the conflict between research goals and patient protection, the adequacy of review procedures, the possibility that more "innovative" therapies will be tried on the poor and minority groups, the morality of using control groups in research, the special problems that relate to prisoners and other confined individuals, and other ethical issues. The majority of the ethical issues discussed by the contributors to this volume apply to all areas of medical research and practice.

It can be debated whether a medical procedure as scientifically and politically controversial as psychosurgery can serve as a useful model for studying the way disputes over medical practice can be resolved. The present author would argue that it is precisely because of the intensity of the controversy and the involvement of so many diverse groups that we can learn so much from the "psychosurgery debate."

CHAPTER 2

Rationale and Surgical Procedures

Elliot S. Valenstein

The Rationale for Psychosurgery

Arguments supporting the practice of psychosurgery may be characterized as either empirical and pragmatic or theoretical. In most instances the two types of arguments are used to reinforce each other, but one or the other may be given greater emphasis.

The empirical-pragmatic argument is relatively easy to characterize, as its justifications for psychosurgery are completely unpretentious. In its purest form, it frankly confesses ignorance about how or why psychosurgery works, maintaining that physiological explanations are pure conjecture at this time. In essence, the argument boils down to assertions that psychosurgery is effective, that alternative treatments are ineffective, and that there are serious dangers in doing nothing. Evidence is usually cited that patients improve significantly after psychosurgery and that the risk of serious complications is slight. Case histories are presented to illustrate that the patients have had long-term, seriously debilitating psychiatric illnesses and that all other reasonable alternatives have been exhausted. Frequently cited in support of the assertion that there are great risks in "doing nothing" are studies indicating that deaths from suicides and other causes related to the psychiatric condition may be quite high. One study (Guze and Robins, 1970) frequently cited in this context reported that successful suicides may be as high as 15 percent in patients suffering from uncontrolled depression. Similarly, it is argued that if the mental illness is left unchecked the patient's mental state and social and economic life may deteriorate to the point of "no return." In a sense, these arguments are much like those given in support of electroconvulsive shock. Here, too, there is no adequate explanation of how the treatment works, but evidence of its effectiveness, the ineffectiveness of other treatments, and the dangers of doing nothing are consistently offered as justifying arguments.

Of course, the empirical-pragmatic defense of psychosurgery has not gone uncontested. Thus, it is asserted that psychosurgery is often performed before all alternative treatments have been exhausted. It is argued that if a patient falls into the hands of a psychiatrist who believes in psychosurgery for certain types of conditions, a quick exploration with drugs and electroconvulsive shock may be all the alternative treatment that is explored prior to referral to a neurosurgeon. Moreover, the dangers of "doing nothing," as expressed in suicide figures, are claimed to be exaggerated or at least unrepresentative of the total group of patients receiving psychosurgery. Lastly, the evidence that patients receive significant benefit from the surgery and that the risks of impairment are slight is challenged.

In contrast to the pragmatic rationale, the theoretical rationale for psychosurgery is based on extrapolations from empirical evidence and hypothesized physiological explanations. Many of the arguments lean heavily on evidence from animal experimentation showing that destruction of particular brain structures sometimes produces dramatic changes in emotional behavior, while stimulation of these same structures (or anatomically related regions in the frontal lobes) can intensify or inhibit those visceral reactions associated with emotional states, such as heart rate, blood pressure, respiration, and hormonal responses. This evidence constitutes the main support for the conclusion that certain brain regions normally play the critical role in modulating emotionality.

Extrapolation from Animal Experiments

Animal experiments demonstrating behavioral and emotional changes following damage to particular brain structures have often led with startling directness to the adoption of particular psychosurgical operations. Only afterward have more physiological explanations been offered. For example, Jacobsen's observations of the emotional changes of monkeys and chimpanzees after ablation of their frontal lobes are believed to have had a direct influence on Moniz's decision to explore the effects of frontal lobotomy on agitated patients (see Chapter 1). Later, when John Fulton was encouraging psychosurgeons to destroy a more restricted region of the anterior cingulate area instead of continuing the "standard" prefrontal lobotomy operation, his argument was heavily based on evidence of behavioral changes seen in monkeys after similar operations (Fulton, 1951). Within a year, several neurosurgeons in Europe and the United States responded to this encouragement. An even more direct connection between animal experiments and psychosurgery was expressed by the late Spanish neurosurgeon Obrador, who wrote that:

> While I was doing neurosurgical practice in Mexico City, in the early forties, I visited Klüver in Chicago . . . who studied the behavior of monkeys after the removal of the temporal lobes by Paul Bucy. I then attempted temporal sections in a few severe psychotic patients [Obrador, 1977, p. xxv].

One can only wonder why anyone would have been encouraged to try the operations on humans in view of Klüver's report that besides the "taming" (which is presumably what interested Obrador) the monkeys exhibited hypersexuality, orality, difficulty in identifying objects presented visually, and increased restlessness.

Other examples have been described more recently. Balasubramaniam and Kanaka, who practice in Madras, India, have described the origin of one of their psychosurgical procedures as follows:

> Until very recently there was no useful method of treating violent and aggressive patients. The only practical way was to keep them tied down. The administration of drugs to quiet them was not consistently useful. The earlier operations of psychosurgery, such as leucotomy, were worse than useless. By removing what remained of inhibition, these operations tended to make patients more irresponsible and unmanageable.
>
> Animal experimentation by pioneers like Cannon and Bard had shown that the rage center was located in the hypothalamus. By means of ablation and stimulation studies, the presence of centers for aggression was confirmed by other workers.
>
> With such excellent physiological studies one may wonder why surgical procedures directed at this area were not considered [Balasubramaniam and Kanaka, 1976, p. 768].[1]

---

[1] Actually, by today's standards these animal experiments would be considered extremely crude, and they certainly did not provide evidence for localization of aggression in any specific region of the hypothalamus of even the cat.

Balasubramaniam and Kanaka explain that the delay was caused in part by the need for adequate surgical techniques, primarily stereotaxic procedures (those procedures are described later in the chapter).

Several German neurosurgeons and neuropsychiatrists have also justified hypothalamic operations on persons who have committed sexual crimes by using the argument that similar brain operations reduced hypersexuality in experimental animals. At an International Neurological Congress in Brussels, Roeder and his associates had an opportunity to see Schreiner and Kling's film picturing the hypersexuality of amygdalectomized male cats and monkeys. (The amygdala is a temporal lobe structure, and this operation was historically related to, but not identical to, that performed by Heinrich Klüver on monkeys.) The film demonstrated highly exaggerated sexual activity directed toward males as well as females and even toward animals of other species. It was also reported at this Congress that this induced hypersexuality could be eliminated by a second brain operation that destroyed the ventromedial nucleus of the hypothalamus. Roeder and his collaborators considered the animal studies "a mine of information for human sexual pathology" and wrote:

> the behavior of male cats with lesions of the amygdalar region in some respects closely approached that of human perversion. The films convinced us that there was a basis for a therapeutic, stereotaxic approach to this problem in man [Roeder, Orthner, and Muller, 1972, p. 88].

It was not long after that they started to perform hypothalamic psychosurgery on some of their patients.

It is clear that demonstrations that selective brain ablations could calm animals or change their sexual behavior frequently provided the initial impetus for exploring the therapeutic effects of various operations on psychiatric patients. It is also clear that these animal experiments were often misinterpreted by clinicians, who apparently had little understanding or appreciation of the number of different changes produced in the experimental animals (see Valenstein, 1973, pp. 326–335). In any event, the many demonstrations that ablation of structures within a particular brain region dramatically altered animals' emotional responsiveness gave support to the conclusion that specific parts of the mammalian brain act as emotional regulators. Thus, specific regions in the frontal lobes, thalamus, hypothalamus, and the "limbic system"[2] of the brain, as well as

---

[2] This system consists of brain structures located in a region that forms an inner border (limbus) underneath the cerebral cortex. The limbic system has often been referred to as the "emotional brain," but lately the justification for assigning emotions to this one system has been questioned.

their interconnecting nerve fiber systems, came to be considered a complex system for regulating emotional reactions (see Valenstein, 1973, pp. 47–63, 266–277). Figure 2.1 shows the location of these structures in the human brain.

Hypothesized Causal Mechanisms

Explanations of how destruction of these brain areas could actually produce the desired changes were (and have remained) extremely vague and have often been based on analogy or metaphors rather than physiological mechanisms. Thus, Moniz argued that psychiatric symptoms were the result of an abnormal stabilization of conditioned neural patterns in the frontal lobes, and he advised that "to cure these patients we must destroy the more or less fixed arrangements of cellular connections that exist in the brain, and particularly those which are related to the frontal lobes" (cited in Freeman and Watts, 1951, p. xvi). It is obvious to anyone with any knowledge of the nervous system that this was an argument based on an analogy, not on any physiological data. Moniz certainly had no evidence of the existence of any "fixed arrangements of cellular connections" or, for that matter, any idea how they might be identified even if they did exist.

In recommending that transorbital lobotomy be performed immediately after electroconvulsive shock, Walter Freeman demonstrated that he had taken over Moniz's pseudo-physiological explanation. Electric shock was used in place of an anesthetic because Freeman believed that the shock would disrupt some hypothesized pathological neural activity; the destruction of the nerve bundles during the transorbital lobotomy would then prevent this neural activity from reforming. The prevalence of these ideas can even be seen in the writings of Norbert Wiener, the "father of cybernetics":

> It may be that, in the future, we can do something better with situations where circulating memories have led to bad traffic jams than to destroy a part of the connections of the brain by a frontal lobotomy or to intervene brutally in all synaptic connections by one or the other varieties of shock therapy [Wiener, 1948, p. 217].

The idea that persisting emotional problems are based on persisting abnormal activity of nerve cells has continued up to the present. As late as 1971, Walter Freeman wrote:

> The most tenable theory would seem to be that the fibers severed in transorbital lobotomy are collaterals of the thalamofrontal projections. It would further seem that these collaterals are highly unstable

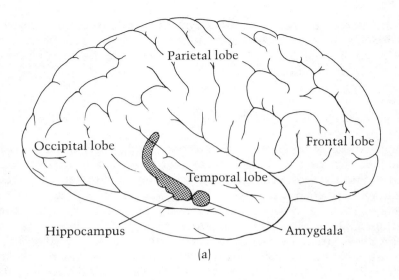

(a)

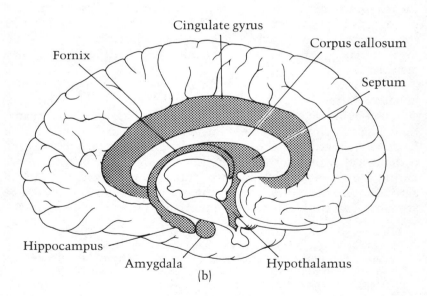

(b)

Figure 2.1 (a) Side view of the brain, illustrating the position of the amygdala in the temporal lobe. The amygdala and hippocampus are below the surface of the cerebral cortex and cannot be seen from the outside. (b) A view of the middle of the brain, showing the brain structures mentioned in the text. The position of some of the structures has been slightly altered in order to show them all on one plane.

and thus unimportant in mental health, but that during the course of a functional mental disorder they become stabilized in their synaptic connections and thus serve to perpetuate the stereotyped thinking disorder and emotional reaction that underlie the psychosis. Thus the original hypothesis of Egas Moniz appears more probable than ever [Freeman, 1971, p. 622].

Throughout the history of psychosurgery, the "metaphorical argument" that stubborn emotional disorders are caused by the fixation of some pathological neural activity, which maintains and exaggerates some emotional state or obsessive idea, has frequently been expressed. One neurosurgeon used the analogy of a stuck phonograph needle, while Sweet recently wrote:

> One thinks of the analogy of the uncontrolled feedback in a public-address system, which then starts to howl. There are as yet no neurophysiologic observations to support the hypothesis of abnormal activity in the limbic or any other specific neural pathways in psychotics [Sweet, 1973, p. 1122].

Sweet clearly indicated that he recognized the limitations of such analogies. But in an even more recent article no such qualification was mentioned when a group of Soviet clinicians offered the following "explanation" of how brain stimulation can produce beneficial results:

> Thus the therapeutic electrical stimulation of the brain's deep structures may lead to destabilization of the stable pathological condition [Bechtereva et al., 1977, p. 587].

There is no doubt that many of the persons who engage in the types of arguments illustrated above clearly recognize that they are only using analogies, even when they do not say so explicitly. Nevertheless, the frequent references to pseudo-physiological explanations tend to create the illusion of a scientific basis that does not in fact exist. Certainly they must give many laymen this impression, particularly when they are couched in neuroanatomical and other technical terms. Such terms as "limbic imbalance" (Brown, 1973) and "diencephalic instability" (Turner, 1973a), although they might conceivably point to identifiable physiological disturbances in the future, at present can be characterized only as "neurologizing" of hypothetical processes.

The need to disrupt, or to reduce the intensity of, persistent ideas and emotions has been expressed with little change almost from the beginning of psychosurgery. This theme is consistent with the belief that patients with exaggerated emotional states—not the "burnt out" chronic schizophrenics—were most likely to be helped by psychosurgery. A report of the first 1,000 prefrontal leucotomy cases performed in England and Wales (Wilson and Warland, 1947) described the best candidates for psychosurgery in language that is not distinguishable from that currently in use:

> A melancholic may be so preoccupied with his sense of failure or ill-health and by his own feelings of guilt about it that he can talk of nothing else. The tension of the urge toward scrupulosity and cleanliness may be so strong in the obsessional that he spends many hours a day carrying out rituals and becomes quite unfitted to lead a normal life [Wilson and Warland, 1947].

The authors of this report concluded that the purpose of the operation was "to break the connection between the patient's thoughts and his emotions. It is to relieve mental tension, to take the sting out of experience." Several years later, in describing the effects of psychosurgery, Freeman and Watts wrote, "The emotional nucleus of the psychosis is removed, the 'sting' of the disorder is drawn" (Freeman and Watts, 1951, p. xiii).

As already noted, the belief that certain anatomical areas are critically involved in regulating the intensity of emotional reactions is supported in part by the demonstrations of physiological and behavioral changes induced by either electrical stimulation or ablation of particular brain structures. The conclusion from a large body of experimental literature is that there are neural circuits traversing regions of the frontal lobes and limbic system (including related thalamic and hypothalamic areas) that either facilitate or inhibit the visceral reactions and mental states characteristic of such emotional states as depression and anxiety. Thus, for example, electrical stimulation at some part of these circuits inhibits visceral responses such as heart rate and respiration, while stimulation at other areas may accelerate or exaggerate these responses. Destruction of the same brain areas often, but not always, has the opposite effect. A number of reviews of the physiological responses to stimulation and ablation of different brain areas have been published (Kelly, 1973; Livingston, 1973, 1975). In general, it has been found that electrical stimulation of the brain sites that are most commonly selected for psychosurgery (lower medial quadrant of the frontal lobes and the anterior cingulum) intensifies the visceral responses that normally accompany emotional states. By destroying these regions, it is hoped that exaggerated and persistent emotional states will be attenuated.

Results of Different Psychosurgery Operations

In spite of the often questionable origins of some psychosurgical operations, conclusions about the changes produced by the surgery are consistent with the physiological events described above. Thus, in the 1973 Presidential Address to the International Congress of Psychosurgery, the best candidates for psychosurgery were described as follows:

> The work to date indicates that functional mental disease is benefitted by surgical lesions only when they [sic] exhibit an excess or exaggeration of normal feelings or thoughts. In other words, there must be an excess of guilt; of depression; . . . or an excess of anxiety and of neurotic fixations. This exaggeration of normal feeling tone or sensory input can be benefitted by surgical lesions resulting in a lowering of such excess down to a normal level. Because of these observations, I believe that psychosurgery of the prefrontal lobes does have a blunting effect, hopefully of a selective nature, on those thought processes and feeling tones which are grossly exaggerated above the normal [Scoville, 1973, pp. 34–35].

More recently, Bridges and Bartlett wrote:

> The contemporary operations appear to restore normal emotional modulation so that excessive swings of depression and extreme anxiety responses are eliminated and normal intensities of emotional experience are restored [Bridges and Bartlett, 1977, p. 256].

It should also be noted that sometimes psychosurgery does not have a dampening effect. In some cases patients have become more irritable and impulsive after operations—an effect attributed to a removal of the inhibitory influence of some parts of the frontal lobes (see Balasubramaniam and Kanaka, 1976, quoted earlier in this chapter). The fact that some patients may show dampened emotions and others a disinhibition is commonly attributed to subtle differences in the brain structures destroyed, but there is little evidence to support this argument. The complexity of the problem of interpretation can be appreciated by the realization that destruction of any region of the brain always produces secondary changes, including the atrophy of nerve cells, at great distances from the site of the operation. There have also been attempts to relate differences in the direction of the results to the premorbid personality of the patient. It is evident that many factors not yet understood contribute to the variability in the effects produced by psychosurgery.

Some idea of the present level of understanding of the physiological basis of psychosurgery can be gleaned by examining differing views on the relationship of psychiatric disorders to specific brain structures. It is clear to anyone familiar with the practice of psychosurgery that individual surgeons have their preferred brain targets. It is generally conceded that if a given patient were referred to different neurosurgeons he or she would most likely be offered different operations (involving different brain targets). This situation, which could be considered an embarrassment to the field, has been rationalized by the hypothesis that the disruption of a given brain circuit at any point along its route may have similar effects on emotionality. Indeed, this possibility was expressed by a number of surgeons in attendance at the Fourth International Congress of Psychiatric Neurosurgery (Madrid, September 1975) after they had heard many similar reports of success following different operations on patients appearing to have identical symptomatology.

It should not be assumed that there is complete agreement among all those performing psychosurgery that all operations are equally effective. Thus, it has been stated by Scoville (1973) that in his hands destruction of the rostral cingulum does not produce beneficial results but that his orbital undercutting operation is appropriate for all patients who can benefit from psychosurgery. Ballantine, however, has consistently reported successful results with the rostral cingulum operation (Ballantine et al., 1967, 1972, 1977; and Corkin, this volume). There is even greater disagreement over the effectiveness of amygdalectomy when performed on patients who do not have demonstrable pathology in this temporal lobe structure.

There is also strong disagreement among those who practice psychosurgery on whether different brain targets should be used for different symptoms. The many statements in the literature arguing that different mental illnesses do not need different operative procedures (Nicola and Nizzoli, 1972; see also Scoville, 1973) stand in sharp contrast to other statements that imply that different brain circuits underlie perceptual, cognitive, and affective disorders and that operations should select targets or combine targets depending on patients' symptoms (Brown, 1973). Turner (1973b) has also argued that the effects of different operations on temperament are predictable and this information can be used for selecting patients for particular operations, resulting in "custom psychosurgery."

The present author conducted a small survey among some of the leading spokesmen in the field of psychosurgery in order to obtain their views on the specificity of different brain targets used in psychosurgery. A statement paraphrased from a 1975 review (Livingston, 1975) of psychosurgery was mailed to a number of neurosurgeons and neuropsychiatrists, who were asked to indicate whether they (1) essentially agreed, (2) agreed, but with some qualification, or (3) did not believe that one could justify the view that different psychosurgical targets were more effective with certain psychiatric disorders. The following statement was mailed:

Based on anatomical and functional considerations, a distinction is frequently made between medial and lateral limbic circuits in the brain. The medial limbic circuit is said to include (among other structures) the medial frontal cortex, the cingulate gyrus, the anterior thalamic nucleus, and connecting fiber systems. The lateral limbic circuit is believed to include (among other structures) the orbital frontal cortex, and dorsomedial thalamic nucleus, the amygdala and connecting fiber systems.

Damage to the medial limbic system often produces states of motor and psychic hypoactivity. Stimulation or irritative disorders on the other hand often produce signs of motor and psychic hyperactivity such as restlessness, anxiety, and irritability. The lateral limbic system appears to be involved in a broad spectrum of disturbances including depression, perceptual and hallucinatory disorders, and uncontrolled aggression.

In broad terms, the types of psychiatric disabilities for which lesions of medial or lateral limbic structures are likely to be most beneficial have been established. Lesions of the medial frontal area, the anterior cingulate region, or closely related fiber systems, are most effective in syndromes characterized by psychic hyperactivity such as seen in patients suffering from tension, anxiety, restlessness, and obsessive behavior. Lesions involving the orbital frontal cortex and closely related fiber systems have been found to be most effective in syndromes characterized by various manifestations of depression. Lesions of the amygdala are most likely to be beneficial in cases where hyperkinetic activity and/or unprovoked assaultive behavior is the major behavioral problem.

Fifty percent of the respondents disagreed completely with the statement and one-half of the remaining responses indicated very significant, but often different, areas of disagreement. A number of neuropsychiatrists and neurosurgeons, who often had a great many years of experience observing psychosurgical patients, indicated that there was no evidence that brain targets should be varied as a function of psychiatric syndromes. Other clinicians, with equally long experience, claimed that there are justifications for varying the brain targets in psychosurgery. With such strong and significant disagreement among those who practice psychosurgery, it can hardly be said that our understanding of the physiological basis of psychosurgery has advanced very far. Nevertheless, despite the considerable uncertainty in many areas, empirical evidence accumulated over the years has produced some clear areas of agreement. There is certainly strong agreement about the usefulness of certain brain targets, and there is also a reasonable consensus on the patients most likely to be helped, although here too there remains some controversy, as will be seen in Chapter 3.

The Evolution of Psychosurgical Procedures

Psychosurgical operations have evolved from crude procedures for destroying poorly defined regions of the frontal lobes to much more precise techniques that make it possible to ablate relatively specific targets in the brain. The original "core" lobotomy technique of Moniz and Lima was not widely adopted, primarily because the anatomical reference points were considered unreliable. Essentially, the "core" technique consisted of drilling several burr holes into the top of the skull and inserting a cutting instrument (leucotome) into the brain. When the leucotome was believed to be in place, a sharpened wire was extruded through a slot in the side of the instrument and the whole tool was rotated, thereby cutting nerve fibers at different places in the frontal lobe (see Figure 2.2).

In contrast, the Freeman-Watts *standard lobotomy* technique, which was introduced approximately one year after Moniz and Lima's first operation, was widely used throughout the world. The technique consisted of inserting a knife into the frontal lobes through trephine holes drilled on both sides of the skull. The locations of the holes were determined by skull landmarks, and for this reason Freeman referred to the method as the "precision technique." The knife was pivoted up and down to make a cut in the desired plane. The holes were placed more or less forward on the skull depending on the severity of the symptoms; if a "standard" lobotomy was not successful, a more posterior "radical" lobotomy was frequently undertaken (see Figure 2.3). Actually, most neurosurgeons devised their own variations on the Freeman-Watts procedure—a state of affairs that led Turnbull (1969) to comment that "no 'standard' operation has ever been performed in so many ways."

In 1948, Freeman introduced the *transorbital lobotomy* procedure —a technique for reaching the frontal lobes by piercing the bone at the roof of the eye socket with a transorbital leucotome, an instrument resembling an ice pick (see Figure 2.4). Transorbital lobotomy deserves special mention because it was the only psychosurgical operation that could be done as an office procedure. No doubt this fact accounts in part for the large numbers of transorbital lobotomies performed (see Chapter 1).

During the late 1930s and 1940s a number of other surgical approaches to the frontal lobe were introduced. In 1938, J. G. Lyerly of Jacksonville, Florida, modified the Freeman-Watts lobotomy pro-

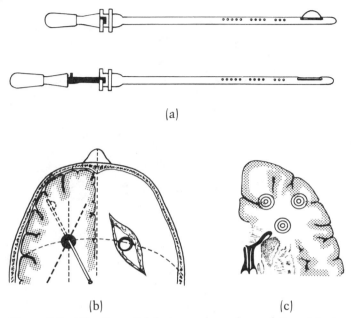

(a)

(b)   (c)

Figure 2.2 The "core" lobotomy procedure of Egas Moniz
and Almeida Lima. (a) The leucotome (knife) with cutting
wire extruded and retracted. (b) The leucotome was inserted
at different angles through a burr hole drilled in the skull.
When the leucotome was in place, the wire was extruded and
fibers were cut by a rotational motion. (c) Sketch of a horizon-
tal slice (parallel to the top of the skull) through the brain,
illustrating the location of three areas of fiber destruction.

cedure. In 1949, Lawrence Pool of Columbia University introduced
his *topectomy* operation, a technique involving the undercutting
and removal of blocks of frontal lobe tissue. This procedure was used
in the frequently cited Columbia-Greystone study. Modifications of
the various lobotomy procedures were introduced in many countries
around the world. What was characteristic of most of these early
lobotomy procedures was that they were designed to destroy brain
tissue in the prefrontal area (in front of the region known to control
speech and bodily movement) and that the majority of the operations were "blind" procedures, meaning that the destruction of tissue was not guided by vision. These operations were also called
"closed" procedures because the brain was not exposed—the knife
being inserted through a small hole in the skull. The wound was
rinsed with a warm saline solution until the bleeding stopped, but
because the surgeon did not have any view of the destroyed area
there was always the possibility of hemorrhage.

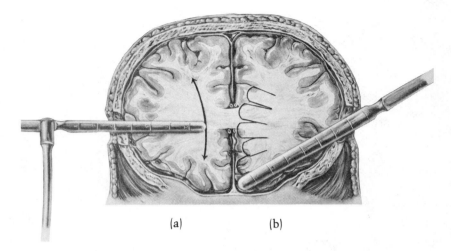

(a)   (b)

Figure 2.3   The Freeman–Watts lobotomy procedure. The leucotome was inserted through holes drilled in the sides of the frontal region of the skull. (a) The position of the leucotome as initially inserted. (b) The rotation of the knife to cut the ventromedial portion of the frontal lobes. The lobotomy was called "moderate," "standard," or "radical," depending on how posteriorly the knife was inserted. [From W. Freeman and J. W. Watts, *Psychosurgery in the Treatment of Mental Disorders and Intractable Pain*, 2nd ed., 1950. Courtesy of Charles C Thomas, Publisher, Springfield, Illinois.]

In 1948, James Poppen of the Lahey Clinic in Boston described an approach to the frontal lobes from the top ("superior" aspect) of the skull. This approach was thought to reduce intellectual impairment by minimizing damage to the more lateral regions while making it easier to destroy those deep, medial structures in the brain that were beginning to appear to be most important targets for best results. In the same year, William Scoville introduced an "open method" for cutting the fibers at the base of the frontal lobes under direct visual guidance. This *orbital undercutting* operation permitted the surgeon to selectively destroy the fibers connecting the deep, medial parts of the frontal lobe with the limbic system, the so-called emotional areas of the brain (see Figure 2.5). The results of Scoville's orbital undercutting operations are summarized under the heading "Surgeon 1" in the Mirsky and Orzack study reported in Chapter 10.[3]

---

[3] Drs. Mirsky and Orzack have respected their agreement not to identify the surgeons whose patients they studied. It is generally known by everyone familiar with the practice of psychosurgery, however, that this procedure (as well as several others) is performed by only one surgeon in the United States. Therefore, a description of the procedure is sufficient to identify the surgeon.

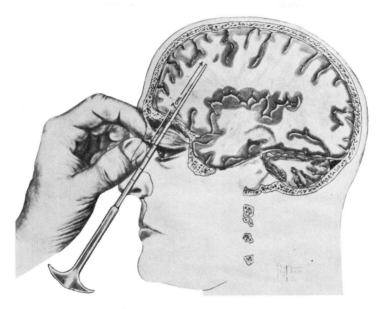

Figure 2.4 The transorbital lobotomy procedure popularized by Walter Freeman. The transorbital leucotome (often referred to as an "ice pick") was inserted (with the aid of a mallet) through the bony orbit above the eyeball. The handle of the leucotome was rotated so that the cutting edge would destroy fibers at the base of the frontal lobes. [From W. Freeman, "Transorbital Leucotomy: The Deep Frontal Cut." *Proc. Royal Soc. Med.*, 1949, *42*, Suppl. pp. 8–12.]

This procedure was adopted with some modification by several other surgeons, including Hirose in Japan. Similar developments leading to other surgical procedures that made it possible to destroy a more restricted medial area in the frontal lobes occurred in Great Britain and elsewhere (see Bridges and Bartlett, 1977).

New Surgical Techniques

Three major changes in psychosurgical operations were introduced during the 1950s and 1960s. One of these was the gradual introduction of *stereotaxic instruments*. Basically, a stereotaxic instrument positions the head in a fixed plane so as to make it possible, with the aid of three-dimensional maps (stereotaxic atlases), to insert electrodes (or other devices) through small holes in the skull into almost

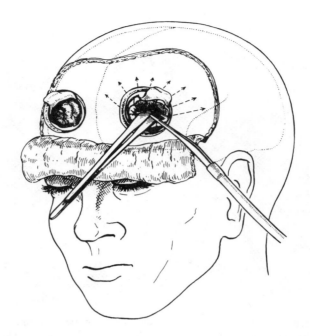

Figure 2.5 The orbital undercutting operation introduced by William Scoville. The frontal lobes are lifted by a spatula inserted through the trephined holes in the frontal pole of the skull, and fibers beneath the orbital (close to the midline) surface are destroyed. [From A. Asenjo, *Neurosurgical Techniques*, 1963. Courtesy of Charles C Thomas, Publisher, Springfield, Illinois.]

any sector of the brain (see Figure 2.6a). Although this technique had been used in animal research since 1908, the first account of its application to psychosurgery was the description by Spiegel and Wycis of Temple University (Spiegel, Wycis, and Freed, 1949) of their use of the stereotaxic instrument to destroy a circumscribed region in the dorsomedial thalamus of psychotic patients. The use of this instrument gradually gained acceptance by those performing psychosurgery, and today most of these operations use some variation of the basic principle of stereotaxic surgery. Gildenberg (1975) has listed over twenty different stereotaxic instruments currently being used by neurosurgeons in the United States and Canada. Stereotaxic techniques made a number of different brain areas accessible to surgical intervention. Without the aid of stereotaxic instruments it is unlikely that any psychosurgical procedures would have been performed on the hypothalamus, thalamus, or amygdala.

Although stereotaxic surgery is also a "blind" or "closed" procedure, the accuracy of its coordinates system justifies placing it in a separate category. Moreover, in current practice, the accuracy of stereotaxic surgery is commonly increased by monitoring the position of the electrodes during their insertion into the brain via on-line X-ray pictures displayed on television screens and, in some instances, via electrical recording information (see Figure 2.6b, c). In the case of posterior hypothalamic operations, the accuracy of the electrode placement may be confirmed by determining the effect of electrical stimulation on blood pressure, heart rate, and respiration prior to destroying brain tissue (Schvarcz, 1977, p. 430). All of this information can be used to complement the stereotaxic atlas coordinates, which are based on average data. In spite of the great increase in sophistication of stereotaxic surgery, there is still a significant amount of so-called "free-hand" psychosurgery currently being performed (Corkill, Ratcliff, and Simpson, 1973; Griponissiotis and Tavridis, 1972; Scoville and Bettis, 1977).

The second major change in psychosurgery involved changes in the method of destroying brain tissue. Initially, all psychosurgery was performed with knives of different shapes designed to either cut through nerve tracts or, in the case of the much lesser used topectomy operation, to remove small cylinders of brain tissue. Later, several neurosurgeons used a suction technique for removing brain tissue or interrupting nerve tracts. With the introduction of the stereotaxic technique, electric current and later radio-frequency waves were more commonly used to destroy relatively circumscribed brain regions. Gradually, the stereotaxic instrument was used in conjunction with a number of different techniques, each of which is believed by its advocates to have some special advantage in destroying tissue. Gildenberg's survey (1975) of neurosurgeons in the United States and Canada revealed that 73 percent of the neurosurgeons using stereotaxic techniques produce brain lesions with radio-frequency waves. Also mentioned by the respondents to Gildenberg's questionnaire were the following methods (listed in order of decreasing frequency of use): cryoprobe (freezing), leucotome, electrolytic (Direct Current), radioisotopes (including the implantation of yttrium seeds), proton beams, ultrasound, balloon cannula (compression), and thermocoagulation. Other neurosurgeons around the world have destroyed brain tissue using injections of alcohol or an inert oil or wax. A great variety of techniques are used, many of them by only a single neurosurgeon.

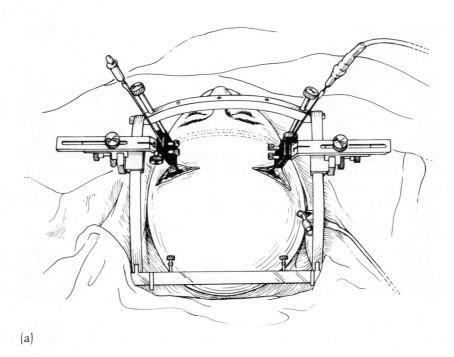

(a)

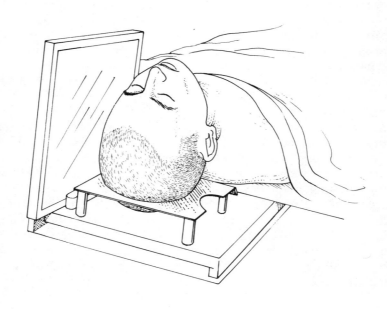

(b)

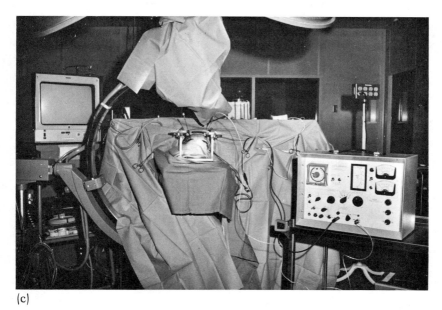

(c)

Figure 2.6 Stereotaxic psychosurgery. (a) The stereotaxic instrument, when used in conjunction with a stereotaxic atlas (brain map), makes it possible to position electrode wires deep in the brain. The use of (b) X-ray and (c) monitoring television screens enables the surgeon to visualize brain landmarks and to monitor the electrode as it is inserted into the brain. [Photograph courtesy of M. Hunter Brown.]

Exploration of New Brain Sites

The third major development that occurred during the 1950s and 1960s was the extension of psychosurgery to brain regions outside the frontal lobes. (See the sketch of modern psychosurgical brain targets in Figure 2.7.) The realization that the most effective targets were the medial and deep (ventral) portion of the frontal lobes tended to draw attention to other brain areas that were anatomically connected to the ventromedial surfaces of the frontal lobes. It was this consideration that was partly responsible for Spiegel and Wycis' selection of the dorsomedial thalamic nucleus as the target for their first stereotaxic surgery on psychiatric patients. Although this target is no longer used, it was selected because several autopsy studies on the brains of prefrontal lobotomized patients had revealed secondary degeneration in the dorsomedial thalamus—a finding that reflects the direct connections between the two areas.

It was the renowned neurophysiologist John Fulton who was most influential in encouraging the exploration for effective brain sites outside the frontal lobes. Disturbed by the evidence of intellectual deterioration in a number of prefrontal lobotomized patients and at the same time encouraged by the evidence from animal experiments of emotional changes following selective destruction of limbic brain structures (see Valenstein, 1973, pp. 47–63), Fulton advised neurosurgeons in the United States and in Europe to investigate the effects of selective damage to either limbic brain structures or those parts of the prefrontal lobes that had neural connections to the limbic system. In his writings and in lectures, Fulton stated that he believed that radical lobotomy as carried out by Freeman and Watts should be abandoned in favor of a more restricted lesion (Fulton, 1948, 1951), and he recommended more circumscribed ablations of the ventromedial quadrant of the frontal lobes or the anterior portions of the cingulum. The cingulum, an important part of the limbic system (see Figure 2.7 and the contribution by Corkin in this volume), had been reported to play a critical role in the emotional behavior of monkeys. Shortly afterward, several neurosurgeons in France, Great Britain, and the United States started to perform anterior cingulotomies on psychiatric patients.

In the early 1950s, neurosurgeons Sir Hugh Cairns in Oxford and J. Le Beau in Paris independently reported favorable results following destruction of the anterior region of the cingulum. Subsequently, many other neurosurgeons have reported success after destroying either specific limbic structures or by disrupting fronto-limbic pathways in regions that were considered to be major crossroads for these fiber connections. Among the principal limbic structures that were selected for destruction were the amygdala, in the temporal lobes, and to a lesser extent thalamic structures such as the dorsomedial, anterior, centromedian, and parafascicular nuclei—areas known to have connections to limbic structures, and also believed (in some instances) to be mediating pain sensation. In addition, selective regions of the hypothalamus, including the posterior regions, the ventromedial nuclei, and the lateral area, have been used, at one time or another, as targets for psychosurgical operations. The anatomical and behavioral evidence and the rationale for exploring these brain regions have been presented in detail elsewhere (Valenstein, 1973).

More recently, several neurosurgeons have developed multiple-target psychosurgical procedures. For example, M. Hunter Brown, a neurosurgeon who has accumulated one of the largest populations of psychosurgical patients in the United States, performs an operation aimed at six targets in the brain (Brown, 1973, and this volume). This procedure involves the partial destruction of portions of the amygdala, cingulum, and substantia innominata on both sides of the

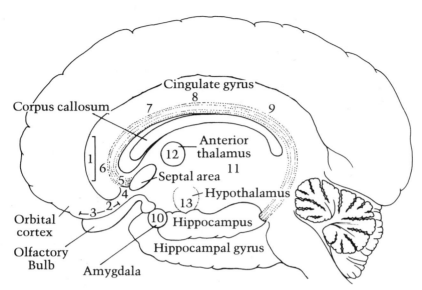

Figure 2.7 Approximate brain targets of psychosurgical operations currently in use. *Frontal lobe procedures:* (1) bimedial leucotomy; (2) yttrium lesions in subcortical white matter; (3) orbital undercutting; (4) bifrontal stereotaxic subcaudate tractotomy; (5) anterior capsulotomy (destruction of fibers of internal capsule); (6) mesoloviotomy (similar to rostral cingulotomy), but lesion invades genu—"knee"—of corpus callosum). *Cingulotomies:* (7) anterior cingulotomy; (8) mid-cingulotomy; (9) posterior cingulotomy. *Amygdalectomy:* (10) amygdalectomy or amygdalotomy. *Thalatomies:* (11) dorsomedial, centromedian, and parafascicular nuclei; (12) anterior thalatomy. *Hypothalotomy:* (13) posterior, ventromedial, and lateral hypothalamic targets.

brain. The results of this operation are summarized in Mirsky and Orzack's contribution under the heading "Surgeon 2" (see footnote 3 in this chapter). In England, one neurosurgeon (Richardson, Kelly, and Mitchell-Heggs, 1976) performs *limbic leucotomy*, a multitargeted operation designed to destroy portions of the ventromedial frontal lobes and the anterior cingulum.

Within the general considerations described in this section, individual neurosurgeons each have their own favorite target, surgical approach, and method of destroying brain tissue. In England, for example, Knight (1965) has used radioactive yttrium seeds to destroy the nerve tracts in the frontal lobe that are located just beneath and in front of the head of the caudate nucleus (see Figure 2.7). This operation, called a *bifrontal stereotaxic subcaudate tractotomy*, has been performed on over 500 patients since its introduction in 1965.

CHAPTER 3

Extent of Psychosurgery Worldwide

Elliot S. Valenstein

In the early 1970s there were many reports that psychosurgery was undergoing a resurgence, but actually there was little quantitative information available. Recognizing the need for this information, the National Commission for the Protection of Human Subjects of Biomedical and Behavioral Research asked the present author to undertake an investigation of the amount of psychosurgery performed each year from 1971 through 1976 (Valenstein, 1977). It was suspected that a valid estimate of the extent of psychosurgery could not be obtained solely from a literature survey as many surgeons who perform these operations probably do not publish any account of them. Moreover, most published articles summarize the results of operations performed over a number of years, making it impossible to determine with certainty the actual number of operations performed each year. It was necessary, therefore, to utilize data from surveys of U.S. and Canadian neurosurgeons conducted by others and to supplement these data with information I obtained from questionnaires mailed to neurosurgeons in selected foreign countries. A comparison of the results of the questionnaire surveys with the information obtained from our literature search confirmed our suspicion that a relatively small percentage of the neurosurgeons performing psychosurgery actually publish their results.

United States and Canada

The primary source of information on the amount of psychosurgery performed in the United States and Canada between 1971 and 1973 was a survey undertaken by Dr. John Donnelly, Chief Psychiatrist at the Institute of Living (Hartford, Connecticut), under the auspices of the Task Force on Psychosurgery of the American Psychiatric Association. A brief questionnaire (Donnelly, 1978) was sent to all active members (as of 1973) of the American Association of Neurological Surgeons and the Congress of Neurological Surgeons. These two organizations include virtually all of the neurosurgeons practicing in the United States and Canada. In total, 1,901 questionnaires were mailed. The questionnaire was designed to determine the number of psychosurgical operations and neurosurgical procedures for pain that were performed for the years 1971, 1972, and 1973 and the number of neurosurgeons performing these procedures. Of the questionnaires mailed, 78 percent (1,481) were filled out and returned.

The responses to the Donnelly questionnaire indicated that 110 U.S. and 19 Canadian neurosurgeons had performed some psychosurgery during the 1971–1973 period. These results are summarized in Table 3.1.

The data summarized in Table 3.1 suggest that the number of neurosurgeons performing psychosurgery decreased over the three years surveyed. Although there are no reliable data available, it is frequently stated by those informed about psychosurgical practices that the number of surgeons doing these operations continued to decline during 1974 and 1975. This opinion is based primarily on what is believed to be the deterrent influence of the public controversy over psychosurgery, and the resulting legislation that has been passed or is pending in several states, as well as the effect of several well-publicized malpractice suits against neurosurgeons performing these operations.

The possibility that the downward trend in the rate of performing psychosurgery may have halted, or may even have been reversed, during the last two years (1977–1978) is raised by Corkin in this volume. Her observations are, however, based on the practice of only one neurosurgeon (H. Thomas Ballantine), albeit one who performs a significant percentage of the psychosurgery done in the United

Table 3.1 Number of U.S. and Canadian Neurosurgeons Performing Psychosurgery

Year	United States	Canada
1971	75	15
1972	71	17
1973	59	12

Note: The total number of different U.S. neurosurgeons indicating that they performed psychosurgery during the three years is 110.

Source: Data obtained from the 1,481 neurosurgeons responding to Donnelly's questionnaire.

States. The slight increase observed in Ballantine's practice seems to be more than counterbalanced by the effect of the California "psychosurgery law" (see contributions in this volume by Grimm and Pizzulli) on the practice of M. Hunter Brown, who had also performed a significant number of the total operations in the United States. Brown had performed between 50 and 60 operations per year prior to 1977, but due to the California legislation he has not done any psychosurgery during 1977 and 1978, with the exception of two cases done with a court injunction (personal communication, March 20, 1979). He reports having had 40 cases on the waiting list when the California law was passed and has since been contacted in behalf of approximately 200 to 250 potential psychosurgical candidates. It is very likely that part of the increase in Ballantine's practice represents people who had first contacted Brown and were referred to Ballantine. Moreover, based on some inquiries, the present author has concluded that many of the neurosurgeons who previously had performed only two or three psychosurgical procedures a year have stopped doing these operations. ("It's not worth the hassle.") Considering all the available evidence, there is little reason to believe that in the country as a whole an increase in psychosurgery has taken place during the last two years; a decrease in both the amount of psychosurgery and the number of neurosurgeons performing these operations is much more likely.

Of the neurosurgeons responding to Donnelly's survey, 7.5 percent reported having done psychosurgery during the 1971–1973 period. If this percentage is used to estimate the number of nonrespondents who may have performed these procedures, the number for the United States would be increased to 141 and for Canada to 25. However, these estimates are probably too high, as Donnelly concluded after examining the names and affiliations of the 420 nonresponding neurosurgeons that it was more likely that the nonrespondents performed much less psychosurgery than those responding.

Table 3.2 summarizes the number of operations performed by the 110 U.S. and 19 Canadian neurosurgeons reporting having done any psychosurgery during the years 1971 to 1973.

The figures obtained from Donnelly's questionnaire can be compared with the results of a survey published by Dr. Philip Gildenberg (1975), Chief of the Division of Neurosurgery, of the University of Texas Medical School in Houston. Gildenberg sent out 2,028 questionnaires to neurosurgeons in the United States and Canada during mid-1973. The wording of the questionnaire was not published, but essentially it requested information from the recipients on whether or not they were currently performing any "stereotaxic and functional neurosurgery." Only 637 neurosurgeons completed and returned the form. This figure represents a return percentage of only 31.5 percent, compared with Donnelly's 78 percent returns. Gildenberg noted that the 637 respondents reported that they were doing a total of about 246 (the respondents' estimates ranged from 228 to 264) brain operations for emotional disorders per year. The procedures included cingulotomies (over 50 percent of the total), frontal leucotomies, dorsomedial thalamotomies, hypothalamotomies, and prefrontal ultrasonic operations. Considering all the information available from questionnaires, the average yearly number of psychosurgical procedures performed in the United States during the 1971–1973 period was probably around 400 and almost certainly below 500. As noted above, the average number of such operations performed per year appears to have decreased after 1973, particularly after 1976.

An analysis of the responses from the neurosurgeons doing psychosurgery revealed that during 1971–1973 approximately 25 percent of the total operations were performed by surgeons doing three or fewer operations per year (see Table 3.3). Approximately 70 to 80 percent of neurosurgeons who performed any psychosurgery at all between 1971 and 1973 performed fewer than three procedures in an average year. Many of these surgeons performed only one operation in a given year. This point is worth emphasizing because many surgeons are convinced that it is not possible to maintain adequate skill if a procedure is performed that infrequently. Some persons have used this argument to advocate the establishment of a few centers where all psychosurgery would be performed.

A comparison of the number of neurosurgeons indicating on questionnaires that they performed psychosurgery with the number of neurosurgeons who can be identified from the published literature proved to be interesting. A thorough search of the relevant literature

Table 3.2   Number of Psychosurgical Operations Performed in the United
States and Canada

Year	United States	Canada
1971	308	22
1972	343	27
1973	321	18
Total	972	67

Note: These numbers are based on the 1,481 questionnaires returned. If it is assumed that the same percentages apply to the 420 neurosurgeons who did not return the questionnaires, the average number of psychosurgical operations for the United States would be increased from 324 per year to 414 and for Canada from an average of 22 to 29 per year.
Source: Data based on the Donnelly survey.

since 1971 revealed only 30 names of neurosurgeons performing psychosurgery. In two of these instances, it was not clear whether the neurosurgeon ever performed brain surgery unless there was evidence of neurological damage. While it is possible that some articles were missed by our literature survey (if they were not published in journals included in the major abstracting services or ever cited in other articles that were included), it is unlikely that the names of more than a few relevant neurosurgeons were omitted. Therefore, at most only 27 percent (30 out of 110) of the neurosurgeons performing psychosurgery publish their results. This percentage is further reduced to only 21 percent if it is assumed that 141 neurosurgeons (a figure including estimates from the nonrespondents) actually perform psychosurgery. It seems evident that a considerable amount of the experience with psychosurgery is not recorded in the archival literature. The present author, for example, became aware of several neurosurgeons who have performed only a few psychosurgical operations and have never published any account of these operations. This was not really surprising or for that matter unusual, as most surgeons do not publish the results of their operations. But because of the controversy over psychosurgery, the situation is worth noting. It is quite possible that the published results might introduce a systematic bias owing to the nonreporting of results achieved by the least-experienced surgeons.

The number of neurosurgeons performing brain operations for intractable pain also cannot be estimated very reliably from the published literature. Donnelly's questionnaire also requested information on whether the respondent had performed surgery for intractable pain. Descriptions of the procedures employed made it possible to distinguish peripheral and spinal cord operations from operations performed on the brain. Donnelly's estimates of the number of brain

Table 3.3 Amount of Psychosurgery Performed Per Year by U.S. Practitioners

Number of Procedures (Per Year)	1971		1972		1973	
	Percent of Surgeons	Percent of Procedures	Percent of Surgeons	Percent of Procedures	Percent of Surgeons	Percent of Procedures
1–3	80.9	28.9	70.4	22.7	78.0	22.4
4–10	10.6	17.1	19.7	22.5	11.8	13.4
11–15	5.4	18.0	4.2	10.2	6.8	16.2
16–20	0	0	1.4	5.8	0	0
21–	4.0	36.0	4.3[a]	38.8	3.4[a]	48.0

[a]One neurosurgeon reported performing between 61 and 80 procedures in 1972, and one reported performing 132 procedures during 1973. If the latter figure is accurate, this individual was responsible for over 41 percent of all procedures that were reported by the respondents for 1973.
Source: Data based on the Donnelly survey.

operations for intractable pain, based on the responses to his questionnaire, are presented in Table 3.4.

Of some interest is Donnelly's finding that many neurosurgeons perform either psychosurgical procedures or operations for intractable pain, but not both. These figures are summarized in Table 3.5.

United Kingdom

Robin and Macdonald (1975) estimated that approximately 200 psychosurgical procedures were performed in Britain in 1974, but this figure was based on general familiarity with the situation rather than on any survey (personal communication). This author's request for information to the Medical Statistics Division of the Office of Population Censuses and Survey in London did not prove rewarding. The reply from this Bureau revealed that no British agency has reliable and comprehensive statistics on the amount of psychosurgery performed (personal communication). The replies to a questionnaire (reproduced in Valenstein, 1977, Appendix 1) mailed by this author to approximately 20 neurosurgeons who perform stereotaxic psychosurgery with some degree of regularity in 15 different surgical units proved more helpful.

The Geoffrey Knight Psychosurgical Unit at the Brooks General Hospital in London performs more psychosurgery than any other unit in Britain. There are eight beds reserved for psychosurgery in this unit, and approximately one operation is performed each week. Geoffrey Knight has recently retired from hospital practice, but the staff at his unit reported that they had done 54, 38, and 46 psycho-

Table 3.4 Number of Neurosurgical Procedures for Pain

	1971		1972		1973	
	United States	Canada	United States	Canada	United States	Canada
Intractable pain only	92	3	97	1	63	1
Intractable pain due to malignancies	20	—	30	1	28	—

Source: Data based on Donnelly's survey.

surgical operations in 1973, 1974, and 1975, respectively. Because the controversy over psychosurgery never reached the intensity in the United Kingdom that it did in the United States, it is likely that these numbers reflect current rates. The neurosurgical group at the St. George's Hospital in London averages about 20 operations a year, while the neurosurgical teams at the Guy's, Maudsley, and King's College Hospitals in London reported that they had performed, respectively, only 1, 6, and 4 operations per year during 1973, 1974, and 1975. Other neurosurgical units performing psychosurgery exist in Birmingham, Sheffield, Edinburgh, Cambridge, Southampton, Plymouth, Bristol, Glasgow, Dundee, Aberdeen, Salford, Manchester, and Derby. The neurosurgeons responding to the questionnaires estimated that between 200 and 250 psychosurgical operations were performed per year between 1973 and 1975 in the United Kingdom. The respondents generally indicated that they believed that the number of brain operations performed for the relief of intractable pain was somewhat less.

Australia

Dr. J. Sidney Smith of the Neuropsychiatric Institute in Rozelle, New South Wales, contacted all "possible surgeons and psychiatrists involved in psychosurgery" in Australia in 1973 (personal communication). Based on the information obtained, Smith estimated that 83 psychosurgical operations were performed in Australia in 1973. Smith believes the rate has remained constant to the present. A report of a recent symposium on psychosurgery summarized much of the history and current practice of psychosurgery in Australia (Smith and Kiloh, 1977). The two main groups performing

Table 3.5 Number of U.S. and Canadian Surgeons Performing Psychosurgery and Operations for Intractable Pain (1971, 1972, and 1973 Combined)

	Number of Neurosurgeons
Intractable pain only	66
Psychosurgery only	78
Both psychosurgery and intractable pain	50

Source: Data based on Donnelly's survey.

psychosurgery consist of neurosurgeons in private practice and those associated with the Neuropsychiatric Institute, a state-financed unit. Both groups are located in Sydney. With the exception of amygdalectomy procedures, most of the operations (primarily "cingulotractotomies") are performed by the private practitioners. It is estimated that approximately 8–12 neurosurgeons perform psychosurgery in Australia. There appear to be many fewer brain operations performed for intractable pain than for psychiatric disorders. Very recent evidence, however, indicates that psychosurgery legislation in Australia has resulted in a decrease in the amount of psychosurgery performed.

India

Psychosurgery in India seems to be completely restricted to the Institute of Neurology of the Madras Medical School. Approximately one-half of the surgical patients are referred from the Madras Mental Hospital, a government facility. There are three neurosurgeons who perform psychosurgical operations, and they constitute one group of colleagues (Balasubramaniam, 1972; Balasubramaniam, Kanaka et al., 1973; Balasubramaniam et al. 1975; Ramamurthi and Davidson, 1975). Since they are at the same Institute and often publish together, it is surprising that their estimates of the number of psychosurgical procedures performed per year varied between 36–61, 24–36, and 26–35 for 1973, 1974, and 1975, respectively. The procedures performed include amygdalectomies (the most frequent), hypothalamotomies, cingulomotomies, and prefrontal leucotomies. Of special interest is the group of 65 patients on whom cingulomotomies were performed for physical dependence on narcotics (see Valenstein, 1977, Appendix 3; Balasubramaniam et al., 1973).

Japan

In 1972 there were three main neurosurgeons (and their colleagues) performing psychosurgery in Japan (Hirose, 1972, 1973, 1977; Narabayashi, 1972, 1973; Narabayashi and Shima, 1973; Sano, 1975; Sano et al., 1972; Sano et al., 1975). The three surgeons were all located in Tokyo in either the Department of Neurosurgery, University of Tokyo; Department of Neuropsychiatry, Nippon Medical School; or the Department of Neurology, Juntendo Medical School. In 1972 approximately 25 psychosurgical procedures were performed, but starting in 1973 an active protest movement (described by one neurosurgeon as "militant psychiatrists and medical students") gradually brought the practice of psychosurgery to a halt. In 1973 approximately 25 procedures were performed. In 1974 the number appears to have been reduced to 15, and, as far as can be ascertained, no psychosurgery was performed in 1975 or more recently.

Czechoslovakia

There are three or four neurosurgeons performing psychosurgery in Czechoslovakia (Nádvorník, Pogády, and Šramka, 1973; Nádvorník et al., 1974; Nádvorník, Šramka, and Patoprstá, 1977; Šramka and Nádvorník, 1975; Šramka et al., 1977). Estimates from two of these neurosurgeons indicate that the amount of psychosurgery performed ranged between 20–47, 40–41, and 50–53 for 1973, 1974, and 1975. Although the numbers are not large, it appears that Czechoslovakia may be the only country of those for which information was obtained that increased the number of operations performed between 1973 and 1975. The estimates of the number of brain operations performed for intractable pain vary too greatly to be considered reliable. The use of brain stimulation for psychiatric disorders and intractable pain appears to have been initiated in 1974. Four to five patients were treated for psychiatric disorders with brain stimulation in both 1974 and 1975, and approximately the same numbers of patients were treated by this technique for intractable pain.

Mexico

Based on only one reply, it is estimated that three neurosurgeons (Escobedo, Solis, and Velasco-Suarez) performed between 10 and 25 psychosurgical operations per year between 1973 and 1975 (Escobedo et al., 1973, 1977). Brain stimulation was used to treat psychiatric disorders in approximately 4 cases between 1973 and 1975.

Other Countries

In addition to the countries mentioned above, it is known that some psychosurgery is currently being performed by at least one neurosurgeon in Spain, Argentina, Poland, France, Germany, Holland, Denmark, Sweden, Switzerland, and Italy. However, it was not possible to obtain estimates of the frequency of these operations in these countries. The one neurosurgeon (Laitinen) who was performing psychosurgery in Finland discontinued this practice in 1976.

Soviet Union

Psychosurgery was outlawed in the Soviet Union in the early 1950s. Although there have been reports (mostly from émigrés) that some form of psychosurgery is currently practiced in the Soviet Union, it was not possible to verify these claims. Kornetov (1972) reviewed the results of 40 prefrontal leucotomies (Freeman-Watts and Lyerly procedures) performed mostly at the First Moscow Medical Institute between 1947 and 1950. The patients were chronic schizophrenics, and, according to Kornetov's brief account of the long-term results, some of them have made excellent recoveries. Kornetov's conclusion implied that at least he believes there may still be a place for psychosurgery in cases of "pernicious schizophrenia." Several recent reports have appeared that indicate that Dr. N. P. Bechtereva and her colleagues at the Institute of Experimental Medicine in Leningrad have used "therapeutic electrical stimulation" (TES) through implanted electrodes to treat intractable pain (including phantom limb pain) and temporal lobe epilepsy associated with aggression or psychiatric disorders such as paranoia and other psychotic thought processes (Bechtereva and Bundzen, 1973; Bechtereva et al., 1975, 1977). Some of these patients had as many as 64 electrodes arranged in 14 different "cables" that were implanted in the temporal lobes. In a few instances, patients were allowed to engage in "self-stimulation"—that is, to control the delivery of stimulation themselves. Stimulation at some brain sites was said to reduce troublesome symptoms and to elevate mood. The neurosurgeons who have collaborated with Bechtereva are A. N. Bondartchuk and O. P. Pissarevsky.

Summary

It is estimated that 141 neurosurgeons in the United States performed approximately 400 operations per year during 1971, 1972, and 1973. There are indications that the annual rate was somewhat lower between 1974 and 1976 and considerably lower during 1977 and 1978. Approximately 75 percent of the U.S. neurosurgeons practicing psychosurgery do not publish their results in the archival literature.

Comparisons with other English-language countries revealed that approximately 200–250 psychosurgical procedures have been performed per year in the United Kingdom and about 83 such operations per year in Australia, at least through 1977. Taking into consideration the differences in populations between 1971 and 1977, psychosurgery has been performed in the United Kingdom at more than twice the rate, and in Australia at more than three times the rate, of that in the United States. Again, adjusting for population differences, Canada has a greater relative number of neurosurgeons who have done some psychosurgery, but the number of operations performed is approximately one-half the number performed in the United States.

PART II

The Psychosurgical Patient

CHAPTER 4

Who Receives Psychosurgery?

Elliot S. Valenstein

Psychiatrists and neurosurgeons who recommend or practice psychosurgery generally agree on the most appropriate patients for these operations. There are, however, some important areas of disagreement, which will be discussed below.

The Major Group

The most appropriate candidates for psychosurgery are patients described as suffering from very intense and persistent emotional responses. The most seriously impaired of these patients are said to be so severely depressed, anxious, or "possessed" by an unfounded fear or thought that their lives are crippled. Particularly in cases of depression, thoughts about suicide and actual suicide attempts are commonplace. Many of the patients are unable to hold jobs, and in some cases of severe obsessive-compulsive disorders the patients may have difficulty leaving their homes or may have to expend great amounts of energy and time repeating a ritualistic behavior over and over again. Often these patients are psychologically crippled by phobias and somatic complaints. In the cases in which psychosurgery is performed for pain symptoms, the pain is described as intense, persistent, crippling, and intractable. Typically, all of these disturbances are claimed to be of long duration and resistant to such alternative treatments as psychotherapy, drugs, and electroconvulsive shock (but see Rachman's chapter on obsessive-compulsive disorders). In contrast to these patients with intense emotional disturbances, who are believed to be most helped by psychosurgery, patients who are described as "resigned," "emotionless," "flat," "burned out," or "lacking motivation to get well" are considered poor candidates for psychosurgical operations.

Although specific symptoms and clinical history vary greatly, the following case history is representative of the type of severe obsessional patient who would be considered a good candidate for psychosurgery. Other typical case histories are presented in the chapters by Corkin and by Mirsky and Orzack in this volume.

Case 1 Severe intractable obsessional neurosis: J.G., Aged 34, female. Referred for treatment of an intractable obsessive-compulsive disorder.

Her symptoms began when she was 23, after an unwanted pregnancy had forced her into an unhappy marriage. A year later, when the baby developed asthma, her feelings of guilt deepened and from that time her symptoms were of such severity that she was unable to cope with even the simplest tasks of everyday life. Her day was totally occupied with checking and rechecking actions such as washing, dressing, and household tasks. She had, for example, to wash her face in a special order—starting with the left side, nose, right side, forehead —up to thirteen times. A similar elaborate system was involved in her bathing, which took her over an hour each day. After washing clothes she had to squeeze them a certain way, repeating the proceedings twenty-two times, the bottom of the bowl was then examined, checking the maker's mark numerous times to make sure the bowl was empty. Cleaning her teeth was a major task, taking over a half an hour. Making a bed, with checking at each stage that the sheets and blankets were exactly symmetrical, might take over half an hour.

Household chores such as washing-up or polishing a table were completely impossible for her, as they took so long and caused her such distress. Her husband and mother were, therefore, forced into running her home and, on medical advice, her two children were at boarding school. The patient felt extreme guilt at her disruption of the family's existence and, at times, felt very depressed and that life was not worth living. Between 1962 and 1970 she was admitted to Severalls Hospital seven times, and received a variety of treatments including ECT, MAOI drugs, tricyclics, major and minor tranquilizers and psychotherapy. During 1968 and 1969 she was admitted on two occasions to the Royal Waterloo Hospital and had a total of five courses of modified narcosis, combined with ECT and antidepressants. After each admission she obtained symptomatic relief for about 2–4 weeks and then relapsed [Kelly and Mitchell-Heggs, 1973, pp. 877–878].

The great majority of the candidates for psychosurgery are referred by psychiatrists who consider the patients' symptoms intractable to other treatments. In a few instances, however, individuals may seek out a neurosurgeon directly, particularly if the surgeon has been featured in a "pro-psychosurgery" article in a popular magazine (see footnote 4 in Chapter 1). Of course, psychiatrists differ in their attitudes toward psychosurgery, and many would never refer a patient for surgery under any circumstances. As a result, "referral channels" tend to become established, consisting of a subgroup of psychiatrists who refer patients to particular neurosurgeons. The different attitudes of psychiatrists toward psychosurgery often reflect other differences in their orientation and therapeutic approaches, which are believed to influence the types of patients that seek them out (see Mirsky and Orzack's contribution in this volume). In some instances, particularly in England, psychiatrists and neurosurgeons participate as a team on the psychosurgical unit of a psychiatric hospital.

The criteria used to establish the intractability of a patient's symptoms and the appropriateness of psychosurgery for those symptoms may vary with different psychiatrists and neurosurgeons. Most psychiatrists referring patients for psychosurgery seem to consider a patient's symptoms intractable if they do not respond to drugs and electroconvulsive shock. Alternative treatments such as behavior therapy (see the contribution by Kazdin in this volume) are rarely considered relevant. The possibility that this may result in premature referrals to a neurosurgeon, particularly in cases of obsessive-compulsive disorders, is raised in Rachman's discussion of these disorders in Chapter 6.

The criteria used for referrals for psychosurgery are only rarely made explicit. Commonly, it is simply stated in the published literature that "psychosurgery is used as a last resort only after all therapeutic alternatives had been exhausted." In the absence of explicit criteria, it is clear that such statements must be taken on faith. One example of explicit criteria is the statement by the psychiatrist Heinz Lehmann describing what he means by a sufficient exploration of alternative therapies:

> Psychotherapy should be administered for at least six months by someone well experienced, not just a first-year resident.

> With drug therapy, the time varies. Antianxiety drugs, such as chlordiazepoxide hydrochloride (Librium) or diazepam (Valium), should be tried for at least two months—but not much longer, because dependency might develop. And the dosage must be adequate. Chlordiazepoxide hydrochloride should be given up to 100 mg/day. If an antidepressant, such as imipramine hydrochloride (Tofranil), is used, the dosage should go as high as 250 mg/day for at least six weeks. If it hasn't been effective by then, it's not going to be. The neuroleptic drugs—chlorpromazine hydrochloride (Thorazine Hydrochloride) or an equivalent—should be given in pretty high dosages, up to 1,000 mg/day. And they should be tried for two or three months without success before giving up on them.
>
> In addition, there should be at least one, but preferably two, courses of electroconvulsive therapy given with 10–15 convulsions per course [Lehmann and Ostrow, 1973, p. 24].

In addition, Lehmann believes that there must also be "clear symptoms of anxiety, depression, or obsessive-compulsive disorder," which have disabled the patient for at least two years. Obviously, not everyone would agree with Lehmann's criteria, but at the very least a clear statement can be useful in starting a meaningful dialogue. Some neurosurgeons add their own criteria to those of the referring psychiatrist. In some instances these include sufficient evidence that the patient will have adequate support from family or friends during the postoperative period (see the contribution by Ballantine in this volume).

Disputed Area

While there may be general agreement among those practicing psychosurgery on the patients most likely to benefit from these operations, there is certainly less agreement about the appropriateness of psychosurgery for other types of patients. It is even feared that psychosurgery may involve considerable risk for some patients who are operated on by other neurosurgeons.

Schizophrenia and Related Disorders

Many psychiatrists and neurosurgeons have concluded that psychosurgery is ineffective in cases where there is serious impairment of thought processes, such as in schizophrenia, particularly if these symptoms are of long standing. Others have argued, however, that even in these instances there may be significant improvement following psychosurgery (see Valenstein, 1977, Appendix 7; Bailey,

Dowling, and Davies, 1973; Flor-Henry, 1975; Lehmann, 1975). Those who dispute the value of psychosurgery for schizophrenia maintain that the operations can normalize abnormal emotional states but not abnormal thinking. Some of the disagreement, though not all, results from the lack of clarity of diagnostic labels used in psychiatry. A number of patients with severe obsessive-compulsive symptoms have thought disorders that may be judged similar to those of schizophrenia. Some patients are diagnosed "schizo-affective" neurotics, a term that implies an emotional disturbance associated with some schizophrenic-like symptoms. Other psychiatrists would diagnose these patients as schizophrenics, thereby implying a thought disorder of psychotic proportions.

It is generally recognized that different psychiatrists and institutions, especially those in different countries, may use particular diagnostic labels with very different frequencies. The difference in incidence of schizophrenia in the United States and United Kingdom, for example, is due almost entirely to differences in diagnostic criteria (Gurland et al., 1970; Kramer, 1969). In the United States, the label *schizophrenia* has become a "wastebasket" category and is used several times as often as in the United Kingdom (and in Europe in general), where more stringent criteria are applied. On the other hand, British psychiatrists have used the diagnosis "affective disorder" (manic-depressive) much more frequently. The problem of characterizing the patients receiving psychosurgery is illustrated most clearly in those cases where there is not even an attempt to assign a diagnostic label. It is not unusual for patients' symptoms to be referred to in the psychosurgical literature by such terms as "emotional illness," "maladjusted states," and similar phrases that are left completely undefined or unexplained. More recently, the awareness of the vagaries of diagnostic labels has resulted in attempts to develop more objective criteria based on the behavioral symptoms that can be more precisely defined and sometimes even quantified (Spitzer et al., 1970).

The disagreement over the effectiveness of psychosurgery for certain types of patients is not all caused by confusion over diagnosis or the use of imprecise labels. Nor is the disagreement restricted to whether or not the thought disorders that are characteristic of schizophrenia improve after psychosurgery. There are also some disagreements on the value of psychosurgery for other diagnostic categories and symptoms. Several psychiatrists and neurosurgeons have noted, for example, that certain symptoms are not only not alleviated by psychosurgery but in some cases may actually be exacerbated by it.

Aggressive Behavior

Quite aside from the social and political controversy (see Chapter 1), the therapeutic value of psychosurgery for aggressive and assaultive behavior has been the subject of considerable dispute. There seems to be general agreement that there are documented cases in which the onset of aggressive behavior has been related to brain pathology caused by a tumor, an infection, or a head injury. There is also agreement that some of these patients have benefited remarkably from brain surgery. There is no such agreement, however, on the effectiveness of psychosurgery for violent patients who do not present clear evidence of brain damage. Vernon Mark, who has performed brain operations (amygdalectomies) on violent, epileptic patients and whose book *Violence and the Brain* was interpreted by many readers as recommending such brain surgery in the absence of evidence of brain damage (see Chapter 1), has more recently written:

> Our claim is that psychiatric neurosurgery to control violence should be limited to cases where the primary cause of the violence is brain dysfunction. . . . Abnormal violent behavior *not* associated with brain disease should be dealt with politically and socially, not medically. . . . we would not approve neurosurgery unless the person's violence could be traced to organic brain disease and could not be treated by nonsurgical methods [Mark and Neville, 1973, p. 767].

Although there may be some question about what constitutes sufficient evidence to trace violent behavior to brain disease, at least the underlying guiding principle is stated explicitly. Neurosurgeons do not all agree on this principle, however, and psychosurgery (amygdalectomy) has been performed on violent patients who did not present convincing evidence of brain damage (Balasubramaniam et al., 1972; Balasubramaniam and Kanaka, 1976; Brown, 1973; Cox and Brown, 1977; Hitchcock and Cairns, 1973; Narabayashi, 1973; Small et al., 1977). Most of these operations have been performed on the amygdala, but Sano et al. (1972) and Sano (1975) in Japan, Schvarcz et al. (1972) in Argentina, Nádvorník et al. (1973) in Czechoslovakia, and Rubio et al. (1977), among others, have reported hypothalamic operations on aggressive patients. Paniagua et al. (1977) have reported performing modified cingulotomies on aggressive patients. Small et al. (1977) summarized the results from fifty-eight patients who received stereotaxic amygdalectomies for the treatment of intractable seizures and/or unmanageable aggressive behavior. The surgeon was Robert Heimburger of the Indiana University School of Medicine. Studies of patients followed from one to eleven years after the surgery led to the following conclusion:

Of the patients receiving surgery primarily for seizures, 50% were considered as improved, both in control of epileptic attacks and overall levels of functioning; 33% of patients with conduct disorders (fighting without provocation and destruction of property were the most frequently described behavior problems) without severe seizure problems showed improvement specifically in behavior, with 25% judged improved in overall functioning. . . .

This study provides evidence that neurosurgical approaches to the treatment of patients with severe epilepsy and/or extremely aggressive behavior which does not respond to other forms of management need not necessarily be associated with evidence of CNS (central nervous system) damage. However, whether the observed improvement was attributable to surgery cannot be ascertained. Such definitive statements cannot be made without a control group (? sham-operated) to demonstrate the natural course of the illness without surgery as the passage of time and many other variables may have contributed. It is possible that psychological aspects of the surgical mystique contributed to the favorable outcome [Small et al., 1977, pp. 410–411].

Even this somewhat conservative endorsement of psychosurgery for aggressive behavior would be criticized by many psychiatrists and neurosurgeons who approve of psychosurgery for other symptoms. Concern has been expressed that psychosurgery may remove some additional controls and therefore exacerbate any combative tendency. Most of this concern, however, has focused on frontal lobe procedures, so it is not clear if loss of control is also a problem following psychosurgery on temporal lobe structures. Those less sympathetic toward the practice of psychosurgery have raised much more serious criticisms. They have pointed to the very serious impairment in the social behavior of animals following amygdalectomies and have claimed that the postoperative evaluations of patients have not been adequate to detect these types of changes. The same criticism has been raised about the posterior hypothalamic operations that are also performed on aggressive patients (Sano et al, 1972; Schvarcz et al., 1972). It is charged that postoperative evaluations have emphasized reductions in aggressive, destructive, rage, and hyperkinetic behavior, but have neglected intellectual and motivational deficits produced by the operations (see Valenstein, 1973, for a more complete discussion). These issues are discussed further in Part III of this volume.

Another issue about which there seems to be considerable disagreement concerns the interface between aggressive and criminal behaviors. It is clear that many, but not all, who are advocates of psychosurgery are opposed to surgery on patients who do not want to change. Thus, one neurosurgeon has recently written:

In conclusion, I wish to mention those types of mental and behavioral diseases which are not benefitted by surgical lesions. They are criminals, constitutional psychopaths and possibly sex perverts. . . . the patient must be acutely suffering with an intense desire to get well and have character integrity. The majority of criminals and psychopaths are constitutionally or genetically lacking in these characteristics and surgical ablations will make them worse rather than better [Scoville, 1973, pp. 34–35].

Bridges and Bartlett (1977) also list "prominent anti-social personality traits" as a counterindication for psychosurgery. Other neurosurgeons, while perhaps not disagreeing on the importance of the patient's motivation to get well, have concluded that criminals, psychopaths, and sexual perverts do benefit from psychosurgery. In Germany, several neurosurgeons have performed psychosurgery (ventromedial hypothalamic ablations) on pedophilic homosexuals and individuals who have committed violent sexual crimes (Dieckmann and Hassler, 1975, 1977; Müller et al., 1973; Orthner et al., 1972; Roeder et al., 1972). Although this operation is viewed as successful by those performing the procedure, others have argued that the amelioration of behavior problems results from a partial "functional castration" and a very significant reduction in all sexual expression (Valenstein, 1973, pp. 328–334). Moreover, some recent tests suggest that there are adverse intellectual and emotional side effects of these operations, the implications of which are not yet understood (Schneider, 1977). It has also not escaped the attention of those concerned with ethical issues that a number of the ventromedial hypothalamic operations are performed on persons either in prison or during a time when they are facing imprisonment. Several neurosurgeons have argued that "functional neurosurgery" should not be performed on persons imprisoned (Laitinen, 1977; Mark and Neville, 1973), but this view has not gone uncontested. M. Hunter Brown, for example, has argued that persons in prison, including those exhibiting behavior characterized as "sociopathic aggression," should not be deprived of the benefits of psychosurgery (see Brown's chapter in this volume and Brown, 1973; Valenstein, 1977).

Substance Abuse and Anorexia Nervosa

There have also been psychosurgical operations performed on patients with symptoms that are not typical of the general patient population. Although the number of patients involved is relatively small, it is important to include this group because it demonstrates some extreme examples of a tendency to treat all behavior problems as medical problems. In Denmark, lateral hypothalamic ablations were made in the brains of very obese patients in order to reduce their appetite (Quaade, 1974; Quaade, Vaernet, and Larsson, 1974). There is no convincing evidence that these operations were successful even in changing eating for more than a few days after the operation. Moreover, the operations are clearly in the tradition of applying a simplified understanding of animal experiments to humans (see Chapter 2). Although lateral hypothalamic destruction has frequently been reported to reduce the amount of food eaten by animals, this change is only one of many that follow damage to this brain area. Because any reasonably thorough reading of the animal experimental literature makes it clear that lateral hypothalamic damage also produces endocrine changes, severe losses in sensory-motor responsiveness, and impairment in motivation in general, such operations on humans have been harshly criticized (Marshall, 1974; Valenstein, 1975).

Excessive eating is only one of a group of so-called substance abuse problems to which psychosurgery has been applied. Alcoholism and drug addiction have also on occasion been treated by psychosurgery (see, for example, Balasubramaniam et al., 1973; Valenstein, 1977, Appendix 3). Some psychiatrists believe that these substance abuse problems share many features with other types of obsessive-compulsive behaviors. Thus, Nádvorník and his collaborators in Czechoslovakia have written:

> Behavioral disturbances manifested by an uncontrollable urge to satisfy the personal needs and to gain a pleasant feeling may well be called hedonia. . . . They imply not only excessive smoking, tobaccoism, but also excessive inclinations to good eating and drinking, lucullianism, and bacchism. Some of the hedonic manifestations, such as toxicomania and alcoholism, disturb the existing social order and sometimes endanger social order to a considerable extent; some others are even criminal, for instance sexual deviations such as pedophilia (love of children as sexual object). Therefore, they are dealt with as subjects for whom Roeder (1966) recommended stereotaxic hypothalamotomy treatment.
>
> Pathophysiologically, all the hedonic manifestations most likely exhibit a close functional mechanism.
>
> . . . The violent feeling of need and the effort to acquire the object of longing are the results of such strong emotional drive that the person is not able to control himself and to refrain. Some of the hedonic manifestations may appear suddenly in a paroxysmal way, and they are so unsuppressible that they are devoted as compulsive hedonias [Nádvorník, Šramka, and Patoprstá, 1977, pp. 445–446].

Psychosurgery has also been used to treat a few anorexia nervosa patients, who refuse to eat enough to maintain their health. Scoville and Bettis (1977, p. 200) have reported that "certain rarer cases of anorexia nervosa have been helped by psychosurgery, mainly in relieving the intensity of their compulsions." Post and Schurr (1977, p. 264) report performing frontal lobe psychosurgery upon seven anorexic patients "with excellent results in six." In two of these patients the follow-up period was short and "the unsuccessful case was a patient who was so ashamed of her increased appetite and weight that she committed suicide." Post and Schurr explain that the latter patient had made several suicide attempts preoperatively.

Demographic Features

The majority of patients receiving psychosurgery are between thirty-five and sixty years of age. In the Mirsky and Orzack study reported in this volume, the mean ages of the patients were fifty-five (Group I) and forty-four (Group II). In the study reported by Corkin in this volume, the average age of the patients receiving operations for psychiatric reasons was thirty-nine; the average age of the patients operated for intractable pain was forty-six and a half. There are, of course, psychosurgical patients both younger and older. Some neurosurgeons have reported good postoperative results with older patients, and others, such as López-Ibor and López-Ibor Aliño (1977), claim that very young patients benefit the most from psychosurgery.

Children

The performance of psychosurgery on children has evoked heated controversy. Questions about how to obtain "informed consent" for operations on children are complex, but not unique to psychosurgery. However, psychosurgery on children does raise unique problems, in light of the growing literature suggesting that brain damage may have very different consequences for children and adults. Several reasons are cited. Some of these reasons involve evidence that many brain structures subserve different functions in the young and the adult. Also relevant is the fact that the young child is acquiring information and problem-solving strategies at much more accelerated rates than the adult. It has been demonstrated repeatedly, for example, that comparable brain damage has a much greater influence on IQ in the young child than in the adult. All of these arguments justify the special concern about psychosurgery on children.[1]

Other factors must also be considered in any discussion of psychosurgery on children. Although it may be possible to present convincing evidence that an adult's psychiatric problem is intractable, it is much more difficult to do so in the case of a child. There are a number of psychiatric and organic problems observed in children that are attenuated or even eliminated later on, particularly around puberty. Quite aside from other considerations, judgments about psychosurgery on children must take into account the fact that the probabilities of "spontaneous improvement" are very different for children than for adults.

Around the world, there has been a significant amount of psychosurgery performed on children younger than fifteen years old. Almost always the circumstances involve a problem of "manageability" (see Chapter 1). A passive, easily cared for mentally defective child is not considered a candidate for psychosurgery. The children who receive psychosurgery are typically described with such words as "destructive," "aggressive," "violent," "hyperkinetic," and "restless" in articles by Sano (1975) and Narabayashi (1972, 1973) in Japan, López-Ibor and López-Ibor Aliño (1977) in Spain, and Balasubramaniam et al. (1971, 1972, 1973) in India (see also Valenstein, 1977, Appendix 3).

The amount of psychosurgery performed on children has been investigated by Valenstein (1977). This investigation covered only the information that appeared in the psychosurgical literature published between 1971 and 1976. (Because of the heated controversy over this subject, it is unlikely that there has been any psychosurgery on children in the United States during the past few years.) After all duplications were eliminated (as far as could be determined), it was ascertained that there were 156 operations on children under fifteen performed between 1971 and 1976 throughout the world. Of these, 17 were performed in the United States. An analysis of the dates of surgery (as far as could be determined) revealed that of the 17 U.S. psychosurgical procedures performed on children under fifteen, only 7 were performed after 1970. Moreover, 2 of the 7 patients had epilepsy in addition to behavior disorders. A comparable analysis revealed that there were 11 U.S. operations on children

---

[1] None of these statements contradicts the evidence with regard to specific functions such as speech that the very young child may display more "plasticity" and better recovery of capacities after brain damage than the adult.

between the ages of fifteen and twenty mentioned in the literature published after 1970.

Minority Groups and Women

Another frequently voiced concern is that a significant number of the patients receiving psychosurgery are minority-group members, women, and the very poor. Valenstein (1977) has investigated the more recent (1971–1976) evidence bearing on these issues. It may provide some clarification at the outset to note that the great majority of psychosurgical patients have been referred by psychiatrists, commonly those in private practice. This fact alone would indicate that the patients are not primarily from the lower socioeconomic class—that their demographic characteristics are more typical of those of middle-class people who seek help from psychiatrists. According to a 1973 American Psychiatric Association report, the typical patient of a psychiatrist is female (62 percent), white (97 percent), and middle-class. Although it was not possible to obtain complete statistics on this question, based on the available descriptions of the patients as presented in the literature and on the institutional settings where surgery is customarily performed in the United States, the patients appear to be primarily from the middle class. Although the demographic information on the psychosurgical patient population collected by Dr. John Donnelly as part of the Task Force on Psychosurgery of the American Psychiatric Association has not yet been fully analyzed, Donnelly's impressions of the data are consistent with the view expressed above (personal communication, 1976). Relevant also are the demographical data presented by Mirsky and Orzack in this volume. These investigators report that approximately one-half of the patients they studied had some education beyond high school graduation and two of them had graduate degrees. Occupations as defined by Hollingshead (1977) were predominantly in the higher categories ranging from clerical and technical (63 percent) to administrative and professional (37 percent).

In an attempt to investigate the charge that black persons may be the target of psychosurgery (Breggin, 1974; Mason, 1973), the author corresponded with those neurosurgeons who have accumulated the largest populations of psychosurgical patients. In addition, the psychosurgical literature was examined in order to determine the patients' race, if specified. The results of the correspondence indicate that the incidence of psychosurgery performed on blacks is very significantly below their proportion in the total population (see

Valenstein, 1977, Appendices, pp. 82–88). This conclusion is also consistent with the views expressed by two black neurosurgeons (see N. Hicks, "2 Black Neurosurgeons Defend Behavior-Altering Operations," *New York Times*, January 8, 1976). The same conclusions appear to apply to Puerto Ricans, Mexican-Americans, and Oriental-Americans. However, the information that can be collected from the literature is inadequate as race is frequently not stated. Where race is mentioned, the most common statement is that "the patients were all Caucasian." One newspaper article that referred to thirteen psychosurgical operations performed between 1968 and 1972 on state patients in Michigan identified two of the patients as black (Cheyfitz, 1976). No other data consistent with this report could be located in the scientific literature or news media. Bridges, who has studied the psychosurgical patients on the Geoffrey Knight Psychosurgical Unit at Brooks General Hospital in London, regards it as unfortunate that not a single black person has had an opportunity to benefit from these operations. Bridges also maintains that because all referrals in the United Kingdom are made through the National Health Service, members of all socioeconomic groups are proportionally represented (Bridges, 1977, personal communication).

The question of the sex ratio of the psychosurgical population is more complicated. Valenstein (1977) analyzed all of the articles on psychosurgery published in the United States between 1971 and 1976 to estimate the sex ratio of the patients. Where it could be determined, patients obviously described several times in different publications were counted only once. The data were divided according to diagnostic category, with the "aggressive" (violent, assaultive, or hyperkinetic) patients collected together in one group and all others in a second group. The majority of the "others" were anxious, depressive, obsessive, and phobic patients. Epileptic patients and those suffering from pain were excluded from this analysis.

The results of the sex ratio analysis revealed that 59 percent of the psychosurgical patients in the "other" diagnostic group were female, while 61 percent of the "aggressive" patients were male. In total, a greater percentage (56 percent) of the psychosurgical patients were female, because the "other" category has approximately nine times more patients than does the "aggressive" category. These results appear to reflect the known sex ratio distribution in these diagnostic categories and therefore do not support the belief that females are being preferentially selected for psychosurgery. In one study, for example, at the New York State Psychiatric Institute, 168 of 203 (83 percent) depressed patients were women. In a study conducted by Raskin (1974), of the National Institute of Mental Health, 71 percent of 555 depressed patients were women. The statement is frequently made in the psychiatric literature that there are approximately three women to every man in the unipolar depressed patient population. A study at the Barnes Hospital in St. Louis revealed that 74 percent of manic-depressed (bipolar) patients were women. It is, of course, possible to develop a more complex argument based on the contention that sex discrimination influences the assignment of diagnostic labels or even accounts for the greater number of females suffering from psychiatric disorders. An examination of this possibility, however, falls outside the scope of this analysis.

Diagnostic Labels and Site of Brain Operation

Tables 4.1, 4.2, and 4.3 summarize the data from the United States and the United Kingdom on the psychosurgical procedures used for patients in different diagnostic categories. This information was abstracted from all articles published between 1971 and 1976 and was included in Valenstein's (1977) report to the National Commission for the Protection of Human Subjects of Biomedical and Behavioral Research. The published articles were perused carefully to determine the probable date of surgery, and, as far as could be determined, all operations performed prior to 1969 were eliminated from the data presented in the tables. The few uncertain cases are not likely to influence the overall statistics. Moreover, articles by the same neurosurgeon or neurosurgical unit were compared in order to eliminate redundancy (again, as far as possible). Therefore, even though the same patients may have been included in several different summary articles, an effort was made to count each patient only once.

As noted in Chapter 2, a great variety of psychosurgical procedures are performed. In order to make the data more manageable, the operations were grouped in the tables according to the general brain area involved. Under the heading "Frontal Lobe Procedure," for example, bimedial leucotomies, orbital undercutting, substantia innominata operations, and various tractotomies designed to partially ablate frontal lobe connections to either the thalamus, hypothalamus, or limbic structures have all been included. Similarly, thalamic operations include ablations of either the anterior, dorsomedial, centromedian, or parafascicular thalamic nuclei. There are some neurosurgeons who would probably argue that such groups violate important distinctions, but in view of the fact that most surgeons

Table 4.1 Diagnostic Labels and Site of Brain Operation (United States)

Diagnostic Label[a]	Total Number of Patients[b]	Frontal Lobe Procedure	Cingulum	Amygdala	Thalamus	Hypothalamus	Multiple Target Sites[c]	Midbrain	Brain Stimulation
Aggression	35			12(34.3%)		4(11.4%)	19(54.3%)		
Neurotic depression	136	9(6.6%)	127(93.4%)						
Psychotic depression[d]	11		11(100.0%)						
Fear and anxiety	4	3(75.0%)	1(25.0%)						
Obsessive-compulsive neurosis	37	9(24.3%)	25(67.6%)				3(8.1%)		
Schizo-affective disorders	7	7(100.0%)							
Schizophrenia and other psychoses	80		32(40.0%)				47(58.8%)		1(1.2%)
Drug addiction and alcoholism	14	1(7.1%)	13(92.9%)						
Pain	379	17(4.5%)	177(46.7%)		120(31.7%)		25(6.6%)	8(2.1%)	32(8.4%)
Psychopathic behavior	6				6(100.0%)				
"Emotional illness"	9		1(11.1%)				8(88.9%)		
"Agitated states of the aged"	2	2(100.0%)							
Involutional melancholia	1		1(100.0%)						
Epilepsy with psychiatric disorders	45			45(100.0%)					

Note: For each diagnostic category, the number and percentage of patients are listed according to target of brain surgery. The articles from which this information was drawn are listed in Valenstein, 1977 (Appendix 4). As far as could be determined, only data from patients operated on after 1970 were included.

[a] Labels are those used in the published articles.

[b] In those cases where authors did not provide a quantitative breakdown of their patients, diagnostic labels were assigned in proportion to the average frequency of usage of these labels for psychosurgical patients.

[c] Multiple target sites include the cingulum, amygdala, substantia innominata, and thalamic structure, in different combinations.

[d] Including manic-depressive syndrome.

Table 4.2 Diagnostic Labels and Site of Brain Operation (United Kingdom)

Diagnostic Label[a]	Total Number of Patients[b]	Frontal Lobe Procedure	Cingulum[c]	Limbic Leucotomy[d]	Amygdala	Multiple Target Sites[e]	Subthalamus (Field of Forel)
Aggression, including self-mutilation	12		2(16.7%)		8(66.6%)	2(16.7%)	
Depression	201	169(84.1%)	2(1.0%)	28(13.9%)	2(1.0%)		
Fear and anxiety	82	58(70.7%)	1(1.2%)	23(28.1%)			
Obsessive-compulsive neurosis	96	50(52.1%)	5(5.2%)	41(42.7%)			
Anorexia nervosa	13	11(84.6%)		2(15.4%)			
Psychopathic behavior	13	7(53.8%)		6(46.2%)			
Schizophrenia and other psychoses	13	6(46.2%)		7(53.8%)			
Drug addiction and alcoholism	13	13(100.0%)					
Epilepsy with psychiatric disorders	36		3(8.3%)		30(83.4%)		3(83.3%)

Note: For each diagnostic category, the number and percentage of patients are listed according to target of brain surgery. The articles from which this information was drawn are listed in Valenstein, 1977 (Appendix 5). As far as could be determined, only data from patients operated on after 1970 were included.

[a] Labels are those used in the published articles.

[b] In those cases where authors did not provide a quantitative breakdown on their patients, diagnostic labels were assigned in proportion to the average frequency of usage of these labels for psychosurgical patients.

[c] Most cingulum operations involve the anterior portion, but one neurosurgeon performs a posterior cingulotomy.

[d] Frontal lobe procedure (medial leucotomy) and anterior cingulotomy.

[e] Multiple target sites include the cingulum, amygdala, substantia innominata, and thalamic structure, in different combinations.

Table 4.3 Comparison of Psychosurgical Procedures in the United States and United Kingdom

	Total Number of Operations[a]	Frontal Lobe Procedure	Cingulum	Limbic Leucotomy[b]	Amygdala and Temporal Lobe	Thalamus	Hypothalamus	Multiple Target Sites	Midbrain	Subthalamus (Field of Forel)	Brain Stimulation
United States	768[c]	6.3%	50.5%	0	6.0%	16.7%	0.5%	13.3%	1.0%	0	5.7%
United Kingdom	479	65.6%	2.7%	22.3%	8.4%	0	0	0.4%	0	0.6%	0

[a] Total operations reported in published articles. Operations performed prior to 1970 and those estimated to have been reported more than once were omitted.
[b] Frontal lobe procedure (medial leucotomy) and anterior cingulotomy.
[c] Includes 379 brain operations for pain.

perform the same psychosurgical procedure for all patients, the broad categories used seem adequate for present purposes. Furthermore, stereotaxic and "open" operations were grouped together, as were those employing different ablation techniques, such as radiofrequency waves, ultrasonic beams, radioactive yttrium seeds, suction, and knife cuts. Lastly, in Tables 4.1 and 4.2 the heterogeneous diagnostic labels were collapsed into groups that were judged not to violate important differences in the symptomatology of patients.

Inspection of Tables 4.1 and 4.2 reveals some differences in the psychosurgical practices between the United States and the United Kingdom. These differences are summarized in a simplified form without diagnostic labels in Table 4.3. It can be seen from Table 4.3 that there is a greater percentage of frontal lobe procedures performed in the United Kingdom, while cingulotomies are more frequently performed in the United States. When cingulotomies are performed in the United Kingdom, they tend to be done in conjunction with frontal lobe operations (bimedial leucotomies), resulting in a combined procedure often termed limbic leucotomy. Excluding limbic leucotomies, there is a much greater tendency to perform multiple-target psychosurgery in the United States. Most of these differences between the two countries can be attributed to a very few active neurosurgeons (sometimes only one neurosurgeon) in one or the other country. For example, Ballantine (see contributions by Ballantine and by Corkin in this volume) has performed the largest number of cingulotomies in the United States, while Brown (see the contributions by Brown and by Mirsky and Orzack in this volume) has performed the majority of the multi-targeted psychosurgical procedures. As far as could be determined from the published literature, neither thalamic nor hypothalamic operations nor electrical stimulation of deep brain structures was performed in the United Kingdom after 1971.

With respect to diagnostic categories, the data confirm the conclusion that, with the exception of operations for intractable pain in the United States, the majority of psychosurgery is performed on patients suffering from depression, obsessive-compulsive disorders, fears, anxiety, and phobias. This trend is less striking in the United States because of the relatively higher number of surgical patients diagnosed as schizophrenic. There seems to have been a relatively lower frequency of psychosurgery for psychotic patients in the United Kingdom in the 1970s, but it is not possible to determine how much of this difference between the two countries results from differences in diagnostic labeling. Lastly, if the published literature correctly reflects the actual practice, there is a much greater tendency for brain operations to be performed for intractable pain in the United States than in the United Kingdom.

CHAPTER 5

Patient Selection

H. Thomas Ballantine, Jr.

The development, application, and evaluation of new surgical treatments give rise to very special problems for society in general and the medical profession in particular. Willard Gaylin (1975) has brilliantly analyzed the issues involved in obtaining "informed consent," in attempting to apply the experimental model to innovations in surgical practice, and in the difficult task of evaluating the results of new surgical treatments. Problems of patient selection for psychiatric surgery are equally difficult of solution; but our own experiences with them over the years may be helpful in clarifying their nature, even if clear-cut answers are not forthcoming.

Clinical Study of Cingulotomy Results

Our interest in the use of stereotaxic anterior cingulotomy for the treatment of psychiatrically disabled patients arose as a result of the report by Foltz and White in 1962. Their "closed" operation was a refinement of the "open" cingulectomy that had first been undertaken in 1948 by Cairns in Oxford, England, and Le Beau in Paris, France. We were especially impressed by the evaluation of Cairns' patients published by Lewin in 1961. Although the procedure described by Foltz and White was much safer and less traumatic for the patient, it could not be determined conclusively that such a limited interruption of cingulate fibers would produce results comparable to those reported by Cairns and his coworkers.

Our clinical study of stereotaxic anterior cingulotomy as an alternative to lobotomy and cingulectomy was begun in April of 1962. At the outset the decision was made to select as candidates for this procedure only those patients who had been intractably and totally disabled by emotional suffering for at least three years despite treatment by psychotherapy, chemotherapy, and electroshock. The majority of our first published series of 15 patients (Cassidy, Ballantine, and Flanagan, 1965–66) were suffering from one form or another of manic-depressive disease, as defined by Cassidy et al. (1957), and had been referred for the procedure by the two senior authors.

The first assessment of postoperative results in these 15 patients indicated "improvement" in psychiatric status in 13, but a "good" result in only 6. The relatively unsatisfactory rate of improvement gave rise to a number of questions, of which the following were considered most important:

1. Had we chosen the lesion sites correctly?

2. Had we interrupted a sufficient volume of cingulate fibers?

3. Were our criteria for patient selection appropriate?

4. Was stereotaxic anterior cingulotomy, under any circumstances, an effective procedure for the treatment of psychiatric illness?

The small number of patients in this first series precluded a judgment as to the efficacy of cingulotomy. We were aware that the amount of cingulate interruption by our procedure was far less than that produced by Cairns, and for this reason—as well as the fact that no adverse effects of the operation had been observed—we resolved to enlarge the lesions in the patients who had failed to improve after one operation and to analyze lesion placement carefully.

In 1970, at the Second International Conference on Psychosurgery held in Copenhagen, Denmark, we reported on our experiences with 66 patients, 40 of whom had been the subjects of a previous analysis in 1967 (Ballantine et al., 1967; Ballantine et al., 1972). Criteria for patient selection with reference to diagnosis, symptomatology, and referral from one psychiatric source remained the same. Twenty-eight of these patients required more than one operation, but we were able to report that 53 of them (roughly 80 percent of the series) were well or at least functioning effectively in society—although some were still in need of psychiatric supervision. These results did not seem to be affected by the age or sex of the patients nor the duration of illness prior to cingulotomy. One of the most reliable indications that a good result could be obtained postoperatively was a history that the patient had at some time been able to function productively.

Our failures seemed to be related to lack of proper postoperative psychiatric care (which could be the fault of either the patient, the patient's relative, or the psychiatrist) and the presence in the constellation of psychiatric symptoms of profound abnormalities of the thought processes, often called "disorders of cognition."

Review of Selection Criteria

By 1970 we were receiving patient referrals from a number of psychiatrists with differing opinions about the types of nonsurgical treatments to be employed and the timing of surgical intervention in reference to the duration of the illness. To alleviate this problem in patient selection, a screening committee was instituted whose members consisted of the operating neurosurgeon, a neurologist, and a psychiatrist with a broad, unbiased knowledge of psychiatric illness and treatment modalities. The two nonsurgeons were involved only in patient selection and never in patient treatment, to assure objectivity in decision making. It was also their task to review again with the patient and next of kin the risks of cingulotomy, to emphasize that it was not possible to predict accurately what degree of improvement the patient might expect, and to make sure, as far as possible, that informed consent was obtained prior to surgery. A final criterion (though not an absolute one) was the identification of one or more persons in the family constellation who would agree to provide environmental and emotional support to the patient in the postoperative period.

Data derived from thirteen years of experiences with stereotaxic anterior cingulotomy were presented to the Fourth World Congress of Psychiatric Surgery in Madrid, Spain, in 1975 (Ballantine et al., 1977). At that time we reported satisfactory postoperative improvement in about 80 percent of those (properly selected) patients suffering from disorders of affect. Independent studies have confirmed the lack of undesirable side effects of the operation, even in those patients who are not helped by the operation (National Commission for the Protection of Human Subjects of Biomedical and Behavioral Research, 1977).

The results of these experiences are now presented in synoptic form in our correspondence with patients and their relatives as indicated in the following form letter:

Dear Mrs. _____:

I am writing this letter in response to your telephone request for information about the cingulotomy procedure that had been proposed as a possible method of treatment for your son.

A "cingulotomy" is an operation that is done on a patient who is suffering from a severe and long-term disabling psychiatric illness, and who has exhausted all other reasonable methods of psychiatric care.

An incision is made in the scalp, just behind the hairline, and holes are drilled in the skull to allow the passage of electrodes into the area of the brain called the cingulum, where heat lesions are precisely placed under X-ray control.

Requirements for the operation are as follows:

1. The patient must be referred to me by his psychiatrist.

2. The patient and his nearest relative must consent to the operation.

3. The patient must agree to return to the care of his psychiatrist for as long as the psychiatrist and/or I feel it is necessary.

4. The patient, his relative, and his psychiatrist should realize that I make a very small "lesion" in the brain and that 30 percent of the patients require a second operation before the anticipated benefit occurs.

5. The patient must submit to examination by a Massachusetts General Hospital psychiatrist and neurologist and myself. All of us must concur that the operation is indicated and that the patient and his nearest relative understand the risks and benefits of the operation.

6. The patient must also agree to undergo psychological tests pre- and postoperatively.

7. Copies of all psychiatric history and treatment are required in this office prior to evaluation.

Regarding #5 above, the following guidelines are used to determine whether or not the operation is indicated:

a. The use of surgical techniques should never be considered unless all other generally accepted methods of treatment such as psychotherapy, drug therapy, ECT, and hospitalization have failed.

b. Surgical treatment should be undertaken only for the relief of suffering and as an attempt to restore a disabled individual to effective functioning in society—never for social or political purposes.

c. In general, the only individuals to be considered for surgery are those who have a prior history of being able to function effectively and who have been continuously disabled and under psychiatric treatment for such a period of time as may be required to determine that the psychiatric illness is refractory to nonsurgical therapy.

If you have any questions, do not hesitate to contact me.

Sincerely yours,

H. Thomas Ballantine, Jr., M.D.

It should now be apparent that surgery is offered to these disabled psychiatric patients only as a last resort. It is a peculiar phenomenon of our times that the term "last resort" seems to be applied only to surgery for psychiatric illness. In truth, however, all surgery should be considered a treatment of last resort; that is, if there is a nonsurgical therapy that entails less risk and can produce the same beneficial result, then, without question, the nonsurgical treatment should be the procedure of choice. It is nevertheless important to emphasize, particularly in reference to surgery for psychiatric illness, the term "less risk." It is becoming increasingly apparent that the chemical substances in use for the treatment of psychiatric patients carry in many instances their own degree of risk. Indeed, some of our patients who have been helped by surgery are still disabled by the neurological abnormalities resulting from the therapeutic use of certain pharmacological agents.

The problem of when, in the course of a patient's psychiatric illness, surgical intervention should be considered is difficult of solution. Should the operation be considered in a disabled patient after one year of total disability, two years, three years, or thirty years? The answer to this conundrum remains a very personal one, which will depend upon the patient, his next of kin, and his psychiatrist, as well as the interaction among them. It would seem, nevertheless, that, if a procedure of little risk and substantial potential benefit can be offered to a patient, it should be done sooner rather than later in order to avoid prolonged suffering, disability, and the ever-present risk of death by suicide, which threatens all chronically depressed patients.

CHAPTER 6

Obsessional-Compulsive Disorders

Stanley Rachman

The contention that psychosurgery is an effective method of treating obsessional disorders incorporates two main claims: (1) that psychosurgery is especially suitable for treating such disorders and (2) that it is most effective in treating chronic and intractable cases. If sustained, these claims would be particularly welcome, offering as they do some hope for those patients who (by definition) are beyond help by other methods. In the course of reviewing the most recent evidence on the effects of psychosurgery on obsessional neuroses, an attempt will be made to evaluate this double claim.

Although there was a short period during which it was believed —or hoped—that psychosurgery might provide an effective way of treating obsessional disorders (Sargant, Slater, and Kelly, 1972), current enthusiasm for these procedures is confined to a small group of advocates. Contemporary advocates are careful to express the view that surgical intervention should be restricted to only the most intractable and chronic cases (for example, Goktepe, Young, and Bridges, 1975, p. 279). The view expressed by Kolb (1973) is representative: "Probably the best results in lobotomy are secured in agitated depressions and in severe obsessive-compulsive reactions accompanied by so much tension that the patient is incapacitated" (p. 653). Unfortunately, the evidence does not seem to bear out this claim with respect to obsessional disorders. If anything, it is the mild cases that respond most, when the treatment works at all.

Is the operation carried out solely on chronic cases? If "chronic" is taken to mean an illness duration of five years or more, then it is not confined to chronic cases. As we shall see, the operation is sometimes performed on patients with an illness duration of two years or less—and, of related significance, on people in their early twenties. Since spontaneous remissions are known to occur in obsessional patients (see Pollitt, 1957), it seems preferable to adopt a strict definition of chronicity when considering psychosurgery. Based on the limited evidence available, a conservative estimate of the spontaneous remission rate for all neuroses, over a two-year period, is ±60 percent (Rachman, 1971). The crude, estimated rate for obsessional neuroses is lower—about 40 percent (Rachman and Hodgson, 1979). In these circumstances, it is difficult to justify performing a major operation on a patient who is not well past the two-year period in which remission is still quite possible. The advocates of psychosurgery would do well to adopt a strict definition of chronicity. The term should be restricted to disorders that have persisted for more than five years.

In order to appreciate the role of psychosurgery in the treatment of obsessional disorders, it is necessary to remember that these operations (Knight, 1964, listed seven variations) were introduced as a cure, not for obsessions, but for schizophrenia. For example, in an early sample reported by Kolb (1973), 60 percent of the patients were schizophrenic and only 10 percent were neurotic (see also Sternberg, 1974; Willett, 1960). The use of psychosurgery was soon extended to include a wide range of disorders from depression to hypochondria (Bernstein, Callahan, and Jaranson, 1975), delinquency, alcoholism, anxiety states, and so on (see Sykes and Tredgold, 1964; Ström-Olsen and Carlisle, 1971). It was even claimed that psychosurgery was marginally helpful in alleviating tuberculosis (Cheng, Tait, and Freeman, 1956).

Imperceptibly, the emphasis shifted, and by 1960 a number of textbook writers expressed the opinion that leucotomy was primarily useful in treating obsessions, rather than schizophrenia. The skepticism about the value of psychosurgery for treating schizophrenia (for example, Willett, 1960) has now spread to its use on obsessional patients (for example, Cawley, 1974; Sternberg, 1974). It need hardly be argued that the use of such radical procedures can only be justified on the grounds of demonstrable success, in the absence of satisfactory alternatives. It is argued here that neither of these conditions is met and that therefore the psychosurgical treatment of obsessional patients cannot be justified at present.

Reasons to Question Psychosurgical Intervention

What are the reasons for the present misgivings about operating on obsessional (and indeed other) psychiatric patients? Psychosurgery is an intervention that carries a slight risk of serious danger for the patient (for example, epilepsy may develop—see below). There is a lack of persuasive evidence that the operation is responsible for therapeutic benefits. Alternative and considerably less dangerous methods are available, including the newly developed behavioral treatments. No serious attempt has been made to explain why surgery should alleviate obsessional disorders; even if there were acceptable empirical proof of its therapeutic value, we would remain in the dark about the causal process. The earlier but now discredited claim that psychosurgery is an effective treatment for schizophrenia is doubly worrying. In the first place, it warns us of our credulity in therapeutic matters, and secondly it reminds us that the recommendation of surgery for *obsessional disorders* is second-hand and atheoretical.

Are we in a position to dispel these misgivings? Unfortunately, we are not; hence those who continue to recommend and use psychosurgery are obliged to provide cogent reasons for so doing. As we shall see, their arguments are largely empirical.

Before presenting the facts and arguments about the effects of psychosurgery, it is worth pointing out that the use of surgical interventions is based upon and helps to perpetuate the notion that obsessional disorders are illnesses. There can be little doubt that acceptance of the alternative view, that obsessional disorders are better construed as psychological problems (see Rachman and Hodgson, 1979), would reduce the likelihood of anyone's proposing a surgical solution. As it would serve no useful purpose to repeat the many reviews of the earliest reports on psychosurgery (see Willett, 1960), this discussion is confined mainly to the most recent claims made on behalf of psychosurgery. To place the matter in perspective, however, it is necessary to preface the discussion by noting that, to the best of my knowledge, no random controlled clinical study of psychosurgery has ever been reported. The most satisfactory reports, all of them of recent origin and discussed here, are those describing the results obtained in prospective studies of patients. Although prospective studies are in general superior to those in which the material is collected retrospectively, this advantage should not obscure the fact that in none of the reported series was any attempt made to compare the effects of psychosurgery with those of conventional treatment, drug treatment, behavior therapy, or other alternative treatments. Additionally, there is no series in which assignment to treatment was determined randomly; that is, selection or rejection for treatment was itself a clinical decision. In none of the reports was the independent assessor, where one was employed, kept ignorant of the type of treatment provided. Of course, one must recognize the problems involved in providing an independent assessment of the effects of psychosurgery. In all therapeutic outcome research it is difficult to ensure that the independent assessors remain ignorant of the type of treatment the patient has received, and in assessing the effects of psychosurgery it may be impossible to achieve single-blind control. Despite its theoretical desirability, the use of a double-blind control procedure would rapidly lead to a depletion of the sample. The fact remains that the evidence of these clinical assessors is open to bias. Other defects of the studies reported so far include the selection and use of inappropriate psychometric tests and the failure to obtain preoperative assessments of function and disorder.

If, in pointing out the shortcomings of the evidence on the effects of psychosurgery, I seem to some to be employing unusually severe standards of evidence, it is because I believe that the more radical and serious the treatment, the greater is the need for full and reliable evidence about its effects.

Therapeutic Outcome Studies

Smith et al. (1976) evaluated the effects of their open prefrontal leucotomy operation (now largely replaced by the stereotaxic technique) on 43 patients, including 5 obsessional patients. "As a result of the operation three patients died, three developed personality changes and one had repeated grand-mal seizures" (p. 731). At the six-month follow-up, 58 percent of the patients were said to be markedly improved, but the obsessional patients did slightly less well than the others. Among these patients the improvement was only slight to moderate. Three of the five patients were improved, one was unchanged, and one was slightly better. The extent of "obsessionality" among the total patient sample was assessed by interviewing the patient and, where possible, an additional informant. On this measure, according to the 34 patients who provided information, obsessionality was unchanged in 56 percent of cases. According to the informants, 67 percent of the patients were unchanged on this criterion. The best results appear to have been achieved with depressed patients (see also Birley, 1964; Post, Rees, and Schurr, 1968). Note, however, that this study meets few of the evaluation criteria listed earlier.

Sykes and Tredgold (1964) carried out a retrospective study of two large series of patients who had undergone a leucotomy. In 29 cases out of 322 mixed cases, epilepsy occurred after the operation. They also found considerable evidence of increases in undesirable behavior, and an overall mortality rate of 1.5 percent. Depending upon finer points of interpretation, one could conclude, as the researchers did, that approximately 50 percent of the 24 obsessional patients were improved after the operation. On a slightly different interpretive basis, one could equally well conclude that 15 out of 24 of the obsessional patients were slightly or not at all improved after the operation. Moreover, their condition at the five-year follow-up had declined slightly in the direction of the preoperative condition. Despite some of their own discouraging figures, Sykes and Tredgold placed a favorable interpretation on much of their information—and one suspects they were a little overenthusiastic. So, for example, they claimed that the operation helped 10 out of 15 of the patients with "skin conditions," 17 out of 23 patients with hallucinations, 38 out of 47 patients with delusions, and 45 out of 73 patients with headache symptoms. These claims of wide-ranging improvements, coupled with the neglect of experimental controls, tend to raise skepticism about the usefulness of psychosurgery in treating obsessional disorders.

The report by Ström-Olsen and Carlisle (1971) followed the assessment and reporting style of Sykes and Tredgold's report, and their conclusions were almost as favorable. These researchers carried out a retrospective analysis of the effects of the stereotaxic operation on 210 patients. "The best results were obtained in the depressions, both recurrent and other forms (56 percent recovered and much improved). Good results were also obtained in obsessional neurosis (50 percent recovered and improved). . . . None of the schizophrenic patients did well" (p. 153). There was some evidence of undesirable behavioral changes occurring after the operation. Sixteen of the patients underwent a second operation, and of these 4 were diagnosed as obsessional. (It is worth noting here that in many of these studies a proportion of patients had more than one operation.)

This retrospective, nonrandom, uncontrolled, partial sample of patients provided slight encouragement for the belief that leucotomy might be of limited value in the treatment of obsessional disorders. On the question of whether or not the operation is best reserved for the most intractable cases, the information that 4 out of the 20 patients in this series were operated on after a duration of illness of less than five years is disturbing. In my own experience, a twenty-one-year-old woman with a mild to moderate hand-washing compulsion of less than two years duration was operated on despite the fact that alternative forms of treatment were readily available. Since she was well motivated and of stable personality, had a good work record, and was reasonably sociable, her prognosis would have been favorable with or without treatment.

Using similar but better criteria, Tan, Marks, and Marset (1971) carried out a retrospective analysis on 24 obsessional patients who had had a modified leucotomy and then compared their outcomes with a matched group of 13 controls who had not had the operation. (Incidentally, the fact that the controls had *not* undergone surgery undermines the basis for comparison between the two groups; presumably there were selective reasons for providing the operation for the one group and withholding it from the other.) Apart from the usual difficulties involved in retrospective analyses, it is unfortunate that only 3 of the 37 patients were interviewed; the rest of the information was coded from the written case notes and then presented to independent assessors. Although this procedure ensures that the independent assessors were ignorant of whether or not the patient had undergone the operation, it does not preclude the possibility that the person who coded the information did so in a way that was nonrandom. Despite these drawbacks, the information is of some interest. Overall, the patients who had the operation did better than the controls, "with respect to obsessions and general anxiety. . . . obsessions were reduced from a severe to a moderate degree of handicap" (p. 163). The relation between depression and outcome is not clear. On the one hand, it is said that "the outcome was rather better in patients who were depressed before operation" (p. 162), but against this is the statement on the next page that "outcome was not associated with pre-morbid personality or pre-operative depression" (p. 163). The reductions in anxiety appeared to occur shortly after leucotomy and then to remain at a fairly low level for some years after. The authors pointed out that "it should be emphasized that most leucotomy patients were not cured at follow-up. As a group their improvement was from a severe to a moderate degree of handicap" (p. 162).

A far more favorable result was claimed by Kelly et al. (1973), who reported an improvement rate of 90 percent for their depressed patients after limbic leucotomy. Of the 40 patients included in this prospective, noncontrolled study, 17 had a diagnosis of obsessional neurosis. Although cured or much improved outcomes are reported for 7 out of 17 patients, by counting the 6 patients who fall into the center of the rating scale (labeled "improved"), Kelly et al. are able to quote an improvement rate of 76 percent. This optimistic picture must be seen against the similar claim of a 66 percent improvement rate of patients diagnosed as schizophrenic—a very unusual result.

These almost entirely favorable results, observed six weeks after the operation, should be regarded with caution as the study suffers from the all-too-common defects of rater contamination, absence of controls, confounded treatments, and the like. Some three years later this team brought the information up to date by reporting a follow-up of sixteen months mean duration (Mitchell-Heggs, Kelly, and Richardson, 1976). Their claims were equally or more enthusiastic but should not obscure the original defects in the study. Before considering the significance of their impressive follow-up data, it must be mentioned that the ages of the patients ranged from twenty-one to sixty-five years. The lower limit confirms that the operation is *not* reserved for chronic cases. Furthermore, roughly 12 percent had an illness duration of less than five years.

If one ignores the flaws in the study's design, it would appear that the operation produced significant and lasting improvements, even if the reason for such improvement is unknown. The authors suggest that "the effects of limbic leucotomy in obsessional neurosis may possibly be achieved, therefore, by diminution of arousal" (p. 237). This vague notion is not supported—and even if it *were* confirmed, there are easier ways of reducing arousal. No one has offered any satisfactory argument showing that psychosurgery has a direct and specific antiobsessional action. Instead, those explanations that are proposed (and all are tentative) suggest that reductions in obsessional problems are *secondary*; but then it must be demonstrated that the *primary* action, be it anxiety-relief or reduced depression, cannot be achieved by easier, nonintrusive means. As the clinical ratings, which show large improvements, were carried out by an informed rater, their value is negligible. The decreases in a range of scores obtained from psychometric tests cannot be dismissed as easily. While it is true that the authors substituted quantity for quality (no reasons are given for the odd, but large, selection of tests), there is no denying the consistency and stability of the results—all pointing in the direction of sustained improvements. Furthermore, the timing of the major changes, occurring so soon after operation, excludes the influence of spontaneous remission effects, as these have a slower time-course. Even though their astonishing claim of an 80 percent success rate for the schizophrenic patients makes one pause, the researchers have at least established that, from a narrow point of view, psychosurgery is worth investigation. Taking a broader view, however, it might be argued that psychosurgery is a redundant and undesirable treatment if there are preferable alternatives.

If one allows the possibility that the operation was indeed followed by clinical improvements, at least as indexed by the test results, then one must discover why. Here it is essential to avoid the error of attributing such changes directly to the operation *per se.* Firstly, one would need to discount the powerful nonspecific therapeutic factors known to influence dramatic interventions, and, secondly, one would need to know the basis of such wide-ranging changes that can include an 80 percent improvement rate for schizophrenia, 89 percent improvement rate for obsessions, and 78 percent improvement rate for depression. Either we are dealing with a treatment of almost miraculously broad powers, or the nonspecific influences contributed heavily to the results. These alternatives assume, of course, that the results are solid; given the nature of the operation, one cannot recommend an independent replication as one would be inclined to do with other forms of therapy.

Even if one discounts the influence of nonspecific factors, the contribution of the postsurgical rehabilitation program may have had a major effect on the results. Although few details are provided in the journal articles describing the results of the trials, elsewhere one of the main authors, Kelly, in association with Sargant and Slater (1972), states that their rehabilitation program "plays an important part in the total treatment programme and usually lasts for 6 weeks" (p. 113). The program appears to include both of the major features of the currently used behavior therapy method—exposure and response prevention. It arranges for "gradual exposure to washing or cleaning situations," along with exposure to familiar environments in which the obsessions are more severe than in hospital, and supplements these with "encouragement from the nursing staff to resist rituals in the interval" (p. 114). What might be expected if the "rehabilitation program" were provided *before* surgery, or *instead of* surgery? A methodical use of exposure and response prevention is capable of producing rapid, large, and enduring improvements in patients with severe obsessional disorders (Rachman and Hodgson, 1979). Lastly, the possible influence of antidepressant medication is not given adequate consideration. It appears that most, though not all, of the patients had tried drugs before undergoing the operation, and one can assume that a high proportion received medication after the operation. Even if these drugs, where used, had been incapable of producing adequate improvements preoperatively, it is unwise to assume that they had no part in the recovery period—alone or in combination with the six-week rehabilitation program.

Bridges, Goktepe, and Maratos (1973) carried out a retrospective three-year follow-up study on 24 obsessional patients and 24 depressive patients who had had a bilateral stereotaxic tractotomy at least three years before. Information was obtained through an interview, to which the patient was accompanied by a relative. Sixteen out of the 24 obsessional patients were said to have benefited from the operation. Although the information was gathered in a direct and methodical manner, the absence of any preoperative clinical or observational information was a serious shortcoming. Moreover, the assessors who carried out the follow-up assessments were aware of the treatment that had been provided. For what it is worth, the depressed patients did as well as, or slightly better than, the obsessional patients. This serves to emphasize the point made earlier that, whatever else it is, psychosurgery of this kind is not a *specific* remedy for obsessional neuroses.

Evidence of serious unwanted effects was also found by the Bridges survey. For example, 5 of the 48 patients suffered fits after the operation. Moreover, 10 of the 48 patients had to have more than one operation (in the series reported by Kelly, 5 of the 17 patients had at least two operations). Despite the statement by Bridges et al. that "no patient reported having become worse since operation" (p. 673), Table VIII (p. 667) shows that for the unsuccessful patients the mean total of weeks per year spent in hospital increased from 26.9 before the operation to as high as 38.6 (that is, nearly 10 months per year) after the operation. These figures give some idea of the extent of the remaining handicaps among this group. In the improved group, the mean total of weeks spent in hospitals declined from 19 before the operation to 8.4 after the operation. Another interesting finding to come out of this study was the observed difference in outcomes between ruminators and patients with overt compulsions; the latter group did significantly better than the ruminators.

In regard to the claim that psychosurgery is particularly effective with chronic, intractable cases, the obsessional patients who did worst had an illness duration of 13.25 years and those who did best an illness duration of 9.75 years (Bridges, Goktepe, and Maratos, 1973, Table V, p. 666). Those patients who had the longest hospital admissions prior to the operation did worst of all (Table VIII, p. 667). In their second, wider review (see details below), Goktepe, Young, and Bridges (1975) found a similar pattern among a larger, mixed sample of patients. Those patients who had the longest hospital admissions (31 weeks) prior to operation did worst—see Table VIII, Goktepe et al., p. 276).

In their wide-ranging review, the same group of researchers reported on 208 patients who underwent subcaudate tractotomy "for intractable psychiatric illnesses" (Goktepe, Young, and Bridges, 1975). They managed to interview 134 patients in this sample and arrived at these conclusions about the clinical effectiveness of the surgical treatments: "Of the diagnostic groups, depressives did best with 67.9 percent in categories 1 and 2 (recovered, minimal residual symptoms), for anxiety this was 62.5 percent and for obsessional neurosis 50 percent ($n = 18$)" (p. 280). They noted a small incidence of adverse psychological consequences following the operation, and the occurrence of epilepsy in 2.2 percent of the cases operated on. Clearly, the results are consistent with those obtained in the first series of patients, reported on by Bridges et al. in 1973. Leaving aside problems of interpretation, the results appear to indicate that roughly 50 percent of the obsessional patients reported clinical improvement after undergoing the operation. As in most of the reports on this subject, the depressive patients appeared to do best. Even if the evidence were interpreted as showing that psychosurgery benefits a proportion of obsessional patients, it cannot be concluded that psychosurgery is especially suitable for managing obsessional neuroses.

Chronic and Intractable Cases

As noted above, Goktepe, Young, and Bridges (1975) found that those patients who were most seriously handicapped *before* the operation did least well after the operation. The least successful patients had spent an average of 31 weeks in hospital prior to the operation, as opposed to the successful cases' average of 19.2 weeks.

In this report, at least, *the most intractable cases did least well.* Evidence pointing in a similar direction can be found in the reports by Sykes and Tredgold (1964), Bridges, Goktepe, and Maratos (1973), and Ström-Olsen and Carlisle (1971). Ström-Olsen and Carlisle reported that the 7 (out of 20) obsessional patients who did *worst* after the operation had illness durations in excess of ten years. As the operations are carried out in order to reduce "long-standing apparently intractable psychiatric illnesses" (Ström-Olsen and Carlisle, 1971, p. 153), this relative lack of success with the most intractable patients is a serious matter. Note that Goktepe, Young, and Bridges (1975) advised that the risks "need to be weighed against the possibility of relieving the intractable illnesses for which the operation is carried out" (p. 279).

The operation in the Goktepe, Young, and Bridges study was not confined to patients with chronic and severe illnesses. So, for example, 2 of the 18 obsessional patients had illness durations of less than two years when the operation was carried out. Of the 208 patients in this series, no less than 42 were under the age of thirty years at the time of their operation. Similarly, in the series reported by Ström-Olsen and Carlisle (1971), 28 percent of 150 patients had an illness duration of less than five years. In Birley's (1964) review of 106 patients, some were as young as twenty-four years of age, and some were operated on after only two years of illness.

In passing, it is worth mentioning that 8 of the patients in a series of 83 obsessional patients studied by Rachman and Hodgson (1979) had undergone at least one psychosurgical operation prior to inclusion in our study. All 8 patients were given a course of behavioral treatment, and in 5 cases the outcome was largely or wholly unsuccessful (an unusually high failure rate for this treatment). These unsuccessful patients had severe and chronic disorders, all in excess of ten years duration, with a maximum of thirty-six years in one case. They all suffered from a range of obsessional complaints, but compulsive hand-washing was pronounced in all cases. In a sixth patient, with a comparably severe hand-washing compulsion, the outcome was reasonably successful (Rachman, Hodgson, and Marzillier, 1970). This comparatively young man had already had one operation and was being considered for a second when the behavioral treatment alternative was attempted. Significantly, his obsessional problems had a shorter history than those of the unsuccessful cases —only four years. Of the two postsurgical patients with problems involving primary obsessional slowness, one did moderately well and the other only slightly well.

Conclusions

Although the earlier psychosurgery operations were dangerous, carrying a mortality risk of at least 1 percent, the newer versions give little cause for concern on this score. It remains true, however, that there is a risk of inducing epilepsy, and an even greater risk of producing adverse psychological effects in a small but significant minority of cases.

A proportion of obsessional patients do experience improvements after undergoing psychosurgery. It remains unclear, however, whether these changes exceed in magnitude or duration those following other treatments, or no treatment at all. The Mitchell-Heggs, Kelly, and Richardson (1976) report suggests that the changes occur far too rapidly to be regarded as spontaneous remissions, but the weaknesses of their study preclude a firm conclusion about the specific value of the operation. It seems most unlikely that the operation produces a specific effect on the course of an obsessional disorder. In any event, there are preferable alternatives.

Although the spontaneous remission rate for obsessional neurosis has been observed to be lower than that for most other forms of neurotic disorder, the rate is not insignificant (see Rachman and Hodgson, 1979). Obsessional patients who receive conventional treatment, or no specific treatment, do not necessarily have a bleak outlook. Of 30 nonleucotomized patients followed up for three months to fifteen years, 21 were judged to be "either free of symptoms or able to carry on a normal life" (Pollitt, 1957, p. 198). More recently, Lo (1967) reported an encouraging outcome of 71 percent improvement in a group of 87 obsessional patients, none of whom had undergone psychosurgery. Cawley (1974) has argued that even though leucotomized patients are sometimes observed to do well after operation, "this is likely to be a comment on the selection procedures for leucotomy rather than on specific effects of the operation" (p. 281). After reviewing the evidence on the effects of physical treatments in obsessional disorders, Sternberg (1974) reached a similar conclusion: "While half the patients with obsessional disorders who have some form of leucotomy may be expected to benefit greatly, these are also the patients who have a better prognosis without leucotomy. Those undergoing operation run a 1.5 to 4 percent risk of dying and 16 percent may be expected to have up to 12 epileptic fits" (p. 303). Ingram's (1961) summary is still applicable: "Many of the factors said to favor the outcome of operation are seen to be the same as those favoring spontaneous improvement. The prominence of affective symptoms, the absence of motor symptoms, and late onset are all held to favor a good leucotomy result; here they are associated with spontaneous improvement" (p. 399).

Alternative Treatments

Although some ambitious claims have been made for *antidepressant drug treatment*, and some of the clinical evidence is indeed persuasive (for example, Capstick, 1975), the qualitative and quantitative data on the results of drug treatment for obsessional disorders are as inconclusive as those on psychosurgery (see Rachman and Hodgson, 1979). However, the prospects are favorable. Depression is a common and important feature of obsessional disorders, and antidepressant medication is moderately effective in reducing depression.

The collection of evidence on the effects of *behavior therapy* has progressed further, and we are in a position to reach clear, if tentative, conclusions. A full discussion of the available information is given elsewhere (Rachman and Hodgson, 1979), but Table 6.1 summarizes this information. On the basis of the present evidence, it is reasonable to conclude that behavioral treatment produces significant improvement in obsessional disorders, and rapidly at that. Clinically valuable reductions in the frequency and intensity of compulsive behavior have been observed directly and indirectly. Significant reductions in distress and discomfort are usual, and physiological changes of a kind observed during the successful treatment of phobias also occur. The admittedly insufficient evidence on the durability of the induced changes is not discouraging; allowing for the provision of booster treatments as needed (see, for example, Marks, Hodgson, and Rachman, 1975), the therapeutic improvements are stable. The successful modification of the main obsessional problems often is followed by improvements in social and vocational adjustment.

With the exception of *symbolic modeling*,[1] which produced comparatively weaker therapeutic effects (Roper, Rachman, and Marks, 1975), no significant differences between variants of behavioral treatment have emerged. Exposure to the relevant provoking conditions, followed by response prevention, appears to be a robust combination, but we are not yet in a position to ascribe particular or

---

[1] Symbolic modeling is a procedure in which the patient repeatedly observes the therapist carrying out the required coping behavior; it is contrasted with participant modeling, in which the patient observes and then imitates the therapist during treatment sessions.

Table 6.1 Effectiveness of Behavior Therapy for Obsessional-Compulsive Disorders

Authors	Sample Size	Exposure and Response Prevention	Control Group	Outcome (As Described)	Follow-Up
Studies Without Experimental Controls					
Meyer et al. (1974)	15	Yes	—	10 asymptomatic or greatly improved	1–6 years
Wonnenberger et al. (1975)	6	Yes	—	5 significantly improved	2 months
Mills et al. (1973)	5	Yes	—	5 significantly improved	Unsystematic
Foa and Goldstein (1978)	21	Yes	—	14 asymptomatic, 4 improved, 3 failures	±6 months
Marks et al. (1976)	34	Plus supplements	—	Significant group results overall	Variable
Catts and McConaghy (1975)	6	Yes	—	All 6 improved	6 months
Heyse (1975)	24	Yes	—	7 failures, 10 much improved	1 month
Ramsey and Sikkel (1971)	4	Yes	—	3 significantly improved	Variable

Studies With Experimental Controls

Study	n		Control	Results	Follow-up
Rachman et al. (1971)	10	Yes	Own control[a] (relaxation)	6 much improved, 4 failures	2 years
Rachman et al. (1973)	10	Yes	Own control[a] (relaxation)	7 much improved, 2 failures	2 years
Roper et al. (1975)	10	Yes	Own control[a] (relaxation)	8 improved, 2 failures	6 months
MRC Trial (Rachman and Hodgson, 1979)	40	± Clomipramine	Own control[a] (relaxation)	Significant behavioral improvements	1 year
Boersma et al. (1976)	13	Yes	Behavioral variants[b]	Average 75% improvement	3 months
Emmelkamp and Kraanen (1977)	14	Yes	Waiting list[c] and variants	Average 75% improvement	3 months
Hackmann and McClean (1976)	10	Yes	Thought stopping[d]	Significant group changes	No
Rabavilas and Boulougouris (1974)	12	Yes	Behavioral variants[b]	6 much improved, 2 failures	No

[a] Relaxation control consisted of 15 sessions of training in therapeutic muscle relaxation.
[b] Behavioral variants consisted of exposure given in unconventional ways, such as in very brief presentation or purely in fantasy, or in the absence of a therapist.
[c] Waiting list control consisted of a no-treatment waiting period.
[d] Thought stopping consisted of instruction in and practice of interrupting unwanted thinking.

essential effects to either element alone. Several explanations of the mechanisms involved have been offered, but none holds sway (Rachman and Hodgson, 1979).

Given these results, it is difficult to justify the consideration of psychosurgery unless and until behavior therapy has been fully tried and failed, and unless and until antidepressant drug treatment (preferably as a supplement to behavior therapy) has also been tried and failed.

Psychosurgery's Inadequate Rationale

In view of the fact that psychosurgery was originally introduced as a method for treating schizophrenia, it is scarcely surprising to find that there is no theoretical rationale for recommending surgery for obsessional patients; at best, it is sometimes argued that the operation will produce general changes (for example, reduced tension) that in turn may yield secondary benefits in the form of reduced compulsive behavior and the like. To the best of my knowledge, no one has even made a serious attempt to trace a specific connection between psychosurgery and the reduction of obsessional-compulsive problems. It follows, of course, that if the rationale for using psychosurgery on these patients is to be an indirect one—that is to say, the benefits are secondary—then it is not unreasonable to look for a rationale of the primary effects *and* of the relation between these effects and the putative secondary benefits. So, for example, if it is argued that the operations reduce psychological tension, one needs to know why; furthermore, the putative relation between reduced tension and an improvement in the obsessional disorder needs to be explained and defended. As mentioned earlier, if improvements in obsessional disorders are secondary to some other change, then it is essential to show that the *primary* action, such as reduced depression, cannot be achieved by other—safer, simpler, nonintrusive—methods.

To return to the opening question of this assessment, it must be concluded, from the present evidence, that neither of the main therapeutic claims made on behalf of psychosurgery is supportable. Psychosurgery is not especially suitable for treating obsessional disorders, and it is not most effective for treating chronic or intractable cases. In one sense, the use of psychosurgery for treating obsessional disorders is a scientific curiosity. Proponents of psychosurgery justify its use on empirical grounds, but on inspection it turns out that this empirically based treatment has an inadequate empirical basis. In the present circumstances, there is little reason to recommend psychosurgery for obsessional disorders.

CHAPTER 7

Organic Brain Disease: A Separate Issue

Vernon H. Mark and William A. Carnahan

The Right of Neurosurgical Patients to Have Treatment and the Myth of Psychosurgery in Patients with Organic Brain Disease (Including Some of the Evidence Relating Behavioral Symptoms to Brain Abnormalities in Patients Who Might Require Neurosurgical Treatment)

One of the most frequent and uninformed criticisms of neurosurgical intervention for the treatment of brain disease in abnormally aggressive patients is that it is necessarily a form of psychosurgery. The word *psychosurgery* has become a symbol that arouses fear and frequently prevents brain-injured patients from seeking surgical treatment. In reality, this term has a number of different definitions. Bertram Brown, formerly Director of the National Institute of Mental Health, has defined it as "a surgical removal or destruction of brain tissue with the cutting of brain tissue to disconnect one part of the brain from another, with the intent of altering behavior even though there may be no direct evidence of structural disease or damage in the brain" (Brown, Wienckowski, and Bivens, 1973). On the other hand, Orlando Andy (1971), a stereotactic neurosurgeon at the University of Mississippi, has defined psychosurgery as "a term which has been loosely used to identify brain operations performed for the treatment of behavioral and related neurologic disorders." The Oregon Legislature (1973) has defined psychosurgery in the following manner: "Any operation designed to irreversibly lesion or destroy brain tissue for the primary purpose of altering thoughts, emotions or behavior of a human being. Psychosurgery does not include procedures which may irreversibly lesion or destroy brain tissue when undertaken to cure well defined diseases such as brain tumor, epileptic foci, and certain chronic pain syndromes" (p. 348).[1]

This latter definition at least makes an attempt to distinguish between patients who have emotional or behavioral disorders with and without recognized pathological or physiological changes in the brain. This has pragmatic importance because surgery in the former group of patients is directed toward isolating or removing abnormal tissue or foci of abnormal electrical discharges. It is not primarily directed toward altering behavior, but toward reversing brain pathophysiology. Strictly speaking, this kind of neurosurgery should not be included under the rubric of psychosurgery.

It is obvious that anti-psychosurgery arguments do not apply when abnormal behavior is related to brain abnormality. With this in mind, it is interesting to note the statement of Peter Breggin (1971c), a spokesman for the anti-psychosurgery movement. His definition of psychosurgery, as quoted by Annas, is "to destroy normal brain tissue to control the emotions, or behavior, or a diseased tissue when the disease has nothing to do with behavior . . . the man is trying to control" (p. 359). It is important to realize that Breggin's definition tries to separate diseased brain tissue from abnormal behavior and is part of the effort to discredit this relationship. This attempt is not surprising since the evidence for an intimate connection between brain dysfunction and behavior abnormalities contradicts the basic premise of the antimedical-psychiatry/antipsychosurgical movement. Breggin and his former teacher Thomas Szasz are spokesmen for this movement whose members apparently believe that human behavior is molded exclusively by the sociopolitical environment (Mark and Ordia, 1976). This belief would lead them to think that biological abnormalities have little to do with the genesis of emotional or behavioral disorders and they are critical

---

[1] Ch. 616 (1973 Oregon Reg. Sess.) (S. Bill 298), amending Rev. Stat. 677, 190 (1971).

when medical (and particularly neurosurgical) techniques are used to treat these disorders.

Risks of Withholding Neurosurgical Treatment

Some critics carry their prohibitions against neurosurgical intervention in symptomatic patients to an extreme.

> One of the present authors (VHM) saw a moribund patient who was originally "treated" and denied neurosurgical attention in the clinic of an outspoken antipsychosurgy psychiatrist (Mark and Ordia, 1976). Apparently, this physician's prohibitions against neurological surgery influenced his resident staff so that they avoided doing even a limited neurological examination on a patient who was complaining of progressive headaches and nausea. They insisted on interpreting the patient's symptoms as a reflection of emotional distress generated by his overbearing and possessive mother. The fundi of this twenty-one-year-old man with advanced papilledema were not examined by the psychiatric resident who saw him two days before he was admitted to our hospital, apneic, with fixed dilated pupils and absent brainstem reflexes. The situation was not made more acceptable when the cause of the patient's problem was found to be a treatable cerebellar tumor.

This case raises some important questions, however. When did this patient stop being a subject for psychotherapy? Most psychiatrists would agree that life-saving neurosurgical procedures should not be deferred in patients who have brain tumors, even when their symptoms are interpreted as emotional in orgin. But who is going to make the decision as to when the patient has crossed the boundary between psychiatry and neurology? The antipsychosurgery psychiatrist in this case waited too long. But is there any way of avoiding an undue delay in therapy, without subjecting the patient to an immediate and thorough neurological assessment?

Some antipsychosurgery psychiatrists might agree to let neurosurgeons care for patients with life-threatening brain tumors. They might even agree to have neurological assessments performed on patients with possible diagnoses of brain tumor. However, most of them would still want to prevent neurologists, and especially neurosurgeons, from treating patients with emotional symptoms who did not have an obvious life-threatening disorder. Unfortunately, this attitude would also interfere with the rational treatment of patients with emotional symptoms whose brain tumors or other pathologies were hard to detect. The case presented by Van Rensburg et al. (1975), illustrates this point.

The patient was a twenty-one-year-old, unmarried white male who complained of episodes of uncontrollable behavior, of which he subsequently had no recollection. Seven years before his admission, he started experiencing attacks, two to three times a day, in which he felt light-headed and compulsively rubbed hands and arms against each other. At the age of nineteen, his attacks changed in character. They commenced with a feeling of intense and indefinable pleasure, after which he had no further recollection of what had happened until ten or fifteen minutes later when he again became aware of his surroundings. He was told that during the period of amnesia he became uncontrollable and did strange things, becoming uncharacteristically violent at times. Normally a mild-mannered man, he assaulted a patient in the bed next to him during his admission to the hospital.

Although diagnostic studies showed some electrical dysrhythmia on brain wave examination and an area of irregular calcification in the middle fossa, contrast studies did not unequivically demonstrate a mass lesion. This patient's symptoms were not controlled by prolonged trials of medical therapy, and a temporal lobectomy was undertaken. At the time of operation, there were no obvious abnormalities on the surface of the temporal lobe. However, on opening the temporal horn, the surgeon discovered a reddish, nodular mass, flecked with gray, which was gritty to the touch of a blunt dissector. It was seen to protrude slightly into the ventricle in the expected position of the bulge of the amygdaloid nucleus. This mass was removed, and directly anterior to it was found a cyst containing about thirty cubic centimeters of clear yellow fluid. Pathological examination showed this tumor to be an intracerebral schwannoma. After its removal, the patient's postoperative course was uneventful, and, at the time the case was written up, twenty-one months after surgery, the patient had not experienced a further seizure and was asymptomatic.

Certainly, to withhold therapy from Van Rensburg's patient would have been a tragic mistake in medical management. The antipsychosurgery psychiatrists might contend that it is rare for a small tumor of the amygdaloid nucleus and anterior hippocampus to cause emotional and behavioral symptoms and temporal lobe seizures. However, the data collected by Falconer (1973) suggest otherwise. Falconer reviewed over 250 of his patients with temporal lobe epilepsy who underwent unilateral temporal lobectomy. Pathological findings in the resected specimens, which included the hippocampus and amygdala were: medial temporal sclerosis in about one-half; harmatomas (small brain tumors) in one-fifth to one-quarter; miscellaneous lesions, such as scars and infarcts, in one-tenth; and nonspecific lesions in the remainder. Interictal aggression was the most common single psychiatric abnormality seen in these patients. Before operation, approximately one-fourth of the patients in each pathological grouping showed prominent aggressive traits.

Relation of Abnormal Behavior to Biological Abnormalities

There is increasing evidence that various types of abnormal behavior are related to biological abnormalities, especially of the limbic brain. This evidence specifically contradicts the notions of the anti-medical psychiatrists that form the basis for their definition of psychosurgery. It is appropriate, then, to describe some of the findings, first, regarding the correlation of abnormal aggressivity with tissue abnormality, and secondly, regarding the correlation of thought disorders with bioelectrical abnormality.

Aggressive Behavior and Limbic Disease

Limbic brain tumors have been associated with abnormally aggressive behavior (Mark and Sweet, 1974). Published reports of such tumors include one by Cushing (1929); one by Alpers (1937); one by Vonderahe (1940); one by Dott, reported by Hill (1944); four by Malamud (1967); one by Reeves and Plum (1969); three by Sweet and his associates (1969); and one by Mullan (1971). The lesion sites were: one inferior posteromedial frontal abscess; one angioma of the temporal pole; one subfrontal meningioma; four invasive, slow growing gliomas (three temporal and one gyrus cinguli); one temporal glioblastoma; three hypothalamic tumors; one glioma of the optic chiasma; and one colloid cyst of the third ventricle. In five patients diagnosed ante mortem, surgical attack on the tumor was followed by cessation of the violent behavior. In other cases, the tumor was a post mortem finding. Recently, Rothman et al. (1976) reported an additional case of a fifteen-year-old boy who exhibited outbursts of violent behavior. He was found to have an ectopic pituitary adenoma compressing the medial surface of the right temporal lobe and invaginating the inferior aspect of the third ventricle.

Patients with cranio-cerebral injuries, especially young men, often go through a phase of hyperactivity and belligerence. In many, the cerebral injury is too diffuse to permit correlation of one specific area of the brain with this symptom. However, McLaurin and Heimer (1965) reported as "restless and combative" seven of twelve patients with contusions of the temporal lobe. In nine of these twelve patients, the diagnosis was verified by open operation, and in the other three, by clear-cut evidence on special radiographic studies.

Temporal lobectomy provided good relief of symptoms in two patients who exhibited violent behavior after significant temporal lobe injury. Both patients had post-traumatic gliosis of the temporal lobe, but neither of them had any seizures (Adams, 1973).

Viral disease of the limbic system, such as herpes encephalitis, may be related to emotional changes and combativeness. Of course, rabies (whose name in French, German, and Italian means rage) has, as the most characteristic of its lesion sites, inclusion bodies in Ammon's horn.

Another category of limbic disease includes the functional derangement of the brain as seen in epileptic patients. By far the most common focal cerebral disorders associated with poor control of destructive impulses and rage are those which also give rise to limbic system epilepsy. Henry Maudsley (1874) had the opportunity to study epileptic patients confined to an asylum and untreated by modern anticonvulsant or ataractic therapy. He described the auras of temporal lobe epilepsy (without anatomical confirmation) and the ictal and interictal violence and assaultive behavior seen in his patients.

The occurrence of abnormal aggressivity in epileptic patients has varied with the group being studied. In some reported series, the clinical correlations of limbic epilepsy with aggression have prompted researchers to remark on the frequent outbursts of anger shown by epileptic patients, often after a minimal provocation. Gastaut, Morin, and Lesèure (1955) recorded paroxysmal rages in 50 percent of their epileptics of the temporal lobe type. Falconer (1958), reporting on fifty patients whose temporal lobe epilepsy was associated with a predominantly unilateral spike focus, found, as the most common personality disturbance in 38 percent, a "pathological aggressiveness occurring in outbursts in an otherwise adjusted individual" (p. 396). Another 14 percent had "an often milder but more persistent aggressiveness associated with a continued paranoid outlook." Rages, called with typical French delicacy "endogenous bouts of impulsiveness," became so severe in thirty-eight epileptic patients of Roger and Dongier (1950) that they had to be confined to mental institutions. Each of these thirty-eight had classical neurological symptoms of temporal lobe epilepsy and evidence of EEG foci in scalp leads from temporal and inferior frontal regions or both.

In light of these facts, one would expect that a feeling of anger might be commonly reported as an aura ushering a frank seizure of temporal lobe epilepsy, and that directed assault might be a frequent symptom occurring during such a seizure. However, in the published accounts the majority of patients who described any emotional component of their seizures classified it as fear. Other emotions, such as anger, sadness, pleasure, and joy, were reported much less frequently. Fear may precipitate attack behavior. Two of our own patients reported experiencing an epileptic aura containing an element of fear immediately before their destructive or assaultive acts (Ervin, Mark, and Sweet, 1969).

Abnormal aggressivity is more frequent as an interictal rather than a seizural phenomenon. For example, Ounstead, Lindsay, and Norman (1966), in a prospective study of a hundred temporal lobe epileptics, found that thirty-six developed repeated episodes of "catastrophic rage" while under their observation. All of these violent patients had other varieties of seizures as well.

Before concluding the evidence relating temporal lobe disease with abnormal aggressivity, it might be useful to review the data generated by Vaernet (1973) of Copenhagen, who found that ablation of the amygdala in hyperaggressive patients without structural or functional abnormality of the brain fails to alter this symptom. Vaernet reported the effects of stereotactic amygdalotomies on thirteen patients with personality disorders, all of whom were abnormally aggressive. He found that the effect of amygdaloid ablation was related to the degree of electrical abnormality recorded in the medial structures of the temporal lobe. All but one of the patients with no electrical abnormality showed no postoperative change in their violent behavior (or any other personality change). Vaernet concluded that "there is hardly any reason to believe that we can make corrective surgery where such behavior abnormalities are part of the patients' inborn pattern of reaction with weak or deficient inhibitory mechanisms."

Professor Norman Geschwind and his colleagues Steven Waxman and David Bear reviewed the psychiatric and neurological literature, including their own contributions, relating limbic system disease to changes in behavior (Geschwind, 1977a; Waxman and Geschwind, 1975; Bear, 1977). They described the behavioral symptoms, in addition to abnormal aggressive behavior, that may be associated with temporal lobe epilepsy—notably, hyperreligiosity, compulsive writing, hyposexuality, and psychosis in patients with chronic limbic epilepsy. Geschwind (1977b) concluded that "we should be wary of describing behavioral changes by means of standard names of other psychiatric conditions. We should treat behavior changes in temporal lobe epilepsy as a phenomenon in its own right. . . . I think it is a real possibility that one day we will ask, not—do the behavioral changes of temporal lobe epilepsy resemble schizophrenia? but rather—are there some aspects of some disorders now called schizophrenia which resemble the changes seen in temporal lobe epilepsy?" (p. 8)

Bear and Fedio (1977) subsequently published a quantitative analysis of interictal behavior in temporal lobe epilepsy, based on investigations carried out at the Clinical Neurosciences Branch of the National Institute of Neurological and Communicative Disorders and Stroke. Patients with unilateral temporal epileptic foci were contrasted with normal subjects and patients with neuromuscular disorders in the evaluation of specific psychosocial aspects of behavior. Eighteen traits were assessed in equivalent questionnaires completed by both subjects and observers. The epileptic patients self-reported a distinctive profile of humorless sobriety, dependence, and obsessionalism. Raters discriminated temporal lobe epileptics on the basis of circumstantiality, philosophical interests, and anger.

Right temporal lobe epileptics displayed emotional tendencies, in contrast to ideational traits shown by left temporal lobe epileptics. Right temporal lobe epileptics exhibited denial, while left temporal epileptics tarnished their image with overemphasis of dissocial behavior. The occurrence of anger, paranoia, and dependence in patients with predominantly left temporal lobe lesions was shown to be statistically significant (P value of less than 0.05). To increase the precision of right–left differentiation, Bear and Fedio employed the analysis of variance to identify those individual items that significantly differentiated the two epileptic groups. (This was done separately for patients' and raters' responses.) The epileptic groups were also contrasted with the control group in this way, and the severity factor distinguished both epileptic groups very significantly from controls (P value of less than 0.001).

The Bear-Fedio study is important not only because it puts the correlation between brain and behavior on a firm statistical basis but also because it tends to confirm the hemispheric distinction between behavioral symptoms. Flor-Henry (1969) was able to correlate the thought disorder occurring in epilepsy with the side of the hemispheric lesion. Our group (Blumer, Williams, and Mark, 1974) subsequently showed that thirteen of fourteen violent unilateral temporal lobe epileptics had structural abnormalities, seen by pneumoencephalogram, only on the left side.

Thought Disorders and Biochemical Abnormalities

The evidence relating specific behavior abnormalities to biological abnormalities has recently been strengthened by two studies conducted by Potkin (1978) that verify the presence of lowered platelet monoamine oxidase activity in chronic schizophrenia. In the first study, a retrospective chart analysis, the mean platelet activity of patients with chronic schizophrenia differed significantly from that of normal controls (P value less than 0.001). Chronic paranoid schizophrenics differed significantly from chronic nonparanoid schizophrenics (P value 0.03). Separate prospective studies confirmed significantly lower values for monoamine oxidase activity in chronic schizophrenic patients diagnosed as paranoid or as having secondary paranoid features, as compared with chronic nonparanoid schizophrenics (P value 0.001). These studies suggested that chronic paranoid schizophrenia may be a separate disorder from the other chronic forms of schizophrenia and that this difference may be related, at least in part, to biochemical characteristics.

Conclusion

In conclusion, there is strong evidence that certain behavioral symptoms may be related to biological abnormalities. These are clearly in a different category from those generated by "functional psychiatric disturbances" and emotional problems related exclusively to environment.[2] These latter symptoms, if severe enough and if resistant to all forms of medical or psychiatric treatment, might influence a patient and a patient's physician to consider neurosurgical treatment; if so, this treatment would be called *psychosurgery.* However, surgical treatment for intractable symptoms related to biological abnormalities should not be considered psychosurgical treatment, but rather *neurosurgical intervention,*[3] differentiated in no significant legal or ethical way from the neurosurgical treatment of aneurysms or spinal cord tumors. It is fatuous to suggest that a disease of the brain must be life-threatening before appropriate diagnosis and treatment are provided. The patient with biological disorders involving the nervous system has the same rights to prompt diagnosis and treatment as any other patient with disease of the bones, gall bladder, or heart. To deny a patient such treatment on the basis of anachronistic philosophical, psychological, sociological, or psychiatric theories is morally and ethically indefensible.

In this chapter we have focused on the biological abnormalities —structural, functional, electrophysiological, and biochemical— that may be related to abnormal behavior. We felt this emphasis was

---

[2] This is not to deny that the interaction between brain and environment plays a role in all human behavior (Mark, in press; Mark and Ervin, 1970).

[3] Neurosurgical intervention refers chiefly to procedures for the treatment of epilepsy.

necessary as a corrective to the arguments suggesting that brain pathology is *never* related to abnormal behavior. But it would be equally misleading to imply that every patient who exhibits abnormal behavior is primarily the victim of some sort of brain disease. Because of the incomplete nature of the medical and neurological examinations carried out on many patients with psychiatric symptoms, it is not possible, at present, to estimate what percentage of these patients have some sort of brain dysfunction. Furthermore, our techniques for detecting brain abnormalities are, as yet, only partly developed. Thus, some patients who do not have any structural abnormality on arteriography, CT scanning, or pneumoencephalography, or electrophysiological abnormality on electroencephalogram or evoked potential recordings, or psychological abnormality on psychometric tests, or psychiatric or neurological abnormalities on clinical examination, may still have a biochemical or other kind of undetected brain abnormality that is at least partially responsible for their abnormal behavior. At the present time, however, when our diagnostic tools are not precise enough to find an abnormality, these patients must be treated in the same fashion as those who have behavioral abnormalities with an apparently normal brain. We have not described these latter patients in detail because they are more properly included in the chapters of those surgeons who specialize in fractional frontal lobe or multi-target operations to relieve the symptoms of otherwise intractable psychiatric complaints. However, some of the legal and ethical considerations of brain surgery in these patients are considered in our chapter on that subject in Part V of this volume.

PART III

Evaluation of Psychosurgery

CHAPTER 8

Review of the Literature on Postoperative Evaluation

Elliot S. Valenstein

Whether they start over legal, ethical, or social issues, most psycho-surgery debates ultimately come down to conflicting opinions about the outcome of psychosurgical operations. If these operations always accomplished what their most enthusiastic advocates claim and never resulted in any impairment, most of the controversy would evaporate. If the converse were always true—that is, if the worst results were typical—psychosurgery would not be performed at all. Obviously, the truth is somewhere in between these extremes, and therefore there is controversy. Of course, even if it were possible to state the precise statistical probability of various outcomes, there would still be disagreement over the course of action. Clearly, personal judgments are involved in any consideration of a trade-off between, for example, a loss of motivation or affect and a gain in "peace of mind." Important as these judgments may be, it is first necessary to obtain evidence—as objective as possible—on the outcomes of psychosurgery. The present chapter summarizes the evidence available in the published literature, and the following chapters present the results of two studies (one retrospective and one prospective) of psychosurgical patients, together with some comments about such studies. It may be argued that these reports do not reflect all the information available or that they draw upon only certain types of evidence and test results and ignore other sources of information. These criticisms notwithstanding, the reports may be considered objective, at least in that their authors had no strong preconceptions as to what they would find nor any personal investment in finding evidence for or against psychosurgery.

The information reported in this chapter was obtained from articles on psychosurgery published between 1971 and 1976. This literature survey was sponsored by the National Commission for the Protection of Human Subjects of Biomedical and Behavioral Research. The core references were obtained through a National Library of Medicine (MEDLARS) computerized search. The core list was considerably expanded by adding all relevant references cited in the articles obtained through the MEDLARS search. Approximately 700 articles that treated some aspect of psychosurgery or related scientific or ethical issues were located.[1] The great majority of these papers did not present firsthand data on the results of psychosurgery. Some of these articles were concerned primarily with the theory and history of psychosurgery. In others, the results of brain operations were discussed only in broad and general terms. Many other articles in this group presented ethical, legal, and sociopolitical views, and these varied in purpose and tone from scholarly presentations of reasoned arguments to emotionally charged polemics by participants in the psychosurgery controversy.

The data on the results of psychosurgery were obtained primarily from 209 articles written by persons having direct contact either with the patients or their records, and containing information on the outcome of a series of operations. Probably with very few exceptions, these *data articles* represent the total number of substantive papers on psychosurgery published anywhere in the world. Fifty of these articles described the results of brain operations on patients suffering from intractable pain, and 6 articles presented information only on electrical brain stimulation. Therefore, the total number of data articles published between 1971 and 1976 that contained information on the results of psychosurgery alone (excluding the opera-

---

[1] This list of references and the reports of the National Commission for the Protection of Human Subjects of Biomedical and Behavioral Research on psychosurgery are available through the Superintendent of Documents, DHEW Publication No. (OS) 77-0001 and (OS) 77-0002. David Marques assisted the author in collecting and collating the information obtained from the psychosurgical literature.

tions for pain and brain stimulation) was 153. Of these 153 articles, 26 presented data on psychosurgery performed in the United States and 39 presented data from the United Kingdom. The remaining articles emanated from other countries. Although all the data articles were written after 1970, several of them included information from patients operated on in the mid to late 1960s.

The information in all the data articles was summarized on record sheets. Descriptions of the patients and their preoperative histories, the types of surgery and their rationale if presented, the postoperative evaluations, complications, and ethical issues were all recorded on forms suitable for later retrieval and collating. This information was summarized and will be presented in the tables that are included in this chapter. In addition, the scientific merit of each data article was rated according to a system described by May and Van Putten (1974).

It is apparent that the ability to obtain a meaningful summary of the effects of psychosurgery from a literature survey is dependent on the reliability, validity, and comprehensiveness of the data that are reported. It was considered most essential, therefore, to examine the way the data have been collected and reported. The first part of this chapter consists of description and commentary on the scientific validity of the data reported in the psychosurgical literature. The second part presents the results of the surgery, including (1) the results obtained from objective tests, (2) the ratings of postoperative changes in the patients' conditions as made (in most cases) by the psychiatrists and neurosurgeons responsible for the treatment, and (3) data on the nature and incidence of complications attributable to the surgery.

Scientific Validity of the Research Data

For obvious reasons, it is usually impossible for neurosurgeons and psychiatrists to use the experimental control procedures that are routinely used in animal research. Understandably, patient care must, and should, take precedence over considerations of research design. The random assignment of subjects to different experimental (treatment) groups, the use of sham operations to control for placebo effects, and other similar procedures routinely used in animal studies are difficult, and sometimes impossible, to incorporate into clinical research without violating patients' rights and, in some cases, even endangering the patients. Some of the scientific shortcomings in the psychosurgical literature probably cannot be remedied without introducing risks to the patients; others, however, might be reduced with no detrimental effects (see Corkin's contribution in this volume).

Measurement Instruments

One criterion that should be used in evaluating the reliability and validity of the information presented on postoperative changes is the extent to which objective and standardized tests are used to evaluate these changes. Granted that clinical acumen and subjective impressions may provide valuable leads, it is nevertheless clear that the results obtained from objective tests are more likely to be replicable, comparable, and free of personal bias. Even where standard tests are not employed, the use of operationally defined criteria that explicitly describe the basis for statements about postoperative changes is clearly desirable.

Elsewhere, I have listed all the objective tests cited in the 153 data articles on psychosurgery (Valenstein, 1977, Appendix 6). This list of tests was compiled liberally, in that it included tests that the authors implied were standardized even when there was no published evidence supporting this assertion. Excluded from the list, however, were patient questionnaires referred to by such terms as "tests of self-scrutiny" and "pleasure ratings" when they appeared to be idiosyncratic to one author and were not stated to have been standardized. The tests were grouped according to categories reflecting their major focus and purpose. The following categories, while somewhat arbitrary, were judged to adequately describe the attributes and abilities that the tests were designed to evaluate: *Behavior Evaluation Tests, Tests of Psychiatric Symptoms or Status, General Personality Tests, Specific Personality Scales* (for example, anxiety, depression, hostility), *Tests of Abstract Thinking, Intelligence Tests, Learning and Memory Tests, Neurological or Psychoneurological Tests* (including perception tests), *Motor Performance Tests*, and *Tests of Language Ability.* Tests having multiple purposes were listed in more than one category. Our purpose in compiling this list was to establish the frequency of use of objective tests for evaluating patients following psychosurgery and to determine if there were any trends in the changes in specific capacities resulting from different psychosurgical procedures.

Figure 8.1 shows the percentage of the data articles that report the results of objective tests. The data are presented for articles from all

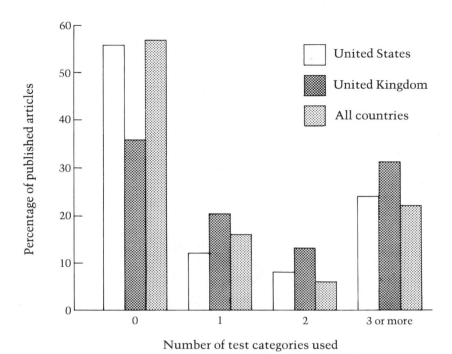

Figure 8.1 Percentage of published articles presenting results of objective tests.

countries combined and also separately for the articles from the United States and the United Kingdom. It can be seen that 58 percent of all the articles present no information obtained from objective tests. Only 70 articles out of the 153 even mentioned the use of any objective tests. Five of the 70 articles referred only to the use of "psychometric evaluation," but did not otherwise specify the tests used; 16 of the articles used only an IQ test. In total, 49 articles reported the use of intelligence tests, but only 27 of these specified the name of the test. A number of articles gave the names of specific objective tests without describing the results other than stating there was no change. The record from the United States was no better than the world average; articles from the United Kingdom generally described the use of objective tests more frequently. Only 25 percent of the U.S. articles reported data from three or more objective tests.

Tables 8.1, 8.2, and 8.3 present data on the use of objective tests analyzed separately by the main brain target ablated during psychosurgery. Table 8.1 lists the results from all articles, while Tables 8.2

Table 8.1 Percentage of Articles Specifying Use of Objective Tests (All Countries)

Target of Operation	Number of Articles	No Test Specified	Behavior Evaluation	Psychiatric Symptoms	Personality Tests
Cingulum	34	44.0%	2.9%	5.9%	41.2%
Amygdala	34	58.8%	8.8%	11.8%	8.8%
Frontal lobe	64	57.8%	0	4.7%	26.6%
Thalamus	15	73.3%	13.3%	0	13.3%
Hypothalamus	25	84.0%	0	0	4.0%
Multiple targets	10	80.0%	0	0	20.0%
Other	14	64.3%	0	0	21.4%

Note: Percentages are calculated separately for each brain target based on the proportion of papers reporting data in each test category. The specific tests included in each test category are listed in Valenstein (1977), Appendix 6.

and 8.3 summarize the United States and United Kingdom record, respectively. The United States record (Table 8.2) suggests some differences in the use of objective tests depending on the brain target of the operation. There were no results of objective tests reported, for example, in any of the articles describing multiple-target or hypothalamic operations. In general, the data in Table 8.2 suggest that the objective tests used are those that are easiest to administer and score. It can be seen, for instance, that general intelligence tests tend to be used more frequently than tests of abstract thinking, even though there has been considerable evidence published indicating that the overall IQ test score did not detect postoperative changes even following the older, more extensive, lobotomy procedures,[2] whereas tests of abstract ability sometimes indicated impairment.

The results presented in Tables 8.2 and 8.3 support the trend seen in Figure 8.1 in that they show that articles from the United Kingdom present the results of objective tests significantly more frequently than those from the United States. Although the differences between the two countries may be somewhat inflated by the tendency of one British group to describe essentially the same objective test results in several articles, the trend remained even when these articles were eliminated from the comparison.

It is important and only fair to point out that there are no readily available objective tests that have proven to be sensitive to intellec-

---

[2] Two studies did report IQ changes following the older lobotomy procedures (Rosvold and Mishkin, 1950; Smith and Kinder, 1959; Smith, 1964) and a few studies have reported deficits in specific subtests of an IQ battery. The vast majority of the studies, however, did not report any postoperative deficits in IQ. A discussion of this issue is presented elsewhere (Valenstein, 1973, pp. 321 and 398).

Table 8.1 *(continued)*

Specific Psychiatric Scales	Abstract Thinking	Intelligence	Learning and Memory	Neurology and Psycho-neurology	Motor Performance	Language
35.3%	23.5%	50.0%	29.4%	29.4%	20.6%	2.9%
11.8%	8.8%	29.4%	8.8%	8.8%	5.9%	5.9%
26.5%	4.7%	28.1%	6.2%	1.6%	3.1%	1.6%
6.7%	0	13.3%	0	6.7%	0	0
0	4.0%	20.0%	0	0	0	0
20.0%	10.0%	20.0%	10.0%	10.0%	10.0%	0
21.4%	7.1%	35.7%	14.3%	0	14.3%	0

tual changes following psychosurgery (see, for example, the contributions by Corkin and by Mirsky and Orzack in this volume). Testing for such capacities as abstract reasoning, facility to switch from one problem-solving strategy to another, and creativity or originality as reflected in "divergent thinking" is not an exact science. There is no agreement on how to measure these capacities even in normal people, and it is certainly conceivable that the testing of psychosurgical patients presents different problems. For example, some psychosurgical patients may reveal abilities when subjected to the challenge of a test situation that they seldom use in everyday life. In other words, the surgery may produce differences in the *probability* of using intellectual capacities rather than a loss of these abilities in any absolute sense. Such "motivational effects," if they did exist, might not be reflected in the performance of patients when tested, but might be evident in the persistence they exhibit in reaching goals in everyday life.

It is clear that we need to explore new ways of testing patients following psychosurgery. Given the shortcomings of the tests presently available, and the consequent lack of meaningful data, there is little justification for the frequent claim in the literature that there were no intellectual changes following surgery. In one extreme case, it was reported that there were "no or little changes in intellect and discrimination ability" following psychosurgery, but the only evidence presented was a sample of a patient's postoperative knitting (Winter, 1972). It may be important to recall in the present context that the use of insensitive tests following destruction of the corpus callosum in the human brain initially led to the conclusion that there was no impairment in conversational facility, verbal reasoning and intelligence, established motor coordination, long-

Table 8.2   Percentage of Articles Specifying Use of Objective Tests (United States)

Target of Operation	Number of Articles	No Test Specified	Behavior Evaluation	Psychiatric Symptoms	Personality Tests
Cingulum	7	43.0%	14.0%	0	28.0%
Amygdala	5	60.0%	0	20.0%	0
Frontal lobe	9	77.0%	0	0	33.0%
Thalamus	3	0	66.7%	0	66.7%
Hypothalamus	1	100.0%	0	0	0
Multiple targets	3	100.0%	0	0	0
Other	—	—	—	—	—

Note: Percentages are calculated separately for each brain target based on the proportion of papers reporting data in each test category. The specific tests included in each test category are listed in Valenstein (1977), Appendix 6.

term memory, personality, sense of humor, and social interactions following surgery. Indeed, no function at all could be attributed to the corpus callosum until it was revealed by the use of appropriate testing by Dr. Roger Sperry and his colleagues. More recently, additional testing has demonstrated short-term memory deficits (Zaidel and Sperry, 1974) and impairment in transfer of learning between different sensory modalities (Goldstein, Joynt, and Hartley, 1975).

Typically, the postoperative results of psychosurgery are reported in terms of categories based on patient interviews, questionnaires sent to relatives, employment record, marital stability, and general information concerning the patients' adjustment. The following description (Ballantine, et al., 1977) of categories used to report postoperative results is representative:

Table 8.3   Percentage of Articles Specifying Use of Objective Tests (United Kingdom)

Target of Operation	Number of Articles	No Test Specified	Behavior Evaluation	Psychiatric Symptoms	Personality Tests
Cingulum	6	33.3%	0	16.7%	50.0%
Amygdala	8	25.0%	37.5%	37.5%	37.5%
Frontal lobe	29	41.4%	0	3.4%	37.9%
Thalamus	0	—	—	—	—
Hypothalamus	0	—	—	—	—
Multiple targets	1	0	0	0	0
Other	1	0	0	0	0

Note: Percentages are calculated separately for each brain target based on the proportion of papers reporting data in each test category. The specific tests included in each test category are listed in Valenstein (1977), Appendix 6.

Table 8.2 *(continued)*

Specific Psychiatric Scales	Abstract Thinking	Intelligence	Learning and Memory	Neurology and Psycho-neurology	Motor Performance	Language
14.0%	14.0%	43.0%	57.0%	57.0%	14.0%	14.0%
0	0	40.0%	0	20.0%	0	0
0	0	22.0%	0	0	0	0
33.3%	0	33.3%	0	33.3%	0	0
0	0	0	0	0	0	0
0	0	0	0	0	0	0
—	—	—	—	—	—	—

Category	Description
5	Patient is well, not taking any medications, no longer under regular psychiatric care, and functioning at 80–100 percent of his ability.
4	Patient feels well, markedly improved since operation, but takes medication, sees psychiatrist occasionally, and is functioning at 80–100 percent of his ability.
3	Patient is not well, but much improved. He is under the frequent care of his psychiatrist, takes medication and psychiatric treatment regularly, and is functioning at 40–70 percent of his ability.
2	Patient is not well, but has improved since operation.

Table 8.3 *(continued)*

Specific Psychiatric Scales	Abstract Thinking	Intelligence	Learning and Memory	Neurology and Psycho-neurology	Motor Performance	Language
50.0%	33.3%	50.0%	16.7%	0	0	0
50.0%	37.5%	25.0%	50.0%	25.0%	25.0%	25.0%
41.4%	3.4%	34.5%	3.4%	3.4%	0	3.4%
—	—	—	—	—	—	—
—	—	—	—	—	—	—
0	0	0	0	0	0	0
0	0	100.0%	0	0	0	0

He is still severely disabled and is functioning at 20–30 percent of his ability.

1   Patient has shown no improvement since operation and/or is 100 percent disabled.

0   Patient is worse since operation.

Information presented in this way is not without value, but it clearly has serious limitations. Because many of the judgments are based on subjective impressions, often from limited samples of the patient's behavior, and from information obtained from people who may not want to offend the physician, there are any number of ways the results may reflect unconscious bias. Such judgments as "the patient is functioning at 80–100 percent (or 40–70 percent) of his ability" are clearly not as quantifiable as the statements imply. A summary of the results of psychosurgery as presented in broad categorical statements about change is presented in the second part of this chapter.

Rating of Scientific Merit

The scientific merit of each of the 153 data articles on psychosurgery was rated according to the scale proposed by May and Van Putten (1974). This rating scale is based on such factors as the use of control groups and standardized tests, the appropriate statistical treatment of data, the independence of the evaluators from those performing the treatment, the duration of the postoperative follow-ups, and other experimental considerations. A rating of 1 is assigned only to studies that have matched control groups, use objective tests, evaluate patients for an adequate period, employ independent testers, analyze data statistically, and do not confound any relevant variables (for example, drug treatment, type and duration of psychotherapy, support from family or friends, and so on). A rating of 6 is assigned to those reports that present only descriptive information on the patients and cite no comparison group. The results are summarized in Table 8.4 for the majority of the data articles. It can be seen from this table that most of the articles on psychosurgery earned a rating of only 5 or 6. Almost 90 percent of the articles from the United States received ratings between 4 and 6. It is unlikely that an animal study with a rating of only 4 would be accepted for publication by the editors of any respectable (refereed) journal. In the case of clinical reports, a rating of 4 is given to studies that have

Table 8.4 Scientific Merit of Articles Based on Experimental Design and Reliability of Data

Country and Number of Articles	May Rating Scale[a]					
	I	II	III	IV	V	VI
United States (45)	0	3.3%	7.8%	16.7%	31.1%	41.1%
United Kingdom (31)	0	3.2%	1.6%	12.9%	50.0%	32.3%
All other countries (104)	0	0	1.0%	9.1%	30.8%	59.1%

[a]I = Well-controlled studies using objective evaluation methods; VI = Descriptive case reports with no control group. See text for details of rating scale.

inadequate control groups to compare with the psychosurgical patients. This inadequate matching may account for many of the differences between patients receiving psychosurgery and so-called "control groups" that are reported in the literature. Not atypical is the following set of selection criteria for psychosurgery outlined in a recent article (Williamson, 1975):

1. The patient must not show any psychotic features.

2. The level of motivation to get well must be high.

3. The patient must desire the operation.

4. There must be strong family and medical support.

Clearly, if any of these variables were not distributed equally between the "surgery" and "control" groups, any comparisons could be misleading.

   In addition to the possibility of a biased selection of patients, articles receiving a rating of 4 usually have important variables confounded in ways that make it impossible to determine whether the postoperative changes should be attributed to the psychosurgery, to an intensification of psychotherapy, to pharmacological treatment, or to the additional effort made by the family and hospital staff. Again, not atypical, is the following comment made in a recent report of the results of psychosurgery.

> The importance of an intensive and long-lasting postoperative rehabilitation in conjunction with psychosurgical treatment cannot be overrated. The fact that this was given to virtually all our patients is presumably a contributing factor to the favorable long-term results [Bingley et al., 1977, p. 297].

When such intensification of rehabilitation is considered together with the fact that the benefits of psychosurgery often do not appear for many months after the operation, it can be seen how difficult it may be to determine the relative importance of the surgery itself.

Placebo Effects

The possibility that the reduction of troublesome symptoms frequently reported in the psychosurgical literature may be attributed to some form of patient suggestibility has, of course, been raised very often. Many patients become convinced that psychosurgery represents their only chance of getting better, and consequently they build up a great anticipation of being helped. Undoubtedly, these psychological factors can influence the results of any treatment. Such placebo effects are known to be very great under some circumstances. In the area of pain treatment, for example, it has been recognized that a very large proportion of the effectiveness of drugs and surgery can be attributed to the patients' attitude toward the therapy (Beecher, 1962). Some of these placebo effects emerge from patient–physician interactions. The combination of a patient who has great confidence in his physician and a physician who believes strongly in the efficacy of his treatment can be a powerful factor in the therapy's success.

Although it is normally impossible to answer the "placebo argument" adequately because of the ethical restraints against performing sham operations, there are several reports of attempts to investigate placebo effects. In 1953, one neurosurgeon at the Oregon Veterans' Administration Hospital reported the following:

> In four separated cases in this series we carried out a control procedure in which the skin incision is made and the bone button removed but no cerebral lesion produced. Each of these patients was included in a group of four operated on at one time, three of whom had a standard anterior cingulate isolation. The four patients were carried as a group through the entire postoperative routine without knowledge on the part of the patients or other hospital personnel that these control patients had not been subjected to the complete surgical procedure. None of these patients showed even slight improvement during this period of control study and all were subjected to cingulate isolation one to three months later [Livingston, 1953, p. 377].

In 1973, a group of Indian neurosurgeons reported the following results obtained in a study of sterotaxic cingulotomies on drugaddicted patients:

> The possibility of "placebo effects" being responsible for the efficacy of surgery was considered and eliminated by the following method. In

three cases, at first only burrholes (skull holes) were done, but the patients were told that "the operation" had been performed. They continued to ask for the drugs and had relief only after the cingulotomy was performed [Balasubramaniam, Kanaka, and Ramujam, 1973, p. 64].

Quite aside from the serious ethical questions that could be raised, the evidence from sham operations can be the most persuasive argument that the beneficial changes have been produced by surgery itself rather than by some placebo effects. In order for the evidence to be convincing, however, it is essential that the patients assigned to the surgery and sham groups be perfectly matched. In the few instances of reports of sham psychosurgical operations, there was inadequate evidence that appropriate controls had been employed to assure against bias in patient assignment. Indeed, in the Oregon study some of the patients in the sham group were assigned on the basis of their having refused to permit surgery to continue (the operations were performed under local anesthetic) after a burr hole had been made in the skull. It is certainly conceivable that such patients had less than the average confidence in the surgery or the surgeon.

It has been suggested on several occasions that the results of psychosurgery that missed the proper brain target provide a form of control for placebo effects. Thus, in an article describing the results of stereotaxic cingulotomy for neuropsychiatric illness and intractable pain, it was reasoned:

> One must also consider the possibility that most manic-depressive illnesses are self-limited; that there may be a "placebo effect" to the operation; that the operated patients are treated differently and more intensively than the others; that the anesthesia could of itself reverse the course of the illness. Ten of the 40 patients in this series benefitted from secondary operation after the first failed. This group tends to refute the "placebo argument" [Ballantine et al., 1967, p. 494].

Here, too, the evidence against placebo effects would have been much more convincing if the information had been more complete. Although it would be difficult to arrive at reliable figures, a careful reading of the psychosurgical literature reveals that there are a substantial number of patients who have undergone several different psychosurgical procedures. For example, one patient included in the study reported by Corkin received a cingulotomy, which was followed by a multiple-target procedure (involving bilateral destruction of part of the amygdala, cingulate, and substantia innominata) five years later, and a second cingulotomy within the same year. Many cases of multiple psychosurgical operations are noted in Corkin's report, as well as in Mirsky and Orzack's, in the following chapter. Some operations that appear to have been correctly placed are unsuccessful—and the converse has also been found. At present, the evidence that the success of the operation is highly correlated with the brain target destroyed is not convincing. However, a partial reporting of the results from successive operations can be misleading.

It should be stressed that the arguments presented here have bearing only on the overall scientific merit of the psychosurgical literature. It is possible that the surgery does produce the benefits and no more impairments than are generally described. The lack of objective evidence, however, leaves open the possibility that the improvement reported in the literature does not adequately summarize all the changes produced by the surgery. Moreover, the absence of adequate experimental controls makes it impossible to determine whether the brain destruction is the most important factor in producing the changes that do occur.

Postoperative Results

Objective Test Results

The postoperative changes following psychosurgery that have been revealed by objective tests are described in detail elsewhere (Valenstein, 1977) and need only be summarized here. The reader who desires more details should consult the original source, where postoperative changes are listed separately for each publication, major psychosurgical procedure, and test category. Also, the contributions by Mirsky and Orzack and by Corkin in this volume describe the postoperative results from a contemporary test battery administered by experienced psychologists. In general, the postoperative changes reported in the published literature are described as improvements, but some deficits have also been reported, sometimes as transient or short-term deficits. An example of short-term or transient deficits in abstract thinking and in a perceptual task (embedded figures) is described by Corkin in Chapter 9.

The most consistent improvements reported are those related to the symptoms typically presented by psychosurgical patients. Thus, depression, anxiety, neuroticism, obsessionalism, somatic complaints, tension, and phobias are reported as reduced after surgery in the majority of the cases. All of the postoperative changes in the results of objective test measures of emotions were viewed as improvements, with the exception of a single report of decreased "impulse control" and increased negativism and belligerence following amygdalectomy.

Deficits are manifested only rarely on objective tests. When they appear, they are usually evident in tests of abstract thinking, learning and memory, and language ability. Under the category abstract thinking, deficits have been reported on tests requiring the categorizing of information such as required in the Wisconsin Card Sorting (Drewe, 1974) and the Goldstein–Scheerer Colour-Forms tests (Bailey et al., 1971; Walsh, 1977). Deficits were also reported in similarities (following a thalamic operation, reported by Jurko and Andy, 1973), block-design, and picture arrangement tests. It should be stressed, however, that these deficits are not normally found. Also, it is not uncommon for the deficits that are detected by objective tests to be relatively short-lived.

Following thalamic operations, which are very infrequently done today, deficits were seen in language tests, in ability to deal with symbols ("word fluency" and "use of tokens" tests), and in performance on psychological tests thought to be sensitive to brain damage (three studies reported deficits either in reproducing figures or in matching faces). Although the evidence could not be considered convincing, there appeared to be a greater probability of finding deficits on objective tests after thalamic operations than after other types of psychosurgery. Also noteworthy were reports in two separate articles of learning and memory deficits following amygdalectomies. None of these deficits are consistently found. At least for the present, therefore, it is necessary to conclude that in spite of all the methodological advantages of objective testing, no one has developed a battery of tests that reveals consistent changes in intellectual capacities following any of the psychosurgical procedures. In our present state of knowledge, it is difficult to determine whether this conclusion reflects more on the inadequacies of the tests or the absence of deficits.

Results Reported by Neurosurgeons and Psychiatrists

As already noted, the results of psychosurgery are most commonly reported in broad categories that are said to reflect the changes in the patient's overall adjustment. Although various authors use three-, four-, or five-point scales, it was found possible to group all of the reported results on the following four-point scale:

I. Excellent results

II. Significant improvement

III. No significant change

IV. Worse

The postoperative results reported by neurosurgeons are summarized in Table 8.5 for the different sites of brain operations and different diagnostic labels. The different psychosurgical operations and the great variety of diagnostic labels have been collapsed into major groupings based on brain region involved and major symptoms.

The overall results of the summary ratings reported by neurosurgeons and psychiatrists appear to be very favorable, especially for the frontal lobe and cingulum operations. Combining ratings I and II (excellent results and significant improvement), it is possible to obtain an estimate of the percentage of patients judged to have improved significantly. It can be seen from Table 8.5 that following either frontal lobe or cingulum operations over 85 percent of the patients received a rating of I or II in most diagnostic categories. Lower success rates were reported for patients diagnosed as schizophrenic (or "psychotic") and for those addicted to drugs. There was a slight trend for frontal lobe operations to be reported as more successful than cingulotomies. This was most evident in the neurotic depression diagnostic category, where 96 percent of the patients received a rating of I or II following a frontal lobe operation, but only 72 percent were assigned these ratings after a cingulotomy. Considering that different persons assigned the ratings and the numbers of depressed patients receiving frontal lobe and cingulate operations were not equal, these results should not be overinterpreted. They may, however, suggest a trend to be explored further.

Although the results reported for other psychosurgical procedures are based on many fewer patients, some trends should be noted. Amygdalectomies for aggressive patients had a relatively low success rate, as only 28 percent of the patients were judged to have improved significantly. Of the epileptic patients with psychiatric disorders who underwent amygdalectomies, 50 percent were judged to have improved significantly. This latter figure is clearly below the success rate claimed for other procedures and diagnostic categories.

There will clearly be a difference of opinion about how much significance should be attached to these overall favorable ratings of the direction of change following psychosurgery. Those opposed to psychosurgery are likely to discount these results entirely on the basis of the subjectivity of the ratings and the fact that the neurosurgeons and psychiatrists responsible for the patients' treatment have assigned the ratings in most cases. Moreover, it has been argued that overall ratings give too much weight to the alleviation of outstanding symptoms, particularly those that are troublesome to others, and give much less weight to the quality of life that remains possible. Such criticisms cannot be dismissed out of hand, but they often are overstated. Considering the fact that this type of criticism has frequently been raised, it is not likely that many neurosurgeons would rate their results as excellent simply on the basis of the elimination of troublesome behavior without considering other aspects of the patients' overall adjustment. It would take overt deceit, not self-deception, to assign a rating of excellent to a patient who spends the days sitting passively and unresponsively at home even if no longer a burden to anyone. In some instances, the criteria for an "excellent result" seem to have been defined quite broadly, if not completely objectively, and include evidence from social workers on the quality of the adjustment to the family, work, and social situations and whether or not the patients appear to display any loss of initiative.

Table 8.6 presents similar data on the postoperative results of the more recent brain operations for pain. The majority of the operations were anterior cingulotomies. The vast majority (over 90 percent) of the frontal lobe procedures were performed by one neurosurgeon, who used an ultrasonic technique (see the contribution by Mirsky and Orzack, this volume). The outcome ratings are generally very favorable, with more than 80 percent of the patients rated as having improved significantly even when examined more than one year postoperatively.

Postoperative Complications

All published reports of physical and emotional complications of different psychosurgical procedures performed after 1965 have been collated and reported in detail elsewhere (Valenstein, 1977, Appendix 9). The intellectual deficits produced by the surgery are generally presented in terms of the results of objective tests and have been summarized above.

The *physical complications* of the surgery reported in the literature include complications probably unrelated to the specific opera-

Table 8.5 Neurosurgeons' Estimates of Outcome of Psychosurgical Procedures (United States)

Diagnostic Labels	Total Number of Patients	Site of Brain Operation	
		Frontal Lobe Procedure	Cingulum
Aggression[a]	55		
Neurotic depression	198	24(3) I = 45.8% II = 50.0% III = 4.2%	174(2) I = 14.7% 11 = 57.6% III = 24.1% IV = 3.6%
Psychotic depression	70	1(1) I = 100%	69(3) I = 88.9% II = 3.2% III = 5.2% III–IV = 2.7%
Fear and Anxiety	385	314(3) I = 16.6% II = 73.2% III = 10.2%	71(2) I = 91.3% II = 3.3% III = 2.5% III–IV = 2.9%
Obsessive-compulsive neurosis	159	67(2) I = 34.4% II = 55.2% III = 10.4%	89(3) I = 62.8% 11 = 24.3% III = 9.4% III–IV = 3.5%
Schizo-affective disorders	32	26(1) I = 38.5% II = 53.8% III = 7.7%	6(2) I = 66.7% III = 16.7% IV = 16.7%
Schizophrenia and other psychoses	233	126(3) I = 5.5% II = 51.6% I–II = 11.9% III = 19.0% IV = 11.9%	56(2) I = 33.9% II = 32.1% III = 33.9%
Drug addiction and alcoholism	19	1(1) II = 100%	18(2) I = 50.0% II = 16.7% III = 11.1% IV = 22.2%
Psychopathic behavior	17		
"Emotional illness"	8		
"Agitated states of the aged"	5	5(1) I = 20.0% II = 80.0%	
Involutional melancholia	10		10(2) I = 90.0% II = 10.0%
Epilepsy with psychiatric disorders	48		

Notes: Information obtained from articles published after 1970. In the vast majority of instances, results of surgery were summarized by neurosurgeons and/or associated psychiatrists and are based on subjective (or poorly defined) criteria.

First arabic numeral refers to number of patients; the figure in parentheses is the number of independent groups reporting results. Roman numerals indicate the judgment of the success of the operation: I = Excellent results, II = Significant improvement, III = No significant change, IV = Worse.

[a] Includes 14 cases of hyperactivity and 2 cases of body rocking (rhythmia).

Review of the Literature on Postoperative Evaluation

Table 8.5 *(continued)*

	Site of Brain Operation		
Amygdala	*Thalamus*	*Hypothalamus*	*Multiple Target Sites*
I = 7.1% 14(2)II = 21.4% III = 71.4%	I = 16.7% 18(1)II = 50.0% III = 5.5% III-IV = 27.8%	4(1) II = 100%	19(1)II = 84.2% III = 15.8%
			I = 66.7% 3(1) IV = 33.3%
I = 100% 1(1)			I = 26.0% 50(1)II = 60.0% III = 12.0% IV = 2.0%
	I = 41.2% 17(1)II = 41.2% III = 17.6%		I = 87.5% 8(1)II = 12.5%
I = 10.4% 48(3)II = 39.6% III = 43.8% IV = 6.2%			

Table 8.6 Neurosurgeons' Estimates of Outcome of Psychosurgical Procedures for Pain (United States)

Follow-up Duration[a]	Frontal Lobe Procedure	Cingulum	Thalamus
More than 1 year	14(2) I = 100%	38(5) I = 37.4% II = 54.6% III = 8.0%	8(2) I = 100%
Less than 1 year	101(3) I = 15.0% II = 74.9% III = 10.1%	152(7) I = 21.3% II = 45.9% III = 32.8%	80(3) I = 21.3% II = 63.7% III = 15.0%

Notes: Information obtained from articles published after 1970. In the vast majority of instances, results of surgery were summarized by neurosurgeons and/or associated psychiatrists and are based on subjective (or poorly defined) criteria.

First arabic numeral refers to number of patients; the figure in parentheses is the number of independent groups reporting results. Roman numerals indicate the judgment of the success of the operation: I = Excellent results, II = Significant improvement, III = No significant change, IV = Worse.

[a] In some instances follow-up duration had to be estimated.

tions, such as hemorrhages and infections. Of more interest are the physical complications such as seizures, weight changes, paralysis, dyskinesias, loss of smell, bladder or bowel incontinence, and endocrine changes (including irregularities in menstrual cycle), which may be the result of surgical destruction of a specific brain structure. *Emotional* and *behavioral complications* are described primarily by such terms as "lethargy" (loss of motivation), generalized or specific disinhibition (volubility, lowered personal standards, carelessness, immature behavior, shoplifting, extravagant behavior, irritability, aggression), increases or decreases in sexuality, and inability to work. The phrase *frontal lobe syndrome* was used during the early "lobotomy era" to refer to a constellation of postoperative symptoms that often included either lethargy or disinhibited behavior in addition to seizures, incontinence, and some loss in capacity for abstract thinking. While these same symptoms may still be seen, they are generally believed to occur less frequently, to be less severe, and often to be relatively transient.

Except for statements from those extremely opposed to psychosurgery, it is generally agreed that the incidence of complications following psychosurgery has been significantly reduced since 1965. The most common physical complication of psychosurgery had been the occurrence of epileptic seizures. Estimates of the incidence of postoperative seizures for surgery performed during the 1945–1965 period range from 10 percent to 50 percent. Summaries of postoperative seizures after 1965 generally indicate an incidence of approximately 2 percent for surgery performed with the aid of

Table 8.6 *(continued)*

Multiple Target Sites	Midbrain	Stimulation	Cortex
14(2) I = 48.0% II = 43.6% III = 7.5%	9(2) I = 100%	6(2) I = 66.7% II = 33.3%	2(1) I = 100%
11(2) I = 63.6% II = 36.4%	35(2) I = 97.1% II = 2.9%	32(3) I = 40.6% II = 28.1% III = 31.3%	

stereotaxic instruments (Goktepe, Young, and Bridges, 1975). Some reports of the larger patient populations give figures as low as 0 percent (Mitchell-Heggs, Kelly, and Richardson, 1977), 0.5 percent (Ström-Olson and Carlisle, 1972) and 1.0 percent (Knight, 1973). The incidence of seizures following nonstereotaxic surgery, however, may be as high as 10 percent (Scoville and Bettis, 1977). The comparison of the incidence of seizures between the "older" and "newer" psychosurgery is somewhat confounded by the tendency of several neurosurgeons to administer anticonvulsant drugs preventively following surgery; but in spite of this practice there seems to be convincing evidence that the occurrence of postoperative seizures has significantly declined. Moreover, bladder and bowel incontinence, which were commonly observed after the older prefrontal lobotomy procedure, are rarely reported in the current literature.

The most common emotional complication reported to occur after current psychosurgical procedures is either some evidence of impulsiveness (and other evidence of disinhibition) or lethargy. The incidence of these emotional complications is about 5–10 percent, but they are usually described as "slight" and "transient." In one recent report of thalamic surgery for intractable pain, the incidence of postoperative lethargy or disinhibited behavior, however, was approximately 50 percent (Rodriguez-Burgos, Arjona, and Rubio, 1977).

The incidence of mortality directly attributable to psychosurgery was approximately 5 percent during the early "lobotomy era." Current estimates of postoperative deaths following stereotaxic psychosurgery are close to zero (Kelly, 1976). For example, in summaries of large patient populations that have had stereotaxic frontal or cingulum psychosurgical procedures, the mortality rate is listed as 0 percent for 345 operations (Ballantine et al., 1977), 0 percent for 204 operations (Brown, 1972a) and 0.2 percent for 660 operations (Knight, 1963). Higher figures (3.7 to 4.5 percent) have been given, however, for stereotaxic operations of other brain regions and for nonstereotaxic procedures (Balasubramaniam and Kanaka, 1975; Peraita and Lopez de Lerma, 1977; Scoville and Bettis, 1977). A search through all of the data articles on psychosurgery performed since 1970 uncovered only 12 deaths attributable to the surgery, and even this figure included a few cases in which it was not completely clear that the surgery was the cause of death.

In summary, data in the published literature suggest that the incidence of all types of complications has significantly declined over the years, but the incidence may vary greatly as a function of brain site and surgical procedure. There appears to be a greater likelihood of motor complications (dyskinesias or partial paralysis) after thalamic operations and, as might be anticipated from a knowledge of brain anatomy, a greater probability of endocrine disorders after hypothalamic operations. Also, the incidence of physical and emotional complications following stereotaxic procedures is lower than following so-called "open," "free-hand" operations. Dr. J. Smith of Sydney, Australia, reviewed the papers published in English on modified frontal lobe lesions performed between 1960 to 1974 and concluded:

> Operative mortality has been reduced to 0.5 percent with nonstereotactic operations and 0.6 percent with stereotactic approaches [Smith, 1977, p. 33].

The technique used to ablate brain tissue (see Chapter 2) may also be a major variable in determining the incidence of adverse side effects. For example, the incidence of complications following anterior cingulotomy was very low after radio frequency destruction of tissue (Ballantine et al., 1977), but after attempted destruction of the same brain region using a "suction technique" the following complications were described:

> One half of our patients had bladder and bowel incontinence which recovered before discharge. Three patients had major, generalized seizures postoperatively without a previous history of convulsions. All were easily controlled on low doses of anticonvulsants. Unusual behavior was observed in several patients. This included flattened affect (57%), confusion (35%), uninhibited facetious speech (30%), dimin-

ished attention span (22%), hallucinations (13%), and automatisms (8.7%). Except for flattened affect all other mental abnormalities were gone by the time of discharge [Wilson and Chang, 1974, p. 65].

Lastly, it must be reemphasized that the results presented are representative of only the published literature. It is possible that the incidence of complications following operations by surgeons performing only one or two psychosurgical procedures a year—a group that usually does not publish the results of operations—may be quite different.

CHAPTER 9

A Prospective Study of Cingulotomy

Suzanne Corkin

For the past five years my colleagues and I have been studying a particular form of psychiatric surgery known as cingulotomy. This investigation is part of a more general program of research in which we are attempting to understand human behavior in terms of the relationship between brain structure and brain function. We have pursued this goal by carrying out detailed evaluations of children and adults with various forms of focal brain pathology due to head injuries, vascular disease, and tumors. These evaluations involve the administration of quantitative behavioral tasks that assess overall intelligence, learning and memory, problem solving, and perception, as well as the capacities of the different sensory modalities and of

The research described here was done in collaboration with Thomas E. Twitchell, M.D., Edith V. Sullivan, Ph.D., and Hans-Lukas Teuber, Ph.D. (deceased). Terry Allard, Robert Cosway, and Susan Stackland assisted us in the study, and Loretta Clement was the statistician. Karen Sauer typed the manuscript, and Mark Hagerty did the graphics. This work was supported by N.I.H. Contract No. N01-NS-62116A, N.I.M.H. Grant No. MH24433, and Grant No. RR-00088 from the General Clinical Research Centers Program of the Division of Research Resources, N.I.H.

the motor system. In addition, qualitative determinations are made regarding the patients' motivation, social adjustment, and emotional status. Our interest in cingulotomy arose from the fact that we would not have encountered a group of patients with such lesions except for this particular neurosurgical intervention. This operation is performed for the relief of chronic, debilitating pain or for the alleviation of severe psychiatric disorders.

Cingulotomy refers to the removal or destruction of brain tissue in an area of the cerebral cortex called the *cingulate gyrus,* and to the interruption of the underlying bundle of nerve fibers called the *cingulum.* This neurosurgical procedure was first introduced in the late 1940s as a possible replacement for the more destructive frontal lobotomy (or leucotomy, in Europe) (Moniz, 1936). It was hoped that cingulotomy would have a beneficial effect on patients with psychiatric disorders without the unwanted side effects of lobotomy, including lack of foresight, undesirable social behavior, blunting of emotions, seizures, and other neurological abnormalities. Apparently, the first operations in the human cingulate region were performed upon a suggestion made by Professor John Fulton, a neurophysiologist from Yale University. In a discussion at a meeting of the Society of British Neurological Surgeons in 1947, he is said to have observed that "were it feasible, cingulectomy in man would seem an appropriate place for limited leucotomy" (Ballantine et al., 1967, p. 489). The reason for expecting therapeutic changes from cingulate lesions is derived from the hypothesis of Dr. James Papez (1937), who saw the cingulum as a major component in an anatomic circuit believed to subserve emotional experience and expression. The notion of such a circuit or ring of structures surrounding the medial wall of the cerebral hemispheres was extended by Dr. Paul MacLean (1958) into that of a *limbic system,* and further modified by Professor Walle Nauta (1958), who stressed the downward continuation of this system into the midbrain and called it the *limbic midbrain region.*

The first clinical reports on the consequences of anterior cingulate lesions in humans came from Dr. J. Le Beau in Paris (Le Beau and Pecker, 1950), Sir Hugh Cairns in Oxford (Whitty et al., 1952), and Dr. Kenneth Livingston in Oregon (Livingston, 1953). Le Beau claimed particular success with agitated and aggressive patients, whereas the Cairns group found their procedure to be most helpful to those suffering from severe obsessional or anxiety states. Livingston did not consider his results in terms of diagnosis or symptoms, but preoperatively all patients had been confined to a neuropsychiatric hospital for the chronically ill, the average period of hospitalization up to the time of operation having been over four years. Of the 72 patients selected for cingulate cortex isolation, 24 were followed for more than two years after operation; 12 of these patients were found improved sufficiently to be discharged from the hospital, and the other 12 were said to have shown definite but less striking improvement. There was one death due to the operation in Cairns' series and one "hospital death" in Livingston's; none of the three neurosurgical teams reported undesirable changes in their patients' personalities or other serious complications due to the operation.

In 1962, Doctors Eldon L. Foltz and Lowell E. White introduced stereotaxic cingulotomy for the relief of intractable pain coupled with anxiety and depression. In this procedure, electrodes were lowered into the cingulate region under X-ray control and electrolytic lesions were made bilaterally. Of the 16 patients who underwent this operation, 12 had good or excellent results, although in some cases the follow-up interval was less than six months. Dr. H. Thomas Ballantine, Jr., of Boston has since modified Foltz and White's technique and has applied it to the treatment of chronic pain and a variety of severe psychiatric disorders. To date this neurosurgeon has carried out 419 such operations in 294 patients. There have been no deaths due to the cingulotomy or to complications arising from it. One woman, however, experienced a brief episode of cardiac arrest when the general anesthesia was administered, and as a result the operation was terminated before the cingulate lesions had been made; she died soon after of a ruptured spleen. The 69 most recent cases in the Ballantine series, operated upon between 1974 and 1978, are the subject of this chapter. They were examined at M.I.T. during that time period, as were 16 additional patients whose cingulotomies were performed before the M.I.T. study began.

The M.I.T. Study: Purpose and Approach

It is important in evaluating a treatment of any disease that those who carry out the investigation have nothing to gain or lose by the success or failure of that therapy. This is particularly true in the area of psychosurgery, which is so controversial and emotionally charged. The study of cingulotomy to be described here is being done at the M.I.T. Clinical Research Center by members of the M.I.T. Psychology Department, and thus this research is geographically, administratively, and financially independent of the referring neurosurgeon and his hospital. Support for this work, which is still in progress and will continue at least through 1980, has come from the

United States Public Health Service and private foundations (see the footnote at the beginning of this chapter).

The goal of this investigation is to evaluate the therapeutic outcome, neurological status, and behavioral test performance in patients who have undergone bilateral stereotaxic anterior cingulotomy (Ballantine et al., 1967) for the relief of persistent pain, which was usually coupled with depression, or for the alleviation of severe psychiatric disease. All patients had been deemed treatment failures prior to surgery. At first, such patients were studied only after operation, in order to dissociate the research endeavor from the process of deciding whether or when the operation should be performed. It soon became evident that many of the patients who were tested had neurological or behavioral deficits; it was not clear, however, whether these predated the cingulotomy or were a result of the brain operation. The only way to deal with this problem was to examine patients both before and after operation and to measure the effects of the surgical procedure by using each patient as his own control. Accordingly, the protocol was modified to include preoperative as well as postoperative testing. The work still proceeds independently of the referring neurosurgeon and his hospital; the patients and their relatives are informed that the role of the research team is that of a neutral party gathering facts about cingulotomy and about the conditions of those upon whom the operation is performed.

The results for Phase I of the study, carried out between 1973 and June 1976, were summarized in a report to the National Commission for the Protection of Human Subjects of Biomedical and Behavioral Research (Teuber, Corkin, and Twitchell, 1977a, 1977b). It was found that some patients were markedly improved following the surgical procedure, whereas others were not helped at all. Regardless of therapeutic outcome, however, there were no lasting neurological or behavioral deficits attributable to the brain operation *per se.*

Phase II of the study, covering the period from June 1976 through November 1977, included a qualitative reassessment of therapeutic outcome in the 34 patients who participated in Phase I. At the same time, 23 new cases were added to the sample for pre- and postoperative interview and examination to assess therapeutic effect, neurological status, and behavioral capacities, including cognitive, motor, and sensorimotor functions (Corkin, Twitchell, and Sullivan, 1979). Phase III, which took place from December 1977 through November 1978, involved the addition of 28 new patients who underwent cingulotomy as well as one-year follow-up studies on others. This segment of the research was just completed, and the qualitative and statistical analyses of the data are still in progress. Consequently, this report will rely in part on the results obtained through November 1977. To date, a total of 55 patients (22 men and 33 women) have been examined both before and after operation; 18 patients (7 men and 11 women) have been evaluated after operation only, because in all but 2 of these cases the cingulotomy was performed before the inception of this study. An additional 12 patients (5 men and 7 women) have been tested preoperatively and now await postoperative evaluation, which is planned for 1979.

Characteristics of the Patient Sample

The group of cases described in this report is probably representative of those who undergo psychosurgery in the United States, but it is not representative of the psychiatric population as a whole. Patients who are referred for cingulotomy are the ones in whom other forms of treatment have failed, leaving the patients with no other hope of relief from their physical or mental suffering. Prior to cingulotomy, most have been hospitalized on one or more occasions, and they have typically been tried on numerous medications, psychotherapy, and electroconvulsive therapy (ECT); occasionally the preoperative therapeutic interventions have included insulin coma therapy (which consists of injecting insulin to produce a deep hypoglycemic coma), Indoklon inhalation therapy (a form of convulsive therapy), drug-induced sleep therapy, and acupuncture. Moreover, some of the patients with chronic pain, in an attempt to obtain relief from their symptoms, have undergone back operations, such as removals of ruptured discs, fusions of vertebrae, exploratory operations, implantations of stimulators, and procedures to cut nerve roots or pain pathways in the spinal cord. In many candidates for cingulotomy the severity of the illness before the operation prevented them from working or from helping with household chores. The preoperative occupations of those who could work included: clerical worker, custodian, dental assistant, factory worker, hairdresser, homemaker, lifeguard, mail handler, nun, organist, patient escort in a hospital, physician, professional gambler, registered nurse, secretary, social worker, and student. Prior to cingulotomy, most of the patients were living at home with spouses or parents, and after operation they returned to the same setting. At the present time about half of the patients come from Massachusetts and half come from out of state. Only 2 patients could be classified as minority group members.

Table 9.1 Preoperative Diagnosis of 85 Cingulotomy Patients

Group	Number of Cases	
	M	F
Pain (N = 26)		
Back or leg	7	10
Abdominal	1	2
Arm	1	0
Head	0	3
Amputation stump	1	0
Thalamic syndrome	0	1
Psychiatric disease (N = 59)[a]		
Depression or probable depression	12	17
Schizophrenia	5	9
Obsessive-compulsive neurosis	2	6
Anxiety neurosis or probable anxiety neurosis	4	1
Hysteria	0	1
Other conditions	0	2

[a] For diagnostic criteria see Woodruff, Goodwin, and Guze, 1974.

These included 1 working-class black and 1 Mexican-American from a middle-class family.

The 85 cingulotomy patients examined to date may be divided on the basis of their primary complaints at the time of operation into two main groups: 25 patients with severe and persistent pain due to disorders other than cancer, and 60 patients with psychiatric diagnoses (see Table 9.1). In the chronic pain group there are 16 cases of back or leg pain, 3 of abdominal pain, 1 of arm pain, 3 of headache, 1 of pain in an amputation stump, and 1 thalamic syndrome due to a stroke. The patients in the psychiatric group were assigned diagnoses on the basis of the criteria listed in the diagnostic manual of Woodruff, Goodwin, and Guze (1974). In each diagnostic category a specified number of criteria must be met for that diagnosis to be made with certainty. If the number of criteria that are met falls within a range slightly below the cutoff, the diagnosis is said to be "probable." Thus, the psychiatric group consists of 29 cases of depression or probable depression, 15 of schizophrenia, 8 of obsessive-compulsive neurosis, 5 of anxiety neurosis or probable anxiety neurosis, 1 of hysteria, and 2 for whom a diagnosis could not be made. Patients who were operated upon for pain differed from those with psychiatric diagnoses in that the pain and concomitant depression had begun later in life and were of shorter duration than the other disorders (see Table 9.2). The pain cases were also older at the time of operation and testing, but there was no difference between

Table 9.2 Age and IQ Data for 85 Cingulotomy Patients: Means and Ranges

Diagnosis	Age of Onset of Illness or Complaint (Years)	Preoperative Duration of Illness or Complaint (Years)	Age at First Cingulotomy (Years)	Age at Time of Present Study (Years)	Wechsler IQ at Time of Operation
Pain [N = 10M, 16F]	34.4 (18–59)	10.8 (2–38)	45.2 (28–76)	46.2 (28–76)	103.5 (76–121)
Psychiatric disease [N = 23M, 36F]	23.8 (3–57)	14.9 (2–40)	38.7 (20–67)	39.2 (20–67)	98.7 (74–127)

the two main diagnostic groups in overall intellectual capacity, as measured by standard tests of intelligence.

Surgical Procedure

All of the patients in the present investigation were operated upon by one surgeon, who began performing cingulotomies in 1962. He applies the following criteria in selecting candidates for cingulotomy:

1. The patient must be referred by a psychiatrist, and psychiatric aftercare must be available to the patient.
2. The patient must be disabled by mental or physical anguish but have a premorbid history of effective functioning. The intent of the surgeon is to restore each patient to a previously healthy state or at least to improve substantially the quality of his day-to-day existence.
3. All other appropriate treatments must have been tried and found not to give a lasting therapeutic effect.
4. The patient must give informed consent.
5. The patient's family must approve the decision to operate and provide a supportive environment for the patient to return to after the operation.
6. The patient must be manageable in a general hospital on a medical-surgical floor. This practical consideration precludes the possibility of performing cingulotomies on violent patients; the neurosurgeon does not perform cingulotomies for social or political control.

In addition to being carefully evaluated by the neurosurgeon, all candidates for cingulotomy must be seen by a psychiatrist and a neurologist who are not involved with the patients' care either before or after the operation. The purpose of these independent assessments is to ensure that the patients who ultimately choose to undergo cingulotomy are in fact appropriate cases for this operation. Accordingly, the psychiatrist reviews the patients' histories and earlier treatment regimens, judging whether other suitable therapies have been given adequate trials. Both the psychiatrist and the neurologist determine whether the patients and their relatives are informed as to the possible risks and benefits of cingulotomy and whether they wish to go through with the surgery. The neurologist also searches for possible neurological causes of the patients' psychiatric illness, such as head injuries, brain tumors, vascular abnormalities, and dementia. If such disorders are suspected or if there is a history of disease affecting the brain, the patients are referred for an electroencephalogram or for a kind of brain X-ray called a computed tomogram (CT scan), in order to determine if it is advisable to recommend cingulotomy. Some brain abnormalities can also be detected in the X-rays obtained in the course of the cingulotomy procedure, described below.

When patients are finally admitted to the hospital for a cingulotomy to be performed, the preoperative work-up includes a complete physical examination including a neurological examination, routine laboratory tests, and a chest X-ray. If the patient is over forty years of age or has a chronic medical complaint, an electrocardiogram is obtained. Medications that are known to interfere with general anesthesia or to affect blood pressure are discontinued prior to the operation.

The surgically imposed brain damage—referred to as brain lesions —involves small areas of tissue in the limbic system, one on the left side of the brain and one on the right side. These lesions are made according to the following procedure: With the patient under general anesthesia, a 2½ in. transverse incision is made in the scalp just behind the hairline, and two openings, each the size of a dime, are made in the skull 1.3 cm to either side of the midline. The dura mater (the tough two-layer covering that supports and protects the brain) is opened, and bleeding is controlled by coagulating the blood vessels in that area. A closed-end ventricular needle is then introduced into the brain to a depth of 2.5–3 cm, the needle is withdrawn, and the scalp wound is sutured in layers. This first insertion of the ventricular needle is to ensure that no subcortical bleeding will be encountered during the remainder of the operation. Next, with the patient still under general anesthesia, a *ventriculogram* is performed. This procedure consists of once again inserting the ventricular needles and injecting air through them into the lateral ventricles (two C-shaped cavities filled with cerebrospinal fluid, one in each cerebral hemisphere) and then taking an X-ray to reveal the outline of the ventricles. Guided by these brain landmarks, the ventricular needles, which are electrically inert except for the distal centimeter, are introduced into the cingulate region. Two adjacent lesions are placed on either side of the midline by applying in each instance a monopolar radio-frequency current of 8 watts for 75 seconds. The duration of the entire surgical procedure is typically two and a half hours.

Following cingulotomy, patients are given bed rest for twenty-four to forty-eight hours, and their preoperative medications are resumed, sometimes at lower doses. Transient side effects of the operation may include headache, fever, nausea, vomiting, incontinence, and unsteadiness of gait. All of these symptoms disappear within forty-eight hours after the operation, except the headache, which is in part caused by the ventriculogram and can last up to a week. Patients are usually discharged from the hospital on the fourth or fifth postoperative day, depending on the severity of the headache and their psychiatric status. The surgeon usually informs the referring psychiatrist of the patient's condition by phone and then sends the hospital discharge summary when it is available.

Once the cingulotomy has been performed, it is important to confirm that the lesions are on target. For this purpose, *computed tomograms (CT scans)* are obtained. This X-ray technique—a noninvasive means of investigating human intracranial anatomy and pathology—produces a series of computed pictures depicting cross sections of the brain (Hanaway, Scott, and Strother, 1977). In the patients who have undergone cingulotomy, CT scans reveal the general location and extent of the lesions (see Fig. 9.1). These lesions appear to involve the cingulate gyrus (cortex and white matter) and probably the genu of the corpus callosum (or anterior body of the corpus callosum). A few lesions have extended into the frontal lobe. It was possible to perform more detailed CT scans in 3 patients, and from these the lesion in each hemisphere was estimated to be 2 cm along the greatest axis and .5 to 1.5 cm perpendicular to the greatest axis.

Experimental Method and Results

For an independent evaluation of the safety and efficacy of cingulotomy, most patients were examined at the M.I.T. Clinical Research Center. Prior to July 1976, some patients were evaluated in the hospital where the cingulotomy was performed, and a few were studied in other institutions or their homes. Patients were typically seen during the week before the operation, from several days to several weeks after the operation, and in follow-up studies at intervals of one to two years. The preoperative and early postoperative

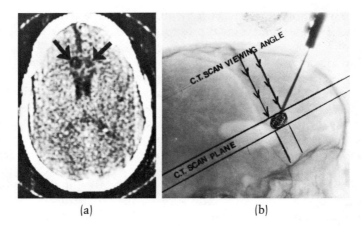

(a)   (b)

Figure 9.1 (a) A CT scan showing the size and shape of a pair of radio-frequency lesions in the anterior cingulate region (indicated by arrows). The angle used in obtaining the CT scan causes the lesions to appear to be anterior to the lateral ventricles. However, on the ventriculogram done during the operation (b), it can be seen that the actual placement was 1 cm posterior to the anterior tips of the ventricles. [Modified from Ballantine et al., 1977, p. 338.]

evaluations were each restricted to one full day, because of the patients' conditions and other demands on their time related to the operation. It was possible, however, to make the follow-up assessments more extensive, and these usually involved a three- or four-day admission to the M.I.T. Clinical Research Center. The specific methods used in these studies and the results obtained with them will be described below according to the three areas of investigation: therapeutic outcome, neurological status, and behavioral test performance.

Evaluation of Therapeutic Outcome

On the basis of information obtained in a review of the patients' records, case histories provided by patients and their relatives, written communications from patients, and telephone conversations with them, it was possible to document each individual's preoperative condition as well as his status at various times after operation. The analysis of therapeutic effect also relied upon separate interviews with the patient and a relative or close friend. In each case, the interviewer began by asking the patient and his relative for permission to tape-record the conversations, a practice begun in 1975. Once consent had been given, it was stated that the M.I.T. Clinical Research Center and its staff were independent of the referring neurosurgeon. It was further explained that the role of the research team was to compare objectively the patient's condition and test scores before and after cingulotomy in order to learn more about the effects of the surgery. No recommendation was made concerning the brain operation or any other form of therapy. Each preoperative interview was directed toward obtaining an account of the patient's history from before the onset of illness to the present. In particular, the interviewer tried to elicit an account of the patient's symptoms, their severity, and the extent to which they intruded upon his day-to-day existence. Thus, the conversations focused on such topics as employment history and participation in household tasks, the quality of relationships with close relatives and friends, hobbies, travel, sleep, sexual behavior, and consumption of food, alcoholic beverages, and drugs. Information was also sought concerning previous treatments and their effectiveness.

The goal of the postoperative evaluation was to determine the nature, extent, and time course of any change in the pain or psychiatric disorder for which the cingulotomy had been performed and to uncover any other alterations in behavior that had occurred since the brain operation. Changes in medication were also noted. The patient and a relative or close friend were questioned directly on these points, and asked to describe symptoms and relate events that illustrated their judgments. It was emphasized by the interviewer that it was particularly important to relate any negative effects of the cingulotomy. In general, the patient's present status was assessed in the same way that it had been before operation, in order to permit comparisons between the two time periods.

In order to supplement the postoperative interviews and to obtain some idea of the patient's condition in between visits to the M.I.T. Clinical Research Center, a plan was initiated in 1977 to request such information by mail. Accordingly, at the time of the early postoperative evaluation, patients and their relatives or close friends were given forms to be filled out and mailed back to M.I.T. at one month, six months, and one year after operation. The same forms have been sent in annual mailings to patients operated on before 1977, and to their relatives, as another way of maintaining contact with them. This sampling by mail of the patients' self-evaluations has elicited a large number of responses and has promoted many patients to write additional letters and cards telling of changes in their condition, their medication, their environment, and so on.

Table 9.3 Therapeutic Outcome at Two Time Periods in 34 Cingulotomy Patients Operated upon Between 1964 and 1976 (Phase I Patients)

Diagnosis	1975–May 1976		September–November 1977	
	Incidence of Improvement	Rating of Improvement	Incidence of Improvement	Rating of Improvement
Persistent pain (N = 11)	9 (82%)	8 marked 1 moderate	10 (91%)	7 marked 2 moderate 1 slight
Depression (N = 7)	5 (71%)	3 marked 2 moderate	4 (57%)	3 marked 1 moderate
Obsessive-compulsive neurosis (N = 4)	1 (25%)	1 slight	2 (50%)	2 slight
Other conditions (N = 12)	6 (55%)[a]	2 marked 3 moderate 1 transient	6(67%)[b]	3 marked 2 moderate 1 slight

[a] 1 undetermined.
[b] 3 undetermined.

With the help of all of the data outlined above, each patient was rated postoperatively as showing marked, moderate, slight, or no improvement; no patient was deemed worse after cingulotomy. These ratings were tabulated in 1976 for the first 34 cingulotomy patients who had been seen in this study; these same patients were reevaluated in 1977. It was therefore possible to compare the incidence of improvement and ratings of improvement for the two time periods, and thereby to assess the reliability of the qualitative evaluation. In this comparison, each patient was assigned to one of four diagnostic groups: (1) pain, (2) depression, (3) obsessive-compulsive neurosis, and (4) other psychiatric conditions (see Table 9.3). The patient's preoperative condition was used as the baseline of comparison for both postoperative periods. The incidence of improvement for the group as a whole was 64 percent in 1975–1976 and 71 percent in 1977; this improvement was marked in 39 and 42 percent of the cases, respectively. In both time periods, the pain cases stood out as showing the greatest therapeutic success. Those with obsessive-compulsive neurosis showed the least improvement, and patients with depression or other psychiatric conditions were intermediate. During the time interval between the two evaluations, 5 of the 34 patients underwent a second cingulotomy, which was followed by improvement in 2 cases but not in the other 3.

Once it was determined that estimates of the success of cingulotomy as a therapeutic tool held up over time, the next task was to

Table 9.4   Relationship Between Diagnosis and Rating of Improvement in 57 Cingulotomy Patients

Diagnosis	N	Number of Cingulotomies		
		1	2	3
Pain	16	9 marked 3 moderate 3 slight	1 none	
Depression or probable depression	19	5 marked 3 moderate 2 slight 1 none	2 marked 1 moderate 1 slight 2 none 1 undetermined	1 none
Schizophrenia	10	1 slight 4 none	1 marked 2 none	1 marked 1 none
Obsessive-compulsive neurosis	7	2 none	1 moderate 2 slight 1 none	1 none
Anxiety neurosis or probable anxiety neurosis	3	2 moderate 1 undetermined		
Other conditions	2	1 marked 1 undetermined		

Source: Corkin, Twitchell, and Sullivan, 1979.

specify more precisely which diagnostic groups benefited most from the surgical procedure. This further analysis could only be done satisfactorily with a larger number of cases; the 34 Phase I patients were combined with the 23 Phase II patients for this purpose.

It seemed desirable to subdivide patients not only on the basis of diagnosis but also according to the number of cingulotomies they had undergone (see Table 9.4). The incidence of moderate or marked improvement was impressive in patients whose primary complaint was persistent pain (75 percent) and in those with depression or probable depression (61 percent). In contrast, the majority of schizophrenics and obsessive-compulsives who had cingulotomies did not benefit from the procedure. Of the 3 men whose diagnosis was anxiety neurosis or probable anxiety neurosis, 2 gave evidence of moderate improvement; the third could not be contacted. The two cases that fell into the remaining category, other conditions, included one woman with temporal-lobe epilepsy, who experienced marked improvement in her psychiatric disorder after cingulotomy, and another whose diagnosis and present status could not be resolved.

If the first cingulotomy fails to benefit the patient or provides only transient relief of his symptoms, he may choose to have a second and even a third procedure. Of the 57 patients, 15 (26 percent) underwent a second cingulotomy and 4 of them (7 percent) a third. The overall success rate declined with each successive brain operation; it was 81 percent after the first, 57 percent after the second, and 25 percent after the third (see Table 9.4).

This objective evaluation of therapeutic success becomes more meaningful when it is illustrated by case histories. Those that follow give brief descriptions of one female and one male patient in each of four diagnostic groups: pain, depression, schizophrenia, and obsessive-compulsive neurosis. In this study, therapeutic outcome was no better for women than for men, although it was found to be in Mirsky and Orzack's investigation (see Chapter 10).

Case 40: 28-year-old married woman tested in hospital on 15 February 1977; admitted to the Clinical Research Center on 2 March 1977.
Diagnosis: Nerve root pain (radiculopathy L4, 5, S1, 2, 3, bilateral, with persistent pain).

This patient was born with a back defect that involved the nerves to the legs (lumbar myelomeningocele). This condition was repaired, and she was able to lead an active and normal life until 1969, when at the age of 21 a minor injury to her back caused a transient weakness of the legs that remitted following conservative treatment with traction and steroids. In 1972, because of recurrent pain in her back and left leg, urinary frequency, and weakness of the legs, she had a myelogram, which revealed a congenital abnormality of her spinal cord (an intraspinal mass with a diastematomyelia and dysraphism of the bone at L5 and S1). An operation on the vertebrae (laminectomy) was performed, and a fatty tumor (lipoma) was resected. The patient improved, was married, gave birth to a child, and graduated from nursing school in 1974. In 1975, she had a recurrence of the back and left leg pain, urinary retention, and a left footdrop. Another operation (laminectomy from L2 through S2) was performed, which revealed two lipomas. These could not be removed, but the nerve roots to which they were attached were dissected free. The patient continued to have pain and became depressed. She was treated with physical therapy, transcutaneous electrical stimulation, and psychotropic medications, without relief. She was admitted to the hospital for cingulotomy by ambulance, totally bedridden.

Neurological examination revealed weakness of both legs, left more than right, a left footdrop, diminution of knee jerks, absence of ankle jerks, and hypalgesia in the right thigh and leg. Vibratory sensation was absent in both feet, and position sense absent in the toes. In addition, she had a mild drug-induced parkinsonism.

Patient had a bilateral cingulotomy on 17 February 1977.

Immediately following surgery the patient was able to walk and was relatively free of pain. On 17 August 1977, six months following surgery, she reported that she was feeling "terrific." She had become involved in several church and civic projects, and she was able to take walks with her son. Although the pain had not completely disappeared, it was less intense and would respond to rest, heat, and Anacin.

Case 18:   47-year-old married man admitted to the Clinical Research Center on 26 February 1974 and readmitted at age 49 on 9 April 1976.
Diagnosis: Persistent pain syndrome.
These were five-year and seven-year follow-up examinations after cingulotomy for persistent pain in a traumatic amputation stump on the left forearm. This case represents possibly the clearest instance of pain as the main indication for cingulotomy: a painful amputation stump without a history of previous escape into illness, depression, or conversion reactions. The patient sustained an accidental loss of his left hand and wrist in 1966. Both he and the hospital records reported that he developed persistent and disabling pain in the stump, which was unrelieved by multiple nerve blocks and many types of drugs. He claimed immediate and complete relief from the stump pain following cingulotomy in June 1969. The patient now works as a hospital maintenance man. He uses a metal hook on his left arm affixed to the previously painful stump.

Neurological examination revealed, aside from evidence of a traumatic amputation of the left hand and wrist, a bilateral hearing loss.

Written communications from both the patient and his wife in 1977 indicated that he was still feeling "great" and working full-time.

Case 33:   27-year-old woman tested in hospital on 1 July 1975; admitted to the Clinical Research Center on 25 January 1976.
Diagnosis: Depression.
Present illness began around the age of 8 or 9, when the patient started to have feelings of low self-esteem. In college she was treated for depression and had to leave at the end of her sophomore year; she has never returned. Treatment had involved multiple hospitalizations, drug therapy, and ECT. She had made one possible suicide attempt.

The patient had a cingulotomy on 7 July 1976 and felt remarkable improvement.

Neurological examination was normal.

The patient subsequently married and had two children. She was busy at home as a wife and mother. Following the birth of her second child, her own mother stated that she had a little "postpartum blues," which did not last long. She has shown no serious symptoms of depression since the cingulotomy.

Case 36:   61-year-old married man admitted to the Clinical Research Center on 18 May 1977.
Diagnosis: Depression.
Patient stated that he had been depressed for twenty-one years, with symptoms of a loss of interest in life, insomnia, anorexia, agitation, and suicidal preoccupations. His wife oftentimes found him moaning and groaning about the house, sometimes shouting obscenities or crying. He had made four suicide attempts. He was admitted to a hospital seventeen times. He had received antidepressant medication and about fifty ECT treatments over this period of time. His longest remission was of five years' duration, according to his wife.

Neurological examination revealed a slight drug-induced parkinsonism and a limp related to a left total hip replacement.

Patient underwent a bilateral cingulotomy on 27 June 1977.

On 27 September 1977, three months following the operation, the patient himself stated that he did not know if the operation had helped him at all. He still stated that he had no enthusiasm, no zest for life, and no happiness. Nevertheless, suicidal thought was much less a problem. He did volunteer work mornings, and in good weather he was able to play tennis with his wife, which he stated was about the only thing he enjoyed. His family seemed to think there had been some change for the better.

The patient returned to the Clinical Research Center for a one-year follow-up on 24 July 1978. He stated that initially he experienced no improvement following cingulotomy. In January 1978, because of continued feelings of depression, he was put on Triavil and felt well. He had noticed that he had no suicidal thoughts, even when depressed. It was the belief of the examiners and the patient that he was improved in terms of the depth of his depression.

Neurological examination at this time was again normal.

Case 48:   62-year-old married woman admitted to the Clinical Research Center on 25 May 1977 and on 18 October 1977.
Diagnosis: Schizophrenia.

Patient stated that she had been ill all of her life, that she was either born with her problem or that it began during the flu epidemic. The world seemed to her to be burning up, even when she was a little girl. She complained of having the shakes all the time, of being unable to concentrate, and of feelings like pins sticking in the left side of her head. Patient had been hospitalized ten or eleven times and had had some ECT as well as psychotropic medication, all without benefit. She appeared anxious, agitated, and somewhat depressed. Her son stated that when she was depressed, she spoke about not wanting to live any more.

Neurological examination revealed a drug-induced lingual-labial dyskinesia, as well as parkinsonism.

Patient had a bilateral cingulotomy on 13 June 1977.

On 18 October 1977, four months post surgery, she felt a little better, less nervous, and was less preoccupied with suicide. Her husband also felt that she was somewhat better and that there was less of the tension and turmoil that she had evidenced earlier.

A follow-up letter from the patient on 13 June 1978 reported that she had experienced no further change in her symptoms. She stated that her whole life had been a "nightmare with nerves." Most of the letter represented an irrelevant repetition of her past history, although there was no mention of the world's being on fire.

Case 53:   39-year-old single man admitted to the Clinical Research Center on 13 July 1976 and on 24 October 1977.
Diagnosis: Schizophrenia.

The patient stated that his problems began sixteen years previously when he became obsessed about darkness and the state of his eyes and head. His spontaneous speech was often incoherent and contaminated continuously by recurrent delusions regarding darkness and his eyes. He also manifested symptoms of anxiety and depression, sleeping all day and often staying up at night watching television. He was hospitalized at least twelve times. He had ECT (approximately 100 treatments) and psychotropic medications, all without benefit.

Neurological examination was normal. The patient appeared very agitated and often hyperventilated.

Bilateral cingulotomy was performed on 13 July 1976.

In the follow-up study on 24 October 1977, the patient reported no improvement. His mother stated that he seemed to have improved initially, but now had difficulty sleeping and remained upset about his condition. The patient stated that he was unable to relax and that he continued to have his obsessions. He felt that he needed another operation because his trouble came back.

The patient underwent a second cingulotomy on 12 December 1977, and follow-up has not yet been obtained.

Case 32: 64-year-old woman admitted to the Clinical Research Center on 8 July 1975 and 5 January 1976.
Diagnosis: Obsessive-compulsive neurosis.

Present illness began years previously when the patient started having obsessions about needles, fearing that any needle that she saw might be poisonous and might hurt someone. More recently she had been obsessed about cesspools, worrying that someone might fall into one at her home, even though it had always been covered. She had developed the habit of telephoning around town and across the country, inquiring of people whether anyone had fallen into a cesspool.

The patient had a cingulotomy on 23 July 1975, without effect.

Neurological examination revealed a drug-induced parkinsonism.

The patient had a second cingulotomy on 16 December 1976. A follow-up letter on 26 December 1978 revealed that the obsessions continued. She was having monthly ECT and continued on a number of medications. Her husband stated that the obsessions were less intense and less bothersome to her. The possibility of automobiles being a source of pain to others had now replaced the concern about cesspools.

Case 38: 29-year-old unmarried man admitted to the Clinical Research Center on 8 and 16 September 1976 and on 23 May 1977.
Diagnosis: Obsessive-compulsive neurosis.

Patient had been incapacitated by his symptoms of the past nine years, which he described in great detail. His major symptoms consisted of six obsessions, involving the need to remain immobile, a concern about his eyesight, concern with stomach and bowels, concern with sex, concern with losing control, and fear of attacking people. He also had a fear of contamination and washed his hands compulsively many times a day.

Past history revealed that he had had several head injuries, one an acute right subdural hematoma in 1970, necessitating a right-frontal craniectomy and later cranioplasty. His right optic nerve was injured at that time.

Neurological examination revealed an agitated man who spoke rapidly and often stammered. He had an optic atrophy on the right.

This patient underwent two cingulotomies, one on 28 September 1976 and one on 3 February 1977, and finally a prefrontal leucotomy on 10 November 1977.

On 3 September 1977 (one year after the first, and seven months after the second cingulotomy) the patient reported that the obsessive thoughts were still present but perhaps less bothersome. There had been no improvement in his fear of contamination, and he had a new fear of losing his interest in sports as a spectator. His mother felt that he did have better control of his temper, and that his speech was less agitated and better articulated.

Written communication from the patient on 25 December 1978 revealed no remarkable change. He commented that many acquaintances felt that he spoke more clearly and perhaps less rapidly than he had previously.

Neurological Examination

Cingulotomy patients were examined neurologically at the time of each admission to the M.I.T. Clinical Research Center. The neurological examination included the standard procedures for evaluation of cranial nerve function (including smell, vision, touch, hearing, and taste), motor function (strength, tendon reflexes, plantar responses, resistance to passive movement, presence or absence of involuntary movements, and so on), coordination, sensation (pin prick, light touch, position, and vibration), and gait and station. Additional tests were used that have been found to detect more subtle abnormalities of posture and movement (see Teuber, Corkin, and Twitchell, 1977a). Of the 85 patients in the series, 26 had a past history of disease affecting the brain, exclusive of their present illness. The disorders included 15 cases of closed head injury, 6 of seizures, 1 of neurosyphilis, 1 of hepatic encephalopathy, 1 of stroke, 1 of retrobulbar neuritis (demyelinating disease), and 1 of herniated disc.

The results of the neurological examinations after cingulotomy showed that 34 out of 85 patients had completely normal neurological status. In 26 patients the neurological abnormalities were movement disorders, specifically drug-induced parkinsonism or dyskinesiae. All of these patients had been on various combinations of psychotropic drugs over a long period. In 20 patients the only abnormalities were related to the primary disease that led up to the eventual cingulotomy. All of these patients were in the pain group, and the neurological deficits were primarily those of root or nerve dysfunction. Of the other patients who showed postoperative neurological abnormalities, 3 were known to have had prior cerebral disease, and in 2 others, who were not examined before operation, the etiology could not be unequivocally ascertained. However, in those patients examined neurologically both before and after cingulotomy, there were no changes in neurological status or new abnormal signs detected, except for one patient who five days after the operation showed an abnormal reflex (grasp reflex bilaterally), which did not persist. There were 2 patients, without an antecedent history of seizures or head injury, who experienced isolated seizures after cingulotomy. In 1 of these cases the seizures were a symptom of abrupt withdrawal of excessive quantities of medication.

Behavioral Testing

Table 9.5 lists all of the behavioral tests that have been given in this study. It was not possible to administer all of the tests listed to all of the cingulotomy patients who have participated in the investigation because the amount of patient time available for research participation was limited. The practice has been to use a particular group of tests that sample a wide range of behaviors. After a year or more, data analyses are performed to determine if there are statistically significant differences between preoperative scores and postoperative ones. As a general rule, tests that have been found to elicit such differences have been kept in the test battery, and others have been dropped so that new tests could be introduced. The Wechsler IQ and Memory Scales and several tasks that were performed more poorly by patients who had received large numbers of ECT treatments (Sullivan and Corkin, unpublished data) were given to all patients.

The main criterion used in selecting these tests was that they sample the capacities of the cingulate region or of the cortical and subcortical areas that are interconnected through this region (see Figure 9.7). Thus, it seemed profitable to search for specific signs ordinarily associated with frontal-lobe or temporal-lobe dysfunction in humans, and to look for the kind of impairment found in monkeys or humans after lesions of the cingulate cortex and other limbic structures. Test items that sampled overall intelligence or personality were also included. All measures were quantitative, permitting an objective description of any changes revealed. Many of these tasks have been used extensively in earlier research done in this and other laboratories, and hence it was possible to fit the results obtained with cingulotomy patients into a broader framework of human brain function (for example, Corkin, 1979).

Table 9.5 Behavioral Tests Used to Assess the Effects of Cingulotomy

Overall Intelligence	*Spatial Capacities*
Wechsler Adult Intelligence Scale	Hidden Figures
Wechsler-Bellevue Intelligence Scales I & II	Body Scheme
	Visual Locomotor Mazes
Cognitive Tests Sensitive to Frontal Lobe Dysfunction	
Wisconsin Card Sorting	*Sensory and Motor Systems*
Verbal Fluency	Two-Point Discrimination
Nonverbal Fluency	Position Sense
Verbal Recency Discrimination	Intermanual Localization
Delayed Alternation Performance	Odor Detection and Discrimination
Porteus Mazes	Grip Strength
Tactual Stylus Maze[a]	Finger Tapping Rate
	Fine-Finger Movements
Memory	Coordinated Tapping
Wechsler Memory Scales I & II	
Continuous Recognition of Verbal Material	*Personality*
Continuous Recognition of Nonverbal Material	Eysenck Personality Inventory
Rey-Taylor Complex Figures	Minnesota Multiphasic Personality Inventory
Faces and Houses[a]	Schalling-Sifneos Personality Scale
Short-Term Recall of Trigrams	
Famous Faces[a]	

[a] Tests given only after operation.

Most of the tests were given before the operation to obtain a baseline performance and then repeated after operation to see if there had been any change; in many cases, alternate forms of the tasks were available for test–retest purposes. The same tasks were given to normal control subjects on two occasions to reveal any gains in performance on second testing due to practice, or losses due to interference from the first session. Where there were such changes in normal subjects, these were taken into account in evaluating the patients' results.

No attempt will be made to describe each test in detail; the interested reader may consult the report by Teuber, Corkin, and Twitchell (1977a) or the other references noted below. The tests have been grouped in Table 9.5 according to the major aspect of behavior that they sample, but it should be understood that such divisions are artificial and that many tasks could have been included in more than one category. The results of testing will be discussed at the end of this section.

Overall Intelligence Preoperative IQ ratings were obtained with the *Wechsler Adult Intelligence Scale (WAIS)* (Wechsler, 1955), and the first postoperative ones with the *Wechsler-Bellevue Intelligence Scale, Form II* (Wechsler, 1946), which served as an alternate form of the WAIS. In subsequent examinations, Forms I and II of the Wechsler-Bellevue were used alternately.

Cognitive Tests Sensitive to Frontal-Lobe Dysfunction The *Wisconsin Card Sorting Test* (Grant and Berg, 1948; Milner, 1963) was a problem-solving task in which patients were required to sort a pack of stimulus cards, and in doing so to shift periodically from one sorting principle to another (that is, from color to form to number); their only clue was the examiner's saying "right" or "wrong" after each response.

Two verbal fluency tests were given: In Thurstone's Word Fluency Test (Thurstone, 1944), which tapped *symbolic fluency*, patients were asked, for example, to write down as many words as possible beginning with the letter *S*. In the other task, which tapped *semantic fluency* (Newcombe, 1969), patients named aloud as many items as possible from a particular class, such as animals. In an attempt to provide a nonverbal analogue of these measures, a *nonverbal fluency* test was devised in which patients were given a number of colored plastic cylinders and squares and told to build as many different structures as possible.

In another test, patients were read a list of words all belonging to a particular semantic category, such as items on a farm, and were then asked some questions to test their memory for content (for example, "Which did I say, rake or plow?") and other questions to test their memory for the serial order of items (for example, "Which did I say first, cart or wagon?"); the latter was a *recency-discrimination* probe.

To perform the *delayed-alternation* task successfully, patients had to predict the location of an object, hidden under one of two cups, as it alternated back and forth between them in a particular pattern, such as right-right-left-left (Jacobsen, 1936; Mishkin, 1957).

Two maze-tracing tasks were used in this study. The *Porteus Mazes* (Porteus, 1965) were printed individually on sheets of paper, and the patients were told to draw a pencil line showing the correct path from the start to the finish, without entering any blind alleys, touching lines, or lifting the pencil off the paper. This was not a learning task but measured the patient's capacity to plan ahead and obey rules. In addition, patients were trained to learn the correct sequence of turns in a *tactual stylus maze* until three successive errorless runs had been achieved or until thirty trials had been performed on each of three consecutive days (Corkin, 1965).

Memory Because the *Wechsler Memory Scale* consists of a heterogeneous group of subtests, heavily weighted with verbal items, the focus of this study was on three individual subtests: memory passages (stories), associated learning (words), and visual reproduction (geometric drawings). In addition to immediate recall of the material, delayed recall of the same items was obtained approximately one and a half hours after the first (and only) presentation (Milner, 1958). Other tests of recent memory included: *continuous recognition of verbal material* (words, nonsense syllables, and numbers) *and nonverbal material* (geometric and nonsense drawings) printed on 3½" × 5" cards (Kimura, 1963; Milner, "Memory," in Milner and Teuber, 1968); copy and delayed recall of the *Rey-Taylor Complex Figures*, shown in Figure 9.2 (Osterrieth and Rey, 1944; Rey, 1942; Taylor, 1969); recognition of black and white photographs of men's *faces and* of *houses* (Yin, 1970); and *short-term recall of trigrams*, composed of three consonants, after 3, 9, 15, and 30-second delays, during which time rehearsal was prevented by having the patients count backwards (Brown, 1958; Peterson and Peterson, 1959). There was also a test of remote memory called *Famous Faces*, in which patients were asked to identify news photo-

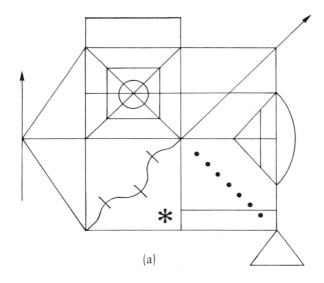

(a)

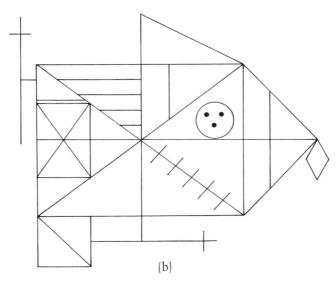

(b)

Figure 9.2 Stimulus materials for Rey-Taylor Complex Figure Test. (a) Taylor figure. [From Taylor, 1969; reprinted with permission of L. B. Taylor.] (b) Rey figure. [From Osterrieth and Rey, 1944; Rey, 1942.]

graphs of public figures from the 1920s through the 1970s (Marslen-Wilson and Teuber, 1975).

Spatial Capacities Three different aspects of spatial capacities were assessed. In the *Hidden Figures Test* (see Figure 9.3), patients had to detect and trace simple geometric figures that were embedded in more complex ones (Thurstone, 1944; Corkin, 1979). The *Body Scheme Test* determined how accurately patients could locate points on their own bodies that corresponded to points indicated on a manikin (Semmes et al., 1963). In performing the *Visual Locomotor Mazes*, patients were given maps that consisted of a three-by-three array of red dots connected by a black line. The floor of the testing room had a similar array of dots about 54 in. apart, and the task was to walk from dot to dot following the path indicated on the map (Semmes et al., 1963).

Sensory and Motor Systems Quantitative measures of various sensory and motor functions were taken to supplement the qualitative ones obtained in the neurological examination. The patient's sense of touch was evaluated in terms of the *two-point discrimination* threshold (the smallest distance between two probes at which the points could be felt as two rather than one), *position sense* (discrimination of small upward from small downward movements of the fingers), and *intermanual localization* (for example, the ability to touch with the right thumb a point on one of the fingers of that hand that corresponded to a point the examiner had just touched on one of the fingers of the left hand (Gazzaniga, Bogen, and Sperry, 1963). The sense of smell was assessed in a detailed examination of *odor detection and odor quality discrimination* (Potter and Butters, in press). The motor tasks included: the measurement of *grip strength* in pounds (Stevens and Mack, 1959), the *rate of tapping* during a 10-second interval, with each index finger alone and with the two tapping simultaneously; a test of *fine-finger movements*, in which a counter was advanced by turning a small knob as quickly as possible; and a sensorimotor task, *coordinated tapping*, in which patients tapped the four sectors of a circle in a particular sequence, both unimanually and bimanually (Thurstone, 1944).

Personality The *Eysenck Personality Inventory* gave three independent scores: neuroticism, extroversion, and a falsification detector (Eysenck and Eysenck, 1968). Preliminary results with this test suggested that it was inappropriate for the cingulotomy group, and it has now been replaced by the *Minnesota Multiphasic Personality*

Look at the two adjacent figures.
One of them is contained in each
of the drawings below.

In each of the following drawings, mark that part
which is the same as one of the adjacent figures.
Mark only one figure in each drawing.

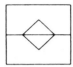 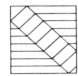 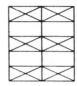 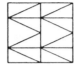

Figure 9.3 Sample of Thurstone's Hidden Figures Test. [From Corkin, 1979.]

Inventory (Hathaway and McKinley, 1967), which measures objectively some of the personality traits that can affect personal and social adjustment. The *Schalling-Sifneos Personality Scale* specifically identifies patients with alexithymia (Sifneos, 1972), who are unable to describe their feelings, have a paucity of fantasies, and are preoccupied with the minute details of events in their lives.

In analyzing the objective test data, the primary concern was to determine whether there were changes in performance that could be attributed to the cingulotomy. The results clearly indicated that on most of the cognitive tasks listed in Table 9.5, the performance of cingulotomy patients was unchanged after the surgical procedure. Thus, the findings to be presented here highlight the exceptions, the tasks on which there were statistically significant differences between the preoperative and postoperative scores. It is too soon to say definitively whether the effects described below are transient or lasting, because the postoperative testing in most cases was done within a few months of the operation. In order to answer this question, these patients are now being tested in a follow-up study, and the results will be reported in future publications. The outcome of the objective personality assessment is also undetermined. The personality scales now in use (the Minnesota Multiphasic Personality Inventory and the Schalling-Sifneos Personality Scale) were introduced into the test battery only within the last year, and there are not sufficient data to present at this time.

Wechsler Adult Intelligence Scale (WAIS) and Wechsler-Bellevue Intelligence Scale, Form II Figure 9.4 illustrates the relationship between changes in overall intelligence and the time of testing. Patients who were examined before operation and then retested in the early postoperative period showed no significant change from their preoperative ratings. In contrast, those who were given their second test more than four months after operation showed significant rises in Full Scale, Verbal, and Performance IQ ratings. These positive changes are probably related to the improvement in the patients' conditions and the concomitant reductions in the amount of medication being taken.

Rey-Taylor Complex Figure Test Cingulotomy was associated with a change in performance on the copying part of this task but not in the capacity to recall the drawing after a one-hour delay. Patients over thirty years of age copied the complex figure more accurately before operation than they did soon after operation, whereas patients under thirty showed no change in the accuracy of their copies (see Figure 9.5). All of these patients will be retested a year or more after operation to document any further changes in performance.

Hidden Figures Test For this task, the results of retesting fewer than five months after operation were again a function of the patient's age (see Table 9.6). Those under thirty years of age, as a group, showed a significant increase in the number of hidden figures detected, whereas patients over thirty showed a significant decrease. A clearer picture of Hidden Figures Test performance is found in the results for a subgroup of 19 patients who were examined at all three testing periods—before operation, less than five months after operation, and later in follow-up study (see Figure 9.6). A comparison of their preoperative with their early postoperative scores revealed no change in the 5 patients under thirty, in contrast to a significant drop in mean number correct in those over thirty. For both groups, the difference between the preoperative and later postoperative results indicated a significant increase in achievement at the time of follow-up examination.

These specific, age-related losses after cingulotomy on the Rey-Taylor Complex Figure Test and the Hidden Figures Test seem to reflect a disorder of visual perception. Although there are no other reports of reduced efficiency in processing complex visual stimuli in animals or humans after such lesions, the neuroanatomical studies

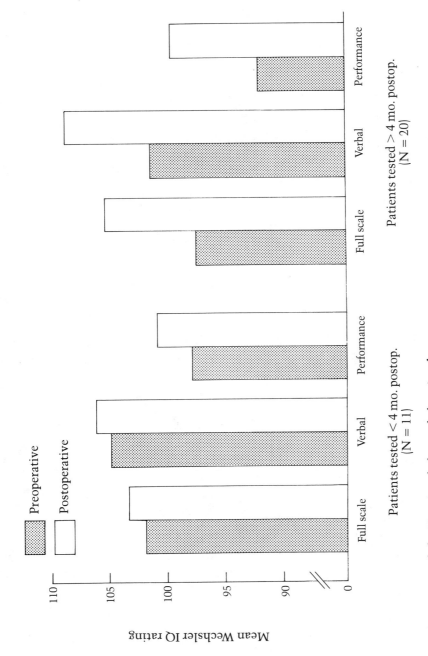

Figure 9.4 Wechsler IQ ratings before and after cingulotomy.

Table 9.6 Number Correct on the *Hidden Figures Test* Before and After Cingulotomy: Relationship with Age

Group	N	Before Operation		Less than 5 Months After Operation		More than 5 Months After Operation	
		Mean	Range	Mean	Range	Mean	Range
Under 30 years old	13	18.1	1–33	21.8	5–40	—	—
	4	16.8	2–26	—	—	19.8	3–33
Over 30 years old	36	16.7	1–44	14.9	0–48	—	—
	3	25.0	3–39	—	—	25.7	9–25

Source: Corkin, 1979.

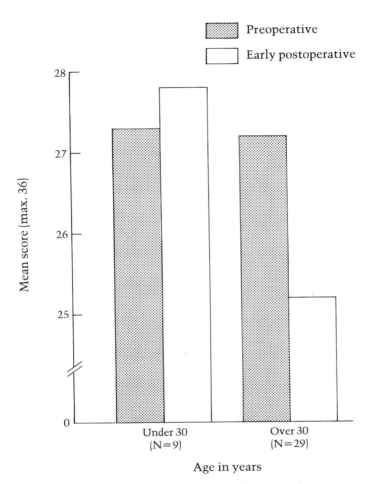

Figure 9.5 Rey-Taylor Complex Figure Test: relationship between age and mean score after cingulotomy.

of Dr. Deepak N. Pandya and his colleagues (Pandya, Dye, and Butters, 1971; Pandya and Kuypers, 1969; Pandya and Vignolo, 1971) have shown that the anterior portion of the cingulate gyrus (area 24) is reciprocally connected with the association cortex of the frontal and parietal lobes, areas of cerebral cortex that in humans and monkeys play a major role in other visuospatial capacities (for example, Teuber and Mishkin, 1954; Semmes et al., 1963; Milner, 1965; Pohl, 1973). The spatial information relayed from these separate

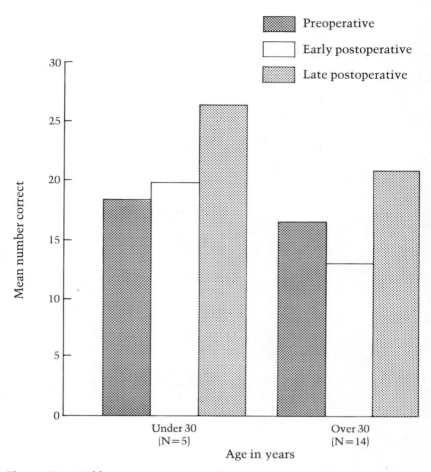

Figure 9.6 Hidden Figures Test: achievement of cingulotomy patients tested three times.

regions may be integrated in the cingulate gyrus, and the drops in performance noted above could represent a temporary disruption of this limbic spatial mechanism.

Interpretation of Results

It is not clear why cingulotomy relieves the mental or physical anguish of some patients but produces no change in the conditions of other patients with the same diagnoses and ostensibly similar

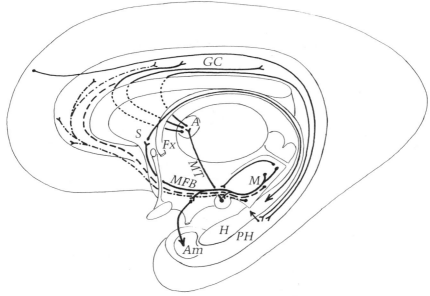

Figure 9.7 Some components of the fasciculus cinguli that are likely to be interrupted by cingulotomy. Quantitatively the most prominent of these pathways is the projection from the anterior nucleus of the thalamus (*A*). Note the initially rostral orientation of this thalamo-cingulate fiber system, a disposition suggesting that lesions in the rostral part of the fasciculus may disconnect from the thalamus most or all of the cingulo-parahippocampal cortex caudal to the lesion. The same holds true for the monoaminergic mesocortical systems: the serotonin system (broken line) originating from the mesencephalic raphe nuclei, and the dopamine system (dot-dash line) arising in cell group A10 of the nigral complex. Also indicated is the fronto-limbic association system extending caudally as far as the parahippocampal gyrus *(PH)*. Other abbreviations: *Am:* amygdala; *Fx:* formix bundle; *GC:* gyrus cinguli; *H:* hippocampus; *M:* midbrain; *MFB:* medical forebrain bundle; *MT:* mamillo-thalamic tract; *S:* septum. [Adapted from Nauta, 1973, by Dr. Nauta and reproduced with his permission from Corkin, Twitchell, and Sullivan, 1979.]

histories. In trying to understand this complex finding it may be helpful to consider factors other than the destruction of brain tissue that could facilitate improvement, either alone or in combination. Just as the causes of psychiatric disease are thought to be multiple in many cases, no single factor being necessary and sufficient to produce a particular disorder, so too can the mechanism of effective treatment involve a number of variables. In the case of patients who have undergone cingulotomy, these may include the presumed alteration in brain physiology, the patients' environments, a placebo (or expectancy) effect, and the natural history of the disorder being treated. These factors will be dealt with in turn below.

Physiological Mechanisms

One explanation of the therapeutic successes that have been seen in some psychiatric patients is a physiological one. The possibility exists that cingulotomy produces long-lasting changes in the levels of certain chemicals that carry messages between brain cells (neurotransmitters, such as serotonin, dopamine, and norepinephrine). These neurochemical events could take place at the site of the cingulate lesion or at some distance from it. Serotonergic and dopaminergic pathways begin in the midbrain and terminate in the region of the cingulotomy (see Figure 9.7). These or other neuroregulatory systems with which they interact could have been altered as a result of the brain operation. Biochemical mechanisms have been implicated in several psychiatric disorders, particularly schizophrenia, in which it is hypothesized that brain dopamine metabolism or activity is excessive (Berger, Elliot, and Barchas, 1978). In depression, as well, norepinephrine and serotonin are thought to be underactive or deficient (Schildkraut, 1978). Although the relationships between neuroregulators and mental disease are poorly understood, there is at least a theoretical basis for implicating biochemical changes in the therapeutic mechanism of the cingulate surgery.

There is also a theoretical basis for attributing the therapeutic effect of the cingulotomy in the treatment of chronic pain to the action of chemical substances in the brain. The recently discovered opiate receptors and endogenous opiates, or endorphins, are concentrated in brain regions involved in pain transmission and emotion —namely, in central grey substances of the midbrain and in the limbic system, particularly, the amygdala (Snyder and Mathysse, 1975). Thus, the internal opiates are ideally situated to influence the central substrata of normal or pathological pain, but the physiological mechanisms by which their role in behavior is exerted, normally or following cingulotomy, is unknown.

Environment

It is likely that environmental factors can influence the clinical course following cingulotomy. This is one reason why the neurosurgeon requires that his patients have a supportive home situation to return to after the operation and that they remain under the care of the referring psychiatrist. It is also the case that a major change in the patient's life situation might have a profound influence on the course of his illness. For example, one patient who underwent cingulotomy was a 27-year-old woman who became depressed after she gave birth for the third time in three years. Her husband, described by her mother as having a serious drinking problem, was said to have been rejecting and brutal to her. The husband apparently assumed that the brain operation would have an immediate therapeutic effect on his wife, and as a result his attitude and behavior toward her improved dramatically right after the surgery. His expectation of improvement in his wife's condition could have been self-fulfilling. The patient was evaluated in the present study twenty-two months after operation. At that time she was off medication and holding a part-time job. Interviews with her and her mother revealed that her relationship with her husband had improved, she had a good relationship with her children, and cared for them competently. Her overall condition was rated as markedly improved.

Environmental factors also appear to have been significant in the case of a 27-year-old male paranoid schizophrenic who received two cingulotomies approximately six months apart. His mother reported that there had been no change in his condition after the first operation, nor after the second until he moved out of his parents' home into a halfway house six months after the second operation. After that he was able to reduce his dose of Thorazine, moved from the halfway house to a youth hostel, and began actively looking for a job and running for exercise. When seen in a follow-up study sixteen months after the second operation, he was deemed moderately improved by the M.I.T. research team and by his family. The purpose of citing these two cases is not to suggest that the therapeutic effects attributed to cingulotomy are solely due to changes in the patients' environments, but rather to indicate that their postoperative clinical course may be influenced by situational variables that interact with changes in the brain produced by the surgery.

Placebo Effect

In trying to evaluate the efficacy of cingulotomy, it is also necessary to deal with the question of placebo effect. That is, does the patient's condition improve because he expects it to, and is the cingulotomy simply a way of giving the patient a strong suggestion? Specifically, it may be asked whether the high rate of improvement in patients with chronic pain, compared with the rate of response in those diagnosed as obsessive-compulsive or schizophrenic, reflects the placebo effects either of the surgery itself or of some other conditions associated with the surgery. The only way to answer this question satisfactorily is to compare patients who have undergone cingulotomy with patients who have received a sham operation. This could be done in the following way. Candidates for cingulotomy would be randomly assigned to one of two groups. The first group would undergo a one-stage cingulotomy in the usual manner. The second group would receive the operation in two stages. In the first stage, burr holes would be made but the dura mater would not be opened and brain tissue would not be destroyed. Six months to a year after this sham operation, the patients would be reevaluated by the neurosurgeon, by the psychiatrist and neurologist who did the independent evaluation preoperatively, and also by the research team at M.I.T. Patients whose conditions had not improved would then receive the second stage of the operation—that is, the bilateral cingulotomy. Doing the procedure in two stages would not entail a greater risk from the administration of anesthesia, because the second stage could be done in an X-ray suite under local anesthesia. The advantages for the patients would reside in the possibility that there might be marked benefit without exposure to the risks associated with brain surgery, such as infection or intracerebral bleeding.

In obtaining informed consent, the neurosurgeon would tell patients what each of the two treatment groups would experience; however, neither they nor their relatives would know to which group they had been assigned. Only the neurosurgeon and the operating room personnel would have this information. The other members of the hospital staff, the Boston psychiatrist and neurologist, the referring psychiatrist, and the M.I.T. group would not. This research procedure in which the individual undergoing treatment and those evaluating it do not know which technique has been used has a precedent in medical research in that it is the usual paradigm of studies that evaluate the effects of drugs.

If drilling burr holes in the skull turns out to be a reliable placebo procedure, one would hope that neurosurgeons performing psychiatric surgery would then implement it in their practices. To do so would not violate the neurosurgeon's responsibility to provide the best available treatment because for certain diagnostic groups, for example patients with chronic pain or depression, the sham procedure might provide maximal benefits with minimal risks. It is even possible that this placebo operation might eventually be reclassified as an active treatment, if a recent report in a related field is replicable. That work on dental postoperative pain suggests that patients who are helped by a placebo have a concomitant release of endogenous opiates in the brain. This condition can be reversed by chemically blocking their action with a specific opiate antagonist (naloxone) (Levine, Gordon, and Fields, 1978). What needs to be shown now is that a similar physiological effect also accompanies the placing of burr holes in the skull.

The proposal to institute placebo operations in the treatment of chronic pain and psychiatric disease raises several problems. One practical consideration is the question of who would pay the bill: Is it fair to expect a patient to sustain the costs of several thousand dollars associated with the procedure? Would the patient's insurer agree to pay it? Another concern is that the performance of sham operations would increase the likelihood that the neurosurgeon would be sued for malpractice. Even though the plaintiff might not ultimately prevail in such an action, the unpleasantness, loss of reputation, and expense associated with a lawsuit are probably sufficient to deter most neurosurgeons from performing the placebo operation. In the context of medical ethics, an obvious worry is that a depressed patient who did not show a placebo response to the placing of burr holes might commit suicide before the second stage of the procedure, the cingulotomy, could be performed.

In response to these arguments, it should be noted that it is not necessary that all neurosurgeons practicing psychiatric surgery perform sham operations. If a few were willing to participate in such an experiment, one appropriate course of action would be to design a sound plan of research and apply to the United States Public Health Service for funds to cover the cost of the operations and of psychiatrists to care for all of the patients who were involved in the study.

It is of interest that Livingston (1953) performed sham operations in four psychiatric patients by simply making an incision in the scalp and removing a bone button. Postoperatively these patients followed the same routine as did his cingulotomy patients, and neither the patients themselves nor the hospital staff knew that the complete surgical procedure had not been carried out. No improvement was seen during the next one to three months, and these patients subsequently underwent cingulotomy. This finding is not definitive, however, because the number of cases is small, and it is not known how they fared after cingulotomy. Moreover, Livingston's patients had been institutionalized for years, and in this respect at least they were not comparable to most of the patients who undergo psychiatric surgery today.

There are two other reports of sham operations that were not successful. Doctors Balasubramaniam, Kanaka, and Ramanujam

(1973) in Madras, India, who perform cingulotomies for the relief of drug addiction, found that burr holes alone had no effect in three such patients, whereas the subsequent cingulotomy did. In Boston, Dr. William Sweet (White and Sweet, 1955, pp. 315–316) inadvertently performed a sham operation (craniotomy) in a woman with facial pain (trigeminal neuralgia), and she too obtained no lasting benefit. These accounts of sham neurosurgical procedures involving institutionalized psychiatric patients, drug addicts, and a case of trigeminal neuralgia, though undoubtedly tantalizing, do not reveal anything about the presence or absence of placebo effects in patients like those described in this chapter. It is therefore essential that a prospective trial be initiated in which candidates for a particular psychosurgical procedure are randomly or alternately assigned either to a lesion group or to a sham-operated group. Until such a study has been done, it will not be known for sure how much, if any, of the therapeutic effect attributed to psychosurgery is due to factors other than the brain lesions *per se*.

Natural History of the Disorder

The proper evaluation of a treatment requires a knowledge of the natural history of the disorders being treated, so that a comparison can be made between the incidence of improvement after the treatment has been applied and the incidence of spontaneous remission. In the evaluation of cingulotomy, it would be useful to know the incidence of improvement in noninstitutionalized patients diagnosed as having chronic pain, severe depression, schizophrenia, obsessive-compulsive neurosis, anxiety neurosis, or hysteria, who do not receive psychosurgery or any other treatment. It is obviously beyond the scope of the research described here to provide an answer to this question. Nevertheless, this same issue is also relevant in studies that evaluate the effects of other treatments of these disorders, such as drug therapy, ECT, and psychotherapy, and it is therefore surprising that the psychiatric literature is nearly void of natural history studies in which an untreated control group was followed over a sufficiently long period of time to make the results meaningful. Studies from the 1930s indicated that 25 to 50 percent of patients with psychoses, particularly schizophrenia, improved without the benefit of treatment other than hospitalization (Bond and Braceland, 1937; Guttman, Mayer-Gross, and Slater, 1939; Hunt, Feldman, and Fiero, 1938; Whitehead, 1938). These statistics were based upon relatively large numbers of cases since this was before the use of psychotropic medications, ECT, and psychosurgery became prevalent. More recently, Dr. Hans J. Eysenck (1965), in a detailed review of studies of the effects of psychotherapy, has concluded that over two-thirds of severe neurotics not receiving psychotherapy recover within two years of the onset of their illness (see also Rachman's chapter in this volume).

The problem in applying such statistics to the patients who undergo psychosurgery is that they are clearly not representative of the total population of psychiatric patients in terms of the length and severity of their illness. It will be remembered from Table 9.2 that among the patients who underwent cingulotomy the preoperative duration of their illness or complaint was on the average 10.8 years for the group with chronic pain and 14.9 years for the group with psychiatric disorders. If these patients had conditions that were self-limiting, a remission would probably have occurred in the years before the brain operation was performed.

Effect of Research on Clinical Practice

There is another question that may have been nagging the reader throughout this chapter: Does the mere existence of an evaluative study such as the one described here increase the likelihood that the procedure in question will be performed? If the evaluation had shown that the cingulotomy was totally unsuccessful and had negative side effects as well, obviously these results would not have attracted more patients. Since the findings were for the most part favorable, however, it is of interest to compare the number of cingulotomies that the referring neurosurgeon performed before this evaluation began with the current number. Figure 9.8 provides the data for such a comparison. The total number of operations carried out during the five-year period from 1966 through 1970 was 162, and from 1971 through 1975 it was 103. This decrease during the current decade was probably due to the social controversy over psychosurgery; in Boston, where these operations were performed, this began in 1972 and peaked in 1974, when the first psychosurgery bill was introduced in the Massachusetts Legislature. At present, it appears that this form of psychiatric surgery is again increasing in popularity, because the number of such procedures done by this surgeon alone rose from 32 in 1975 and 1976 combined to 57 in 1977 and 1978 combined. Nevertheless, it would be presumptuous to attribute this increase in patient flow to the research described here. Rather, there are two other factors that are probably responsible to a

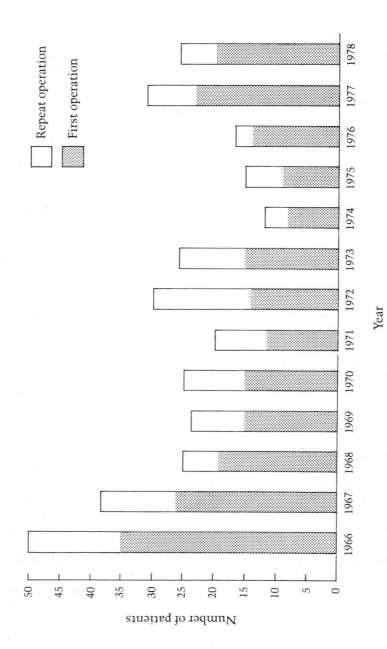

Figure 9.8 Number of cingulotomies performed by one neurosurgeon between 1966 and 1978.

great extent for the rise in the number of operations. The first is the report of the National Commission for the Protection of Human Subjects of Biomedical and Behavioral Research (1977), which did not recommend, as it could have, that psychosurgery be prohibited, but instead stated the conditions under which it would be appropriate to perform psychosurgical procedures. At the same time, several out-of-state psychiatrists who had referred patients for cingulotomy observed that their patients benefited from the operation, and they subsequently increased the number of referrals they made.

Future Research Plans

As this ongoing research progresses, the number of cingulotomy patients evaluated and the length of the follow-up interval will increase. These circumstances will permit the study of other interesting variables that it would have been premature to examine to date. Accordingly, future analyses will deal with the time course of any changes in the patient's condition in relation to the date of the operation. An attempt will be made to understand why some patients respond immediately to cingulate surgery, whereas in others a favorable response does not occur for several months. Another aim will be to tabulate the incidence of improvement for different diagnostic groups according to the length of time that has elapsed since the operation. The results obtained will make it possible to say with greater certainty whether the positive effects of cingulotomy are lasting.

The global, qualitative ratings of therapeutic outcome will soon be supplemented by quantitative ones. A psychiatric rating scale will be filled out for each patient by a research psychiatrist before operation and at various intervals after operation (Spitzer et al., 1970). This instrument will provide scores that indicate the severity of psychiatric symptoms, such as depression-anxiety, social isolation, and grandiosity, as well as scores that indicate the effectiveness with which patients carry out different roles, such as wage-earner, housekeeper, and parent. The therapeutic effect of cingulotomy may then be measured quantitatively in terms of changes in percentile scores obtained by the patients at different points in time.

In order to measure the extent of the relief experienced by patients with chronic pain who undergo cingulotomy, the McGill Pain Questionnaire (Melzack, 1975) will be given before operation and then repeated at all postoperative evaluations. This research tool consists of twenty sets of words that describe the sensory, affective, and evaluative properties of pain. Patients are asked to choose the word in each group that best describes how they feel, and from these responses a numerical rating is obtained. They also rate the intensity of their pain on a scale from 0 to 5. By thus quantifying separately the psychological and physical components of pain, it should be possible to provide a more adequate description of the therapeutic mechanism.

Future reports based on this investigation will also present data for unoperated patient control subjects who have been evaluated according to the same protocol as have the cingulotomy patients. These control patients will include those referred for cingulotomy who for various reasons have decided not to go through with the procedure; those with severe, chronic pain who have been deemed treatment failures elsewhere but have not been referred for psychiatric surgery; and those with psychiatric disorders that have been treated with massive doses of ECT or that for other reasons have been judged to be severe and intractable.

Conclusions

On the basis of five years of research in which 85 patients who underwent cingulotomy were examined, it can be concluded first of all that no patient showed the severe adverse effects that had been associated with prefrontal lobotomy. In fact, there is so far no evidence of any lasting neurological or behavioral deficits after cingulotomy. In addition, this surgical procedure was followed by improvement in the condition of many of the patients, though not all of them. Specifically, those with chronic pain or depression showed a high rate of therapeutic success, whereas those with schizophrenia or obsessive-compulsive neurosis did not. These conclusions must be guarded, however, because at this point in the study the length of the follow-up interval is short in many cases and because the behavioral test results are still incomplete. Moreover, it is not understood why cingulotomy is effective in some cases and not in others, or what brain mechanisms or other factors are responsible for the improvement when it does occur. Our future research will address these issues.

CHAPTER 10

Two Retrospective Studies of Psychosurgery

Allan F. Mirsky and Maressa Hecht Orzack

The suggestion that a retrospective evaluation of the safety and efficacy of psychosurgery be conducted under the sponsorship of the National Commission for the Protection of Human Subjects of Biomedical and Behavioral Research was made by an ad hoc advisory group to the National Commission that was convened in June 1975. This study was deemed necessary in view of the wording of Public Law 93-348, Section 202 (c) of the Congress of the United States. Among other things, this law created the National Commission and assigned it a number of tasks, including investigating the safety and efficacy of psychosurgery.

We wish to thank our colleagues and staff for their help in carrying out these studies and in preparing this manuscript. In particular, Marcia Kornetsky contributed greatly with her gentle competence and insight. Deborah Orzack and Stafford McLean provided much help as our lab persons-of-all-work. Anne Pomerantz, Howard Wheeling, and Cheryl Grady, all graduate students, also helped us to achieve our goals. We also thank our cooperating surgeons and psychiatrists, whom we cannot name, and our participating patients, without whom we would have had no study. Our thanks also go to Charlotte Johnson, who held the lab together through both studies as our administrative assistant and secretary. Finally, we acknowledge with gratitude support from Contracts N01-HU-6-2114 and NIH 278-76-0064, and grant K5-14,915 (Research Scientist Award to A.F.M.) from NIMH, ADMHA.

Research Plan

Within the context of investigating psychosurgery, our research team at the Boston University Medical Center hoped to conduct a pilot study to (1) determine the utility and value of a retrospective study of operated cases and (2) gather some preliminary information concerning the benefits and/or hazards of psychosurgical treatment. The specific goals were to:

1. Assemble, coordinate, and supervise a clinical evaluation team including representatives of the disciplines of neurosurgery, clinical neurology, psychiatry, psychology, and social sciences.
2. Develop a detailed evaluation protocol, which would specify procedures to:
   a. Identify at least two and no more than four surgeons who would participate in the study by making available to the evaluation team the medical records of their patients who had been referred for psychosurgery and by contacting selected patients to request their cooperation.
   b. For each of the surgeons, obtain populations of at least 20 and not more than 30 patients sufficiently homogeneous with respect to presenting behavioral problems, locus and size of lesion, and other significant variables in order to permit valid and reliable results.
   c. For each patient, obtain from records (to the extent possible) information on:
      (1) Age, sex, race, and socioeconomic status;
      (2) Nature and duration of symptoms, including preoperative emotional status;
      (3) Nature and extent of previous treatment;
      (4) Preoperative intellectual and cognitive functioning;
      (5) Preoperative clinical neurological status;
      (6) Preoperative educational, employment, social adjustment, and health status; and
      (7) The surgeon's and/or referring physician's postoperative evaluation (including the rationale for such evaluation).
3. Select and enlist patients in accordance with the protocol requirements.
4. Interview the patients and their families to determine the factors surrounding the decision for surgical procedures, and their evaluation of outcome and present status, including education, em-

ployment, social adjustment, and health status. In addition, information that might be lacking on the medical reports regarding preoperative status could be obtained during such interviews.

5. Test patients with an appropriate battery of tests to evaluate present neurological, intellectual, perceptual, cognitive, and emotional status.

6. Secure an appropriate number of controls—these controls being persons for whom psychosurgery was recommended but not performed.

In addition to these formal work scope goals, there were a number of recommendations made by the Commission, including the use of Dr. A. Earl Walker, a prominent and widely respected neurosurgeon, as the person to make the initial contacts with the neurosurgeons. Because of the difficulties in obtaining the requisite number of patients (to be detailed below), the work scope was modified to specify a total of "less than 40 . . . but more than 30 subjects." The report to the Commission presented information on 27 operated patients and 8 controls, for a total of 35. The difficulties in obtaining patients for the *pilot study* stemmed from the brief time of the contract, eight months, over which the data gathering phase could actually take place (all but two patients were seen between March and May of 1976). Four months were necessary to complete Institutional Review Board (IRB) approval procedures, contact and make necessary arrangements with the three cooperating neurosurgeons, assist them in obtaining informed consent statements from their patients, obtain records from the surgeons, and make contact with the patients and arrange for their travel to Boston for the study. This was true despite the fact that planning for the study began as early as July 1975. This left only four months for actual data collection and compiling the report to be presented at a hearing of the National Commission. All the information about the pilot study contained in this chapter can be found in the Report to the National Commission (Mirsky and Orzack, 1977).

The two surgeons in distant states were contacted only after our consultant, Dr. Earl Walker, had spoken with at least seven other neurosurgeons located closer to Boston. No attempt was made to study their cases because they reported having done too few operations during the 1968–1972 study period (six surgeons) and/or they were not interested in participating (one surgeon). One surgeon declined to sign an informed consent statement, designed to inform him of the possible risks, in terms of identification, of his participating in the study. It was at this point that we requested an extension of time to include the years 1965–1974.

Although the three neurosurgeons who agreed to participate in the study were extremely cooperative, there were delays of several weeks in each of two instances due to vacation plans or the fact that all concerned underestimated the difficulty and time involved in sending out the initial requests to examine records. Our third surgeon reported to us that he had finally to close his office for a week in order to get the letters out.

The securing of control subjects presented unexpected problems. Our initial plan called for such subjects to be provided by leads from the surgeons themselves, from cases for whom surgery had been recommended but declined. Except for one surgeon, this proved to be a virtually nonexistent group. All three surgeons reported instead that they are sought out by persons who are desperate for relief from various symptoms; two of the surgeons also reported that they refuse to operate if certain patient and/or family criteria are not met. Together, Surgeons 1 and 3 could not come up with as many as 5 cases over the years who had declined the recommended operation. Surgeon 2 had 20, but most of those were not acceptable for other reasons.

After some consultation, we sent a letter to all members of the Massachusetts Psychiatric Society, and within a few days we had made contact with a group of appropriate control patients—that is, unoperated patients with depression and/or obsessive-compulsive behavior that was resistant to treatment and of long duration. Near the end of the pilot study, we learned of a local clinic whose chief psychiatrist could provide us not only with control cases but with an estimated population of 150 operated patients from Boston or the local New England region. Subsequent to the submission of the report to the National Commission, we made arrangements to test 25 of these cases, and the data obtained from the completed tests are included in this report. We shall refer to these cases as the *follow-up group*.

Research Methods

Selection of Neurosurgeons

The three surgeons selected in the pilot study and the fourth surgeon (who operated on the follow-up group) agreed to sign informed consents and to make available to us all their records on cases operated during the period 1965–1974. Each surgeon (as far as the cases in-

Table 10.1 Classification of Patients by Diagnosis and Surgeon (Pilot Study and Follow-up Study Combined)

Surgeon	Depression	Obsessive-Compulsive	Depression-Obsessive	Schizo-phrenic	Schizo-phrenic-Affective	Pain	Total
I	3	1		3	1		8
II	3	1		2	1		7
III	4				1	5	10
Other			1		1		2
IV[a]	5	2	12	2	4		25
Total	15	4	13	7	8	5	52
Controls	4	2		2			8

[a] Patients from this group were used exclusively in the follow-up study.

cluded in this study are concerned) performs a distinctive type of psychosurgery. Surgeon 1 does only orbital undercuttings, which sever fibers in the inferior surface of the frontal lobe; Surgeon 2 performs multi-target bilateral stereotaxic operations, using radio-frequency or other lesions to destroy areas in the cingulate gyrus, amygdala, and substantia innominata of the diencephalon. Usually four to six targets are lesioned in a patient. Surgeon 3 performs only "prefrontal sonic treatment" (that is, using focused ultrasonic energy) either unilaterally or bilaterally. All the cases of Surgeon 4 (follow-up group) received a bimedial prefrontal leucotomy, in which a superior approach is used to cut fibers (white matter) in the frontal lobes. Two cases operated by two other surgeons appear in Table 10.1. These patients received an anterior prefrontal leucotomy, an older but still used procedure that severs fibers in the anterior frontal lobe through a more lateral approach than that utilized in the bimedial leucotomy.

Selection of Operated Cases

The initial letters requesting permission for us to obtain patients' records were sent to the patients at our direction by the participating surgeons. Surgeon 1 sent letters to all his patients who were operated on during the time period discussed above. Surgeons 2 and 3 sent letters to those patients who were judged by the surgeon to have diagnoses comparable to the patients of Surgeon 1.[1] The responses

---

[1] This requirement led us to select persons diagnosed primarily as depressed or obsessive-compulsive. Consequently, the patient pool was considerably reduced in the case of Surgeon 2 (see Table 10.2).

Table 10.2   Patient Contact and Follow-up Summary (Pilot Study)

Surgeon	Number Operated On, 1965–1974	Number of Letters Sent	Number of Replies	Full Participation
I	32	23	19	8
II	156	19	15	7
III	193	150	58	11
Other	Unknown	—	—	2

were sent to us. Once a patient's file was available, we asked three psychiatrists to make a diagnosis based on the preoperative record. Our requirement for including a patient was that at least two out of the three diagnoses be in essential agreement. After this step, the patient was contacted and a visit to Boston was scheduled if the patient appeared suitable and was willing. Most patients elected to bring a companion (usually a spouse or relative), thus allowing us to question this person concerning the pre- and postoperative status of the patient, the nature of the contact with and information from the neurosurgeon, and so forth. Vigorous follow-up attempts (phone calls or a second letter) were made for every patient to whom a letter was sent. Table 10.2 summarizes the patient-contacting activities for each of the three surgeons. The cases in the follow-up study are presented separately in Table 10.3

In the pilot study we attempted to ascertain the reasons for refusal in every case. Of the 8 cases who wished no further participation, 5 checked the item "for personal reasons," one indicated "too busy,"

Table 10.3   Breakdown of Patient Sample (Follow-up Study)

	Records Seen	Records Not Seen	Totals
No reply	—	19	19
Participants	25	—	25
Refusals[a]	9	4	13
Inappropriate diagnosis[b]	7	—	7
Deceased	7	12	19
Others	5	—	5
Remaining to be tested	1	—	1
Totals	54	35	89

[a] 9 patients allowed us to see their records, but refused to participate further; 4 patients did not allow us to see their records.

[b] Refers to patients who had either an organic involvement or a strong component of pain that we felt was inappropriate for this study.

Table 10.2 *(continued)*

Wished No Further Participation	Records Only			
	No Time to Test	Unable to Reach	Phone Interview	We Rejected
2	0	2	4	3
1	2	1	2	2
5	32	3	4	3
—	—	—	—	—

and two indicated that they "wished not to be reminded of the operation." The number (and percentage) of refusals in the pilot study was small, thus lending confidence to the belief that we were not missing a significant proportion of the operated cases.

In the follow-up study, a total of 89 letters were sent to patients. Out of this total, 54 patient records were seen; 9 persons refused to participate in the study for their own reasons; 7 were judged to be inappropriate because their primary diagnosis was intractable pain with or without concurrent psychiatric problems; 7 were deceased; and 5 were unable to participate for other reasons. This group of 5 consists of the following individuals: (1) an elderly patient who is blind; (2) an elderly patient who agreed to participate in her home, but not in Boston; (3) a patient whose surgery predates the study; (4) a patient who is suffering from senile dementia and is confined to a nursing home. The fifth was a patient who remains to be tested. Of the remaining 35 patients, whose records were not seen, 19 did not reply even after repeated follow-ups by the participating psychiatrist; 4 refused to participate at all; and 12 were deceased. We were able to obtain only statistical information on the 12 deceased patients.

The composition of the cases in the pilot study, including controls, is shown in Table 10.1. This table reveals the preponderance of diagnoses of depressive or affective illness for the patients in both studies (as well as a sprinkling of some with schizophrenic symptoms as the primary diagnostic label). The choice of patients in the pilot study, however, was determined largely by the cases operated on by Surgeon 1. After having selected his cases to begin with, we sought to obtain subjects with similar diagnoses from the files of the other two surgeons, in order to minimize heterogeneity between surgery groups.

We had no reason to believe, in our dealings with the four surgeons whose cases are discussed in this report, that there were cases being concealed or that the surgeon was not being completely honest and open with us. In fact, the usual offer from the surgeon was to throw open his files completely and to provide names and addresses of all operated patients. Our own protocol, as dictated in part by the Institutional Review Board and the National Commission, prevented us from accepting this offer. Constraints of time also (in the case of the pilot study) prevented us from seeing more than a small number of subjects. As discussed later in the report, independent verification of the surgeons' lists of operated cases proved impossible.

Selection of Control Cases

For controls, we sought patients in whom the primary diagnosis was obsessive-compulsive or recurrent affective illness, but did not exclude those in whom schizophrenia was also present. The quality of the available records of the control cases is in general much poorer than that of the operated patients' records. Often, we had only a brief summary of the psychiatrists' notes or records. This is in contrast to the operated cases, for which detailed pre- and postsurgical information of a diagnostic nature was available, including (in some instances) reports of psychological testing, notes from prior hospitalizations, and descriptions of other therapies as employed or reported by the referring psychiatrist.

The Test and Interview Battery

All but three of the patients were tested in Boston. This testing lasted two to three days and consisted, for the most part, of standard psychiatric, psychological, social work, neurological, EEG, and neurophysiological procedures.

Psychiatric Examination   All patients were administered the *Spitzer-Endicott Psychiatric Status Schedule (PSS)*, a machine-scored version of a semi-structured psychiatric interview, which yields scores on various factors such as subjective distress and behavioral disturbance and for which norms have been derived from various psychopathological populations. All of our psychiatrists were trained in the use of the *PSS*. In addition, the *Spitzer-Endicott Problem Appraisal Scale (PAS)* was filled out once by the psychiatrist and twice by the social worker. The psychiatrist's and one of the social worker's ratings addressed current functioning; the other filled out by the social worker estimated preoperative status as compared with optimal status. The patient was also asked to fill out the *Hopkins Scale (HSCL-80)*, an assessment of current function'ng, and the *Profile of Mood States (POMS)*, addressed specifically to current mood. A *drug questionnaire* to assess drug intake and alcohol consumption was also administered. The psychiatrist also gave a global rating of each patient.

Social Worker's Evaluation   The social worker administered several forms: a *Social Adjustment Scale (SAS)*, a measure of pre–postoperative change (based on information from both the patient and an informant); a *questionnaire* designed to answer specific questions about the patient's preparation for the surgery (based on individual interviews with both the patient and the informant); and two *estimates of preoperative function*, as compared with the person's optimal functioning, one three years prior and one immediately prior to surgery. These latter categories were discontinued as it proved difficult to obtain accurate information about them. The questioning of the control subjects was suitably modified. *Demographic data* were also obtained from the records.

Psychopharmacological Assessment   A separate review was made by a psychopharmacological consultant of each patient's records and interviews to assess the nature and quality of preoperative, postoperative, and current psychopharmacological therapy.

Psychological Tests   The following procedures, designed to assess a variety of cognitive and motor functions, were administered to all subjects: The *Wechsler Adult Intelligence Scale* (for assessing current intellectual function), the *Wechsler Memory Scale* (a test that yields a memory quotient designed to be comparable to the IQ), the *Porteus Maze Test* (a measure of visual-spatial and planning abilities), the *Wisconsin Card Sorting Test* (a test of the capacity to categorize and sort, and to shift set or plan), the *Benton Visual Retention Test* (a test of the accuracy of visual-spatial memory), the *Continuous Performance Test of Attention (CPT)* (a measure of sustained visual attention and vigilance, in which the subject is required to press a response lever for certain "critical" stimuli), *tapping speed*, and *hand dynamometer* (strength of grip).

Neurological Examination   All patients were subjected to a routine but thorough clinical neurological examination by a neurologist. His findings were entered on a form that permitted scoring of both individual symptoms and global functioning.

EEG Examination This consisted of a standard clinical examination that included waking and sleep recordings (if possible), hyperventilation, and photic stimulation. The records were read by an electroencephalographer and then ranked by us on a 0–4 scale, on which

0 = normal;

1 = normal plus drug-induced fast or slow activity;

2 = moderately abnormal, with some excessive slow activity, asymmetry, and the like;

3 = abnormal due to presence of spike focus; and

4 = abnormal due to presence of multiple spike foci.

Neurosurgical Evaluation Copies of all operative records of study cases were sent to a neurosurgeon for his evaluation and comment. Special note was to be made of any complications or unusual operative circumstances that could be adduced from the surgeons' notes.

Our *test battery and interview schedule in the follow-up study* was essentially the same as in the pilot study, with a few modifications. (1) We added the *Hidden Figures Test* as modified by Teuber and a *new version of the Continuous Performance Test.* (2) There were some changes in format of the questionnaire administered by the social worker in order to obtain more information. (3) The *Problem Appraisal Scale (PAS)* was given four separate times instead of twice. This meant that the patient and the informant were interviewed both for past and present assessments. We also deleted the *Social Adjustment Scale.* (4) Neurological exams and clinical EEGs were given only to patients who had any indication or history of seizures; there were five such patients in all. (5) No consulting neurosurgeon was used.

Research Findings

Classification of Cases

Since the number of cases in the pilot study contributed by any single surgeon was small, we chose to ignore surgery type and instead to classify cases according to outcome. This was done on the basis of two interviews, one by the social worker and one by one of

Table 10.4 Outcome Groups (Pilot Study)

Very Favorable Outcome (VFO)		Less Favorable Outcome (LFO)	
Case Number	Surgeon	Case Number	Surgeon
123	1	109[a]	1
125	1	122	1
211	1	207	1
103	2	213	1
107[a]	2	219	1
113[a]	2	118[a]	2
124	2	126	3
209	2	217[a]	3
222[a]	2	112[a]	Other
104	3	127[a]	3
224	Other	233[a]	3
220	3	129	3
114	3	203[a]	3
226	3		

Note: The 27 patients were classified into 14 VFO and 13 LFO cases on the basis of two independent interviews. The classification reflects basically the patient's evaluation of the degree of relief obtained from the symptoms, his or her current status, and willingness to undergo the operation a second time.

[a] Patient had prior psychosurgery.

the authors (A.F.M.). The classification reflects basically the patient's evaluation of the degree of relief obtained from his/her symptoms, his/her current status, and his/her willingness to undergo surgery a second time. Patients were thus classified into four categories: (1) very much improved or "cured"; (2) slight to moderate improvement; (3) no improvement; and (4) worse. These classifications were made independently of the results of the other testing of the patients. In the classification of the 27 pilot study cases, there were two disagreements—both over whether the improvement was very much or moderate. The differences were resolved by discussion and review of the information. Since the number of cases per category would otherwise be too small, the outcome was dichotomized into very much improved versus all other outcomes. We labeled these groups Very Favorable Outcome (VFO) and Less Favorable Outcome (LFO), respectively. This dichotomization yielded 14 VFOs and 13 LFOs. The case composition of the two groups is presented in Table 10.4.

In the follow-up study, we used a more complex—and we hope, more informative—evaluation procedure. After the patient's visit, three evaluations were made at a staff meeting. Evaluated were (1) improvement: current symptomatology compared with the reported previous symptomatology; (2) functioning: a rating of the adequacy

Table 10.5 Ratings of Patients' Improvement, Functioning, and Support Systems (Follow-up Study)

Case Number	Diagnostic Label	Improvement	Functioning	Support System
	Group I (Most Improved)			
906	Schizophrenic	2	2	2
933	Obsessive-compulsive	2	1	1
953	Depressive/Obsessive-compulsive	2	4	3
961	Depressive/Obsessive-compulsive	2	3	4
962	Depressive	2	2	1
965	Depressive/Obsessive-compulsive	2	3	1
970	Depressive/Obsessive-compulsive	2	3	4
981	Depressive	1	1	2
985	Schizophrenic	1	2	3
986	Depressive	2	2	3
988	Depressive	2	2	1
994	Schizo-affective	2	2	1
992	Depressive/Obsessive-compulsive	1	1	1

Key to Ratings: Improvement: 1 = very much improved, 4 = no improvement, through 7 = very much worse. Functioning: 1 = no limitation of activities, through 6 = total limitation. Support System: 1 = excellent, through 5 = poor.

[a] Patient had prior psychosurgery of the same type.

[b] Patient had a prefrontal leucotomy and then a cingulotomy.

of the patient's current functioning; and (3) support system: a rating of the quality of the patient's support at home or elsewhere.

Improvement was rated on a scale of 1 to 7, ranging from very much improved to very much worse, with 4 signifying no improvement. The psychologists, psychiatrists, and laboratory technicians were given no information about the patient's preoperative history prior to a staff meeting. At that time, the social worker's presentation of the patient's history served as a baseline from which to rate the patient's improvement. In addition to changes in psychopathology, we assessed the development of minor, or more pronounced, unfavorable personality traits if these were in evidence. As a way of summarizing our evaluations, we pooled the two most improved categories (1 and 2) into Group I (13 cases) and the balance of the cases (3–5) into Group II (12 cases). The composition of these two groups is presented in Table 10.5, which also shows the ratings of functioning and support systems.

Functioning was rated on a scale of 1 to 6, ranging from no limitation to total limitation. These ratings refer to the level of interference by the patient's symptoms with day-to-day activities. Judgments of this factor were made on the basis of ability to carry through daily activities, relationships with family, and performance

Table 10.5   *(continued)*

Case Number	Diagnostic Label	Improvement	Functioning	Support System
	Group II (Least Improved)			
901[a]	Depressive/Obsessive-compulsive	5	4	4
905	Depressive/Obsessive-compulsive	3	3	3
914	Depressive	3	4	3
935	Schizo-affective	4	4	5
942	Depressive/Obsessive-compulsive	4	4	4
957	Schizo-affective	4	4	5
963	Schizo-affective	3	4	4
964	Depressive/Obsessive-compulsive	4	4	1
968[b]	Depressive/Obsessive-compulsive	3	4	2
973	Depressive/Obsessive-compulsive	3	3	2
975	Obsessive-Compulsive	3	3	2
990[a]	Depressive/Obsessive-compulsive	4	5	5

of the person's major life role. The *support system* was rated on a scale of 1 to 5, from excellent to poor. Factors taken into account for this rating were living arrangements (level of stability and organization of family and neighborhood when known or type of institutional setting when applicable); stress of reality factors (finances, burdens of responsibility, and so on); and, most important, level of emotional support from significant persons and professionals. We are aware that these three assessments may be interrelated, indeed very highly correlated (note the correlation between ratings in Table 10.5). Nevertheless, we attempted to separate out current functioning from improvement by basing our judgments on different factors, such as day-to-day activities and performance of work role, as described above. Most other studies do not do this, but base their improvement ratings on both current functioning and change from prior status. We considered improvement as relative to the preoperative condition and functioning of a comparison to normal individuals.

Table 10.6 presents the demographic and certain other descriptive characteristics of the two outcome groups and the control subjects in the pilot study. As can be seen from the table, the two outcome groups are reasonably similar on these measures and do not differ

Table 10.6 Demographic and Other Characteristics[a] of Outcome Groups and Controls (Pilot Study)

	Very Favorable Outcome (VFO), N = 14	Least Favorable Outcome (LFO), N = 13	Control, N = 8
Age (at testing 4/76)	49 (29–69)	48.4 (29–67)	45.4 (30–62)
Sex	2 M, 12 F	8 M, 5 F	3 M, 5 F
Occupation (presurgery)			
Higher executive or professional, administrative personnel	5	7	6
Clerical or never worked	9	6	2
Education			
Professional training or some college	7	8	7
High school graduate	7	5	1
Time (years) from first symptom to most recent surgery	17.5 (4–45)	22.0 (5–40)	—
Time (years) from most recent surgery to present examination (4/76)	5.3 (2–9)	4.9 (2–9)	—
Time (years) from first symptom to present examination (4/76)	22.4 (10–49)	26.9 (10–47)[b]	19.4 (12–31)[b]
Marital status			
Never married	2	4	3
Presently married (first)	5	4	4
Presently married (second)	1	0	1
Previously married (divorced, widowed, etc.)	1	1	0

[a] All patients were white.
[b] Data unavailable for one person in LFO and Control group.

sharply in any respect from the controls. Worthy of note is the fact that there are significantly ($p < .05$) more women in the VFO than in the LFO group; that the patients are all white; and that the patients are predominantly middle-aged.

We attempted to analyze changes in occupational, educational, and marital status after surgery, but our analysis revealed relatively little change in these variables. Two VFO patients resumed their education after surgery and one was married. Three VFO cases improved their occupational level, one retired, and the one who was married quit her job. One LFO case improved occupationally, and one took a less demanding position after surgery. It should be noted that these educational, occupational, and marital variables are commonly used as indices of psychosocial adequacy and adjustment. Their failure to indicate substantial change in this instance may reflect, in part, the fact that 17 of the 27 operated cases were female and most of them occupied a homemaker role. Changes in this status were rare.

In the follow-up study, Group I, which included those patients who were judged as showing most improvement, was composed of 2 males and 11 females; Group II, which included those who were judged less improved or worse, was composed of 5 males and 7 females. Group I was older, with a mean age of 55; Group II had a mean age of 44. The two groups did not differ significantly in educational level. Approximately half of the subjects had a high school diploma or less, and half had some education beyond high school graduation, including graduate degrees in two cases. Occupations as defined by Hollingshead (1977) were predominantly in the higher categories, ranging from clerical and technical workers ($N = 12$) to administrators and professionals ($N = 7$).

Prior to surgery, only 4 of the 25 patients in the follow-up study were working full- or part-time. Seventeen could not work due to their illness, and 4 were dependent spouses, students, or retired. After surgery, 8 were employed full- or part-time; 17 were dependent spouses or unemployed. In Group I, 10 patients felt the postoperative limitations on their work were due to factors other than psychopathology, such as family responsibilities or retirement. Three were limited because of their illness. In Group II, 10 patients were limited in work because of continuing psychopathology. In general, there seemed little clear-cut evidence of any contributory physical illness.

Psychiatric and Social Work Ratings (Pilot Study)

Since the various scales and forms administered by the psychiatrist and social worker and self-administered by the patient covered the same ground, it is not surprising that they tended to yield much the same result: The Very Favorable Outcome Group (VFO) appeared healthier than the Less Favorable Outcome Group (LFO). The *Hopkins* and *POMS* data tend to support this finding. The VFO group appeared significantly healthier than either the LFO or control group on the following *POMS* items: tension-anxiety ($p < .05$), friendliness ($p < .05$), and depression ($p < .05$). The *Hopkins Scale* revealed

Table 10.7 Psychiatric and Social Work Ratings (Pilot Study)

	Present Functioning				
	No Illness[a]	VFO	LFO	Control	p
PSS Measure					
Behavioral disturbance	41.0	_42.8_	50.8	59.3	<.05
Impulse control disturbance	45.0	45.3	47.5	_52.6_	<.05
Grandiosity	47.0	47.0	47.0	_54.1_	<.01
Retardation	43.0	43.8	48.4	_53.5_	<.05
Daily routine	37.0	_41.7_	50.1	53.1	<.05
Speech disorganization	45.0	_45.5_	51.4	66.4	<.05
PAS Measure					
Suicidal thoughts		1.0	1.2	_2.0_	<.01
Obsessive-compulsive		1.8	1.5	_4.1_	<.001
Speech disorganization		1.0	1.2	_2.1_	<.05
Leisure problems		1.4	2.1	_2.9_	<.05
Overall severity		_2.5_	4.8	5.0	<.001
Depressed mood		_1.9_	2.9	3.0	<.05
Suspicion		1.0	1.4	_2.1_	<.05
Hallucination		1.0	1.0	_2.0_	<.05
Anger		1.0	1.5	_2.3_	<.05

Note: On the PSS measure, higher scores indicate greater pathology. On the PAS measures, 1 = none, 2 = slight, 3 = mild, 4 = moderate, 5 = marked. Underscore denotes disparate groups.

[a] Score values are derived from the original normative data and indicate no pathology on a particular measure.

greater depression ($p < .05$) and tendency to panic in the LFO and controls than in the VFO subjects and a suggestion of greater schizophrenic tendencies in the LFO cases and controls. It is important to recall that the classification of outcomes was made independently of the results of these tests; hence, the test results corroborate the outcome classification.

On a number of measures from the *PSS* and *PAS* (Table 10.7), both operated groups appear healthier than the controls. This is true, apparently, for impulse control, grandiosity, and retardation on the *PSS*, and for seven of the nine *PAS* variables in Table 10.7. On some measures, however, the LFO group resembles the controls rather closely: named, behavioral disturbance, daily routine, and speech disorganization on the *PSS*, and overall severity and depressed mood on the *PAS*. Significant results were evaluated, usually, by means of a one-way analysis of variance. Since the *PSS* was administered by the psychiatrist without consultation with the social worker or psychologists, the results provide more support for the VFO–LFO patient classifications.

These findings raise the question whether the VFO group was less psychiatrically ill to begin with—that is, before surgery. The *PAS* scores derived from the patients' and companions' estimates of preoperative functioning suggest that this was probably not the case. Although there was significantly greater ($p < .05$) grandiosity in the LFO cases, there was significantly more ($p < .01$) depression in the VFO cases, preoperatively. This latter finding indicates that the VFO group was more depressed than the LFO group prior to the operation, and hence shows a greater improvement after the operation. Several findings bear this out: the *PAS* estimate of present functioning (Table 10.7) shows significantly better functioning with respect to overall severity ($p < .001$) and depressed mood ($p < .05$) in the VFO than in the LFO group. In addition, the *SAS*, which assesses change in social adjustment based on information from both the patient and companion, indicates greater ($p < .001$) overall change in the VFO than in the LFO group.

The questionnaire administered by the social worker to both the patient and the companion was designed to reveal the nature of the information available to the patient and family and the decision-making process at the time of surgery. This questionnaire also probed the patient's current feeling about the operation and specifically asked whether or not the patient would undergo the procedure again. Much of the information obtained from this questionnaire went into the classification of cases—VFO and LFO groups in the pilot study, and Groups I and II in the follow-up study—used throughout this report. Here we shall address the issue of the communications that took place before surgery about the surgery's potential benefits and risks—noting, along the way, any striking differences or similarities between the findings of the pilot study and those of the follow-up study.

The "typical" experience of a patient will be described in narrative form, with exceptions noted where the VFO and LFO groups differed. Some data from Table 10.6 are incorporated in this narrative.

> The patient is a married white female, with some college education, who is in her late forties. Her illness dates back sixteen or more years, and she has usually had at least one hospitalization and one course of electroshock therapy. If her illness was classified as pain or headache, she received many analgesic and probably narcotic drugs. She has also received tranquilizer and antidepressant drugs, and most often, psychotherapy. The operation was suggested or recommended by a psychiatrist, usually, and was described to her in at least superficial terms. Moderate benefits were promised by the surgeon and expected by the patient. No promises were made concerning exactly when the benefits would be forthcoming. The surgical risk was explained as minimal to none, and the patient was told that she would probably not be made worse, nor would her intellect suffer. There was slightly more recall of explanations of serious risks by patients in the VFO group.

There seemed to be no alternative to surgery at the time it was being considered, and usually no other types of psychosurgery were discussed. The patient and informant generally felt free to question the surgeon as much as they wished. The patient herself (usually after consulting with spouse or family) made the decision to have the operation. Three of the LFO cases (only) reported (or recalled) some family disagreement as to whether the surgery should be performed. However, there was little pressure from family members or other sources. If improvement came, it was within a year or less. (Note here that both the patient and the informant see significantly more ($p < .001$) overall beneficial change if she is a member of the VFO as opposed to the LFO group. This highly significant difference comes through in every change measure.) There are few if any regrets expressed, although more ($p < .05$) of the informants of the LFO cases (6 of them) express regrets than the informants of the VFO cases (only one). The VFO cases would almost unequivocally have the operation again, but there are more reservations and qualifications among both the patients and informants of the LFO group.

Since this is a description of a typical case, it fails to indicate the variability in some of the measures. However, this narrative would apply in large measure to most of the patients. A difficulty with the description concerns the remembered interaction with the surgeon at the time of preoperative evaluation. Many patients report being so ill (including being so heavily medicated) at the time that they have faulty or little recall of what the surgeon told them. Often the patient describes having been desperate for help and willing to accept any risk if there were some chance of relief. This report tends to agree with the surgeons' reported experience noted earlier and relates to our problems in obtaining persons for whom the operation was recommended but declined.

Psychiatric and Social Work Ratings (Follow-Up Study)

Table 10.8 is derived from an analysis of the *Psychiatric Status Schedule (PSS)*, which was administered by the psychiatrist in the follow-up study. In this table, the scores from the two outcome groups are compared with each other and with the scores from the three groups used by the New York Psychiatric Institute in its original standardization (Spitzer et al., 1970). These include the Washington Heights outpatients, who have been sick for two or more years and are still in therapy; the Fountain House patients, who have had multiple hospitalizations; and the Washington Heights group of normal controls. The data show that Group I (the most improved) patients have scores on these scales commensurate with those of the Washington

Table 10.8 Psychiatric Ratings of Outcome Groups and Comparison Populations (Follow-up Study)

	Group I	Group II	F Ratio for Group I Versus Group II[a]	Washington Heights Normals[b]	Washington Heights Outpatients[b]	Fountain House Patients[b]
Total score	37.15	50.27	15.73***	33.52	45.42	41.54
Subjective Distress	39.54	53.27	14.90***	35.75	45.55	43.89
Behavioral disturbance	40.00	50.09	8.58**	42.12	46.00	46.46
Impulse control disturbance	46.46	51.91	2.71	45.56	47.60	46.52
Reality testing disturbance	44.85	49.09	3.64	44.48	47.29	46.26
Summary role score[c]	47.91	59.11	14.95***	42.12	49.43	58.19

Note: Ratings are from the PSS measure; higher scores indicate greater pathology.
[a] Superscript ** = $p < .01$; *** = $p < .001$.
[b] From Spitzer et al., 1970.
[c] The summary role score is an average of the role scores obtained.

Heights normal group. The Group II (the least improved) patients, however, appear to be as sick as or sicker than both of the patient comparison groups. Each of these scores is a summary or second-level score made up of several component first-level scores. For example, the summary role score is an average of the role scores obtained, and the summary score of subjective distress is composed of scores of depression/anxiety, daily routine, leisure time, social isolation, suicidal self-mutilation, and somatic concern. As in the pilot study, these scores support our clinical dichotomy.

The clinical dichotomy in the follow-up study is supported further by ratings of both patient and informant on the *Problem Appraisal Scale (PAS)*. Both preoperative and current behavior were rated. The comparisons are presented in Figures 10.1, 10.2, and 10.3. As seen in Figure 10.1, there are no significant differences between outcome groups on any assessment of the patient's *preoperative* behavior. The ratings by patients and informants are similar. Ratings of *current* behavior, however, as shown in Figure 10.2, differ extensively for the two outcome groups. Group I patients consider themselves better sleepers, better adjusted in their social relations with family and others, less depressed, less obsessive-compulsive, less withdrawn, and less angry than do the Group II patients.

It is important to note here, in light of the fact that this is a retrospective study, that there is a high correlation between the informants' and patients' ratings on the majority of items on the scale. However, as shown in Figure 10.3, a few symptoms were rated differently by patients and their informants. The informants did not see the Group I patients as less obsessive-compulsive, less withdrawn, and less angry, but saw them as having less grandiosity and having less phobic-anxiety than the Group II patients.

The two self-rating scales, one a symptom scale and the other a mood scale, also support the clinical dichotomy of the two groups. On the *Hopkins Scale,* the improved group is characterized as less anxious, less depressed, less obsessive-compulsive, less sensitive to the interview, and showing less schizophrenic tendencies. On the *POMS* they reveal less anger, less depression, more vigor, less confusion, and more friendliness.

In the follow-up study, we questioned the patients about new symptoms or changes in behavior and found that these were experienced by a large number of patients. Five patients suffered seizures postoperatively (2 in Group I and 3 in Group II), and 5 reported some sort of pain syndrome, mainly severe headaches. One-third of the patients and a slightly larger number of relatives mentioned new characteristics of apathy or lethargy, such as poor housekeeping or

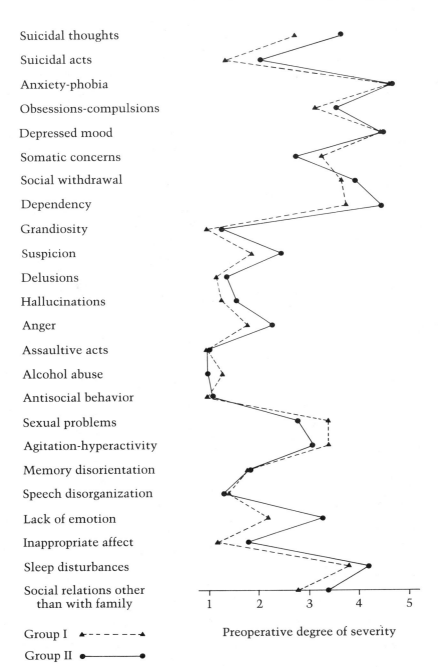

Figure 10.1 Comparison of Group I patients' and Group II patients' Problem Appraisal Scale (PAS) ratings of their preoperative functioning.

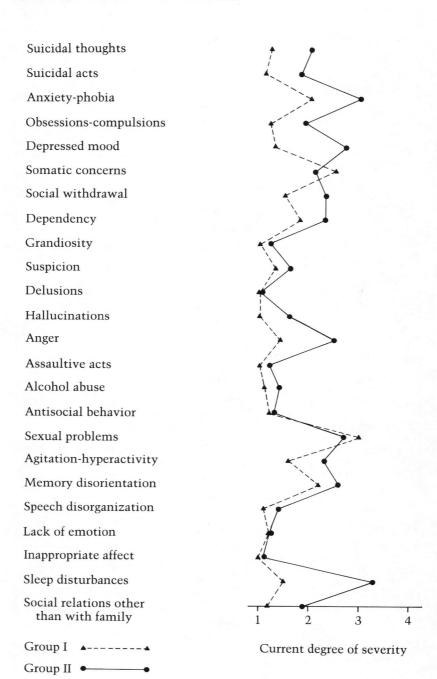

Suicidal thoughts
Suicidal acts
Anxiety-phobia
Obsessions-compulsions
Depressed mood
Somatic concerns
Social withdrawal
Dependency
Grandiosity
Suspicion
Delusions
Hallucinations
Anger
Assaultive acts
Alcohol abuse
Antisocial behavior
Sexual problems
Agitation-hyperactivity
Memory disorientation
Speech disorganization
Lack of emotion
Inappropriate affect
Sleep disturbances
Social relations other
than with family

Group I ▲--------▲
Group II ●————————●

Current degree of severity

Figure 10.2 Comparison of Group I patients' and Group II patients' Problem Appraisal Scale (PAS) ratings of their current functioning.

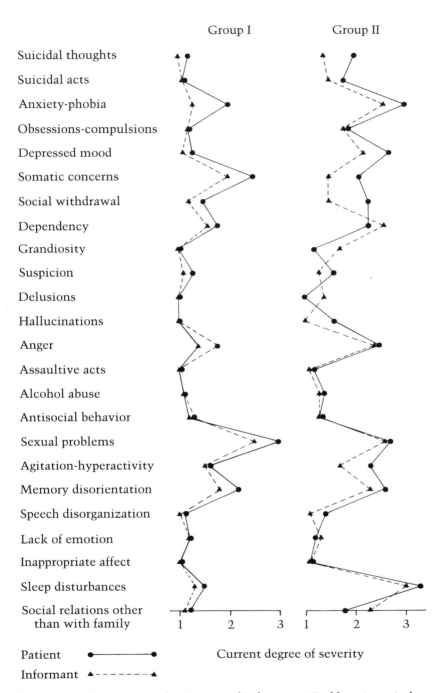

Figure 10.3 Comparison of patients' and informants' Problem Appraisal Scale (PAS) ratings of patients' current functioning.

poor personal habits. Half of the patients in the follow-up study (irrespective of outcome) specified symptoms of disinhibition, such as excessive weight gain or swearing, as did two-thirds of the relatives. One patient reported memory impairment, while 6 relatives felt that such impairment existed. Out of 8 patients in Group I who reported new symptoms, 5 saw the level of impairment resulting from these symptoms to be minimal and 3 saw it as moderate. In Group II, also with 8 patients, 4 felt impairment to be minimal and 4 moderate.

Comparison of the Pilot Study and Follow-Up Study

There appears to have been a somewhat higher incidence of undesirable side effects in the follow-up study than in the pilot study. However, it is not certain whether this finding reflects the differential effects of the bimedial leucotomy or the more vigorous questioning (in terms of support levels and current functioning as well as improvement) of patients in the follow-up study. Moreover, the follow-up cases were older and often appeared easily fatigued, fragile, or cantankerous. It was often necessary to modify the testing schedule (for example, to hold five two-hour sessions rather than two five-hour sessions) and to remind the cases of appointments by telephoning them to awaken them in the morning. It is doubtful whether this group would have been able to travel 3,000 miles, as did some of the subjects in the pilot study.

Another imponderable complication in the comparison between studies is the fact that 10 of the 27 operated patients in the pilot study (seven LFOs and three VFOs—see Table 10.4) had a prior experience with psychosurgery; in 7 cases this was with the same surgeon who performed the procedure of concern in this study. Presumably, there must have been at least partial, if temporary, relief afforded by the earlier operation, and some of the material in the interviews attests to this. Surgeon 2 considered the second operation a matter of course. The effects of this earlier experience on patient and informant attitudes are difficult to assess, since it is not clear whether it tended to result in more positive or negative expectations. In the follow-up study, 3 of the Group II (least improved) cases had had prior surgery, and none of the Group I (most improved) cases; see Table 10.5.

A thorough and detailed analysis of other therapies is difficult, either because of incomplete records or faulty memory on the part of patient and informant. Consequently, the precise dosages of drugs, length of treatment (either pharmacological or psychotherapeutic), exact number of hospitalizations, numbers of ECT treatments, and so on were often unavailable. Nevertheless, in the pilot study we found that most patients had had trials with many other psychiatric treatments over the seventeen to twenty-two years (on the average) that they had suffered from their illness prior to psychosurgery. These treatments include minor tranquilizers; major tranquilizers; antidepressants of various types; sedatives; lithium; stimulants; analgesics and narcotics for pain; hospitalization with or without insulin coma or electroshock therapy; intermittent, regular or intensive psychotherapy; and miscellaneous other treatments. Significantly ($p < .05$) more VFO than LFO cases had taken MAO inhibitors (antidepressants) prior to surgery.

In the follow-up study, we found many of the same results but were able to pinpoint pretreatment more exactly because most of the patients had extensive clinical records. Most of the patients had undergone 15–36 ECT, but the number ranged from 0 to over 100. Again, we found it so difficult to ascertain preoperative medication that we settled for current medication. Since the average length of time for the patients between first symptom and operation was eight years, all of them had undergone other therapies, which they found either useless or providing only temporary relief.

Psychological Test Scores

The majority of the scores yielded by the battery of tests indicated no significant differences among groups. The only significant differences that were found in the pilot study are presented in Table 10.9. The individual significant findings must be viewed cautiously, since so many comparisons were made. However, the findings can be interpreted as follows. The perseverative error on the *Wisconsin Card Sorting Task* indicates a tendency to continue to sort the stimulus cards according to a previously correct sorting scheme (that is, color, form, or number), and to fail to shift when the examiner's response indicates that the prior scheme is now incorrect. Both operated groups appear to make larger numbers of errors (slightly more in the VFO), suggesting some inability to adapt easily to the test requirements. In this, they differ significantly from the controls. The *Continuous Performance Test (CPT)* error of commission reflects a tendency to respond inappropriately (and possibly impulsively) to noncritical stimuli in this vigilance-type task. The significant result here appears to be due to the poor performance of the LFO group. On

Table 10.9 Psychological Test Scores (Pilot Study)

	VFO, N = 14	LFO, N = 12	Controls, N = 7	p
Wechsler Adult Intelligence Scale				
Verbal IQ	117.5	109.0	108.9	—
Performance IQ	111.1	103.1	99.4	—
Full scale IQ	115.8	107.4	105.4	—
Wechsler Memory Quotient	119.5	101.8	111.3	—
Wisconsin Card Sorting				
Perseverative errors	29.9	24.1	7.0[a]	<.05
Continuous Performance Test				
Errors of commission	6.6	33.4[a]	15.7	<.05
Benton Visual Retention				
Perseverative errors	0.1[a]	0.8	1.1	<.05

[a] Significantly different from both other groups.

the *Benton Visual Retention Task*, the perseverative error is a measure of the subject's tendency to repeat portions of a previously presented stimulus card. The LFO and control groups appear to make more errors of this type than the VFO group.

In addition, Table 10.9 presents some descriptive intellectual data. Two general characteristics appear. The VFO group is somewhat brighter than the other two groups, although not significantly, and has somewhat higher memory functioning. Also, all groups tend to have higher verbal than performance IQs and memory. For 11 of the subjects in the pilot study, preoperative IQ test scores were available. A comparison was made of the amount of changes in the VFO and LFO groups taken separately and combined. These data are presented in Table 10.10. The data in Table 10.10 indicate an overall improvement in Full Scale IQ postoperatively ($p < .05$), but this is contributed primarily by the LFO group, all of whom showed an increase in Full Scale IQ. In the VFO group, 3 patients improved and 3 obtained worse scores postoperatively.

Very few of the psychological test findings in the pilot study were confirmed in the data of the follow-up study. These results are presented in Table 10.11. It is still true that the group with the better clinical outcome (Group I in the follow-up study) appears brighter and may have better functioning than the other group. No other differences between the groups were found on the *Wisconsin Card Sorting Test, Benton*, and *CPT*. However, as in the pilot study, the clinically improved group tends to make more perseverative errors than does the less improved group.

Table 10.10 Pre- and Postoperative WAIS Scores (Pilot Study)

	VFO[a]	LFO	Total
N	6	5	11
Preoperative full scale IQ	111.7	104.0	108.2
Postoperative full scale IQ	116.2	111.6	114.1
p value of t test	n.s.[b]	p < .001	p < .05

[a] Three subjects obtained higher and three lower scores postoperatively.
[b] Not significant.

Table 10.11 Psychological Test Scores (Follow-up Study)

	Group I, N = 13	Group II, N = 12	p
WAIS			
Vocabulary score	13.85	11.92	<.05
Verbal IQ	114.39	104.50	<.05
Full scale IQ	111.31	103.92	>.05
Wechsler Memory Quotient	121.92	106.50	<.05
Porteus Maze			
Cut corners	1.50	.54	>.05
Wisconsin Card Sorting			
Sort shifts[a]	2.69	2.63	n.s.
Perseverative errors	17.46	10.09	n.s.
Continuous Performance Test FPX[b]			
Omission errors	2.46	1.91	n.s.
Commission errors	2.54	4.18	n.s.
Mean time to respond (MS)	482.50	475.54	n.s.
Continuous Performance Test DPX[c]			
Incorrect	2.07	13.36	>.05
Mean time to respond (MS)	489.92	441.82	<.05
Benton Visual Retention			
Perseverative errors	1.46	1.22	n.s.

[a] A shift in the criterion used to sort the stimulus cards.
[b] FPX = fixed-paced task.
[c] DPX = dynamic-paced task.

Results of Neurological and EEG Examination

No significant differences were found in neurological status between the two outcome groups in the pilot study. Positive neurological findings were in fact rare and almost invariably attributed by the neurologist to other disease processes. Similarly, no differences were found in the average degree of EEG pathology among the three groups. Four subjects in the VFO group had EEGs that were not considered normal, 2 of which showed a spike focus. The others were normal or showed changes attributable to medication. The LFO group contained 3 subjects with abnormal EEGs, one of which showed multiple spike foci. The others were normal or showed possible evidence of drug-related changes only. No spike foci were seen in the control group, although the EEG in 3 of the subjects was classified as at least borderline abnormal. The remaining subjects showed possible drug-related changes or were normal. Seven presurgical EEGs have been located. Four subjects have EEGs classified as normal at both pre- and postsurgical examinations; one with a postsurgical spike focus shows a focus presurgery; one subject with a moderately pathological EEG presurgery shows a less abnormal record postsurgery. In one subejct only was there evidence that a normal EEG presurgery became moderately abnormal postoperatively. The number of cases is too small to indicate whether any particular operation is associated with risk of developing a pathological EEG. Nevertheless, it can be noted that in the 3 subjects in this report who have had an additional psychosurgical procedure prior to the one of interest in this report, one had a normal EEG (following transorbital leucotomy plus prefrontal sonic lesion), one shows evidence of possible drug-induced changes only (following cingulotomy plus orbital undercutting), and one shows a moderately pathological record (following cingulotomy plus a multiple-target stereotaxic procedure). One additional note: 4 of the 13 subjects in the LFO group were left-handed, whereas only 1 of the 14 subjects in the VFO group was left-handed.

There were no substantial differences in outcome of the neurological and EEG examinations between the pilot and follow-up studies. In the latter, only 4 patients, those with a history of seizure disorders postsurgery, were seen by the staff neurologist and underwent clinical EEGs. Generally, the neurological findings were normal. For 3 patients, however, the EEGs were abnormal, consistent with the diagnosis of seizure disorder. Two of these patients are on anticonvulsant medication and are seizure-free. The third patient reports developing seizures eight years after surgery. The staff neurologist considered this disorder to be of uncertain relationship to the surgery and possibly "potentiated by alcohol withdrawal." This patient is under the care of a neurologist who diagnosed postsurgical seizure disorder continuing after medication was prescribed. He noted there was a question as to whether the patient took the prescribed medication. A CAT-scan revealed postfrontal lobotomy changes but was otherwise normal. The fourth patient had a single seizure following surgery. She is now entirely seizure-free and off anticonvulsants, and her EEG record is within normal limits. In addition, another patient reported to us during the interview that she had convulsions twice after using marijuana. She never received any treatment for these.

Discussion

This project was conceived initially as a pilot study with two major purposes: (1) to determine the feasibility of a retrospective approach to studying the effects (specifically, the efficacy and safety) of psychosurgery, and (2) if possible, to acquire some information about the benefits and/or hazards of psychosurgery. We will discuss the second issue first.

Benefits and/or Hazards of Psychosurgery

The Balance of Evidence   From a consideration of the results of the two studies, it is apparent that 14 of the 27 subjects in our pilot sample (the VFO group) and 13 of the 25 in the follow-up group (Group I) have derived considerable benefit from their psychosurgical operations. It should be noted that the standards on which we based our division of cases into VFO and LFO groups (or Group I and Group II) are stricter than those used in most evaluations published in the psychosurgical literature. Had we included cases showing slight to moderate benefit, the proportion of "improved" cases would have been 21/27 or 78 percent in the pilot study and 19/25 or 76 percent in the follow-up study. This would be in agreement with at least some of the published studies. However, our dichotomy appears to have substantial validity as evidenced, in both studies, by the patients' own (and their informants') statements in several interviews, the standardized psychiatric and other interview material, the self-rating scales, the relatively low use of psychotropic drugs by patients in the improved groups, and the general willingness of these patients to undergo the procedure a second time. That the behavioral improvement may be relatively permanent is attested by the fact that five years (on the average) elapsed between surgery and our examination in the pilot study and eight years between surgery and the follow-up study.

On the other hand, the other 13 cases of the pilot study sample (the LFO Group) and 12 Group II cases in the follow-up study had outcomes ranging from worse to only moderate benefit. On a number of measures it was difficult to distinguish the LFO cases in the pilot study from the controls. These subjects (and the informant-family members) expressed more reservations about undergoing the procedure again. The same holds for Group II in the follow-up study. In this connection, we note that 10 of the 27 cases in the pilot study and 3 of the 25 in the follow-up study had had an operation prior to the one that brought them into the study.

In both groups of subjects, the decision to undergo the operation seems to have involved at least a fair degree of discussion with the surgeon and the psychiatrist or other physician who recommended it initially. The period of time over which the subjects suffered from some psychiatric illness ranged from 4 to 45 years in the pilot study (for the operated group as a whole). Since the mean is over 17 years (Table 10.6) it does not appear that surgery was considered prematurely. Similarly, in the follow-up study the patients reported illness durations ranging from 4 to 23 years and averaging 10.52 years. It should be noted that these figures are based on the patients' first contact with a professional about their psychiatric problems. Their actual illnesses may have predated this by a considerable time.

Factors Associated with a Successful Outcome What can be gleaned from the data concerning the presurgical characteristics of patients who had a very favorable outcome? The following characteristics emerge, which may possibly merit further evaluation. In the pilot study, the VFO group showed greater evidence of depression preoperatively than the LFO group, and this is the symptom that appears to change most with surgery (interview data). The only other characteristic that emerges is an indication of less grandiosity in the VFO group, possibly an index of less schizophrenic-like pathology in this group.

The findings of the follow-up study, however, do *not* provide confirmation for the special susceptibility of the depressive symptomatology to surgery. We could not, in multiple analyses, confirm that affective disorders respond more favorably to surgical intervention than schizophrenic or schizo-affective illness. Unfortunately, our sample of cases is still too small to determine whether there is a particular surgical procedure that is more likely than any other to benefit intractable depression, nor can we conclude that there is a single diagnostic entity or cluster of symptoms that is most likely to be benefited by surgery. Various alternatives suggest themselves to account for the differences between the pilot and follow-up study results. One is that the perseverance or stability of specific psychiatric symptoms (or the reliability of diagnostic labels) is weak. Depression may change to obsessive-compulsive disorder, which may in turn change to schizophrenic-like symptoms. Possibly, according to this line of reasoning, the only persistent and reliable variable to consider is psychic pain or distress. And for reasons that still elude us, approximately 50 percent of persons afflicted with chronic psychic distress are benefited from some form of destruction of brain tissue.

There are two predictors of outcome that are seen to hold for both the pilot and follow-up studies. One of these is sex. Combining the data from both studies, we found that the chance of a favorable outcome (VFO or Group I) for a female patient was two out of three; for a male patient it was one in four. Stated in another way, in the VFO-Group I combined cases, females outnumber males by six to one; in the LFO-Group II combined cases, females and males are represented equally.

We are not certain how to interpret this finding, but there are numerous possibilities. Each of these is suggested by at least one patient interview. It may be that the homemaker role, which so many of our female patients occupy, is more conducive to a good recovery than the (possibly) more stressful role of wage earner. Many of our female patients grew up in an era when it was not acceptable for a woman to work after she was married. Alternatively, it is conceivable that the successful-outcome male patients are too busy to take time off from successful careers and occupations, and hence are less likely to respond to invitations to be studied. Since more women suffer from affective disorders than men, more women patients were included in the sample, thus skewing the data for statistical purposes. Also, the men may have been sicker prior to surgery. A less sanguine interpretation is that they are less willing than women to discuss their past illness, or to request time off from an employer from whom the prior illness (and brain surgery) may have been concealed. More than one of the patients in the follow-up study spoke of the stigma of a "lobotomy" and how important it was to keep this information hidden from personnel offices, job interviewers, and the like. Finally, there is the possibility that there is something about the female brain—its anatomy, chemistry, or physiology—that renders it more likely to show the kind of change after surgery that we interpret as a favorable behavioral outcome. Goldman has provided evidence that in at least young male and female monkeys there are sex differences in behavioral effects after experimental lesions (Goldman et al., 1974), and Lansdell has shown that the effects of temporal lobe removals in female epileptic patients are different from those in male patients (Lansdell, 1968).

A second predictor of outcome (identified, of course, retrospectively) is prior experience with psychosurgery. Patients with a less

favorable outcome are more likely to have had a prior surgical procedure (the chance is 40 percent, or 10 in 25) than those with a more
favorable outcome (the chance is 11 percent, or 3 in 27). These data
are based on the pooled samples of the two studies. The information
is understandable, perhaps, if one assumes that the operation produced some prior benefit or relief from distress in these persons,
although not of a permanent nature. This suggestion stems from
interview data, in fact.

Some postsurgical characteristics of the subjects who experienced
major benefit merit comment, but the picture that emerges is by no
means entirely consistent. The VFO and Group I cases showed greater evidence of what might be viewed as cognitive loss: (1) there was
a trend for VFO and Group I patients to make the most perseverative
errors on the *Wisconsin Card Sorting Task*, despite the fact that they
appeared somewhat brighter and appeared to have somewhat better memories (Tables 10.9, 10.10, and 10.11). This measure of the
ability to shift "set" in a flexible way has been shown to be sensitive
to frontal lobe damage (Milner, 1963); (2) the VFO subjects did not as
a group show the highly significant rise in IQ seen in the LFO group,
presumably due to practice and/or amelioration of psychiatric
illness; and (3) on electrophysiological measures from frontal locations, there was some indication of reduced capacity to show the
characteristic cerebral electrical activity *(Contingent Negative
Variation)* that usually accompanies the presentation of a stimulus
requiring a response (Tecce, Orzack, and Mirsky, 1978).

Not all of the findings conformed to this pattern of greatest "deficit" in the improved VFO patients; the error scores on the measure
of visual attention *(CPT* task) suggested that the least accurate (and
possibly most impulsive) performers were in the less-improved LFO
groups, followed by the controls, with the improved VFO group
performing best. Nevertheless, these findings suggested that the
VFO subjects were performing in certain ways below the expectation created by their somewhat higher IQs compared with the LFO
cases.

These speculations raised the possibility that recovery from the
severe and crippling psychiatric illnesses from which these patients
suffer may in some cases be made at a price—the loss of certain
cognitive capacities. We suggested in our discussion of the pilot
study data (1977) that, in some way, this loss permits the patient to
function in a more effective and less troubled way. It also follows,
we suggested, that recovery is less likely to occur if some cognitive
loss is not sustained. However, the psychological test data from the
follow-up group, shown in Table 10.11, appear to provide relatively

little support for the cognitive loss–behavioral recovery hypothesis. Nevertheless, there remains a suggestive trend in the data. The follow-up study was not precisely a replication of the pilot study, to be sure, but it was similar enough to encourage the belief that similar principles (if indeed there are any) should be operating. We obviously need to study more cases to determine whether there is any real merit to the hypothesis.

Some Undesirable Effects of Psychosurgery   A number of patients, in whom outcomes ranged from moderately to extremely successful, reported with some poignancy the necessity of having to conceal the fact of their prior psychosurgery. In some cases, this deception was necessary in order to obtain a desirable position. One supposes that the public image of the patient who has undergone brain surgery for psychiatric illness may be largely conditioned by the film "One Flew Over the Cuckoo's Nest," and by similar distortions. Consequently, considerable fear, doubt, and suspicion could surround any person who admitted to having had such a brain operation—and could conceivably prevent that person from attaining desirable goals. In our pilot study, we witnessed, or rather precipitated, a very moving life event. A young woman who had been married for nearly two years had informed her husband about her brain surgery only after receiving the letter from us requesting participation in the study. The letter from us apparently precipitated her revealing this information to him for the first time. When the couple came to Boston to be interviewed, the husband had had the new knowledge only for a matter of ten days. He commented frequently about his wife's sunny disposition. The unfortunate side effect of having to conceal and live with knowledge of prior major psychiatric treatment is not unexpected, and is undoubtedly related to the aura of fear that may surround any person who is known to have had a major mental illness.

Another unfortunate side effect of psychosurgery was expressed by at least one patient in the following way (paraphrased): "I know that there is something wrong with my brain since I have had the operation. As a result, I tend to blame my failure at being able to learn and my other difficulties or failures on the operation. It's a crutch that I wish I didn't have." This patient was mildly depressed, in our judgment, and her depression may have colored this statement. However, the feeling expressed in this statement could also represent an internalization of the limited expectations that the rest of the world has with respect to mental patients generally, and those who have undergone psychosurgery specifically. It would be of interest to be able to explore these issues further.

Some other issues emerged in the follow-up study or were somehow crystallized in our thinking from a more amorphous state in the pilot study. We will mention these briefly. Some are promissory notes for future investigations or papers, some are mentioned because they seem important to remark on in the context of this chapter and book, and some are responses to criticisms that have been raised about our pilot study.

Evaluation of Outcome

Some who have read our prior report (1977) or other evaluations of the outcome of psychiatric surgery have been extremely critical of our assessment procedures because of the postoperative state of some of the patients. While it is true that some of these patients live extremely limited or marginally adequate lives, life for them is still far better in many cases than it was prior to surgery. One of the follow-up cases was apparently, at one point, headed for a career in mathematics and science; she now operates a newsstand. Nevertheless, this is a superior existence, in our view, to the repeated hospitalizations interspersed with suicide attempts that characterized the years prior to surgery. As our social worker points out, although walking with crutches is severely impaired locomotion in an absolute sense, compared with being bedridden it is a marvelous enhancement of capacity. One must recall, in short, the level from which many of these patients started.

We have leaned heavily, in our evaluation of the outcome of psychosurgical procedures, on the patient's own assessment of the effectiveness of the operation. Routinely, we asked the patient, "If you had to do it all over, would you have the operation?" and "Would you recommend the operation to other people?" Questions such as these led to a free and open discussion of the patient's view of the efficacy of the procedure. Usually, there was reasonably close agreement between the patient's view, the informant's view, and the objective tests of the patient's status. However, since it was subjective pain and distress that led the patients to obtain psychiatric care in the first place, and ultimately brain surgery, it seemed reasonable that the patient's own view should be weighed heavily in our evaluation. This self-evaluation was the basis from which the professional staff developed its assessments of improvement. Assessments took into account new symptoms, informant's report, recent exacerbations of illness, current drug therapy, and so on. In the event of disparity between the reports from the patient and informant, we tended, for the most part, to rate the degree of improvement as less. Thus, any discrepancy in the information resulted in a bias toward judgment of less improvement. It is not clear that this is necessarily the most objective way of proceeding. However, there may be no completely satisfactory solution except to present multiple outcome measures, and the ultimate report of all of our patient information must do that. It might also prove worthwhile (we have not yet attempted this) to study the cases with marked discrepancies (in terms of outcome measures) to see in what ways they differ from other cases we have studied. In any event, the number of cases in which there were discrepancies in the information was small.

The Referral Network

Early on in our planning of the pilot study, one of our informal consultants advised us to study what he referred to as the "referral network." By this he meant the process, the persons, and the institutions involved in the provision of service for psychiatric illness. The concept of the "network" had little meaning until we began to study patients who had received treatment from a local clinic, in our follow-up study. From interviews with a number of patients it became apparent that many of them had been treated by one or another member of the same group of psychiatrists; that they had been hospitalized at one or more of the same group of local institutions; and that they were referred ultimately to the same psychiatrist at one local clinic, who arranged, eventually, for the surgical procedure to be performed. The referral network appears to have the following characteristics: There are certain psychiatrists in the Boston area who are more likely than others to use organically oriented therapies in their treatment of patients. They frequently recommend the use of electroshock therapy, as well as psychotropic medications. They tend not to be psychoanalytically oriented and appear to eschew membership in the Boston Psychoanalytic Institute. On the other hand, they are more likely to be members of the Boston Society for Psychiatry and Neurology and, most likely, the Society for Biological Psychiatry. The patients treated by these psychiatrists appear to belong primarily to certain ethic and religious groups. Their expectation of therapeutic transactions with a physician do not, by and large, include delving deeply into innermost feelings, past events, wishes, fantasies, and dreams. From interviews with such patients, it seems clear that many of them would have found and would find it difficult to accept such dynamically oriented or insight therapy. They expect to receive pills when they are sick, and in the event the illness is very persistent and grave, an operation is not unexpected.

We are not in a position to reach any conclusions with respect to the success rates of organically oriented versus dynamically oriented treatment in psychiatry. Our sample of cases is small and it is highly selected in any case. Furthermore, the dichotomy we have drawn between organic and dynamic treatment is probably exaggerated; many, if not most, dynamically oriented psychiatrists use psychotropic medications, and most organic therapists provide at least supportive psychotherapy to their patients. Some of our cases report having had extensive courses of psychotherapy, in fact. In terms of the specific treatments that are recommended and provided, psychosurgery and psychoanalysis, and to some extent electroconvulsive shock therapy, are likely to differentiate most sharply between the two kinds of psychiatric approaches. One of us (A.F.M.) recalls vividly an interview with a senior psychoanalytically oriented clinician who reported how ineffective all efforts to treat an obsessive-compulsive female patient had been, and how he felt personally unable to refer her to the organic "network" for psychosurgery even though he felt she might benefit from it. Such referral, in fact, did take place somehow. The patient underwent the operation and received considerable benefit from it.

Our study of psychosurgery has introduced us to two referral networks in the Boston area. It would be valuable to investigate this sociological-medical phenomenon further, in terms of the relationships among mental illness, patient and societal expectations about treatment and sociological factors.

The Question of Selection Bias

We have been criticized for using the surgeon to furnish us the patients. Indeed, there was no other way for us to obtain the names. As noted before, the surgeons were most cooperative and offered to throw open their files to us. Unfortunately, we were forced to refuse their offer. Efforts to verify or cross-check the surgeon's list with the hospital record were usually unsuccessful. Only one surgeon's records were made available to us in this manner. This was apparently due to the slowness or reluctance of the administrative personnel of the hospital to release the information—and not, obviously, to the surgeon's wish to conceal data. Indeed, the only hospital operating room list we have obtained was released at the surgeon's insistence.

It has been suggested that the surgeons influenced the case selection. It must be noted, however, that any study design or plan that required the surgeon to serve merely as a passive supplier of names and addresses would not succeed. Many of the patients, in both studies, called the surgeon (or in some cases their psychiatrist) to ask whether or not they should participate. One of the surgeons had in fact modified the original permission letter because he thought it too cold and impersonal. Another added a personal note to each letter. In the follow-up study the referring psychiatrist actually telephoned the patients urging them to participate. We encountered no evidence that any of the cooperating surgeons or psychiatrists placed more pressure to participate on patients with good rather than with poor outcomes. The refusal rate in general appears to be low.

The selection of cases, as noted in a number of places in this report, depended primarily on the design we wished to follow (that is, comparing affective with schizophrenic-type illnesses) and not on any overt or obvious selection by the surgeon. In communications both before and after publication of the pilot study in 1977, surgeons have generally expressed disappointment that more of their patients were not to be studied, and in general gave the impression of being most eager to have the thorough and independent evaluation of their cases that our team could provide.

If there is any lingering doubt about bias in our sample, it does *not* appear to relate to the reluctance of the cooperating surgeons to open their files. Instead, it has to do with patients who have not answered our letters requesting their participation, or who have refused to participate. Are we justified in assuming that the same proportion of "cure" exists in the sample that we cannot contact? Conceivably, it could be higher. Or, this group may represent a population of persons for whom the operation was a dismal failure. A prospective study, unless it were done on some sort of captive population, would have no more success in reaching such cases in extended follow-up than our retrospective study.

The Feasibility of a Retrospective Study of Psychosurgery

Our experience with these studies leads to the conclusion that retrospective studies are indeed feasible, although they have certain limitations, some of which we did not anticipate. On the positive side of a retrospective study is the fact that a patient can be seen several years after the treatment. To do this in a prospective study would involve enormous expenditure of funds to keep a team together to test patients over a long term. On the negative side is the fact that a retrospective study cannot study the same individual pre- and postsurgery. This is a serious problem, particularly (for example) in view of the suggestion that cognitive loss may be related to recovery from illness. A prospective study, on the other hand, is handicapped by having to test highly medicated, sick, distressed persons prior to the surgical insult. We admit that our attempts to estimate preoperative function are undoubtedly not completely successful. The stress surrounding the period when the operation was being discussed probably interferes with the effective recall of events, particularly by the patient. As noted, many patients report this. Our protection against gross distortion in recall is the interview with the informant and the use of the available records.

Summary

Under the auspices of the National Commission for the Protection of Human Subjects of Biomedical and Behavioral Research, and the National Institute of Mental Health, a pilot study and a follow-up study were undertaken to investigate the feasibility of retrospective investigations of the efficacy and safety of psychosurgery and to contribute some information concerning the benefits and/or hazards of psychosurgery.

To accomplish this, 52 persons who received psychosurgical operations during the period 1965–1974 were studied. In addition, a group of 8 unoperated control cases with psychiatric illnesses similar to those of the operated cases were also studied. The operated patients were provided through the cooperation of four neurosurgeons. All cases were evaluated by a team of investigators from Boston University Medical Center and Boston State Hospital. The team included psychiatrists, psychologists, social workers, neurologists, electroencephalographers, and other experts in the area of psychiatric and neurological research and practice.

The primary symptoms of the majority of the patients included depression or affective illness, obsessive-compulsive behavior, phobias, acute anxiety, and chronic pain. These symptoms were usually present in varying combinations and were accompanied in some cases by a diagnosis of schizophrenia. The patients were on the average in their late forties or early fifties, had had their symptoms on the average of seventeen to twenty years, and had received a large variety of other psychiatric therapies (usually with little or no lasting benefit) before undergoing surgery. The prior treatments included other psychosurgical treatment in 13 cases. Of the 52 operated cases, 35 were female and 17 were male; all were white.

We conclude the following:

1. The large majority of patients were adjudged to have had adequate preparation by and discussion with a physician before the operation, including a fairly adequate review of the risks and benefits.

2. Twenty-seven of the cases (in the pooled sample) were adjudged to have improved markedly. This we determined on the basis of subjective relief of symptoms as reported by the patient and a spouse, family member, or close friend. The assessment was supported by the results of independent psychiatric and psychosocial evaluations. This very favorable outcome was not accompanied by detectable neurological deficit.

3. Twenty-five of the cases showed less improvement, varying from slight or moderate benefit to worse (three cases). Their symptoms were ameliorated temporarily or only to a slight degree by the surgery. However, there was no significant evidence of neurological deficit attributable to the operation.

4. The results of the pilot study suggested that the symptom of depression was especially amenable to psychosurgery in these patients, and that the greatest change in those with very favorable outcomes was in that symptom. This was not confirmed in the follow-up study; in the combined sample of 52 cases, preoperative diagnosis did not predict successful outcome.

5. There was little evidence of overall cognitive or intellectual deficit attributable to the psychosurgery, although this is difficult to assess considering the distressed state of the patients prior to surgery.

6. The two studies suggest also that retrospective research on this problem is feasible, and that further research may help to illuminate the question of which patients may receive benefit from psychosurgical intervention.

The fact that some patients eventually have psychosurgical treatment is probably a function of the limits of current psychiatric knowledge, or at least of the application and utilization of available knowledge. The resort to surgery in medicine generally means that there are no effective treatment alternatives available. One of our surgeons put it succinctly when he noted that he saw only psychiatry's failures, and none of its successes, on the operating table. This judgment may be too harsh, however, since the nature of the illnesses for which psychosurgery is now recommended may defy our understanding and therapeutic efforts for some time to come.

CHAPTER 11

The Psychosurgery Evaluation Studies and Their Impact on the Commission's Report

Stephan L. Chorover

The Commission's Report

In August 1976, the National Commission for the Protection of Human Subjects of Biomedical and Behavioral Research issued its initial report on psychosurgery. As noted at the time in one widely read and highly respected scientific journal, both the tone and content of the report were "surprisingly favorable" (Culliton, 1976). In order to understand what the surprise was about, it is necessary to recall that the National Research Act of 1974 (Public Law 93-348), which created the Commission, had come close to carrying an amendment banning all psychosurgery in the United States. As finally enacted, the law specifically mandated that the Commission should conduct an investigation of the use of psychosurgery in the United States in order to determine the circumstances, "if any," under which its continued use might be appropriate.

The establishment of the Commission was partly a sign of growing public apprehension over the potential for abuse inherent in powerful new forms of psychotechnology (see Chorover, 1973,

1979), and this particular mandate reflected the existence of a controversy that had been triggered several years earlier by various proposals to employ brain manipulation as a means of social control.[1] As a matter of fact, the earlier appearance of a number of reviews (for example, Valenstein, 1973) and criticisms (for example, Chorover, 1974) of psychosurgical theory and practice had created a climate conducive to skepticism about the safety and efficacy of psychosurgical procedures and about the scientific and social propriety of what I have elsewhere termed "the pacification of the brain" (Chorover, 1976). Thus, as the Commission set to work, in the aftermath of the Indochina War, ghetto uprisings, and other events of the turbulent sixties, "there was a strong bias in Congress against such brain operations. And it is probably fair to say that several, perhaps most, of the 11 members of the commission approached their study of psychosurgery with a negative bias" (Culliton, 1976, p. 299).

There was thus ample reason to be surprised when—only two years later—the Commission issued a report that fell only slightly short of endorsing psychosurgery.[2] More specifically, although the initial report prompted some criticism, which led to a number of revisions, the final version, issued in May 1977, continued to refer to psychosurgery as a legitimate (albeit "experimental") biomedical and behavioral procedure that "can be of significant therapeutic value in the treatment of certain disorders or in the relief of certain symptoms" (DHEW, 1977, p. 26329).[3] More to the point, the Commission, terming psychosurgery a "potentially beneficial therapy," recommended its continuation under certain procedural safeguards.

The recommended regulations did not please those observers who had been particularly concerned about the potential use of psychosurgery as an instrument of social control. For example, it was proposed that a potential subject's status (for example, that of a minor child, a prisoner, or an involuntarily confined mental patient) should not *de facto* prohibit him or her from undergoing psychosurgery. Commenting that (1) "Fairness requires that individuals not be denied access to potentially beneficial therapy simply because they are involuntarily confined or unable to give informed consent" (p.

---

[1] A few of these are cited in my chapter on the problem of violence (Chapter 16) in this volume. For a more extensive discussion, see Chorover, 1976, 1979.

[2] Indeed, the unexpected tone of the report led one periodical to misleadingly headline its account: "Congress [sic] endorses psychosurgery" (*The Nation*, October 23, 1976).

[3] All quotations from the Commission's report are taken from the final version, which was issued on March 14, 1977. While reconsidered at subsequent meetings and revised somewhat in the light of comments and criticisms, the report remained essentially unchanged in respect to the points mentioned here.

26330) and (2) that "the Commission does not wish categorically to deny children the possible advantages" (p. 26331), the report also asserted that "the misuse of psychosurgery can be prevented by appropriate safeguards" (p. 26329) and hence proceeded to stipulate various circumstances under which experimental psychosurgical procedures upon human subjects (including children, prisoners, and involuntarily confined mental patients) could be and should be allowed and, indeed, ought to be encouraged.[4] In effect, therefore, the latter stipulation does give the Commission's endorsement to the further use of psychosurgery under certain circumstances and thus does appear, as some critics have observed, to open the way for the systematic use of certain classes of children, prisoners, and mental patients as experimental subjects in officially sanctioned programs of psychosurgical research.

Under the circumstances, it becomes pertinent to ask: What, precisely, was it that caused the Commission members—contrary to their own and the public's expectation—to issue a report that, in general, treats psychosurgery so favorably? The answer is not hard to find. Indeed, when he was asked this question, the chairman of the Commission is reported to have replied:

> We looked at the data and saw they did not support our prejudices. I, for one, did not expect to come out in favor of psychosurgery. But we saw that some very sick people had been helped by it, and that it did not destroy their intelligence or rob them of feelings. Their marriages were intact. They were able to work. The operation shouldn't be banned [Kenneth John Ryan, quoted by Culliton, 1976, p. 299].

What, precisely, were the data that the commissioners "looked at" that dispelled their "prejudices" and led them to make recommendations so favorable to the continuation of surgical practices that had generally come to be regarded as scientifically unfounded and socially threatening? The answer seems to be that the data in question were obtained mainly, perhaps wholly, from two studies of the "safety and efficacy" of psychosurgery conducted by two separate teams of scientists and clinicians working under special contracts from the Commission. The first team, headed by Allan F. Mirsky and Maressa H. Orzack of Boston University, was commissioned to conduct a *retrospective* study of the safety and efficacy of

---

[4] Specifically, Recommendation (6) read: "The Secretary DHEW is encouraged to conduct and support studies to evaluate the safety . . . and efficacy of [specific psychosurgical] procedures in relieving specific psychiatric symptoms and disorders, provided that the psychosurgery is performed in accordance with [the Commission's] recommendation" (DHEW, 1977, p. 26331).

psychosurgery (hereafter referred to as the B.U. study); the second, headed by the late Hans-Lukas Teuber and Suzanne Corkin of the Massachusetts Institute of Technology, was given additional support by the Commission to accelerate and expand a study (hereafter called the M.I.T. study) already under way, which ultimately included some *prospective* as well as retrospective components. According to the Commission's summary account,

> Both studies, drawing upon interviews and objective tests, provided evidence that (1) more than half of the patients improved significantly following psychosurgery, although a few were worse and some unchanged, and (2) none of the patients experienced significant neurological or psychological impairment attributable to the surgery. The investigators in one study suggested that the risks of the psychosurgical procedures that were performed may be less than the risks of continuing electroconvulsive treatments over long periods of time.
>
> These studies appear to rebut any presumption that all forms of psychosurgery are unsafe and ineffective. The Commission finds that there is at least tentative evidence that some forms of psychosurgery can be of significant therapeutic value in the treatment of certain disorders or in the relief of certain symptoms. *Because of this finding* and the belief that the misuse of psychosurgery can be prevented by appropriate safeguards, *the Commission has not recommended a ban on psychosurgery* [DHEW, 1977, p. 26329, emphases added].

If it is presumed that this summary means what it says, there is no mystery about the grounds on which the Commission reached its recommendations. However, claims about the safety and efficacy of psychosurgery are a constant feature of *The Psychosurgery Debate*, and prudence would appear to warrant a more careful examination of both the passage that the investigators took from making their observations to drawing their conclusions and the path that the Commission followed in interpreting those conclusions and translating them into procedural recommendations. In my view, the former passage is not nearly as short and the latter path not quite as direct as the Commission's summary of the matter appears to suggest.

In order to substantiate this contention, it is necessary to examine the data and the reports that were presented to the Commission and to ask whether there is any real sense in which the two studies provide a proper scientific foundation for the recommendations they are required to support. In my opinion, it is particularly important that this be done in the present context because there is still much room for serious skepticism about the safety and efficacy of psychosurgery, and because the Commission's recommendations regarding psychosurgery are being considered in this volume as a possible model for handling other controversial public policy questions in the area of mental health. Accordingly, my analysis will focus on the B.U. and M.I.T. reports in the form in which they were presented to the Commission, and not the more recent versions presented in this volume.[5]

The B.U. Study

As the authors suggest at the start of their account, the B.U. study was plainly conducted under the most intense time pressure. In the original report to the Commission (Mirsky and Orzack, 1976) reference is made to the "extremely rushed, if not frantic conditions" under which it was done. This needs to be borne in mind because it may help to explain certain otherwise inexplicable facts about the procedures employed, the data obtained, and the conclusions reached in the study, and because it highlights the fact that this was no ordinary clinical investigation. More to the point, the investigators evidently knew that this was a "study of high mental health relevance, the outcome of which may help to shape future national health policies," and they quite properly and prophetically pointed this out to some of their prospective informants (Mirsky and Orzack, 1976, p. 122). In view of the latter consideration, it is not surprising that every effort was made during the initial planning stages of the study to ensure that it would yield valid and reliable results. And because the work plan was clearly defined (B.U., pp. 206–207), it is pertinent to note that there are certain discrepancies between what was initially envisaged for the study and what was eventually done.

Selection of Patients

From the account given (B.U., pp. 206–207) of the original agreement between the Commission and the investigators, it is clear that the initial intention was to examine between 40 and 120 psychosurgery patients. More specifically, the agreement stipulated that

---

[5] Copies of the original reports were obtainable at the time of writing from the Commission: Westwood Building, 5333 Westwood Avenue, Bethesda, MD 20016. For the most part, they are similar to the ones presented in this volume. Thus, except where significant differences are notable, I will, for the reader's convenience, refer to page numbers in Chapter 10 of this volume for citations to the B.U. report.

separate groups of 20 to 30 patients were to be obtained from each of two to four surgeons and that each group would be "sufficiently homogeneous with respect to presenting behavioral problems, locus and size of lesion, and other significant variables in order to permit valid and reliable results" (B.U., p. 206). In other words, the original intention was to select and enlist subjects in such a way as to permit the investigators to make systematic comparisons of the safety and efficacy of psychosurgery across a reasonable sample of patients who had been suffering from particular disorders and who had received psychosurgical treatment at the hands of different neurosurgeons.

In my opinion, these are scientifically reasonable stipulations. But—even under the most propitious circumstances—the best-intended effort to adhere to them would be fraught with many and varied practical problems. Laboring, as they were, within the extremely short period time allotted by the legislatively mandated timetable of the Commision, it is wholly understandable that the B.U. investigators were unable to meet them. Which is simply to say that at a point well before the start of the data-gathering phase of the study, the investigators were evidently confronted by a direct—though not inescapable—contradiction between the need to adhere, on the one hand, to scientifically reasonable methods of procedure and the need to adhere, on the other hand, to the mandated time-table of the Commission. What they chose to do at that point must be considered in the light of their evident awareness that the outcome of the study was bound to have an influential effect upon the shaping of social policy in an extremely controversial domain. Granting, therefore, that "valid and reliable results" of the stipulated kind could not possibly be obtained within the period imposed by the original contract, it is necessary to note that one possible way of resolving the problem would have been to simply report to the Commission that the job that needed to be done could not be done under the prevailing time constraints and that it was necessary, therefore, either to seek an extension of the time limit or to terminate the project forthwith. However, a somewhat different course was taken. Scarcely three months from the date the final report was to be submitted—and before most of the data were collected—a decision was made to "modify the work scope" (B.U., p. 207). With the benefit of hindsight, it may be seen as the first of several fateful choices each of which was more congenial to the administrative requirements of the Commission than to the procedural demands of scientific probity.

In the context of ensuing events, this initial procedural modification had some far-reaching social policy consequences. Indeed, the decision to bypass some very real and serious practical difficulties involving the selection and participation of patients paved the way for the eventual submission of a report that—falling far short of original intentions—included only 27 psychosurgery patients and 8 unoperated "controls."

But the small number of subjects turns out not to be the only nor even the most problematical aspect of the sample of psychosurgery patients examined in this study. To make matters worse, the 27 psychosurgery cases were "drawn" (in a fashion never fully described in the report) from the rosters of five different neurosurgeons, each of whom practices a different form of psychosurgery. Moreover, far from being "homogeneous with respect to presenting behavioral problems . . . and other significant variables," the 27 came bearing a bewildering array of diagnostic labels, including: schizophrenic (2), pseudoneurotic schizophrenic (3), psychoneurotic schizophrenic (2), psychoneurotic (2), chronic depressive anxiety state (5), schizo-affective (2), manic-depressive (3), obsessive-compulsive (1), depressive (2), and various intractable pain states with attendant anxiety, addiction, and depression (5).[6] As indicated in Table 10.1 (B.U., p. 209), different neurosurgeons contributed different numbers of cases to the study (8 cases from Surgeon 1, who "does only orbital undercuttings"; 7 cases from Surgeon 2, who "performs multi-target bilateral stereotaxic operations, using radio-frequency or other lesions to destroy areas in the cingulate gyrus, amygdala, and substantia innominata"; 10 cases from Surgeon 3, who "performs only 'prefrontal sonic treatment' . . . either unilaterally or bilaterally"; and 2 cases "operated by two other surgeons" who performed "anterior prefrontal leucotomy," B.U., p. 208). Finally, in what the original report refers to as "another imponderable complication" of the sample, it developed that 10 (or almost 40 percent) of the patients who were eventually included in the study had actually received two or more psychosurgical operations. What is not understandable, to me at least, is the fact that the report suggests, without the benefit of supporting data, that the reason why some patients with a less than favorable outcome undergo further psychosurgery is that the previous operation produced some prior benefit or relief. This is, to put it mildly, a gratuitous suggestion in view of the data presented and in the light of the more familiar claim that psychosurgery is a treatment of last resort.

As the foregoing example illustrates, the B.U. report tends to deal with certain complex questions in a simplistic way. Moreover, it

---

[6] This compilation is drawn from Table 2 in the original report (Mirsky and Orzack, 1976, p. 7).

tends to give the benefit of the doubt to interpretations that provide a more, rather than a less favorable evaluation of the safety and efficacy of psychosurgical treatment.

As the concluding part of the account in the present volume implies, the B.U. study has been criticized on various grounds. Obviously, the small size of the sample and the large variety of patients included in the study are grounds enough for questioning the legitimacy of any substantive conclusions drawn from it. I will presume that those facts speak for themselves and, accordingly, turn here to an examination of the path that the investigation followed *after* the decision was made to proceed with the retrospective study within the limitations already described.

To begin with, it deserves notice that the ultimate inclusion of subjects in the study depended upon a process in which the operating surgeons played a key initial role. The surgeons selected by the investigators were asked, in turn, to select the patients who would, if they consented, be included in the study. From the information available, it is not clear what the surgeons were told about the criteria they should use in selecting patients. Nor is it clear, for that matter, whether any additional factors influenced the choice of patients they ultimately did select, but it is instructive to note that, in the cases of the three surgeons who ended up referring the majority of patients, the number of solicitation letters sent to patients represented an inconstant and perhaps nonrandom fraction of the total number of operations allegedly performed during the relevant period (1965–1974). Consequently, in each cohort, the number of patients seen and studied was a still smaller proportion of those who had been operated on. It is evident from Table 10.2 (B.U., pp. 210–211; cf. Table 1 in Mirsky and Orzack, 1976) that in the cases of Surgeons 2 and 3 (who accounted for more than 60 percent of the original sample), only about 5 percent of the patients actually operated on during the relevant period were eventually examined. I cite this figure, not so much to suggest (as some critics properly have) the possibility of bias (conscious or otherwise) in selection procedures of this kind, as to point out that these circumstances raise serious questions about the representativeness of the patient sample. They render irrelevant the assertion that "[t]he number (and percentage) of refusals . . . was small" and contradict the more significant claim that "we were not missing a significant proportion of the operated cases" (B.U., p. 211; cf. Mirsky and Orzack, 1976, p. 6). I am not nitpicking; the importance of these misleading assertions becomes apparent when one recalls that the Commission justified its own finding "that some forms of psychosurgery can be of significant therapeutic value" partly on the grounds of the otherwise unqualified assertion that in the contracted studies *"more than half of the patients improved significantly following psychosurgery"* (DHEW, 1977, p.26329, emphasis added).

The B.U. study actually raises many more questions than it answers regarding the safety and efficacy of psychosurgery. And, as already noted, many of those questions appear to be traceable to problems inherent in the patient selection procedures. A final example may suffice to make the point. It is indicated in the report that a concern (obviously justifiable in itself) about the protection of privacy of the psychosurgery patients led the investigators to decide that it would be wholly improper for them (and, by extension, for the Commission) to obtain access to patient records without first getting permission from the patients themselves. Yet in weighing the ultimate consequences of the small size and heterogeneity of the subject sample produced by this decision, together with the difficulties inherent in retrospective studies, against the need of the Commission for valid and reliable data, I think a case could be made for having proceeded quite differently. The point is that this was another of those procedural decisions that, in view of the prevailing time constraints, may be seen as possibly fateful. For when the investigators found themselves, at the outset of the data-collection phase of their study, faced with the fact that their sample was bound to be very small and very heterogeneous, again, they were forced to make a further choice. In their own words, "Since the number of cases . . . contributed by any single surgeon was small, we chose to ignore surgery type and instead to classify cases according to outcome" (B.U., p. 214).

Evaluation Procedures

Since one of the avowed purposes of the overall project was to obtain and analyze a large amount of data supposedly indicative of the patients' outcome and present status, in order retrospectively to evaluate the safety and efficacy of the psychosurgery that had been performed in specific kinds of cases, it may be counted as truly remarkable that the investigators chose to classify the patients into just two outcome categories, *irrespective* of the "presenting behavioral problems, locus and size of lesion, and other significant variables" (B.U., p. 206) and without regard to psychological and neurological test data, which were initially (and quite properly) presumed to be required for valid and reliable results.

The original report to the Commission was quite explicit on this extremely important point:

> Outcome was decided on the basis of the social work interview—questionnaires and an independent interview of the principal investigator. Outcome was evaluated on the basis of the patient's answers to questions such as "Do you feel you benefited from the operation?" "How did you benefit?" "Knowing what effect it had, would you have the operation again?" Answers which led to a classification of "very much improved" or "cured" included: "It saved my life" or "I would be dead now if not for the operation" or "It was like being born again." Other answers, leading to a less favorable outcome classification included, "It helped for awhile, but then my trouble started again," or "It was no help," or "I got worse"....
> ... Since the number of cases per category would otherwise be too small, the outcome was dichotomized into very much improved or "cured" versus all other outcomes (Mirsky and Orzack, 1976, p. 14).

The patients' own evaluations of outcome, then, provided the grounds on which the investigators based their categorization of the 27 operated cases into 14 with "very favorable outcome" (VFO) and 13 with "less favorable outcome" (LFO). Since this categorization forms part of the basis, in turn, for the Commission's conclusions that "more than half of the patients improved significantly following psychosurgery," and "that some forms of psychosurgery can be of significant therapeutic value," it deserves close attention.

It is necessary, in this connection, for me to make something explicit that I hope most readers will already understand. My intention is *not* to criticize the authors of the B.U. study for resorting to "subjective judgments." They had no other choice. And I most definitely wish to dissassociate myself from those who, according to at least one account, have accused the investigators of bias in a manner that "impugns the integrity of a group of highly respected scientists with well-known reputations for sound and scholarly research" (Memorandum, dated December 8, 1977, from Deputy Director, Division of Extramural Research Programs, National Institute of Mental Health to Associate Director for Extramural Programs, Alcohol, Drug Abuse, and Mental Health Administration, Public Health Service, Department of Health, Education and Welfare). The authors of both reports are friends and esteemed colleagues; in my view, their integrity is beyond question. However, it is plainly necessary for me to scrutinize their methods of procedure and to stress at this point that in their decision to employ an "interview-questionnaire" format as the basis for evaluating the safety and efficacy of psychosurgery the investigators effectively moved their project out of the domain of neuropsychological research and into a realm of survey research where serious methodological questions of a procedural and evaluative nature abound. My point here is not that such a move is unwarranted or that they—as biologically oriented psychologists —are not entitled to make it. On the contrary, it is that in making such a move one is obliged to adhere to prevailing research standards and methods of procedure. In the case of survey research, and specifically in the use of questionnaires or interview procedures, it is a notorious fact that the answers one obtains tend to depend in subtle and complex ways upon the kinds of questions one asks and upon the way one phrases and poses them. Do the sample questions offered by the investigators (and quoted above) provide adequate assurance that attention was paid to the serious semantic and contextual (let alone the statistical and sampling) problems that pervade the field of attitude measurement and associated areas of social psychological research? I do not think so.

In support of their use of "interview data" to classify the patients into VFO and LFO groups, the authors of the B.U. study remark that each patient was invited to bring an informant who had some knowledge of his or her preoperative and postoperative status. They also say that "Usually, there was reasonably close agreement between the patient's view, the informant's view, and the objective tests" (B.U., p. 238). However, no evidence to support this contention is provided in either the original report or in the account presented in this volume. On the contrary, the latter plainly states that "The 27 patients were classified . . . on the basis of two independent interviews. The classification reflects basically the patient's evaluation of the degree of relief obtained from the symptoms, his or her current status, and willingness to undergo the operation a second time" (B.U., Table 10.4, p. 215). How valid, reliable, and representative are the judgments of the sampled psychosurgery patients? In view of the assurance about the agreement between patients' and informants' views, a reader might conclude that there is little reason for concern on this point. But in the report to the Commission—to which case histories for all but one of the patients (103) are appended—I was able to find only five instances in which an informant's opinion was mentioned. There were only two explicitly documented cases. In one of them (222), "generally the friend reported less preoperative pathology and less postoperative improvement" than did the patient. In the other (122), "a discrepancy between the subject's self-report and other evidence" was noted. In that case, the patient's mother saw his condition as "improved," while according to "the subject's self-report he is as badly off now as he was prior to surgery." Thus, despite the assertion that there is close agreement between patient and informant judgments regarding "safety and effi-cacy" (see also Figure 10.3, p. 227), the actual data that are presented leave this question largely unresolved.

It is interesting to note that the report takes a somewhat inconsis-tent view of the effects of psychosurgery upon global psychological functioning. On the one hand, Item 5 in the list of conclusions states that

> There was little evidence of overall cognitive or intellectual deficit attributable to the psychosurgery, although this is difficult to assess considering the distressed state of the patients prior to surgery (B.U., p. 243).

On the other hand, the text itself says

> The VFO . . . cases showed greater evidence of what might be viewed as cognitive loss (p. 236).

While it is perplexing that the latter evidence was apparently deemed unworthy of being cited in or of influencing the aforemen-tioned conclusions, I believe on the basis of a close reading of the report itself that the data obtained overall were consistent with the latter passage. It also seems likely to me that those patients who suffer the greatest degree of cognitive and intellectual impairment are most liable to be influenced by any bias that happens to be inherent in an interviewer's questions about safety and efficacy and are hence most likely in the present instance to have ended up in the VFO category. In other words, it seems plausible to me that if psychosurgery produces cognitive losses, the decision to base the outcome categorization upon the "patient's evaluation of the out-come," combined with the tendency to pose questions about "safety and efficacy" in rather loose and inadvertently biased terms, may have led to findings that grossly overestimated the incidence of suc-cessful outcomes. More to the point, this interpretation helps to explain the otherwise rather curious finding of "the greatest degree of cognitive and intellectual impairment" in those patients who ended up in the "most improved" group. It must also be noted, in this connection, that "[v]ery few of the psychological test findings in the pilot study were confirmed in the data of the follow-up study" (B.U., p. 230) and that, in particular, there were in the follow-up study fewer differences between the two groups on tests ostensibly related to cognitive functioning, intellectual status, or capacity for judgment. I do not know what to make of this disparity except to say that it calls into question the reliability of the original results upon which the Commission based its important and controversial rec-ommendations.

Before turning to a necessarily much briefer consideration of the second study upon which the Commission based its findings, I must comment on just one more aspect of the first. The investigators make an effort in the present volume (p. 235) to explain a fact that went largely ignored in the original report to the Commission—namely, that among the psychosurgery patients in the VFO category, there are six times more women than men! I doubt, quite frankly, that the explanation of this fact lies in "the female brain," in the "homemaker role," or in any of the other conditions suggested, however tentatively, to account for it. My own belief—based upon the most serious consideration of which I am capable—is that the explanation lies mainly in a complex, historically rooted, network of relationships between women and men, a network in which connections between different diagnostic categories, social expectations, and professional perspectives overlap and alternate and combine and thereby determine the texture of the whole (see Chorover, 1979). In short, I mean to suggest that the sources of the observed 6:1 ratio should be sought just as seriously and energetically in the minds of mental health professionals as they are in the brains of mentally ill patients. I also believe that they will ultimately be found to lie (if we are ever to really find them) at the interface between professionals and patients (considered singly and collectively as individuals) and within the broader social context of which all individual thoughts and actions are necessarily a part.

The M.I.T. Study

Since the cases for this study all received the same type of surgical operation [bilateral stereotaxic anterior cingulotomy (Balantine et al., 1967)] by the same neurosurgeon, and since slightly more than half described in the report to the Commission (Teuber, Corkin, and Twitchell, 1977b; hereinafter cited as M.I.T. I) were studied both pre- and postoperatively, it might be expected that the findings of this investigation would be simpler, more straightforward, and easier to interpret than those of the B.U. study. Yet, as the principal author of the report remarked in his submission to the Commission, the effort to find any specific effects of the cingulate lesions had turned out to be more baffling than any task he had previously encountered in thirty years of research on the effects of brain injuries in human beings (M.I.T. I, p. 1). One reason for this, also noted in the report, is that the length of follow-up study that was possible within the timetable imposed by the Commission was "much too brief, for the majority of cases, to permit definitive conclusions" (M.I.T. I, p. 12).

Research Findings

Despite the inconclusiveness of the study's data, the Commission was presumably impressed by the following pair of findings:

1. "Neither the formal testing, nor the more qualitative assessments through history review and detailed interviews, reveals any uniform side effects or obvious 'costs' of the operation in the 34 cases studied" (M.I.T. I, pp. 16–17).

2. Nine of eleven patients previously suffering from severe, prolonged, and otherwise intractable physical pain (mostly radiculopathies and other conditions yielding low-back pain) reported "conspicuous and generally lasting relief" following a single bilateral anterior cingulotomy. In numerous cases, this outcome was corroborated by one or more of the patient's relatives (M.I.T. I, p. 37).

The latter is, as the report to the Commission states, "a remarkable outcome" (M.I.T. I, p. 39), and it has since been further supported by findings obtained in 23 patients who received cingulotomy for intractable pain (Corkin, personal communication). Yet, as the report points out, the complete or near complete relief obtained in these "pain cases" stands "in striking contrast to the [outcome in] other subgroups with cingulotomy in this general series" (M.I.T. I, p. 39). Since the use of neurosurgery for the relief of pain due to physical injury or disease is not generally regarded as psychosurgery, since brain surgery *per se* is not (and has not been) the subject of controversy in the present context, since the legislative mandate to the Commission was wholly silent with respect to the study of neurosurgical treatments for pain (see Public Law 93-348), since the Commission's own report states that "there is no agreement in the medical or scientific community as to whether brain surgery for relief of pain should or should not be considered psychosurgery" (DHEW, 1977; p. 26319), and (most pertinently) since the Commission's own definition of psychosurgery emphasizes its goal as "changing or controlling . . . behavior or emotion" (DHEW, 1977, p. 26318), the results of cingulotomies performed for pain have questionable relevance for the investigation of psychosurgery.

Had the Commission decided, however, to regard the "pain cases" as a separate category (as the M.I.T. group did, to some extent), the *only* data on psychosurgical cases available from the M.I.T. study would have been the data provided by a heterogeneous group of 23 chronically disturbed patients having a wide range of "overlapping" and "often inconsistent," "arbitrary and sometimes contradictory" diagnoses. Moreover (as in the B.U. study), almost half (10) of these patients had been subjected to at least two psychosurgical procedures (half of those had three operations). Overall, perhaps the fairest thing that could be said about the entire group of 23 is that (in contrast to the "pain cases") there appears to have been a very varied outcome. Thus, of 7 cases "presenting primarily with depression," 5 were said to be "successes." However, 3 of the 7 had sustained at least two operations at intervals of one to seven years, and *none* of those deemed to be "successes" in the present study had been followed for more than a year after the most recent cingulotomy. Three of 4 cases bearing the diagnosis of "obsessive-compulsive" stated "emphatically that they were unchanged by the operation." (One of them had received three cingulotomies.) The remaining patient, seen a year after a second cingulotomy had been performed (following another one about a year earlier), reported her condition as only slightly improved. Finally, in a residual subgroup consisting of 11 cases with "multiple and somewhat arbitrary diagnostic labels," almost half of whom had had more than one operation, a "rough count" was said to "yield the following balance: striking improvement in two. . . ; transient improvement followed by a drop to preoperative status (in one). . . ; partial improvement in two. . . ; and no change or worse now, in the remaining six," two of whom were evidently too sick to be tested postoperatively (M.I.T. I, p. 53).

Considering the fact that many patients in this study evidently relapsed within a year or so after surgery and were deemed to require another operation, it is significant to note that most of the patients were seen within a relatively short time after their first, or most recent, cingulotomy. Since reoperation within a year or so is not uncommon among all but the "pain cases" in both studies, and since reoperation is most reasonably understandable as evidence that the previous operation failed to provide effective or lasting relief, it seems prudent to conclude that, at best, any "success" obtained may be a relatively transient and fragile affair. It is moreover evident that the patients' attitudes toward the operation and its effects may undergo rather dramatic changes over time. One case in point is that of a woman who was 20 at the time of operation. Now, several years later, she alleges that she was inalterably changed from an energetic, high-achieving, creative young woman who was undergoing a difficult period of adolescent adjustment into a person who tires easily, lacks energy, has difficulty concentrating, is subject to unexpected seizures and "blankouts," is unable to experience emotions as strongly as she once did, and is permanently disabled and unable to keep a job or otherwise support herself. It is of course impossible to tell whether such alleged changes are "real" and, if so, whether they are a direct result of the cingulotomy. Nevertheless, claims of misdiagnosis, failure to provide adequate treatment, and failure to exhaust all possible modes of standard treatment before causing irreversible damage through inappropriate and excessive ECT and psychosurgery are far from rare as long-term sequelae in this complicated field.

This necessarily brings us back to the fact that the investigators reported no "lasting effects of the cingulotomy *per se* on the 24 behavioral tasks sampled" in the study (M.I.T. I, p. 8). Combined with the aforementioned finding that repeated analysis of life history data and of interview material did not disclose any obvious "costs" of cingulotomy in the patients studied and that (with the "pain cases" included) "the patients as a group show a slight gain" (M.I.T. I, p. 7), the conclusion would appear to follow that cingulotomy produces therapeutic effects without "losses" or, more specifically, without the undesirable behavioral side effects so often ascribed to the more massive frontal lobotomies.

Rationale and Testing Procedures

Since one may fairly conjecture that the finding of no "obvious costs" in the M.I.T. study, together with those of the B.U. study, strongly influenced the Commission's recommendations, it must be asked what these findings really mean. Is it possible, for example, that a failure to find significant behavioral effects following a particular brain lesion may have something to do with the nature and scope of the methods used to search for them? According to the M.I.T. report, the behavioral tests used were "chosen to sample behaviors thought to be dependent upon the integrity of the areas that [the cingulum bundle] interconnects" (M.I.T. I, p. 26). However, on closer examination this turns out to be a rather problematical assertion. To begin with, the relevant connections are multiple and complex. As the report points out, the usual rationale for interrupting the cingulum bundle is derived from the view of it as a component of the limbic system, which includes a ring of structures surrounding the medial wall of the hemispheres (including cingulum and fornix, hippocampus and amygdala, as well as various subcortical structures, notably the septum and the mammillary body regions of the hypothalamus, the mammilo-thalamic tract, and the anterior thalamic nuclei). There is also a downward continuation of the "limbic system" into the central grey substance of the midbrain and an upward projection to cingulate and orbito-frontal cortex (Nauta, 1958; Nauta and Domesick, 1979).

Instead of adhering to this view of the limbic system as essentially a circuit (a view that has been generally accepted since Papez's [1937] original description of it), the M.I.T. study was predicated on the much narrower proposition that the cingulum bundle is essentially a pathway interconnecting the frontal and temporal lobes: "Thus," the investigators write, "we set out to search for signs ordinarily associated with frontal lobe or temporal lobe dysfunction and to look for impairment found after lesions of cingulate cortex." Moreover, tests "sensitive to any lesions of the cerebral convexity, regardless of locus, or to changes in overall intelligence or personality" were also included in their test battery (M.I.T. I, p. 26). One basic difficulty is that there are, as a matter of fact, no tests known (even now) to be specifically sensitive to the effects of cingulate cortex lesions in human beings. Such lesions are exceedingly rare, since they are—as the authors point out—"unlikely to arise from any other source, except for the sake of this particular therapeutic attempt on the part of some neurosurgeons" (M.I.T. I, p. 12). Another difficulty is that there is no *a priori* reason to believe that tests sensitive to frontal and temporal insult to the convexity of cortex would be sensitive also to the effects of cingulate lesions. Finally, the usual presumption about the limbic system as a whole is that it is somehow mainly involved in the mediation of emotional experience and expression; yet, a review of the two dozen behavioral tasks actually included in the M.I.T. test battery reveals that there were *none* that might even remotely be called tests of affect, motivation, or emotionality. Indeed, all of the tests except one are best characterized as mainly "cognitive" or "motor," including tests of sensation, perception, linguistic and nonverbal fluency, categorization, memory, and dexterity. The single exception was a "personality inventory," which appears to have been included as an afterthought and was administered in a rather cursory fashion to less than one-third of the patient sample. The results showed no "pattern in the data related to time of testing or to the presumed therapeutic success or failure of the surgical procedure" (M.I.T. I, p. 73). As a matter of fact, the authors of the report themselves suggest that their choice of this test was inappropriate for their sample (M.I.T. I, p. 73). Under the circumstances, it is significant to note that the single most important negative conclusion drawn from this study —namely, that "for this group of patients . . . no lasting additional deficits in behavioral capacities can so far be identified after the surgical procedure" (M.I.T. I, pp. 10–11)—was arrived at without the benefit of any test data even remotely relevant to the notion that the cingulum bundle is a crucial component within an anatomic system subserving emotional experience, expression, or affect.[7]

Conclusions

In concluding my critique of the B.U. and M.I.T. studies, I will make no effort to restate the points that I have tried to make. Nor will I try to adduce any further evidence of the inadequacies of these studies as bases for the conclusions that the Commission actually reached. I will, however, make one concluding remark.

There appears to be a rather striking difference between the kinds of decisions that scientists are likely to make when following the intrinsic demands of their professional disciplines and those they are likely to make when adhering to the dictates of external authorities or agencies. Put another way, the kinds of errors to which we scientists are normally prone in the course of our efforts to describe what is actually the case are not the same as the kinds of errors we are likely to make while trying to serve the interests of public policy makers. In my opinion, the essential difference is that as scientists we are generally prepared to accept (and hopefully to withstand) the rude shock of discovering that we have been mistaken. Indeed, we are supposed to welcome it as a form of enlightenment when our scientific beliefs about the world and its contents are shaken by a rationally-organized and intellectually persuasive argument based upon carefully assembled and analyzed facts. But the mistakes of political organizations (and those we are liable to make in their service) are much more difficult to undo. As I have tried to show elsewhere, this is largely because political organizations are more closely tied to the exercise of *power* than to the pursuit of *meaning* (Chorover, 1979). Yet, in any society, power and meaning are tightly

---

[7]The failure to give serious consideration to affective aspects of human experience is, unfortunately, a general characteristic of contemporary neuropsychological studies of this kind. In a review presently being prepared, I discuss this problem and propose that the limbic system, as a whole, is essentially involved in the mediation of relationships between cognitive and expressive aspects of affective experience. If this notion is correct, then the kinds of tasks most likely to reveal effects following lesions of the limbic system in human beings would presumably be those with a clear-cut combination of cognitive, motor, and affective components, and the kinds of deficits most likely to appear, according to this hypothesis, would be those reflecting a breakdown of relationships between cognitive and motor aspects of behavior in affectivity charged situations.

coupled in a reciprocal feedback loop. Accordingly, those of us whose work lies at the interface between behavioral science and social policy must somehow come to understand that the decisions we make in our laboratories are often influenced by—and in return have an effect upon—the world of social affairs of which scientists and nonscientists alike are a part. Neither the scientists who undertake the investigation that has foreseeable social policy implications nor the agencies that support such research can claim to enter upon their respective roles free of potentially influential social preconceptions. On the contrary:

> The myth of scientific objectivity notwithstanding, we bring to our professional labors a set of commitments—disciplinary, theoretical, political, ethical, religious, etc.—of which we are, at very best, only partially aware. These commitments are normally of little practical moment when other animal species are being studied . . . [but] may have profound consequences . . . when we study *human* behavior and the results are perceived as bearing on current public policy issues [Peterson and Somit, 1978, p. 18].

Which is to say, finally, that the work we do and the way we come to do it are mutually interconnected to each other in ways that inevitably influence the results we get and uses to which they may be put.

CHAPTER 12

Response to Dr. Chorover's Critique of the Psychosurgery Studies

Allan F. Mirsky and Maressa Hecht Orzack

Dr. Chorover's criticisms of our study can be summarized, essentially, under four headings: (1) since there was inadequate time to do a well-controlled, well-designed study, no study should have been done at all, (2) the sample, although possibly not biased, is too small and selected to be representative; (3) we tended to apply simplistic and incorrect resolutions to difficult problems when they arose in the execution of the study; and (4) we were basically out of our depth in doing social science research when we should have stuck to our area of competence—that is, neuropsychological research. In response to these criticisms, it is fair to say that there is probably no one who has read the first of our studies—that is, the report to the National Commission—more thoroughly than Dr. Chorover. However, it is clear that he has not read as carefully the chapter that we have prepared for this volume.

It is also fair to say that Dr. Chorover has probed every soft spot in our research and correctly called attention to these problems. On the other hand, it is our belief that he has made some incorrect judgments or drawn some inappropriate conclusions from what we wrote. Without going over every one of the criticisms point by point that Dr. Chorover raised, we wish to discuss some of the major points of contention as summarized above.

First, with respect to the issue of time, we tried to document the difficulty of obtaining subjects for this work and some of the experimental compromises that we were forced to make because of this. Clearly, some of the neurosurgeons we approached were unenthusiastic about the prospect of having their patients studied. So far as we can discern from subsequent conversation and contact with some of these surgeons, the concerns grew more out of the widespread worry that most surgeons and many physicians now have about malpractice suits than out of any fear that the horrible results of their psychosurgical practice would now be revealed for all the world to see.

We were presented with a problem and chose to face it squarely: The National Commission had been assigned the responsibility by Congress of making a recommendation with respect to the further practice of psychosurgery in this country. The National Commission could have made a recommendation on the basis of the literature in this field, which is generally acknowledged to be of poor quality. Dr. Valenstein's review speaks to this. Moreover, there is the suspicion of bias, since the research is frequently done by the operating surgeons themselves. On the other hand, the Commission could make recommendations on the basis of new research conducted under its own aegis. It seemed to us—and we think this is still true—that it was far better for the Commission to deliberate on the basis of partial information gathered independently than on the basis of no new information at all. The data gathered by the Teuber–Corkin group and our group made at least a start in this direction. Dr. Chorover and others seem to have forgotten that our study was a pilot study and that it was not claimed, nor is it now claimed, to be a definitive answer to the perplexing questions that have plagued this field.

The second criticism raised by Dr. Chorover is that we had a sample that was too small and selected to be valid. There is the implied suggestion that somehow we were hoodwinked by the neurosurgeons into seeing only their best cases and that the horrible failures were confined to mental hospitals or somehow sequestered from our view. From our interactions and interviews with the surgeons, we can only reaffirm that, far from withholding information, they were all very open with us, offered us more information than we were ethically able to use, and in general (unless one assumes that they went through elaborate efforts to doctor their files) made information fully and freely available to us.

We have tried to document in both of our reports the reasons why we saw only a small number of cases. However, the point may be worth restating. The cases that were provided by the first surgeon dictated to us the diagnostic sampling that we were perforce required to see in the caseloads of the other neurosurgeons. We attempted, in other words, to see primarily cases with a diagnosis of affective illness and/or obsessive-compulsive illness, after having seen the first surgeon's cases. Surgeons thereafter who provided us with large numbers of cases were willing, even eager, for us to see all of their cases. We still receive correspondence from one of these surgeons who is concerned lest we not see large and more representative samples of the kinds of persons that he has operated. However, it was again time and money that forced us to focus on a smaller sample of patients than we had hoped to see and to restrict the diagnostic groups to the ones listed. Dr. Chorover probably views the diagnostic label issue with more concern than we do. It is well known in psychiatry that the particular way in which a patient's symptoms are described may vary considerably from alienist to alienist and that diagnostic labels are not fixed, God-given categories. Consequently, one cannot take too seriously his allegation that we looked at a very heterogeneous population of persons with mental illness. One of the characteristics of the psychosurgery case is a confused diagnosis. If he chooses to criticize us on the basis of lack of expertise in social science research, it is perhaps then not inappropriate to suggest that his expertise in the area of psychodiagnosis is at least as much in question as ours in social science research. We will return to this issue later.

To the criticism that we have tended to resolve complex problems in a simplistic and incorrect way, it is difficult to formulate an answer. This is a very damaging global criticism, and if we believed it to be an accurate reflection of our work we would not have submitted it to the National Commission nor to this volume. An example, perhaps, of what Dr. Chorover means is given by his criticism that we do not document the agreement between the patient's judgment of surgical outcome and that of the informant. The agreement between the ratings of the subjects and the ratings of the informant is, however, documented thoroughly in the chapter in this volume, and the reader is referred to it. Furthermore, our own evaluation of the subjects' outcome was in excellent agreement with the measures obtained from the Spitzer-Endicott and the other psychiatric evaluations. These are standardized tests not constructed by us but used by the research community extensively. We really do not understand Dr. Chorover's criticism here.

The issue is raised that we were out of our depth in doing social science research. Specifically, it is suggested that our questions biased the subjects' answers. This is a difficult criticism to refute. Our staff was large and we considered everyone's opinion in making our outcome judgment. It should also be pointed out in fairness to our consultants that they are expert in the area of evaluation and the outcome of therapy. It is perhaps necessary only to mention the collaboration of Dr. Douglas McNair, who has devised some of the most widely used methods for evaluating effects of psychiatric therapy. Moreover, the fact that all of our independent measures agreed so consistently among themselves, as well as being in agreement with the self-rating of the patient, lends credibility to the results we have discussed.

Several other issues are worthy of comment: There is the assumption that the missing group—the patients who failed to respond or refused to participate—consisted entirely of failures and that therefore we grossly exaggerated the percentage of persons who were helped by the several psychosurgical procedures that we studied. Clearly, some of the missing group consisted of failures. On the other hand, it was also clear from conversation with some patients that they could not participate because they were living full and busy lives; for them to interrupt those lives and take five days out to come to Boston for our purposes was simply not feasible. Others indicated that the period surrounding the operation was one of great personal misery and they did not wish to relive that experience; nevertheless, they seemed to be functioning well now. It is important to remember that there is always the possibility of a type 2 as well as a type 1 error. We felt it important to provide the Commission with some new information based on neuropsychological study of patients, whether favorable or unfavorable in terms of future use of psychosurgery. Clearly we are expert in dealing with the area of neuropsychological deficit.

A final point: Dr. Chorover notes that he is perplexed about the fact that, on the one hand, we stated in our conclusions that there was no evidence of overall cognitive or intellectual deficit attributable to surgery, while on the other hand stating in the text itself that the very favorable outcome cases show greater evidence of what might be viewed as cognitive loss. There is a difference, we would aver, between a trend or a suggestion of a finding and a solid result that warrants being cited as a conclusion of the study. Of the very many cognitive measures we looked at, we saw only a few that fitted the hypothesis that cognitive deficit was somehow necessary for a favorable outcome. Moreover, if the results of the second study were read carefully, it could be seen that this hypothesis was not con- firmed. There is no real disparity and no reason for Dr. Chorover, in our view, to reach his alarmist conclusion.

Dr. Chorover is a friend and colleague whose judgment we respect. Nevertheless, we are in substantial disagreement over his interpre- tation of the validity and value of our studies. We suspect, based in part on his previous writings on what he has referred to as "the pacification of the brain," that he might be critical of any results that did not condemn psychosurgery unequivocally.

PART IV

Conceptualization of Psychiatric Disorders

CHAPTER 13

Some Conceptual Tools for Appraising Psychosurgery

Michael H. Shapiro

There is an epidemic of talk about psychosurgery. The reasons for the unusual attention paid to this comparatively rare procedure seem to be these: (1) the difficulties in defining the nature of the mental or physical disorder,[1] if any, that causes the anomalous behavior, thought, or feeling sought to be altered by the surgery; (2) the difficulties in assessing the benefits and deficits, such as they are, produced by the surgery; (3) a general reluctance to tamper with anyone's identity, personality, or autonomy in a potentially significant and irreversible way; and (4) a general fear that psychosurgery may be used as a tool of political mind control.

The first reason suggests the governance of something called a *disease model:* If a disease is present, this may justify certain therapies; if there is no disease, there is no reason for—and there is a good reason against—the use of the physician's knife, drill, or medi-

---

[1] For convenience, "disorder," "disease," "illness," and "abnormality" are used interchangeably, as is frequently done among health care professionals. I recognize that these terms technically are not synonymous, but I do not think any issues considered here are affected by my usage. Where appropriate, the terms should be understood to encompass the concepts of "trauma," "lesion," and the like.

cine. There are, however, those who reject the necessity and perhaps even the relevance of invoking a disease model. For them, the justification for surgery or other therapy may lie simply in the conclusions that certain forms of behavior and mental functioning are odd, harmful, or maladaptive, and that the therapy will, on balance, improve the patient's functioning. They are guided, it might be said, by a *behaviorist model*, which embraces concepts like "maladaptive behavior" or just plain "dangerousness." (On behaviorism generally, consult Bandura, 1969.) In view of such disputes, it seems reasonable, in appraising psychosurgery, to investigate the very idea of a "model" and its role in the justification of therapy.

The other reasons cited for the strong interest in psychosurgery suggest the importance of constructing conceptual tools to describe and evaluate as precisely as possible the actual effects, wanted or feared, of psychosurgery or any other *organic therapy*—that is, a therapy that acts directly upon the brain's structure or electrochemical properties. (Nonorganic therapies of course require assessment also, but they will not be considered here.)

In discussing the conceptual tools in this chapter, I will begin with an explanation of some different kinds of autonomy and their relevance to appraising psychosurgery and other organic therapies (see Shapiro, 1975, pp. 725–733 and n. 121). This will involve an account of the distinction between the "effectiveness" and the "intrusiveness" of therapies, and a description of certain autonomy dilemmas. Next, I will discuss the notion of "therapy by impairment"—a concept that may aid the cost–benefit analysis required in assessing psychosurgery. Finally, I will review the models we use (1) to describe, explain, and predict matters of empirical fact, including behavior, mental functioning, and the physical properties and processes of living organisms; (2) to morally or legally evaluate conduct or states of affairs; and (3) to justify or proscribe the taking of particular actions in response to (or in anticipation of) other actions or to states of affairs. (Consult Engelhardt, 1975, p. 127.) The kind of empirical information that is to be fed into the resulting conceptual system is described at some length elsewhere in this volume. I do not intend in this essay to describe in detail particular physical or mental disorders thought to justify psychosurgery; nor to define generally what is meant by "physical disorder" or "mental disorder"; nor to review the empirical evidence offered in defending or attacking psychosurgery. *What I mean to do is discuss the very systems of thought —the "conceptual maps"—that instruct us in how to describe and judge therapies: our models and their constituent or affiliated concepts.* These abstract "guidance systems" are necessarily involved

—implicitly or explicitly—in any rational estimate of the merits of psychosurgery. A full analysis of such systems (a model of models) includes an account of what questions to formulate in making such an appraisal, and thus is a statement of the terms in which the psychosurgery debate should be pursued. It will be for the reader to undertake the final integrative stage of analysis: combining models and empirical data to judge the propriety of particular forms of psychosurgery in specified circumstances. If decisive resolution of the debate remains beyond us, we will at least have put the issues properly.

Interpretations of "Autonomy"

External autonomy refers to freedom from having one's decisions overruled by another—whether "another" is the government, a physician, or anyone else. It is, by other names, freedom from coercion or substitution of judgment, or just plain "freedom" or "liberty." *Internal autonomy* refers to one's intellectual, emotional, and physical capacities to pursue his interests; or, somewhat more narrowly, his capacity for rational self-direction. In this sense, persons who are, say, physically able and highly intelligent are more autonomous than the infirm and the dull. What the two forms of autonomy have in common is simply this: Both are measured by one's total opportunities to do things if one tries, and these in turn are functions of both internal capacities and freedom from human interference. (I will not consider other possible meanings of autonomy; for example, those relating to features of the physical world or social and economic status.) The connection between organic therapy (including psychosurgery) and these forms of autonomy seems plain: External autonomy is compromised by coercive therapy or by denial of access to therapy. Internal autonomy may be enhanced in some respects and diminished in others by the effects of various therapies.

We might also wish to relate autonomy to the very nature of our wants and preferences, but giving a precise account of that relationship would be problematic. (Such "preference-related autonomy" might be viewed as an aspect of internal autonomy.) Which of our wants "enslave" us, and which "enhance" us? Which of our wants should we want (see Fried, 1973), and which should we want excised —perhaps by therapy?

It is, of course, arguable that the term *autonomy* has, in the definitions above, been stretched too far. But I will leave this interpretative problem now, and simply suggest that autonomy is well enough understood for present purposes by linking it to our opportunities and capacities to do what we prefer and to prefer what we do. (In general, see Project, 1968, pp. 1421–1422; Katz, 1969, p. 771; Henkin, 1974; Dworkin, 1976; Shuman, 1977, p. 126.) The various conflicts among a person's own interests, and between his interests and those of others, will remain whatever our terminology.

One example involving different strands of autonomy might be instructive here—the case of Edmund Kemper, a convicted mass murderer. He has filed several unsuccessful petitions in the Solano County Superior Court to compel the Department of Corrections to allow him to undergo psychosurgery.[2] His first petition stated, "I have led a very violent life and wish to stop the violence while I can" (O'Neill, 1977). Perhaps Mr. Kemper in effect believed that his internal autonomy would be enlarged by deleting urges that, in some sense, he preferred not to have. Perhaps he also thought that his external autonomy would be enlarged—that is, that proof of the neutralization of his drives would eventually result in his release (see Delgado, 1977a, and this volume). Indeed, that prospect might in general be an important rationale for such proposed surgery (see Brown, 1975, and Brown, 1977). If therapy does in fact effect wants, it would of course also affect preference-related autonomy.

In what ways are the various forms of autonomy compromised? Limitations on external autonomy may appear in the form of laws and their enforcers. They may also appear in the form of private coercive actions or conditions that impair external autonomy—for example, therapy imposed by physicians or relatives. Limitations on internal autonomy are more difficult to characterize and assay. Disease models may purport to describe some impairments of internal autonomy, but the incorporeal qualities of the psyche make for a quite uncertain application of such a model. Still, disease models, coupled with (or containing) a general catalogue of capacities to think, feel, and strive, might well aid in explaining internal autonomy, in applying that concept to specific persons, and in evaluating the effects of organic therapies. Organic therapies, as already suggested, may in some respects augment and in other respects

---

[2] Regulations of California's Department of Corrections forbid any psychosurgery on prisoners (Title 17, California Administrative Code, Section 3343, undated; see parallel provisions in California Department of Corrections Administrative Manual, Chapter 6400, Article 3, Section 6420 (b) (1), undated). This seems inconsistent with state statutes that establish procedures by which a prisoner may be permitted, with his informed consent, to undergo psychosurgery (California Penal Code, SS2670-2680; Deering, 1978).

attenuate internal autonomy. The following sections deal with the designing of concepts for identifying and appraising such therapeutic outcomes.

The Impact of Organic Therapies on Autonomy

In assessing the impact of therapy on personal autonomy, it is useful to distinguish between the therapy's "effectiveness" and its "intrusiveness." The distinction can be explained by considering some examples of possible therapeutic results. (The explanation is in terms of effects on mental functioning and behavior, and not of the physical invasiveness of the therapy's administration.) Assume that someone is suffering from a severe case of depression of a form thought to be caused principally by electrochemical malfunctions of the brain (Mendels, 1973; Grenell and Gabay, 1976). We have a choice of therapies. We might use antidepressant drugs, stimulant drugs, electroconvulsive therapy (ECT), or psychosurgery (see Freedman, Kaplan, and Sadock, 1975, chap. 31; AMA Evaluations, 1977, pp. xxxiv, 498; see also Klerman, 1975, pp. 1003–1004). (Some work only, or best, on certain forms of depression, or are useful, if at all, mainly for short-term treatment (see AMA Evaluations, 1977, pp. xxiv, 498); and they do not all enjoy the same degree of scientific support or clinical favor. We can ignore such matters for the present purpose of conceptual analysis.)

If the antidepressants work as they are intended to, the depression will, in a sense, simply disappear after a time: the patient will just report that he has been restored to his prior condition—whatever it was—minus the depression (see Cole and Davis, 1975, pp. 1941–1942; Ulett, 1972, p. 303). If stimulants are used, the depression may briefly be masked by a "foreign" or "abnormal" state of mind—the euphoria that can be induced by such drugs (see AMA Evaluations, 1977, pp. xxxiv, 498; Ulett, 1972, p. 303; Klerman, 1975, pp. 1003–1004). ECT may also restore the prior normal mood, but with some risk of temporary memory deficits (Kalinowsky, 1975, pp. 1971, 1972). Finally, psychosurgery may eliminate the depression (see Hirose, 1972, p. 294; Hetherington, Haden, and Craig, 1972). Such surgery, however, will irreversibly destroy some brain cells. It is not known precisely what the cascading effects of this destruction might be, but some observers express concern about a "blunting" of emotional (affective) capacities—a concern not generally associated with antidepressants or ECT. There is also some concern about possible intellectual deficits. (The competing views are outlined in the National Commission's Report and Recommendations, 1977, and in the appended study by Valenstein, 1977.)

This review of some *possible* therapeutic outcomes suggests certain comparisons. The antidepressants may be effective in dissipating the unwanted mood. Their effectiveness does not seem to depend upon producing unusual or abnormal states of mind, irreversible or transient. (There are some unwanted effects, perhaps less serious than those associated with some other organic therapies, but we will disregard them here for purposes of exposition. (Consult Freedman, Kaplan, and Sadock, 1975, chap. 31; see, however, AMA Drug Evaluations, 1977, p. 476.) Contrast this with the stimulants, which may be *both* effective *and* intrusive. That is, they may produce fairly rapidly a state of mind that is probably not normal for the patient, and that, though possibly pleasurable in some sense, may be dysfunctional and even dangerous (see Cole and Davis, 1975, p. 1948). Psychosurgery may also be effective, but its mental intrusiveness remains the subject of sharp dispute. Given such dispute among medical and other authorities, it seems proper for policy-making purposes to view psychosurgery as posing a serious risk of intrusive action.

We are now ready to consider some partial definitions of *effective* and *intrusive* (Shapiro, 1974, pp. 262–269, 284–288; Shapiro, 1975, 745–746, n. 162). The notion of *effectiveness* need not long detain us, though it is not the most precise of concepts. All we need to say here is that if a therapy is effective, it diminishes, abolishes, or "covers over" the unwanted mood or thought processes. (Such outcomes, of course, are a matter of degree.) *Intrusiveness* seems to depend on a number of criteria. (Few, if any, are necessary for applying the term, although some may be individually sufficient if present in strong measure, and some may be jointly sufficient.) They include: (1) the relative abnormality (for a given person) of the induced psychic state; (2) the possibility of resisting such mental changes once the therapy has been administered (a criterion that, like some others, overlaps with "effectiveness"—it would be difficult, should anyone wish to try, to resist the mental effects of antidepressants by an exercise of will); (3) the scope of the induced change (a slight decline in anxiety is not quite as global as massive euphoria); (4) the extent to which it is possible to resist acting in ways impelled by the therapy; (5) the rapidity of onset of the effects; (6) the duration of the effects; and (7) the potential irreversibility of the effects. (This list is not intended to be exhaustive.) The conceptual overlap between effectiveness and intrusiveness is obvious, but so are the differences. Perhaps the most appropriate caution concerning these concepts is to suggest that they designate continua, and that one should speak of *relative* degrees of effectiveness and intrusiveness—just as we speak of relative degrees of autonomy, or of impairments caused by disease. Any organic psychiatric therapy in current use does not indeed seem to be a mix of effectiveness and intrusiveness.

Application of the Effective/Intrusive Distinction to Organic Therapies

The task of applying the concepts of effectiveness and intrusiveness began with the very process of defining them, so what follows is both application and additional specification of meaning. It also continues our exploration of the various facets of autonomy.

What a person will do or think or feel is a function of (1) his basic capacities and dispositions, both mental and physical, (2) his environmental circumstances (including social and economic status), and (3) his preferences. (We need not inquire here as to the rationales for these preferences.) The first two—capacities and environmental circumstances—determine his *opportunity set* (or *attainable set*): what he can in fact do or think or feel under existing conditions. His preferences (or *preference rankings*) over a *field of choice* within which his opportunity set is included theoretically account for his actual decisions. (On this choice-theoretic terminology, see Newman, 1965, pp. 8–10, 13–16.)

We may use these distinctions in describing and assessing the effects of psychosurgery and other organic therapies (Shapiro, 1974, pp. 301–307). For example, we can consider the effect of certain drugs upon a person's opportunity set—that is, what can be attained by him. Phenothiazines (a class of antipsychotic drugs) may help repair disordered thought processes and so increase one's opportunity set in that respect by restoring internal capacities. But in some cases "reactivation or aggravation of psychotic processes may be encountered," as may certain psychomotor and other disorders (*Physicians' Desk Reference*, 1978, p. 1615 (Prolixin); consult also Davis and Cole, 1975, p. 1936). Both sets of effects obviously may impair opportunities.

Tricyclic antidepressants may dispatch some depressions, but "can aggravate schizophrenia or convert a depression into a mania" (AMA Evaluations, 1977, p. 476), thus working intrusively as well as effectively for some patients. It seems proper, then, to hold that as a result of certain therapies, internal autonomy may in some respects be enhanced and in other respects diminished, depending upon the post-therapeutic status of a given patient's opportunity set.

If psychosurgery "blunts" emotional (affective) or cognitive capacities (Valenstein, 1973, p. 352), one's opportunity set may be diminished in those respects. But overall the set may be enlarged because the surgery's control of, say, depression or obsessive-compulsive neurosis restores the patient to greater net functionality (Kalinowsky, 1975, sec. 31.7).

If medication or psychosurgery in some way diminishes certain violent drives, it seems plausible to conclude that in some sense one's preferences have been changed (though it also seems plausible to think that conscious preferences for violence might never have existed and that the treatment nullified nonconscious impulses). As remarked, however, it may be hard to say whether a certain induced change in preferences enhances or diminishes autonomy.

The point of such observations is simply to stress the different ways in which therapy may enhance or impair opportunities and alter preferences; and to emphasize that an "aggregate" analysis of advantages and disadvantages must be pursued in making therapeutic choices. Such an analysis must take account of enlargements and diminutions in opportunity sets, and of changes in preferences and drives. If psychosurgery can cause a partial "reconstruction" of a person's identity, it seems both appropriate and necessary for the parties involved to insist upon this sort of detailed assessment of the effects of such surgery upon the internal determinants of human behavior: mental and physical capacities, and preferences. With somewhat less urgency, the same demands apply to any organic therapy. (This is not to say that nonorganic therapies should escape such scrutiny entirely; in certain cases, they too may be somewhat intrusive.)

To review: Internal autonomy will be enhanced by an effective therapy that neutralizes or controls the crippling aspects of a disorder. But to the extent that the therapy is intrusive, internal autonomy *may* be diminished. If the therapy dulls certain aptitudes or capacities (for example, by a sedative effect), the impairment of internal autonomy *in that particular respect* seems fairly plain, although on balance we might well want such an outcome (for example, in order to mask anxiety). If the therapy alters preferences, the effect on autonomy depends upon whether such preferences bind us or increase our opportunities—a problem of characterization already encountered. Whether a patient is, as a net result, better off after therapy requires a difficult "moral addition" of the positive and negative aspects of the therapy. Autonomy of any sort is of course a matter of degree (as is "competence").

Categories of Mental Functioning

In characterizing the effects of organic therapy, it may be useful to construct a categorization (a "taxonomy") of mental functioning. One could, for example, divide mental functioning into cognition (a product of intellect, reasoning power, reflection, memory); emotion or feeling (including mood—elevated or depressed, rage, anxiety); sensation and perception; "drives," "appetites," "conation" (striving), or impulses to action (see McNeil, 1970, pp. 27–37). This listing is hardly complete, but it is suggestive. (The categories of course overlap and are connected with each other in a complex mental "ecosystem.") Adequate analysis of psychosurgery, or any organic therapy, should as precisely as possible assess changes in opportunities and preferences by specific reference to these categories and subcategories of mental functioning. The concepts of effectiveness and intrusiveness should also be used with such a classification in mind.

An Autonomy Dilemma

Suppose that a patient is suffering from a severe obsessive-compulsive disorder that greatly interferes with his functioning, and that all reasonable therapies other than psychosurgery have failed to produce noticeable improvement. Assume it is thought (at least by his physician) that the disorder can be remedied—if at all—only by psychosurgery (see Valenstein, 1977, p. 37; Scoville, 1971, p. 54). The patient is nevertheless competent and capable of making informed decisions about whether to accept therapy. (Mental disorder is hardly an all-or-nothing proposition, as is evident from the complexities just noted in the classification and description of mental functioning, and from the fact that mental impairments seem frequently to be matters of degree.)[3] Assume also that the patient, although seriously incapacitated by the disorder, refuses treatment by surgery. Finally, assume, for the sake of argument, that the surgery does not cause significant emotional or intellectual deficits.

---

[3] *Winters v. Miller,* 446 F.2d 65 (2d. Cir. 1971); *New York City Health and Hosp. Corp. v. Stein,* 335 N.Y.S.2d 461, 70 Misc. 2d 944 (1972).

If he is forced or hornswoggled into surgery, his external autonomy
—freedom from substitution of judgment—is obviously compromised. Yet the therapy, under our assumptions, may promote his internal autonomy—his mental and physical capacities to pursue his
interests generally. His opportunity set, considered as a whole, may
thus be enlarged. (One might also urge that his external autonomy in
general is of greater value to him after his improvement.) For some
observers, then, the coerced therapy may appear justified. But this
purely utilitarian argument will not satisfy everyone. The man has
been "forced to be free," and for some (like myself), good consequences do not in all cases justify such intrusion upon individual
competent choice. On this view, external autonomy is presumptive-
ly prior in importance to internal autonomy (Shapiro, 1975, pp. 733–
737). (For some observers, the presumption might be overcome in
cases where external autonomy is substantially useless because of
grave impairment.) Because the purpose here is to *join* the issue and
not to settle it, I will forgo additional argument concerning this
priority. Contemporary writings on the collisions among the interests of justice, fairness, liberty, and utility abound (Rawls, 1971;
Nozick, 1974).

Other autonomy dilemmas arise because most therapies may produce both benefits and deficits (see the preceding discussion of effectiveness and intrusiveness). These problems are exacerbated when
the proposed therapy is experimental. (See Perkoff in this volume for
a discussion of the term *experimental* as used in medicine.) If a
therapy is experimental, this means that (1) we cannot confidently
list all its major effects or (2) if we can, we remain unable confidently to assign probabilities to these outcomes.[4] (Some "established"
therapies may satisfy these conditions also!) A given patient, when
presented with such a therapy, must gamble more heavily than if his
treatment were better understood. (A parallel dilemma exists where
the patient is not competent to make decisions concerning the therapy in question. The substitute decision maker—a parent or guardian, or the court—is then faced with resolving the difficulty.)

Therapy by Impairment

My reason for discussing the paradoxical term "therapy by impairment" is to call attention to the necessity of doing careful cost–
benefit analyses of the *net* effects of organic psychiatric therapies

---

[4] For another formulation, see Oregon Revised Statutes S426.700(2).

in general and psychosurgery in particular. (Some of what is said below applies, with varying degrees of force, to therapy for physical diseases.) Despite the use of negative terms like "impairment" or "diminution"—neutral terms are hard to find—I do not aim here to condemn organic therapy of any sort. As is evident from my earlier remarks, the task addressed by this paper is to try to contribute toward care and precision in thinking about organic therapy.

Some adverse outcomes of therapy may be in the form of certain kinds of "side effects." For example, antibiotics may cause anaphylactic shock. Cancer chemotherapy may kill healthy cells as well as malignant ones—a kind of "overbreadth." Antidepressants may produce dizziness (Cole and Davis, 1975, p. 1946). Phenothiazines may produce tardive dyskinesia—involuntary facial/oral movements (Davis and Cole, 1975, pp. 1934–1935). But none of these effects are part of the "logic" of the therapy. Anaphylactic shock is not a contributory factor in the killing of bacteria, nor an inevitable consequence of such destruction. Dyskinesias are not a necessary accompaniment to the control of psychosis. Sedation might be helpful to a depressed patient, but it is not essential to nor an inescapable outcome of eliminating the depression. One can imagine—and await the development of—pharmacological therapies whose target objectives are achieved without such major adverse effects.

Suppose, however, that some concededly disordered condition has an *aspect* or *property* that might be valuable. Consider a person who displays bizarre associations of concepts, "flight of ideas," odd syntheses, and a low threshold of sensitivity to environmental stimuli. (Not all these processes are among the usual targets of psychosurgery. All, however, are treated, with varying degrees of success, by organic therapies.) One facet of the syndrome might be the possibility of generating useful new ideas or perspectives. But if the underlying condition is expunged by therapy, so also is its valuable aspect. Our quandary exists because what we *do not* want is closely bound up with what we *do* want, and *both* are diminished by therapy. Note that the cost of therapy—if indeed it is a cost—is not a "side effect" unrelated to the purpose of therapy. The cost here is borne because the very point of therapy is to delete or alter certain patterns of thought and feeling that, though disordered, may have some desirable properties. Although we may not directly intend the loss of such properties, we nevertheless proceed knowing that controlling the disorder entails that loss.

Of course, some "losses" are intended. The whole point of treatment is to arrest certain tendencies that characterize the disorder. But, to the extent that these dispositions have a valuable aspect, the therapy's effects—perhaps undesired but nevertheless foreseen—include the loss of a beneficial capacity. It may well be that the syndrome under attack is such that it prevents any significant benefit from its favorable characteristics. The actual application of a creative bent associated with it might be thwarted by inappropriate mood or thinking. But these are possibilities, not certainties, and one must assess the prospect of genuine losses from, say, a slowing of ruminative thought patterns or lessened responsiveness to environmental stimuli. We cannot tell what worthy contributions may be forgone by abating the "excessive" rehearsal of ideas and feelings, or by any other repair of a thought, mood, perceptual, or motivational disorder (see Arieti, 1967, Part III; Offer and Sabshin, 1974, pp. 123–124; McNeil, 1970, pp. 32–33).

I stress again that the potential loss is not simply a side effect or the result of therapeutic "overkill," like memory loss resulting from ECT; nor is it just a relatively minor incident of some particular healing act, like cutting the skin in surgery. Losing your memory is not a necessary antecedent of elevating your mood, and boring a hole in your skull is not conceptually connected with obliterating obsessive thought patterns. But when a disorder has a serviceable aspect, eliminating the disorder eliminates that aspect and its effects: that loss is a necessary consequence of the intended workings of the therapy. What is lost is part of, or a property of, the very condition that is supposed to be palliated. The loss might be considered unfortunate, but is nevertheless accepted as an inevitable concomitant of controlling the disorder. The salutary attribute cannot be severed and preserved while the malady is cured.

Let us continue this analysis by considering the following description of the effects of extensive frontal lobe surgery. (The procedure is evidently no longer in use, and the example is offered here only as an aid to the analysis.)

> It was my impression that the beneficial effects of frontal lobe surgery, when they occurred, were attributable to a diminution of affect, or emotion, associated with memory. This procedure seemed most beneficial in patients whose pathologic behavior resulted from faulty anticipation of future events, reflected in painful emotions such as anger and depression. The effect of surgery was the patient's reduced concern for the future—a concern based on faulty memories. . . . Thus it was patients in whom painful affect was the outstanding feature —those suffering depression, severe obsessive-compulsive neuroses, intractable phobias, or intractable pain—who showed the most significant clinical improvement from this operation. The surgery altered brain function and produced the behavioral effect on the patient of living more for the present moment [Heath, 1971, p. 21].

This extract suggests the reference made earlier to intended losses. Although in some cases we may regret the loss of a possibly advantageous feature of a disorder, here the losses seem directly intended. What on one view might be a useful aspect is instead regarded as an integral part of the problem—perhaps even the main constituent of it. Thus, the "diminution of affect" (see Valenstein, 1973) may be precisely what is desired, and not simply a regretted but expected outcome. It is part of the "cure." Anyone wishing to pursue this distinction between intended and regretted effects might consult Freeman and Watts, who discuss surgical alteration of what they call "[t]he consciousness of the self by the self" (1942, p. 192). Scheflin and Opton (1978) comment on this extensively. (Again, I use these observations only to aid in constructing conceptual tools. The procedures described by Freeman and Watts are apparently not used now.)

It thus seems fair to speak (a bit loosely, perhaps) of "therapy by impairment" (see Scheflin and Opton, 1978, using different terminology), particularly where the enfeebling of something fairly called a "capacity" seems to be exactly what is wanted, rather than a reluctantly accepted inevitability. The distinction is of course difficult to draw because of the melding of the good and bad facets of the same disordered condition, and because of the problems in discerning what facets are indeed good or bad. Use of the phrase "therapy by impairment," moreover, requires an accompanying explanation indicating that even with an expected impairment the patient may be better off (or not worse off) because other native or acquired capacities not closely connected with the disorder may become more available for use after therapy.

Additional insights into the concept of therapy by impairment can be gleaned from various reviews of the basic forms of mental disorder. I emphasize that the burden of my argument is not to extol disorder, but to urge that we watch for any potentially valuable qualities that may attend it. Certain descriptions of schizophrenia are particularly instructive. One observer notes the "proliferation of psychic productions" and "increased sensitivity and heightened responsiveness to sensory and emotional stimulation" associated with schizophrenia (Lehmann, 1975, p. 891). Another observer refers to the possibility that "some schizophrenic experiences, once detached from the whole picture, can be definitely seen as an enlargement and enrichment of human life" and suggests that aspects of schizophrenic thinking "can open new horizons and lead to new paths of feeling and understanding." He stresses, of course, that "the world of schizophrenia is not to be recommended" and that "as a rule the patient is unable to exploit his potentialities" (Arieti, 1974, pp. 378–379). (On the use of psychosurgery for schizophrenia, see Brown, 1975; Scoville, 1971, p. 54; Valenstein, 1977, pp. 37–41.)

To conclude, let me reiterate that in any case of anomalous ideation, mood, or drives, one must consider whether there are desirable aspects of the illness—aspects that might be regarded as useful capacities. The attenuation of such a capacity may either be an intended part of the cure or the unwanted result of annulling a condition and so also its attributes and effects, favorable and unfavorable. It is conceivable that a patient might deem the price of controlling an illness too high if it entailed significant diminution of such a capacity. A rational decision would then be either not to treat at all or to select a relatively less intrusive treatment even if it were less effective than others.

Perhaps the problem of therapy by impairment can be managed to some extent by adjusting the *degrees* of a therapy's intertwined benefits and harms, rather than proceeding on an all-or-nothing basis (though it seems difficult to tailor psychosurgery in this way). It bears reemphasis, however, that the very identification of a "therapeutic" result as a benefit or detriment is a perilous one, as is the process of "summing up" the consequences of a given procedure. These difficulties, and the uncertainties involved in distinguishing disorder from normality in the first place, may in some instances thrust the terms "therapy" and "impairment" into a partial merger. (Consult Gaylin, 1975, pp. 16–17, for examples of impairments in physical therapy; in those cases, however, it seems clear that the net outcomes are beneficial.)

Models as Guides for Description, Evaluation, and Justification of Actions

Readers of this volume are likely to have been assaulted repeatedly with the word *model*—as in *disease model, psychological model, criminal punishment model, therapeutic model,* and so on. My project here is to explain briefly what models are, describe certain categories of them, and discuss what use models might be in appraising psychosurgery or any organic therapy. As before, the commentary is intended to further our efforts at conceptual cartography.

What sort of entity is a *model?* For our purposes, we can regard a model as an abstract set of instructions: it is a guide for thinking and decision making.[5] Thinking about problem behavior requires (1) empirically describing, explaining, and predicting behavior; (2) making moral and legal evaluations of behavior and of states of affairs, actual or predicted; and (3) justifying or proscribing private and governmental actions taken in response to such behavior and states of affairs—in particular, therapeutic actions. These are strikingly different though obviously interconnected enterprises. The models that purport to guide us in pursuing these tasks must therefore be described and distinguished.

Three types of models are relevant to our purposes: (1) *descriptive models*,[6] (2) *evaluative (ascriptive) models*,[7] and (3) *action-justifying models*. These models aid us in answering the following kinds of questions: (1) What happened, or will happen, and why? What persons might commit what kinds of acts? (2) What persons were culpable or innocent, what actions were right or wrong, what consequences were good or bad—and why? As to predicted actions and consequences, what are the answers to these same questions? (3) What responsive actions are required or permitted, if any, given these evaluations and descriptions (for example, punishment, treatment, or preventive detention), and why? Given our purposes, any action-justifying model must rest upon descriptions and evaluations, and all evaluations relate in some way to descriptions. This sequence of models, then, might be thought of as arranged in a series of three concentric circles. The first contains instructions on matters of description, explanation, and prediction. The successive larger circles contain instructions on how to carry on the enterprises of evaluation and action-justification, respectively, given the prior application of the instructions in the smaller included circles.[8] Con-

---

[5] For other and more rigorous uses of *model*, see Papandreou (1962) and Papandreou (1958). For a comparison of *model* with *theory*, see Papandreou (1958). See also Siegler and Osmond, 1974, p. xviii.

[6] "Description," when used alone, should be understood to refer not only to empirical reporting of events and processes but also to their explanation and prediction. Complex scientific languages are "descriptive" in the sense used here, even though the observational referents of many of their terms may be difficult to specify.

[7] "Evaluative" and "ascriptive" are used interchangeably here. Legal evaluation models may closely track or subsume moral evaluation models, but there is no need to elaborate on that now. For convenience, readers may take "evaluation" (or "ascription") to comprehend both matters of law and morals. "Action-justification" should be understood to refer to both government and private conduct.

[8] Depending upon our purpose, action-justification can precede evaluation, and vice versa. We might, for example, say that a person ought to do something and then conclude that he would be morally praiseworthy if he performed his duty. (We might then go on to justify giving him a medal.) Because we are appraising therapeutic action, it is appropriate to view the action-justification model as the "largest."

sider this simplified potential entry in a comprehensive action-justifying model (I express no opinion on its merits): "If (a) a person's anomalous thought, feeling or behavior—for example, depression or episodic violence—are the result of conditions $X_1, X_2, \ldots X_n$, then (b) that person is neither morally nor legally responsible for his conduct. (c) It would therefore be wrong to punish him. (c') And it would be both proper and obligatory to treat him, with or without his informed consent." The hypothesis in (a) is a descriptive one. The moral evaluation in (b) rests upon the application of moral principles within the evaluation model to the posited facts in (a). The judgment in (c), foreclosing certain action, derives from the application of another set of moral precepts, this time within the action-justifying model, to the evaluation in (b). The same holds for (c'), a conclusion that certain action is justified.

It is apparent, even from this very abbreviated example, that many models compete for recognition as *the* or even *a* governing set of instructions for each function—description, evaluation, and action-justification. Punishing may compete with curing, followers of different descriptive paradigms may do battle (Kuhn, 1970), and so on.

This overview requires elaboration. We should now investigate further the attributes of our hierarchy of models—construed as collections of basic rules, descriptions, hypotheses, and the like, that instruct us in matters of description, moral ascription, and action-justification. In the course of this exercise we will focus particularly upon disease models. It will become apparent that *disease model* can refer *either* to descriptive, evaluative, or action-justifying models. (The term is thus "normatively ambiguous.") Indeed, probing the nature of these quite different forms of disease model can be a particularly illuminating way of explaining the basic tripartite categorization of models tendered here, as well as of exposing the huge equivocality of the term disease model (Engelhardt, 1975, pp. 126–127). After completing this initial investigation, we will briefly apply the resulting conceptual scheme to psychosurgery and other organic therapies.

Descriptive Models

Descriptive models direct us in formulating and verifying useful empirical propositions, particularly by positing the existence of verifiable causes in general and then (in submodels) aiding us in finding specific causal explanations and in predicting effects. Suppose, for example, that we observe and are puzzled by the fact that someone's limbs are moving or shaking randomly and without apparent purpose. He reports that the movements are indeed involuntary. A disease model may contain as a postulate a proposition to the effect that certain anomalous bodily motions evidence or constitute a "disease" of some sort—the definition of "disease" in general and of certain diseases in particular being contained in the model. A hunt through the model may yield a rule that enjoins us to look for some damaged area or system in the brain to locate a cause; or to find an undamaged portion whose destruction would halt the random movements (Valenstein, 1973, p. 203). The disease—which might be named Parkinson's disease—may then be controlled by reference to rules (still within the descriptive model) telling us what to do *if* we wish to cure or arrest a disease. In the case of Parkinson's disease, we may, as suggested, be told to destroy certain healthy brain tissue to stop unwanted movements—the damaged portion of the brain (or other part of the body) remaining undiscovered. (Or, more likely, we will be advised to use certain drugs to control the symptoms (AMA Evaluations, 1977, chap. 71).) The model (or submodel) is thus incomplete in its explanation of the cause of the disease. (The fact that the therapy here does not entirely "fit" the disease by attacking its causes as well as its effects is not sufficient to condemn it, unless other reasonably available therapies offer a better fit—see Shapiro, 1975, pp. 712–722.) Such incompleteness saddles us with having to destroy healthy tissue, should we decide to venture brain surgery. This of course carries with it a risk of loss of normal brain function (Valenstein, 1973, p. 203).

Models for the description, explanation, and prediction of mental and behavioral anomalies are in general also incomplete. The etiology of emotional or thought disorders is still a puzzle, although theories positing the involvement of particular neurotransmitters are thought to hold much promise (Akiskal and McKinney, 1975).

A *descriptive* disease model, then, serves to order and organize our chaotic observations of human conduct and appearance. It might announce, for example, that thought, emotion, and behavior occur in recognizable repetitive clusters (M. S. Moore, 1975, p. 1491) and that a notion of disease can be founded upon the existence of some of these aggregations. (Other interpretations of "disease" might also be included in the model.) "Disease"—or references to specific diseases —would then serve approximately the same logical descriptive-explanatory-predictive functions that more precisely defined theoretical terms like "electromagnetic field" serve in the physical sciences. Contrast a model of this sort with a behaviorist descriptive model, which dispenses with notions of disease and simply focuses on describing how living beings behave under varying conditions, and how behavior is shaped by arrangement of different environmental contingencies.

Evaluative (Ascriptive) Models

After incorporating some descriptive model, an evaluative model would add rules concerning the determination of moral or legal culpability, the rightness or wrongness of actions,[9] and the goodness or badness of various states of affairs. Perhaps a body of utilitarian rules would inform such assessments. Or the model might instead embrace a set of "formalistic" moral rules not focusing on utilitarian appraisal of consequences (Frankena, 1973, pp. 14–17). An evaluative disease model (not a descriptive one) would contain rules announcing (for example) that if certain conduct were caused by mental disease, such conduct should be considered non-culpable or less culpable than similar conduct by healthy persons. An evaluative behaviorist model might, however, be partly self-annihilating. It could decree the ascription of personal moral responsibility to be irrelevant or meaningless and wave us on to its related action-justifying model dealing with behavior therapy for those engaging in "maladaptive conduct." But even if customary moral terminology were not used, a utilitarian standard informed by descriptions of adaptive behavior would seem to be implicit within a behaviorist model. That standard would, quite simply, announce that "adaptive" behavior does more good than "maladaptive behavior" and is therefore right. The model, however, is a rather sparsely populated one when compared with evaluative disease models.

Action-Justifying Models

Action-justifying models subsume both descriptive and evaluative models. They contain principles that state what ought to or may be done or avoided, *given* certain descriptions, empirical hypotheses, and moral and legal evaluations of persons and their

---

[9] Actions evaluated within this model do not belong within an action-justifying model as understood here; the latter is reserved for actions taken in response to earlier actions or situations, or to avert or deal with future actions or situations. Thus, someone's actions might first be adjudged legally culpable under an evaluative model, and punishment might then be justified as a response under an action-justifying model.

actions. Action-justifying models and evaluative models are both concerned with species of moral judgment (or "evaluation" in a broad sense), but they serve different functions. The former tell us what actions to take (if any) *in response* to or in anticipation of certain *other* actions that have been evaluated via the latter. Action-justifying models also instruct us on what to do, if anything, about various existing or potential conditions.

Consider, for example, a punishment model. This model would direct us to inflict certain penalties on those—and only those—who had violated the penal laws, and not just to "treat" them in order to "cure" their criminality (if it bid or allowed us to try that at all). It might also require that violators found to be nonculpable because of mental disorder (in accordance with an included evaluative disease model) should be dealt with only by way of treatment. Such a punishment model would, then, incorporate an action-justifying disease submodel, telling us what to do to offenders whose conduct is found to be the result of certain disorders.

A "therapeutic state" model would displace punishment entirely and deal solely with treatment of offenders—and perhaps even of nonoffenders—thus melding with the traditional mental health systems. Under a disease submodel, certain forms of therapy would be justified on a showing of mental disorder that results in dangerousness or disability, or possibly even on a showing of mental disorder alone. Under a behaviorist submodel, behavior therapy would be authorized for persons engaging in maladaptive behaviors of certain kinds.

It is once again apparent that rival systems vie for recognition as operative models and submodels. A punishment model may compete with a therapeutic state model, different forms of punishment models may compete with one another, and therapeutic state models may contend among themselves. Thus, within a punishment model, sanctions might be justified solely by reference to their beneficial effects—like deterrence, incapacitation, rehabilitation, and moral education. A competing punishment model might instead announce that an analysis of such consequences would be irrelevant, and that punishment should be inflicted solely on the basis of moral desert.

Varieties of Constituent Models

Now that we have glanced at the three major categories of models, let us venture some additional comments about their submodels.

Disease models may be either descriptive, evaluative, or action-justifying. And they may be "physicalist" or "psychological" ("mentalist"). (See Blaney, 1975.) A matter of particular importance is that descriptive and ascriptive disease models do not stand primly alone: they are generally constructed with a view toward justification of therapeutic action (Engelhardt, 1975, pp. 126–127, 137). That is, it may be expected and intended that a descriptive disease model will be implanted in an evaluative model, which in turn is to be included in an action-justifying model. One should stress here that action-justifying models serve not only to justify actions but also to condemn them. If the action-justifying disease model is used properly, for example, it not only permits or requires therapeutic actions, but, under appropriate conditions, decrees that they should *not* be undertaken. For example, the absence of disease or of a threat of it would foreclose any therapeutic actions. One might expect, however, that a properly eclectic or "mixed" therapeutic action-justifying model could specify the appropriate occasions for certain forms of "behavior modification" programs without violating the basic tenets of a disease model (see Kazdin, 1978, and in this volume).

A *psychological* descriptive model is one that couches its descriptions of events and processes, its causal hypotheses, and its predictions in the language of psychology, using primarily "mentalist" terms (for example, psychodynamic concepts). A *physical* or *biological* descriptive model would, instead, correlate behavior with descriptions framed in physical terms: neurotransmitter concentrations, lesions, and the like. But there is, I think, no theoretical barrier to construction of a blended model combining both physicalist and mentalist terms. Whether physicalist and mentalist descriptive models include disease submodels depends on the subject matter involved.

An examination of *social models* can aid in reviewing the analysis of our triad of model types. In its descriptive mode, a social model focuses mainly upon the environmental causes of behavior. Such a model, as one might expect, is likely to be tailored for use in both an evaluative model and an action-justifying one. The evaluative social model may be intended to attenuate traditional concepts of personal moral responsibility by announcing that certain environmental factors (a gravely disadvantaged upbringing, for example) can be inconsistent with a fair ascription of moral culpability for specified kinds of action. A "rotten social background" might thus (in such a model) exculpate as effectively as a case of insanity or automatism (La Fave and Scott, 1972, chap. 4). (A "rotten social background" defense was chanced unsuccessfully in 1973 in *U.S.* v. *Alexander.*)[10] An action-justifying social model might concentrate upon both governmental and private programs for social betterment and public welfare as means of reducing crime. There is certainly no reason, however, why models of this sort cannot include as useful tools an assortment of descriptive psychological or biological submodels, including disease submodels.

Applications to Psychosurgery

The last task of this commentary is briefly to apply our collection of conceptual tools to the problems of appraising psychosurgery. This may aid in explaining why some observers view the practice unfavorably.

We are properly uneasy about invading the body by surgery. Unless explained, cutting looks like mayhem, and boring into the "executive organ" (Brody, 1973) appears even more alarming. One expects the explanation to be a medical one, and so we listen for an account describing either a physical disorder or a mental one. We listen further for a causal hypothesis linking the disorder to unwanted mental functioning and behavior. And finally we await an exposition of another causal hypothesis—one that claims the surgery to be effective in achieving the therapeutic goal. The last hypothesis, one would hope, would appear in a form detailed enough to enable us also to assess the relative intrusiveness of the surgery.

Although there seems to be no decisive argument against employing organic therapies for maladies described or explained solely in psychological terms (Durell, 1973, p. 5), those favoring certain forms of brain surgery are likely to be heavily influenced by physicalist causal models (for example, Mark and Ervin, 1970). So, the likeliest starting point for justifying psychosurgery is some notion of physical disorder. But here we encounter difficulty from the outset. Quite apart from the problem of showing certain mentation and behavior to be the "product" of disease of any sort, physical or mental, we are confronted with the stunning gaps in our knowledge of the brain —its structure, chemistry, and electrical properties. If psychosurgery is for mental and behavioral anomalies caused by brain disorders, what is the nature of these disorders? If we can find, through implanted electrodes, brain sites correlated with aggressive impulsives or abnormal "spiking" on an electroencephalogram (EEG), we

---

[10] *U.S.* v. *Alexander,* 421 F2d 923 (D.C. Cir. 1973).

may have the *beginnings* of a physical interpretation of the person's disorder. We cannot always do this, however, and even when we can, the correlations may be weak or relatively uninstructive: aggression may not always be associated with EEG abnormalities, and EEG abnormalities may not always be associated with aggression (Valenstein, 1973, pp. 258–260).

But why bother with a notion of physical disorder at all? If destruction of brain tissue does indeed improve mentation and behavior, perhaps the surgery should proceed whether or not we have verified the existence of a specific physical disorder of the brain. Some surgeons may indeed hold this view, as suggested by Valenstein (1973, p. 222): "[I]t seems apparent that Dr. Narabayashi [in dealing with behavior problems] is not destroying a specific abnormal brain focus, since he tends to aim for the same target in all patients."

Thus, psychosurgery does not at present seem to be a straightforward application of any therapeutic model that embraces a physicalist causal submodel to explain mental and behavioral problems.

If we take the alternative route of holding that mental rather than physical disorder is what justifies surgery, we are then confronted with a notion so vague and variable that psychiatric diagnosis may sometimes look more like rolling dice than forming scientific hypotheses (see Spitzer and Fleiss, 1974; Morse, 1978). While one need not embrace the full Szazsian conclusion that "mental disorder" is dangerous gibberish (gibberish because the term is meaningless; dangerous because the concept purports to authorize abusive medical action), his attacks on the use of the concept do score points (Szasz, 1974). (For a commentary on Szasz, see M. S. Moore, 1975. In general, consult Morse, 1978.)

If neither physical nor mental disease models provide an entirely satisfactory basis for justifying psychosurgery, it may be tempting for its advocates to become functional behaviorists of sorts, and to dispense with the notion of disorder. The focus would then be on the objectionable or dysfunctional character of behavior, and on the relative efficacy of psychosurgery in appropriately altering it.

Some efforts to apply the ideas of effectiveness and intrusiveness to psychosurgery and other organic therapies were begun earlier, and elaborated upon in the section on "therapy by impairment." I do not intend to apply the data gathered in recent years on the outcomes of psychosurgery to the intellectual maps I have been trying to outline. The reader should consult other entries in this volume and certain recent works that are instructive on these matters (National Commission, 1977; Valenstein, 1973; Shuman, 1977). It remains much in dispute whether psychosurgery's relative effectiveness in ameliorating mental or behavioral anomalies supports its use, and whether its relative intrusiveness is such as to weigh against it. Two competing appraisals of psychosurgery still stand in full battle dress: the belief that psychosurgery increases *net* capacities with minimal or undetectable losses, and the belief that it constitutes a kind of ruinous "trespass on the mind" (see Scheflin and Opton, 1978). Because of the differing values these beliefs may represent, the battle could continue even if there were agreement on all sides on what actually happens, as a matter of raw fact, following surgery.

Let us focus now on the connection between moral or legal evaluation and the ultimate justification of psychosurgery or other organic therapy. Suppose that we are governed either (a) by an evaluative disease model, which contains certain rules for moral and legal exculpation or mitigation, or (b) an evaluative behaviorist model, which contains an instruction not to bother ascribing personal culpability at all. Under the evaluative disease model, we may decide that certain persons are relatively nonculpable because it is thought that their conduct was the product of some disease, physical or mental. (Looking ahead to the application of an action-justifying model, we would expect such persons to merit little or no punishment.) If the disease is physical—particularly a brain disorder—the exculpatory pressure may be greater than if the disease were a mental one. (I will not try to explain here why that might be so.) To the extent, then, that harmful behavior is "explained" within a physical disease model, there is a push toward exculpation or mitigation. (Our action-justifying model might then decree organic therapy for disease.) Further, the more we know about the biological bases of behavior and the workings of organic therapy, the more diseases we are likely to recognize (invent?) and the more potential therapeutic targets we will have (see Gardner, 1974). Disorders defined within a mentalist model may of course also exculpate or mitigate and open the way for greater therapeutic opportunities within an action-justifying model.

Within the relatively meager evaluative behaviorist model, there is probably no well-worked out culpability theory. (In a pure behaviorist action-justifying model, the only "punishment" concept to be found is one having to do with how behavior therapists should structure reward and punishment schedules, and that has nothing to do with criminal punishment based upon moral desert.) One would surely expect an impetus to treat when the very concepts of culpability and moral desert are thought to be irrelevant or meaningless (see Kadish and Paulsen, 1975, pp. 151–155; Wootton, 1963).

In general, then, evaluative disease models that serve to exculpate or mitigate in certain cases pave the way for justification of therapy, and so also do evaluative behaviorist models that exclude notions of disease and culpability and concentrate upon the analysis of adaptive and maladaptive behavior under a utilitarian standard. In short, when little or no culpability is assigned, under whatever model, one's thoughts turn to therapy.

A caution should be added here on the interplay between culpability ascriptions and the ultimate justifications for punishment or therapy. A finding of culpability under an evaluative model, followed by a justification for punishment under an action-justifying model, does not necessarily foreclose therapy—no rational action-justifying model contains an absolute moral proscription against providing criminals with behavior-altering treatment. The processes of rehabilitation, the inducing of mental and behavioral changes by organic therapy, and the techniques of behavior therapy seem quite different, but I cannot pursue these distinctions here. (See, however, Delgado, 1977a, 1977b, and this volume.)

Some closing remarks on the application of action-justifying models to psychosurgery seem to be in order. The process of justifying or proscribing actions requires descriptions—here, of conduct and its causes. It also requires certain moral evaluations of individual conduct, or, at the least, of particular states of affairs. But if our descriptive models are incomplete, any evaluative or action-justifying models that include such descriptive models are ill-informed. This is illustrated by the difficulties we encounter in trying to use the concepts of mental and physical disorder to justify psychosurgery. Because of the present weakness of the physical disease model in accounting for behavior and the near-legendary difficulties in using the concept of mental disorder, there may be some tendency to embrace—at least implicitly—a semibehaviorist action-justifying model. In such a model, the prime justificatory concept would be "maladaptive behavior," or perhaps "dangerous behavior." But these are exceptionally imprecise concepts, and when applied they may call into question whether we are indeed engaged in an intelligible discourse. Action-justifying concepts are supposed to aid us in saying "when" and "when-not." The concept of disease is *both* an authorizing tool *and* a limiting tool. But replacement concepts—for example, behaviorist ones—may be so vague that decisions are left largely unguided. "Dangerous" is a dangerous term to adopt as the principal tool for justifying therapy, particularly psychosurgery and other organic therapies.

CHAPTER 14

The Sociopsychological Model and Behavior Therapy

Alan E. Kazdin

Traditionally, psychiatric disorders have been viewed as diseases. Where organic pathology is evident, as in the case of some psychotic disorders, there is no dispute about the appropriateness of the view that there is a "disease process," as the term is ordinarily used in medicine. Yet, the disease view has been extended to those disorders for which no clear organic pathology is evident—that is, functional disorders. With these disorders, the absence of clear physical disease has led to the notion that there is "mental disease," or psychological dysfunction analogous to physical disease. Abnormal behavior is regarded as a product of pathological psychological processes.

The disease view has had a major influence on all facets of the "mental health" professions, including the search for specific disease entities, the treatment of individuals who are diagnosed as mentally ill, and the model of delivering psychological services. The disease view is so deeply entrenched in contemporary psychiatry and clinical psychology that one cannot easily discuss psychological problems or aberrant behavior and their amelioration without drawing upon the terminology of the disease view. For example, "patients" who have some form of "psychopathology" are seen for "treatment" either on an "outpatient" or "inpatient" basis. Each of these terms and many others that could be generated reflect the disease model of deviant behavior.

Many writers have rejected the disease model as an appropriate characterization of problems that individuals bring to treatment (for example, Laing, 1967; Szasz, 1961). Prominent among the alternative approaches is the sociopsychological model (Ullmann and Krasner, 1969). This model views psychological disorders as behavioral problems and examines the social context in which these behaviors are likely to develop.

There are many factors that have given rise to a sociopsychological model of abnormal behavior, aside from criticism of the disease model. One impetus has been recognition that detection, diagnosis, and treatment of abnormal behavior vary drastically from the model used in physical medicine. Defining and diagnosing abnormal behavior entail a number of social considerations and value judgments that extend beyond the boundaries of merely detecting disease. Investigation of many of these factors has stimulated views that give greater weight to the social conditions in which problem behaviors arise than to disease processes within the individual.

Another impetus for the sociopsychological model has been the development of effective psychological treatment techniques—particularly, *behavior modification* techniques, which are based upon the assumption that deviant behavior is learned and can be altered through new learning experiences.[1] Behavior modification refers to the application of principles from scientific psychology for the purposes of changing deviant behavior and psychological dysfunction. The techniques have effected therapeutic change in a number of problem areas and, hence, have promoted the role of learning in conceptualizations of the development and amelioration of deviant behavior.

The sociopsychological model and behavioral treatment methods that are subsumed under it represent multifaceted topics. A detailed account of these topics is beyond the scope of the present chapter. For present purposes, it is important to provide an overview of the model and to illustrate the assumptions and general approach toward psychiatric disorders. The model provides the conceptual basis for treatment techniques. The treatment techniques warrant more

---

[1] The terms *behavior modification* and *behavior therapy* occasionally are distinguished in the literature. However, since this distinction is not consistent and is invoked very infrequently, the terms will be used interchangeably here.

detail because they represent alternatives to more intrusive interventions such as psychosurgery. Thus, much of the chapter will be devoted to treatment techniques for psychiatric disorders to which psychosurgery is most frequently applied. Finally, the limitations and restrictions of contemporary behavioral treatment techniques will be discussed.

The Sociopsychological Model

The sociopsychological model can be characterized by a relatively small number of assumptions about the nature of psychiatric disorders and the principles that govern behavior. The model can be represented by describing how psychiatric impairment is viewed in general, without considering specific disorders.

Abnormal Behavior as a Social Phenomenon

Behavior is labeled and diagnosed as mental illness on the grounds of social criteria. Individuals are diagnosed as mentally ill or psychologically disturbed because they are not functioning adequately in everyday life. Their behaviors are either disturbing to themselves or to others around them. Whether a behavior is disturbing may depend upon the social context in which the behavior occurs and hence the evaluation of that behavior. Deviance is defined by the normative standards for performance and a judgment that these standards are in some way violated.

Although deviant behavior occurs throughout society, not all of it is labeled as mental illness and comes to the attention of mental health professionals (see Srole et al., 1962). Presumably, facets such as bizarreness, intensity, and dangerousness contribute to labeling the behavior as deviant and indicative of mental illness. The very labeling of behavior as deviant has a significant effect, according to the sociopsychological model, inasmuch as it helps crystallize forms of deviance that might otherwise be transient (Scheff, 1966). Labeling individuals as mentally ill influences how they are viewed by others and how they view themselves. These changes in perception are not innocuous influences but themselves contribute directly to the perception and actual performance of deviant behavior on the part of the individual identified as mentally ill (see Farina et al., 1971).

Learned Basis of Behavior

An important tenet of the sociopsychological model is that most behavior is learned. Whether behavior is labeled as deviant or normal, it follows the same laws and principles of learning. Abnormal behavior, according to the model, does not differ qualitatively from normal behavior. In the absence of objective organic signs of impairment or dysfunction, abnormality can be profitably conceptualized and treated as learned behavior. (Ullmann and Krasner, 1969).

Conceptualizing abnormal behavior as learned in much the same way as normal behavior brings to bear scientific findings from the psychology of learning. Indeed, the sociopsychological model relies upon the psychology of learning both as an explanation of the development of behavior and as the basis for generating specific treatment techniques to effect therapeutic change. Different types of learning have been delineated, among them *classical conditioning, operant conditioning,* and *observational learning.* These are not the only types of learning that can be distinguished in psychology. However, these forms of learning and their interrelationships have been relied upon heavily in explaining the development of behavior and in generating specific treatment techniques. If deviant behaviors are conceptualized in terms of problems in learning, then distinct courses of action can be recommended for treatment.

Traditionally, psychiatry has diagnosed deviant behaviors in terms of specific disease entities. Even where there are no signs of organic impairment, the search has been for diseases—mental diseases. One reason for attempting to distinguish disease entities is to discover etiology and treatment methods for the disorders. The sociopsychological model attempts to formulate maladaptive behaviors in terms other than disease entities but with the same purposes in mind. Deviant behavior is conceptualized in terms of particular learning experiences or the absence of particular learning experiences. Problem behaviors are interpreted as reflecting avoidance reactions (for example, phobias), deficits in responding (for example, lack of social skills of psychiatric patients), bizarre behavioral patterns (for example, self-abusive behavior of autistic children), control of behavior by socially inappropriate or censured stimuli (for example, attraction to socially inappropriate sexual objects), behavioral excesses (for example, hyperactivity), and similar concepts. Formulation of problems in these terms suggests the learning experiences that need to be provided to ameliorate behavior.

Behavioral Problems Versus Illness

As already mentioned, traditionally psychiatric disorders have been viewed as illnesses. The illnesses are viewed as distinct entities recognizable by certain constellations of symptoms. This approach obviously reflects the medical approach to physical diseases. Diseases usually have a common set of recognizable symptoms. One or a few symptoms or perhaps the combination can be used to diagnose the disorder. The search for distinct disorders in psychiatry has led to a host of problems. For example, professionals frequently disagree over how to diagnose particular patients' symptoms (Zubin, 1967). Also, many different psychiatric disorders seem to share similar symptoms (for example, Katz, Cole, and Lowery, 1964). Finally, the search for specific diseases has not greatly enhanced treatment. Specific treatments are not available for the vast majority of psychiatric disorders.

The sociopsychological model deviates rather sharply from the traditional approach within psychiatry. Rather than attempting to diagnose general conditions or states, the model focuses upon specific behaviors. For example, neurotic individuals would not be treated with global treatments such as psychotherapy that attempt to ameliorate the general conditions assumed to underlie their neuroses. Rather, treatment specifies those stimuli that evoke anxiety for a given client and consists of techniques designed to reduce anxiety in the presence of these stimuli. Treatments derived from the sociopsychological model tend to be recommended for concrete and specifiable conditions. This does not necessarily mean that the treatments focus upon superficial behaviors or attempt to trivialize significant psychological problems. Rather, global problems as defined by the client or professionals are analyzed to address concretely the changes that need to be made in treatment.

Relationship to Traditional Models of Behavior

The sociopsychological model has developed as an alternative to major positions traditionally adhered to within psychiatry. The two dominant models have been the intrapsychic and biological models of psychological dysfunction.

The *intrapsychic model*, the more recent view, has traced psychological problems to disturbed psychodynamic processes. These "diseased" processes may reflect conflict, unresolved tensions, or repression of socially censured impulses. Problem behaviors that are identified as abnormal are considered to result directly from these underlying psychological processes. Psychoanalytic theory, as espoused by Freud, has exerted the greatest influence on the intrapsychic model in contemporary psychiatry. However, psychoanalytic theory and its variations represent only one of many different intrapsychic theories of abnormal behavior. Each of these positions takes a disease view of aberrant behavior. Since the aberrant behavior is viewed as a symptom of an underlying psychological disturbance, it is the underlying disturbance rather than the aberrant behavior that is assumed to be the most appropriate focus of treatment. Psychoanalysis and psychotherapy often are viewed as ways to unravel the intricate psychic processes and thereby rectify the individual's performance.

The sociopsychological model grew largely as an alternative to psychoanalysis and the intrapsychic model of abnormal behavior. These models diverge sharply, particularly in their assumptions about the factors that contribute to behavior and their approaches to evaluating therapy techniques. The sociopsychological model attempts to treat maladaptive behavior as such and to evaluate procedures designed to ameliorate specific client problems. Intrapsychic processes that are based upon inferential leaps and clinical interpretations tend to be avoided. The strong commitment of sociopsychological treatment techniques to empirical research has required operationalization of client problems and the treatments with which they are altered.

Aside from the intrapsychic approach, much of psychiatry has been deeply committed to a *biological model* of abnormal behavior. Essentially, this model views abnormal behavior as a function of biological substrates. Behavioral aberrations and psychological symptoms are considered to be the result of physical anomalies or dysfunction. Biological approaches cover many different areas of research, including genetics, biochemistry, neurology, and other fields that may help uncover these organic bases of abnormal behavior. Indeed, many advances have been made. The biological bases of psychiatric disorders have been clearly established in the case of organic psychoses, specific forms of mental retardation, and certain other disorders.

Treatments within the biological model have included surgery, electroconvulsive shock, insulin treatment, drugs, and others. Certainly, the advent of psychotropic drugs has had the greatest impact on patient care in the last twenty-five years. Many drugs are available to alleviate anxiety that inhibits the functioning of neurotic patients, to reinstate favorable affect in individuals whose depression is acute, and to reduce psychotic symptoms or hyperactivity.

The sociopsychological model does not conflict directly with the biological model or treatments of abnormal behavior. Disorders for which biological causes and treatments have been identified are certainly within the domain of biological approaches and disciplines such as medicine. The sociopsychological model focuses primarily upon those disorders not yet known to have a clear biological basis or treatment. Even for disorders with demonstrable biological components, the possible relevance of the sociopsychological model is not necessarily ruled out. Behavior modification techniques may effectively alter problem behaviors independently of their origin. The original cause of a disorder does not necessarily limit the type of intervention that will be effective. (Also, effective treatments for a disorder do not necessarily reveal the original cause.) Thus, the etiology and treatment of a disorder may be independent.

The efficacy of treatment for a given problem must be determined empirically. Treatments from the sociopsychological model have successfully treated diverse behaviors. Occasionally, the treatments are used in conjunction with biological interventions (for example, drugs). The effects of treatment procedures need to be evaluated on the basis of their evidence rather than on the theoretical model of deviant behavior from which each technique was derived (see Kazdin and Wilson, 1978).

In general, the sociopsychological model departs from the biological model in explaining the nature of many problems of living that are currently in the domain of psychiatry. The disease model is rejected for psychological dysfunction in general in favor of looking at learned behaviors, response deficits, and so on. The sociopsychological model is concerned with developing effective treatments and as such does not necessarily rule out biological or other sorts of interventions. Proponents of the sociopsychological model are mainly interested in psychological interventions but view the verdict on effective treatments to be in the realm of experimental evidence rather than theoretical orientation. Because of the similar commitment of biological approaches to empirical evaluation, there is no incompatibility or necessary competition among different sorts of treatment.

Although concerns about treatment efficacy represent a compatibility between biological and sociopsychological models, efficacy is not the only dimension on which treatments are evaluated. The sociopsychological model is interested in treatments based upon learning. The treatments generally are not intrusive or irreversible in their effects, as biological procedures such as psychosurgery may be. For this reason as well, proponents of the sociopsychological model tend to advocate behavioral treatments as alternatives, whenever possible, to more intrusive and less well-researched techniques.

Behavior Modification Techniques

The primary basis for assuming that maladaptive behaviors are learned is that this assumption has been extremely useful in generating treatment procedures. Actually, the sociopsychological model has not made major advances in understanding the etiology of behaviors that are seen in psychiatric treatment. If etiology refers to original causes of behavior—the frequent meaning of the term in psychiatric circles—then little firm data are available for any model of psychiatric disorder. On the other hand, the *contemporary* causes or sources that sustain behavior can be more readily identified. These latter causes refer to contemporary factors in the individual's life that may sustain deviant behavior and serve as the basis for developing new behaviors.

The sociopsychological model has generated several effective behavior modification techniques that focus upon the individual's current functioning. These techniques include many procedures that are well researched. Behavioral techniques draw upon experimental psychology, particularly the psychology of learning, to generate specific forms of treatment. Although the treatments are well investigated in their own right, experimental laboratory research has provided a heuristic base. Another unifying theme among the diverse behavioral techniques is a strong commitment to experimental evaluation of treatment. In the final analysis, the experimental evaluation of a given technique must serve as the basis for claims of efficacy. Behavior modification has been committed to evaluation perhaps even more than to the derivation of new techniques.

Behavior therapy techniques have been used for diverse forms of neurotic reactions, psychotic behaviors, childhood problems, mental retardation, hyperactivity, obesity, alcoholism, delinquency, and several other behavioral disorders (see Kazdin and Wilson, 1978). It is not possible in this chapter to enumerate or describe the techniques and the specific problems within each disorder that have been treated. For present purposes, it is more important to evaluate the evidence for behavioral treatments of anxiety, obsessions and compulsions, and depression. The reason for this delimited focus is that the bulk of psychosurgery for psychiatric disorders has focused upon these problems as a "last resort" technique. Although anxiety has received considerable attention in behavior modification, obsessive-compulsive disorders have received relatively little controlled treatment research, and depression even less. Nevertheless, it is useful to appraise the available evidence that would attest to the viability of behavior therapy as an alternative treatment procedure.

Anxiety and Phobic Reactions

Behavior therapy techniques have been applied very successfully to anxiety reactions. The reactions usually consist of avoidance and fear responses to specific sorts of situations or stimuli, such as the fear of heights, open spaces, or social situations, but extend to many other problems as well, such as insomnia, sexual dysfunction, and psychosomatic disorders, in which anxiety may be implicated.

Several different behavior therapy techniques exist for the treatment of anxiety. The best known is *systematic desensitization*, a technique developed in the 1950s by Wolpe (1958). Systematic desensitization usually begins by training clients to deeply relax individual muscle groups until a general state of relaxation can be achieved. After relaxation training, formal treatment begins. This consists of pairing a state of relaxation with the presentation of anxiety-provoking cues. Typically, the cues are presented by instructing clients to imagine a series of scenes. The scenes are presented in a hierarchical fashion beginning with those that elicit little or no anxiety and continuing through the hierarchy to the most anxiety-provoking scenes. The purpose of treatment is to associate the anxiety-provoking stimuli with relaxation so that the stimuli no longer evoke anxiety responses. This is accomplished by ensuring that only small doses of anxiety-provoking stimuli are presented while the individual maintains deeply relaxed throughout treatment.

Although desensitization usually is conducted with imagery, the procedure may be used *in vivo* as well. With *in vivo* desensitization, patients learn how to apply relaxation in the actual situations that provoke anxiety. As with the imagined stimuli, *in vivo* events are graded according to the extent to which they provoke anxiety and are presented gradually in an hierarchical fashion. Although both desensitization with imagery and *in vivo* are effective, the *in vivo* procedure tends to effect greater therapeutic change (for example, Crowe et al., 1972; Sherman, 1972).

The outcome research for systematic desensitization has been impressive. Indeed, comprehensive reviews of the research have uniformly endorsed desensitization as a highly effective technique in overcoming anxiety (for example, Leitenberg, 1976; Paul, 1969). A wide range of anxiety-based disorders has been treated, including relatively circumscribed as well as more global problems and single as well as multiple phobias. Several investigations have compared desensitization with other therapy techniques (Kazdin and Wilson, 1978). Although desensitization has been more effective than psychotherapy, and no treatment, alternative behavior therapy techniques exist that are more effective than desensitization in treating anxiety-based disorders.

Reinforced practice, another behavioral treatment technique, consists of overtly practicing behavior in anxiety-provoking situations to overcome anxiety. The procedure attempts to encourage individuals to engage in increasing amounts of contact in the environment with the stimuli or situations that produce anxiety. In this sense, the procedure resembles *in vivo* desensitization, although no relaxation is used to help minimize anxiety. Also, in reinforced practice the therapist relies heavily upon instructions to encourage initiation of the behaviors, consistent feedback for client performance, and praise for progress. Research has demonstrated that reinforced practice is superior to no treatment and to systematic desensitization in effecting therapeutic change (for example, Barlow et al., 1970; Crowe et al., 1972).

Modeling is yet another technique for the treatment of anxiety reactions. Modeling as usually conducted consists of exposing the patient to someone else (a model) who can perform the desired behaviors without experiencing anxiety. By merely observing a model engage in the responses that were associated with avoidance behavior, either on film or in a live demonstration, the patient learns to perform the desired response. As with desensitization and reinforced practice, the behaviors that are performed, in this case by the model, are ordered in a graduated or hierarchical fashion. Outcome research has shown that modeling with either a live or film model is effective in overcoming anxiety reactions (Rachman, 1976; Rosenthal and Bandura, 1978). The effects of treatment can be markedly enhanced by a variation referred to as *participant modeling,* or modeling with guided participation. In this procedure, the client not only observes a model perform the desired responses but, after observing the response, makes an attempt to perform the response as well. In a sense, this procedure combines modeling and reinforced practice into one treatment. Research has demonstrated that participant modeling is more effective than desensitization or modeling without participation (for example, Bandura, Blanchard, and Ritter, 1969; Röper, Rachman, and Marks, 1975).

Flooding is a very effective treatment of anxiety-based disorders and has been well investigated. Flooding consists of exposing the client to the maximum intensity of anxiety-producing situations. Unlike systematic desensitization, reinforced practice, or modeling, flooding does not present the fear-producing situations in a graduated fashion. Rather, the client is exposed to the full intensity of the fear-provoking events. For example, a client who fears open spaces would be exposed to the relevant situations either in imagination or *in vivo* to maximize anxiety. Exposure to the feared stimuli is continued for prolonged periods at one time (for example, an hour) until anxiety and physiological arousal subside. Exposure, either in imagination or *in vivo*, is repeated until anxiety is eliminated. Although both variations of flooding are effective, exposure to the fear-provoking stimuli in real life is more effective than exposure in imagination (for example, Stern and Marks, 1973; Watson and Marks, 1971).

The treatments just described are the major techniques currently available for treating anxiety. The range of clients treated with these techniques is rather large and encompasses both outpatient and inpatient populations. The research on these techniques is voluminous and has been amply reviewed in the behavior modification literature (for example, Kazdin and Wilson, 1978; Leitenberg, 1976; Marks, 1975). Each of the procedures has been shown to be very effective in controlled experiments. A relatively consistent pattern in the literature is that variations of the above techniques that involve actually performing in everyday situations are more effective than imagining the feared stimulus or seeing a model engage in the desired performance. However, these latter procedures are sufficiently effective to warrant use in their own right. Occasionally, clients are given "homework" assignments or specific recommendations to complete various tasks outside of treatment to provide *in vivo* experiences and, hence, to enhance the effects of therapy. This appears to accomplish the intended goal.

An important point should be noted in passing about the focus of behavior therapy techniques for anxiety. The bulk of the research has focused upon specific and relatively circumscribed fears. The primary purpose of this focus has been for experimental evaluation of treatment effects. The specificity of focus facilitates evaluation of patient progress and comparisons among patients receiving different treatments. However, the specificity of focus in much of the research should not be construed as meaning that behavior therapy must be directed at narrowly circumscribed problems. Indeed, there is no evidence that the effectiveness behavior therapy depends upon the specificity of focus. Many clients treated in research or case applications evince anxiety to multiple sources of stimuli. Also, treatment for specific sources of anxiety often results in reductions in anxiety across several areas of maladaptive functioning that have not been treated directly.

Obsessive-Compulsive Disorders

Obsessive-compulsive disorders have remained refractory to modification by a wide range of psychiatric and psychological techniques. No doubt this is precisely why psychosurgery has been attempted as an alternative. Until recently, obsessive-compulsive disorders have received scant attention in the behavior therapy literature.

Obsessive-compulsive disorders ordinarily are viewed as anxiety-based. Hence, the treatments applied have been those with demonstrated efficacy in altering other anxiety-based problems, such as phobias. The extensions of procedures used with phobias have demonstrated that obsessive-compulsive disorders are more difficult to change. For example, systematic desensitization, which has proven highly effective in reducing fear, has not been effective in overcoming obsessions.

Quite recently, significant inroads have been made with behavior modification techniques that effectively alter obsessive-compulsive rituals. These rituals include constant checking (for example, of doors, gas, and water taps) and cleaning (for example, excessive hand-washing), slowness (for example, repetition of movements that interfere with the completion of tasks), and others. A technique that appears to be very effective for the treatment of compulsive rituals combines *response prevention* with exposure to the actual situations and stimuli that trigger compulsive acts. Response prevention consists of restraining individuals from performing their ritualistic behaviors. For example, applications with compulsive patients in a hospital setting arrange to have nurses supervise the patients to prevent the compulsive behavior (for example, repetitive hand-washing or checking things). When prevention can be achieved by interruption or distraction or even very occasionally by physical restraint, the exposure treatment is begun. Exposure consists of introducing the patients gradually to those situations that have been associated with the rituals.

Although there have been a large number of case applications, an increasing number of controlled investigations also have demonstrated the efficacy of response prevention and other variations of exposure treatments. For example, one series of investigations compared the efficacy of participant modeling, *in vivo* flooding, and modeling plus flooding in overcoming compulsive rituals (Hodgson, Rachman, and Marks, 1972; Rachman, Hodgson, and Marks, 1971). For each group, response prevention was included by encouraging individuals not to engage in rituals outside of the treatment sessions. In treatment, the patients were encouraged to approach stimuli that precipitated the rituals, to observe the therapist in the presence of these approach stimuli, depending upon the specific treatment, and to avoid performing the compulsive rituals. Modeling with *in vivo* flooding and response prevention reduced compulsive rituals at the end of treatment. These effects were generally maintained up to six months of follow-up (Hodgson et al., 1972).

The extent of information available on obsessive-compulsive rituals does not approach the evidence available on phobias and avoidance reactions, highlighted earlier. However, controlled outcome studies with seemingly intractable and chronic patients suggest that an effective treatment is emerging. At present, response prevention appears to be a crucial component, which can be effectively combined with other procedures such as flooding or participant modeling (Chesser, 1976; Rachman and Hodgson, 1980). These techniques have been effective in inpatient settings, where the bulk of research has been done, but in outpatient treatment as well.

Most of the research on obsessive-compulsive disorders has treated individuals who suffer from compulsive rituals. Less research has focused upon those who have obsessive thoughts without concomitant overt behavioral signs such as rituals. Consequently, fewer procedures can be offered as specific treatments for obsessive ruminations. Preliminary research suggests that interrupting obsessive thoughts with neutral or pleasant images or thoughts, as well as having patients continue their obsessive thoughts for prolonged periods, are both effective (Emmelkamp and Kwee, 1977). However, the techniques are not sufficiently well established or replicated to endorse strongly a particular technique at this time.

Depression

Behavioral techniques have been applied to depression, but the vast majority of reports have been case studies and hence do not permit conclusions about the efficacy of various techniques. A few isolated investigations have suggested effective techniques, although these do not constitute a large body of evidence at this point. A few promising leads warrant mention in passing.

A technique referred to as *cognitive therapy* has recently been demonstrated to be effective in treatment of neurotic depression (Rush et al., 1977). Cognitive therapy is sometimes viewed as a variation of behavior therapy that helps the client examine his or her cognitions and beliefs associated with the disorder. The treatment is based upon the assumption that an individual's affective response is partially determined by the way he or she structures experience. The depressed patient views him or herself, the world, and the future negatively. Treatment critically examines the distorted thinking processes. In addition, patients are assigned tasks (for example, identifying self-statements, validating one's interpretations of experience) to perform to help resolve problems and handle situations that they previously regarded as insuperable. Rush et al. (1977) compared cognitive therapy with tricyclic pharmacotherapy for outpatient treatment of depressed patients. Both techniques were found to reduce depressive symptomatology. However, cognitive therapy was more effective after treatment and up to a six-month follow-up. Recent replications have supported the efficacy of cognitive therapy relative to different forms of psychotherapy and behavior therapy (Morris, 1975; Shaw, 1977).

Other studies have examined the incidental effects on depression of treatment directed toward other problems. For example, Hersen et al. (1973) experimentally evaluated the effects of an inpatient behavior modification program for neurotic patients. The program provided incentives to the patients for interacting with others, performing activities such as attending occupational therapy, and completing self-care tasks. It was found that the treatment not only changed the specific behaviors focused upon directly but also reduced depression. The presentation and withdrawal of incentives—and the related changes in activity level and participation in the hospital routine—were systematically associated with changes in depression. Other treatment programs have reduced depression even though depression was not focused upon directly. For example, treatment procedures for obsessive-compulsive rituals, mentioned earlier. have shown reductions of depression following treatment (e.g., Hodgson, Rachman, and Marks, 1972).

A large number of case reports have focused upon behaviors that are associated with depressed affect. For example, depressed patients may perform relatively few routine activities in their everyday lives, often engage in self-defeating obsessive thoughts, show low skill levels in social situations, and show deficits in expressing affect in general. Case reports have shown that improvements have been brought about by developing skills and activities in everyday life and by eliminating competing thoughts, affect, or complaints (Lewinsohn, 1975). The focus upon select aspects of depression as a treatment strategy to alter the affect state is based upon theory and experimental research on the characteristics of depressed clients and possible antecedents of depression.

At this point, little firm evidence can be offered for a viable treatment technique for depression. Cognitive therapy procedures appear to be effective; yet controlled outcome research has been too scant to draw conclusions. Moreover, the case studies reporting behavioral techniques, although not reviewed here, have suggested a number of promising techniques that warrant investigation (see Leitenberg, 1976).

Limitations of Behavior Modification

Although the outcome evidence for behavioral techniques has been promising, it is not without limitations. Leaving aside the more specific substantive issues within the field, there are important general limitations of contemporary research in behavior modification.

Etiology of Disorders

Behavioral techniques assume that many deviant behaviors are learned and hence can be altered through additional learning experiences. Well-controlled investigations have clearly demonstrated that behavior can be altered without a full understanding of its development. The efficacy of behavioral techniques does not necessarily attest to the nature of the etiology. Indeed, behavioral techniques are frequently applied to medical disorders (for example, cardiac arrythmias, hypertension, pain) even though learning interpretations are not invoked to account for the problem.

Although disorders can be treated without a firm understanding of their etiologies, the procedures used to modify psychological functioning cannot be fully understood independently of the theory of development and maintenance of the behavior to which they are directed. The absence of clear inroads into the etiology of various disorders constitutes a limitation of contemporary research in behavior modification. Theories are available to explain the development of various disorders, and some of these have begun to be actively tested with clinical populations (for example, depressed patients). Although many theoretical formulations have been advanced, few of these have been adequately tested. Hence, understanding of the nature and development of many problems has lagged far behind treatment. This condition has parallels in many medical treatments as well. And, as in medicine, one can expect significant treatment advances when the etiology of a disorder is unraveled.

Range of Applications

The breadth of applications of behavior modification techniques probably has not been approached by other techniques. In addition to the traditional areas within psychiatry and clinical psychology, the techniques have been applied extensively to education, community and social problems (for example, pollution, energy, conservation), gerontology, medicine, and other areas (for example, Kazdin and Wilson, 1978). Of course, the evidence varies considerably both in quality and quantity across each of these areas.

The applicability of behavioral treatments has been facilitated greatly by the use of treatments that often are readily disseminated and conducted by nonprofessionals. For example, treatment of anxiety-based disorders such as phobias often can be conducted by patients themselves. Systematic desensitization can be conducted by the patients themselves in their everyday situations and produce effects equal to those accomplished in ordinary outpatient treatment (for example, Rosen, Glasgow, and Barrera, 1976). In addition, many problems such as conduct disorders in children can be treated by the parents or others with whom the children have contact (for example, Patterson, 1974).

Despite the broad applicability of behavioral treatments, insufficient evidence exists for many disorders to make claims about the efficacy of a given technique or the relative efficacy of alternative treatments. One problem in evaluating the results of outcome research in behavior therapy and in communicating these results to others is that behavior therapy research focuses upon specifiable classes of behavior rather than global states or diagnosed conditions. For example, behavior therapy does not treat "psychotic disorders" as such. Hence, no conclusions could be made about the efficacy of behavior modification for a psychosis, as a general condition. On the other hand, considerable research has demonstrated that social skills, irrational speech, hallucinations, delusions, and functioning in the community all can be altered with behavioral techniques (Hersen and Bellack, 1978).

Durability of Treatment Effects

In the area of psychotherapy in general, there has been a paucity of follow-up data. The issue of follow-up has achieved increased attention in recent years as more effective treatment techniques have emerged. With firm evidence that therapeutic change can be achieved, the question of durability of these changes assumes greater significance.

In contemporary therapy research, follow-up evaluation of treatment effects are still reported infrequently. Also, the available evidence suggests that durability of treatment effects may be a function of both the problem focused upon and the treatment technique. As with the outcome data, follow-up data are uneven across problem areas. For example, evidence suggests that anxiety can be treated with marked effects that are maintained up to one- and two-year follow-up assessments (for example, Paul, 1967; Paul and Shannon, 1966). On the other hand, with other disorders such as obesity and cigarette smoking, treatments tend to produce effects that are transient or of such small magnitude at follow-up as to be of little significance. Even with the sparse evidence available, it is clear that treatment effects are not likely to be automatically maintained after the intervention is terminated. This is particularly true for institutionalized patients whose treatment programs have been restricted to performance in the facility itself (Kazdin, 1977).

Behavior modification has concentrated heavily upon the technology of changing behavior. At present, the technology of maintaining these changes appears to differ from the technology of effecting change. Thus, considerable research has turned to techniques that can be added to treatment to extend the durability of therapeutic change when behaviors are not likely to be maintained. Utilization of booster sessions, training individuals who live with the client, training individuals to manage their own behavior to sustain therapeutic changes, and several other techniques are under investigation for maintaining treatment changes (for example, Marholin, Siegel, and Phillips, 1976; Stokes and Bear, 1977).

Behavior Therapy and Psychosurgery

Certainly, a major issue concerning the use of psychosurgery is whether all the viable alternatives are explored prior to surgery. Psychosurgery often is resorted to only after seemingly all other treatments have been tried. However, the rules for applying other treatments prior to psychosurgery still vary on a case-by-case basis.

In light of the evidence with select disorders, behavior therapy would seem to be one of the alternatives that should be tried before resorting to surgery. Several considerations support this recommendation.

Behavior modification has placed considerable emphasis on empirical research and experimental validation of treatment. Many techniques currently available have been studied extensively. Variations of treatment that enhance therapeutic change have been evaluated along with comparisons among different techniques. For example, one area where this research has made major inroads is the treatment of anxiety, where several procedures are available that are known to be generally effective.

Not all behavior therapy techniques or problems for which they are used have been thoroughly researched. Indeed, some of the problems for which psychosurgery has been used are precisely those on which the behavior therapy research has been meager. However, the void in areas such as obsessive-compulsive disorders and depression is now beginning to be filled. Even the preliminary results in these areas warrant serious attention as treatment alternatives. Aside from direct studies, many behavior therapy techniques have been shown to be effective for problems not reviewed in this chapter and might be extended to disorders treated with psychosurgery. In these cases, techniques already known to be effective for one problem at least provide viable leads for applications to areas where research has not advanced as far.

Another consideration that would favor use of behavior modification as a viable alternative pertains to the risks associated with treatment. Although all treatments have some conceivable risk, grossly different risks would be expected from behavioral and surgical interventions. Psychosurgery has been associated with postoperative complications and side effects including death, epileptic seizures, impulsiveness, lethargy, impaired memory, and several others reviewed in a previous chapter. The actual risk of these complications may be quite small, and of the complications that do occur, many may be transient. Yet the potential effects are serious even if their incidence is low.

The complications and side effects of behavioral treatment are not well documented. This, of course, does not attest to their absence. Yet, even in cases where side effects are reported, they do not approach the severity of problems associated with surgery. For example, when procedures are used that expose individuals to high levels of anxiety-provoking stimuli, such as flooding, patients occasionally have shown signs of stress (for example, nightmares) between treatment sessions (see Barrett, 1969, Emmelkamp and Wessels, 1975). Yet procedures that expose clients to high levels of anxiety are not essential for effective behavioral treatment since there are more palatable alternatives.

A major advantage of behavior therapy techniques is that both the procedures and their effects are reversible. If untoward side effects are evident during therapy, alternative treatments can be implemented immediately. The ability to alter procedures in the process of treatment enables behavioral interventions to avoid complications more readily than surgical interventions. The flexibility of treatment is a decided advantage in effecting therapeutic change in the individual case.

A final consideration in recommending behavior therapy as a viable alternative to surgical interventions pertains to the duration of treatment. It is extremely difficult to specify durations required for behavioral treatment because duration may vary as a function of the specific problem, ancillary client variables, the techniques, and a host of other factors. As a general rule, behavior therapy techniques need not be conducted for a prolonged period before their effects are apparent. Traditionally, psychotherapy has required very intensive and prolonged treatment, sometimes amounting to a matter of years and hundreds of sessions (for example, psychoanalysis). In contrast, behavior therapy usually requires only a matter of weeks and less frequent sessions within that period. Also, prior to completing treatment, the efficacy of treatment can be evaluated to ensure that behavior is changing in the direction of the desired outcome. The relatively brief treatment period and the ability to measure progress over the course of treatment make behavior therapy a viable treatment alternative.

CHAPTER 15

Causes and Treatments of Mental Disorders

Elliot S. Valenstein

It seems only natural that the cause of an illness should greatly influence the choice of treatment. Thus, an illness caused by a bacterial infection would normally be treated by an appropriate anti-bacterial agent, just as a disorder caused by a hormonal deficiency usually requires hormonal administration. However, even in the cases of "physical illness" the relationships between causes and treatments are often more complex than they may appear to be at first. A duodenal ulcer may have to be treated physically, but if environmental pressure and internal tension have contributed to the formation of the ulcer, physical treatment alone is not going to be very effective in the long run. From this point of view, the ulcer is not a cause, but a symptom. It may become necessary, therefore, to consider other factors, such as the patient's gastric acidity levels, eating, drinking, and smoking habits, personality, life style, and other potentially contributory "causes." Even resistance to bacterial invasion may be influenced by some physiological concomitant of stress, and hormonal deficiencies may be caused, or at least exacer-bated, by eating habits. The growing awareness of these multidimensional aspects of all diseases has no doubt been largely responsible for the recent interest in "holistic medicine" (Cousins, 1979; Pelletier, 1979).

With mental disorders, the situation is many times more complex. Not only are the causes of psychiatric disorders less well known and the subject of much dispute, but even where there is some agreement about the cause, there may be considerable differences of opinion about the effectiveness, or appropriateness, of different treatments. The grounds of disagreement go even deeper. For example, in spite of the increase in the use of objective, behavioral criteria to define different mental disorders, there is still disagreement about the primary characteristics of the disorders. Is schizophrenia primarily a cognitive, emotional, or perceptual impairment? The incidence of use of the diagnostic label "schizophrenia" can vary between institutions and between countries. Lastly, there is disagreement on whether mental disorders are "diseases" at all, and whether the "patients" are "patients" or "clients," whether "treatment" is "treatment," "counseling," or "therapy" and whether it should be "performed" or "allowed to occur" in a medical setting. These issues are much too complex to be treated exhaustively in a short chapter, but perhaps the raising of some of the different viewpoints on causes and treatments of mental disorders will set the stage for a useful dialogue.

Multiple Causation

It is essential to recognize from the outset that all mental disorders[1] have multiple causes. Constitutional factors always interact with life experiences to produce maladaptive behavior. People will be predisposed to respond in different ways even if they are all subjected to the same extreme environmental conditions. Predispositions to respond in particular ways vary not only because of the role of experience in shaping personality, but also because of genetically determined constitutional differences. Alcoholism, for example, may be an acquired pathological behavior pattern that is influenced by cultural factors, but there is considerable evidence of a genetic contribution to individual differences in the initial acceptability of

---

[1] In order not to get bogged down, I have elected to use the term "mental disorders," which may not be completely neutral but prejudges the questions under discussion less than "psychiatric disorders" or "deviant behavior." For similar reasons, I will refer to the person with the mental problem as the "patient."

alcohol as well as to differences in metabolic and other physiological responses to alcohol that predispose some individuals more than others to drink excessively. Similarly, Bergman and Escalona (1949) suggested that the large differences in sensitivity to such stimuli as sounds, odors, and tastes that exist even among infants may underlie differences in vulnerability to psychological damage, though some children with extreme sensitivities may "turn their handicap to unusual advantage."

It should be unnecessary at this time to defend the view that constitutional factors may underlie differences in predisposition to develop a given personality characteristic or differences in vulnerability to various diseases. There is a mistaken belief, however, that it is inherently undemocratic and pessimistic to employ explanations involving constitutional factors. The fact that hypothetical biological differences have on a number of occasions been used to justify undemocratic positions should not be considered an adequate reason to ignore real differences that may help us to understand how certain disorders develop and to place us in a better position to prevent or alleviate them. Interestingly, when Roger Williams (1956) described the great range of anatomical and physiological differences between individuals and went on to suggest that "biochemical individuality" may explain differences in predisposition to develop all kinds of disorders, including mental problems, his thesis was considered quite controversial. In about two decades, this idea has become so widely accepted that it is almost a commonplace. Williams was not referring to those extreme cases of "inborn errors of metabolism," but to the fact that there are large individual differences in every biochemical measure, including the enzymes, neurotransmitters, and hormones, which together comprise the chemistry of our brains. The majority of us are, to a greater or lesser extent, either above or below average levels on any biochemical determination. All of this tends to increase the significance of the statement, attributed to an early physician, that it may be "more important to know what sort of patient has a disease than to know what sort of disease a patient has."

Nevertheless, it is only in very extreme cases (if in any at all) that it is justifiable to speak of a psychiatric disorder being *determined* by constitutional factors. A genetic predisposition may or may not be realized depending on environmental circumstances. Even though it is generally recognized, however, that the influences of genetic and environmental factors are never independent of each other, it is still possible to argue about the *relative* importance of constitutional and environmental contributions to mental disorders. Unfortunately, it is often overlooked in such arguments that *there is no logical reason why the relative importance of genetic (constitutional) and experiential contributions should be the same for all mental disorders.* Thus, there are many people who would argue that genetically determined constitutional predispositions play a major role in schizophrenia[2] and in so-called "bipolar depression" (Mendlewicz, 1977; Dorus et al., 1979) but believe that such factors are much less important for many other mental disorders.

Unfortunately, many of the most influential people who have written about the causes of mental disorders, or the appropriate "models" for conceptualizing them, have taken very extreme positions. While it is certainly the most dramatic and possibly also the most effective way to draw attention to a single aspect of a complex problem, the discussion of mental disorders as though they had unitary causes or were one-dimensional issues has produced a great amount of unproductive controversy. In most cases, the spokesmen of single-factor theories have addressed important issues, but by exaggerating the importance of "their factor" and rejecting all others they tend to make their readers believe, mistakenly, that they must make a choice.

Different Models of Mental Disorders

Although there are several ways of grouping the various explanatory "models" of mental disorders, it may be most helpful to arrange them according to the relative importance they assign to factors that are within or outside the patient. Those theories that postulate genetically determined biological factors to be primarily responsible for mental problems stand at one end of the scale. While not necessarily denying the importance of the environment, these theories assume that factors within the individual play the major role in the organism—environment interaction. Evidence indicating an inheritable factor is frequently used in support of biological theories, as are data suggesting biochemical differences in patients with certain disorders, the effectiveness of pharmacological therapies, and the dem-

---

[2] Even those who believe that the evidence of a strong genetic contribution to schizophrenia is very compelling recognize that this factor does not operate alone (Kety et al., 1968). If genes *determined* schizophrenia, the concordance rate between monozygotic twins would be 100 percent rather than the 50 percent that has been found. While still supporting the existence of a genetic factor in schizophrenia, the concordance rate between biological relatives is lower when children are adopted at early ages into "normal" families.

onstrations that certain drugs can produce symptoms similar to those found in mental disorders. The validity of drawing conclusions from some of this evidence will be discussed briefly below.

On the other end of the scale are those theories that assign the major role to forces outside the person. Some of these theories assert that the various mental disorders are in reality nothing more than labels, or "metaphors," used to describe behavior and thought processes that are deviant in a given culture. Thus, Scheff, a sociologist, has argued that we should not prejudge the issue by using certain labels:

> The medical metaphor "mental illness" suggests a determinate process which occurs within the individual: the unfolding and development of disease. It is convenient, therefore, to drop terms derived from the disease metaphor in favor of a standard sociological concept, deviant behavior, which signifies behavior that violates a social norm in a given society [Scheff, 1963, p. 438].

This "metaphor" argument often takes the position that the medical model of mental disorders may be used as a political weapon, with psychiatrists acting as an instrument to control deviants who have the potential to disturb the equilibrium of society and its power relations. This form of the argument will be discussed in the following section of this chapter.

Other theories at this end of the scale may accept the reality of mental disorders but assert that they exist only within the network of people that has created and continues to maintain the behavior patterns and thought processes characterizing the disorder. It is argued, therefore, that the patient cannot be treated apart from the group. Treatment must consist of group therapy or "network therapy."

Distributed throughout the middle of the scale are a great variety of "psychological theories" that locate the mental problem within the patient but argue that its origin can be found in earlier interactions with the environment. Most of these theories emphasize early social interactions within the family; but with the introduction of so many new "psychological theories" within the last fifteen years, there are hardly any descriptive statements that would include all of them. Most of these theories reject the "medical model" of mental disorders, at least to the extent that the model requires the therapist to have a medical degree. The increased use of tranquilizing and antidepressant drugs, as well as the antipsychotic ("neuroleptic") drugs commonly administered to schizophrenics, has complicated the question of lay therapy. The more responsible lay therapists have some working relationship with physicians in order to refer patients for neurological examinations, if not also for the prescription of drugs. Although the majority of psychoanalysts are physician-psychiatrists, Freud's book *The Question of Lay Analysis* is frequently cited to illustrate that the founder of the movement did not believe it should be a specialized branch of medicine (Freud, 1927). What Freud's attitude would have been after the introduction of many psychoactive drugs is not at all clear.

Biological variables may or may not be stressed in psychological theories. The various forms of psychoanalytic theories, for example, maintain that the major dimensions of personality and the conflicts that create mental disorders are shaped by the resolution of biological drives and primitive anxieties within a family structure embedded in a given culture. Other theories distributed along this middle area of the scale give much less credence to the resolution of biological drives and stress the interactions between people—usually between the child and its family. Thus, Gregory Bateson and his colleagues have hypothesized that schizophrenia represents a child's attempt to escape from an environment of mutually contradictory messages (double-bind communications), as, for example, when a mother verbally expresses her love to a child but communicates something else in her behavior and facial expressions (Bateson et al., 1956). The child is thus placed in a "damned if I do and damned if I don't" conflict, much like Pavlov's dogs when they were no longer able to differentiate the essential cues. R. D. Laing (1967) also believes that schizophrenia is a mental state "that a person invents in order to live in an untenable situation." He maintains, however, that this state can be insightful, a "hyper-sanity," and that with proper guidance it can become a "mental voyage" capable of solving the feeling of alienation that is usually at the root of the problem.

Lidz and his colleagues maintain that schizophrenia results from family conflicts that impair the child by depriving it of nurturance and other essential experiences (Lidz, Flick, and Cornelison, 1965). There may be open conflict between the parents ("marital schisms"), or one parent may passively yield to the unreasonable demands of the other ("marital skews"). Both conditions are hypothesized to be potentially schizogenic because they interfere with the identification of the child with the parent of the same sex—a condition assumed to produce a weak differentiation between self and non-self ("ego boundary") and cognitive impairment (Lidz, 1968). Other theorists, such as Wynne and Singer, have stressed communication problems and have sought the explanation of schizophrenia in what they claim to be the vague and inconsistent speech pattern of some parents (Wynne, 1968).

These theories, which emphasize the parental role in the development of schizophrenia, are interesting, but there are very little supporting experimental data (Hirsch, 1979). It has not proven possible, for example, to distinguish schizophrenic and control families with appropriate blind techniques. Moreover, it has been argued that any differences in the behavior of the parents of schizophrenics could just as easily be explained as a result of the abnormal behavior of their child rather than the cause of it, or even as evidence of a genetic factor.

In contrast, those behavior therapies that evolved out of the operant conditioning laboratory have been relatively less concerned with schizophrenia and psychoses in general. Instead, they have concentrated, although not exclusively, on phobias, anxiety, obsessive-compulsive behaviors, sexual deviancy, and so-called "substance abuse" problems such as smoking, drinking, and excessive eating. These behavior theories usually assert that troublesome behaviors have been learned (as a result of having been rewarded in the past) and that they can be unlearned. In general, behavior therapists focus their efforts on developing techniques to modify overt behavior, rather than searching for causes of mental states (see, for example, the contribution by Kazdin in this volume).

Psychiatry as a Socio-Political Weapon

It is not a very large step from the position that mental disorders are not real diseases, but "metaphors" used to stigmatize and control "deviants," to the conclusion that psychiatry is often used as a political weapon, which can curtail civil liberties because it is above the law. So, for example, Thomas Szasz has written relentlessly about psychiatric injustice, namely the misuse of the disease model to deprive deviants in our society of their civil liberties without due process of law. Szasz claims that in the past, deviants were labeled witches and heretics, but today we use the pseudoscientific labels of psychiatry to accomplish essentially the same purpose. Thus, Szasz gives his numerous books such titles as *The Myth of Mental Illness* (1961), *Psychiatric Justice* (1965), and *The Manufacture of Madness: A Comparative Study of the Inquisition and the Mental Health Movement* (1970), and writes:

> The term "mental illness" is a metaphor. More particularly as this term is used in mental health legislation, "mental illness" is not the name of a medical illness or disorder, but is a quasi-medical label whose purpose is to conceal conflict as illness and to justify coercion as treatment [Szasz, 1961, p. xviii].

Szasz is a psychiatrist, but ironically he is probably the person most frequently cited by the so-called anti-psychiatry movement. Members of this "movement" maintain that most "treatment" of mental disorders is part of a conspiracy to isolate and control individuals who are either troublesome, inconvenient, or embarrassing to the power structure. Szasz maintains, for example, that mental illnesses are "myths" created by the "mental health industry" for their own enrichment and for the convenience of others.[3] Most psychiatric treatments, especially if they involve involuntary commitment or the use of such physical interventions as drugs, electroconvulsive shock, and psychosurgery, are primarily discussed as civil liberty issues. Whatever the shortcomings of this view, there can be little doubt that it has sensitized people to the potential, and actual, use of psychiatry as a political weapon. (See, for example, "The Serbsky Treatment," *Psychology Today*, June 1977, Vol. II, pp. 38–44, 87, for a discussion between the psychiatrist E. Fuller Torrey and the Soviet dissident Vladimir Bukovsky; Medvedev and Medvedev (1979); Grimm, this volume; and Szasz, 1963, for a discussion of the commitments of Ezra Pound and General Edwin Walker in U.S. government hospitals.)

That social and political outlook has influenced psychiatric judgment cannot be questioned. An almost unbelievably straightforward example of the transforming of a social problem into a medical disease was provided by one Dr. Samuel Cartwright in the last century (cited by Chorover, 1979, pp. 149–151). About ten years before the Civil War, Cartwright (1851) explained in a report to the Louisiana Medical Association that the reason slaves ran away was because of a "disease of the mind," which he called drapetomania (from the Greek *drapetes*, meaning absconding or running away). Drapetomania is still listed in some medical dictionaries as "the insane desire to wander away from home" (*Dorland's Medical Dictionary*, 1957).

More current support of the belief that psychiatry and politics are often closely linked has been presented by Braginsky and Braginsky (1974). These authors describe experimental data purporting to demonstrate that psychodiagnosis is influenced by a patient's social class and political ideology. They report that patients' views tend to be on the average more politically radical than those of the population at large. In fact, their testing indicated that psychiatric patients held views closer to the "New Left" philosophy than even Columbia University students, a group that previously had scored the highest on this measure. Moreover, Braginsky and colleagues report that

---

[3] With reference to schizophrenia, it has been said in reply that if mental illness is a myth, it is a "myth with a genetic basis and a pharmacological treatment."

when mental health professionals were asked to view videotaped interviews between a doctor and a "bogus mental patient" (enacted by a college senior) they judged the "patients" to have more severe psychopathology if they expressed "New Left Radical" rather than "Middle-of-the-Road" political views. Ironically, the "patients" were judged most "sick" if they expressed views against the mental health profession.

In addition to the claim that psychiatry often serves as an instrument of political repression, psychiatric hospitals have been accused of providing a means of getting rid of those who have difficulty adjusting to society. Thus, Bruce Ennis (1972), a lawyer active in the American Civil Liberties Union, has written in the Preface to his book *Prisoners of Psychiatry* that:

> The most important function of mental hospitals is to provide custodial welfare. They used to be called insane asylums, but before that they were called, more accurately, poorhouses. Almost all mental patients are poor, or black, or both, and most of them old.
> Less than 5 per cent of these patients are dangerous to themselves or to others. Indeed, the incarceration of mental patients cannot be justified by their threat to the community at large. Studies have shown that they are less dangerous than the "average" citizen. They are put away not because they are, in fact, dangerous, but because they are useless, unproductive, "odd," or "different" [Ennis, 1972, pp. vii–viii].

Although it could be argued that such descriptions of the "political" and "custodial" role of psychiatry are exaggerated and somewhat out of date, there are few informed people who would deny that they are addressed to real problems that still exist. That involuntary commitment on psychiatric grounds is a potentially dangerous practice has been documented many times. Nevertheless, it is necessary to ask if we are prepared to do away with this practice entirely, as Szasz and others would insist. Is there no possibility for a compromise? Should we not refine the laws in all states so that commitments are limited and closely monitored in order to accommodate a depressed patient who is suicidal or a patient whose behavior is so irrational or irresponsible that the consequences for his family could be disastrous? Szasz views suicide as a personal right, a civil liberty that should not be denied; others argue that some suicidal thoughts may be produced by abnormal brain biochemistry and that temporary protection should be imposed.

The view that mental disorders are all myths and all treatment is coercive has to be regarded as an exaggeration and a gross oversimplification of a complex, multidimensional problem. To the extent that such views are accepted uncritically, however, every innovative therapeutic development—be it a new behavior modification technique or pharmacological treatment—is greeted with great suspicion and tends to be dismissed reflexively as simply another means of coercing and controlling patients. Moreover, a strong commitment to the position that mental illnesses are myths and not "real" diseases often creates a closed-minded attitude toward suggestions of possible causes of mental disorders. Biological causes are especially likely to be rejected. It might be well for those who seem to believe there is something inherently evil in every attempt to find a biological cause of a mental disorder to recall that many of the patients in the "lunatic asylums" at the turn of this century were suffering from a vitamin deficiency (pellagra) or a form of neurosyphilis that was diagnosed as "general paralysis of the insane." It might also be recalled that Parkinson's disease, which is now generally acknowledged to result from a biochemical deficiency in the brain, was considered at one time to be a conversion hysteria by Charcot, one of the greatest figures in French medicine (Valenstein, 1978).

Actually, Szasz seldom gets involved with evaluating the validity or efficacy of a treatment, as he is concerned almost exclusively with questions of coerciveness in their application. In this respect, his views are in many ways quite similar to those of the laissez-faire liberals of the eighteenth century, but opposite to the views of present-day liberals. "The government that governs best, governs least" is a slogan Szasz seems to want to adapt to "the therapist who treats least, treats best." Surprising as Szasz's views may seem at first, they follow directly from his commitment to maximum freedom with no coercion:

> I believe we could clarify our thinking about psychosurgery if we compared it to abortion. In both cases, a surgical intervention is performed on a person's body not for the purpose of curing a disease but for some other purpose: in one case, for removing an unwanted fetus; in the other, for removing unwanted feelings or behavior.
>
> The analogy between abortion and, say, lobotomy yields some surprising results. Liberals, who are notoriously fuzzy-headed about medical matters, are apt to be for abortion but against lobotomy. I find it difficult to see, however, why one woman should have the right to hire a doctor to destroy the fetus in her womb, but another woman, or a man, should not have the right to hire a doctor to destroy part of her, or his, brain [Szasz, 1977, p. 10].

After indicating that he does not feel people should be prevented from committing suicide, Szasz concludes:

> In short, I am wholly in favor of free trade in psychosurgery between consenting adults. Insofar as other critics of psychosurgery favor banning lobotomy (or any other psychosurgical procedure), I oppose them

just as vehemently as I oppose those who favor banning abortion, heroin, pornography, or schizophrenia [Szasz, 1977, p. 10].

Szasz is not explicit about whether he believes "free trade" in psychosurgery between consenting adults is the rule or the exception. Those who perform psychosurgery, however, are quite explicit in stating that their procedures for obtaining consent are above reproach (see, for example, Ballantine in this volume).

Labels: What's in a Name?

Most psychiatrists believe that mental disorders cannot always be diagnosed from overt behavior. This fact produces a situation in which underlying processes can be inferred and then used to justify various diagnostic labels. Speaking with some irony about the ability of the mental health professional to penetrate below the surface, William Ryan has written:

> They detect the deep depression behind the most cheerful and sanguine faces. They perceive the boiling hostility that lies deep within the psyche of the sweetest, friendliest of persons; and they can spot the latent homosexuality which motivates the most exuberantly heterosexual young bachelor [Ryan, 1976, p. 153].

Once they are applied, labels are difficult to shake loose. Rosenhan (1973) has written about the "stickiness of psychodiagnostic labels" and has provided evidence that "once a person is designated abnormal, all of his other behaviors and characteristics are colored by that label." Rosenhan's "pseudopatients" gained admission to psychiatric wards by reporting to the admitting physician that they had heard voices, which were unclear, but seemed to be uttering the words "empty," "hollow," and "thud." The "pseudopatients," with one exception, all were given the diagnostic label "schizophrenia" on admittance. Immediately after being placed on a ward, the "pseudopatients" behaved completely normally and spoke to patients and staff members as they might talk to people under normal circumstances. Nevertheless, much of this perfectly commonplace behavior was considered evidence of psychopathology. Personal histories that most people would consider to be well within the range of normal experience were translated into psychopathological jargon. Rosenhan cites from one of the psychiatric "histories" written about one of the pseudopatients:

> This white 39-year-old male . . . manifests a long history of considerable ambivalence in close relationships, which begins in early child-

hood. A warm relationship with his mother cools during his adolescence. A distant relationship to his father is described as becoming very intense. Affective stability is absent. His attempts to control emotionality with his wife and children are punctuated by angry outbursts and, in the case of the children, spankings. And while he says that he has several good friends, one senses considerable ambivalence embedded in those relationships also [Rosenhan, 1973, p. 253].

It proved impossible to be sane in an insane place. As Rosenhan described it:

> Having once been labelled schizophrenic, there is nothing the pseudo-patient can do to overcome the tag. The tag profoundly colors others' perceptions of him and his behavior [Rosenhan, 1973, p. 253].

Obviously, the application of labels can have a significant effect on the persons to whom they are applied. Persons designated as mentally ill may incorporate this external judgment into their self-perception, at which point they tend to conform to the role assigned to them. Thomas Scheff, whose own point of view is reflected in his substitution of the phrase "rule-breaker" for patient, has described this process as follows:

> The more the rule-breaker enters the role of the mentally ill, the more he is defined by others as mentally ill; but the more he is defined as mentally ill, the more he enters the role, and so on. This kind of vicious circle is quite characteristic of many different kinds of social and individual systems [Scheff, 1966, p. 92].

Scheff considers labeling to be the single most important cause of the persistence of deviance (mental illness). The "patient" assumes the role of a mentally ill person. Other writers have proposed that mental disorders be considered within the "game playing" model of human behavior (Szasz, 1960). While the role playing by mental patients may mostly be involuntary, simulation of psychotic states is by no means unknown (Sadow and Suslick, 1961). In either case, it follows that if abnormal behavior is being maintained by labels, their removal—and the concomitant changes in self-perception, role playing, and also in the expectancies of others—should lead to an improvement in behavior. Where a physician has confidence a treatment will be effective and this confidence is successfully conveyed to the patient, the change in expectancies of both parties is likely to influence the course of the disorder, as Beecher (1961) reported a number of years ago. Undoubtedly, this process may underlie some of the improvements that are attributed to "placebo" effects.

Labels that imply that a disease is the cause of a behavioral problem can have significant consequences on a patient's outlook as well as on the attitude of family and friends. A person who has a disease may rightfully assume a "sick role" and as a consequence be excused from some responsibilities, not be held responsible for his condition, and be treated by someone else, usually a physician, rather than having to help himself. In some respects, the patient is often relieved to learn that he has a disease. This point is probably best illustrated by people with a drinking problem. There are several "models" that have been used to discuss alcoholism (Siegler, Osmond, and Newell, 1974), but most commonly it has been "explained" either as a "moral problem," a "weakness of character," or a disease based on some constitutional predisposition to drink alcohol in excess and to become dependent on it. Obviously, whichever model is accepted will have major consequences on the alcoholic's self-perception and the attitudes of others.

"Labeling theories" have been referred to by various names such as "societal reaction theory" or the "sociological model." While they may give slightly different emphases, it has been pointed out that all these theories share a common attitude toward the behaviors categorized as mental illness and also toward the impact of labels. These shared attitudes have been summarized by Jane Murphy:

> (i) these behaviors represent deviations from what is believed to be normal in particular sociocultural groups, (ii) the norms against which the deviations are identified are different in different groups, (iii) like other forms of deviation they elicit societal reactions which convey disapproval and stigmatization, (iv) a label of mental illness applied to a person whose behavior is deviant tends to become fixed, (v) the person labeled as mentally ill is thereby encouraged to learn and accept a role identity which perpetuates the stigmatizing behavior pattern, (vi) individuals who are powerless in a social group are more vulnerable to this process than others are, and (vii) because social agencies in modern industrial society contribute to the labeling process they have the effect of creating problems for those they treat rather than easing problems [Murphy, 1976, p. 1019].

Murphy has discussed psychiatric labeling from a cross-cultural perspective and has reported that similar kinds of behavior are considered symptomatic of mental illness in very diverse cultures. Studying several cultures, but particularly that of Eskimos living on a Bering Sea island and the Yorubas, a West African coastal people, Murphy concluded that explicit labels for insanity seem to exist in all cultures. Although not all cultures have words for all the psychoses and neuroses described in Western psychiatric literature, and although symptoms may be colored by the cultural backgrounds, most of the basic patterns are known. Murphy studied the evidence for the universality of schizophrenia and noted that the major symptoms ("a pattern composed of hallucinations, delusions, disorientation, and behavioral aberrations") seem to be present in all cultures and therefore concluded:

> Rather than being simple violations of the social norms of particular groups, as labeling theory suggests, symptoms of mental illness are manifestations of a type of affliction shared by virtually all mankind [Murphy, 1976, p. 1027].

Cross-cultural studies make it difficult to maintain the extreme view that mental illness is only deviant behavior as *arbitrarily* defined by a particular culture. This is not to deny that particular cultures may regard as abnormal certain behavior that would not be so regarded in other cultures. There does seem, however, to be agreement in all cultures on a common constellation of behaviors that justify a label conveying the sense of being "crazy."

The use of cross-cultural studies to support a biological explanation of mental illness, however, cannot be justified, as it is possible that there are basic social processes operating in all cultures that tend to produce similar symptomatology in deviant individuals. It would also be a mistake to conclude that cross-cultural studies refute the influence of psychiatric labels. In addition to the influences already mentioned, there is much evidence to suggest that labels can serve to exaggerate deviances by transforming them into illnesses or grouping together, as one disease entity, behavior problems that have very different underlying causes. Several examples could be used to illustrate this danger. For example, it has been noted that prior to 1960 the use of such diagnostic labels as "minimal brain dysfunction," "hyperactive," or "hyperkinetic" for children was relatively rare. It is not that there were not always difficult children (mostly boys) who displayed distractibility, short attention spans, and restlessness, but the popularization of these labels has resulted in the identification of much greater numbers, and, moreover, they are now thought to have a medical problem. Although some of the children so diagnosed may have so-called "soft" (suggestive, but not convincing) neurological signs, the main indices of the minimal brain damage (MBD) or hyperkinetic syndrome are the behavioral patterns listed above. While any reasonable consideration of these behavioral patterns must lead to the realization that many different causes might account for them, the wide-scale adoption of the label MBD has produced estimates that between 5 and 10 percent of prepubertal boys suffer from some brain dysfunction and that many of these need medical treatment (Wender, 1971). Indeed, there are several estimates that over 200,000 children are treated with amphetamine-like drugs (Stroufe and Steward, 1973).

According to many authorities on MBD:

> The most compelling evidence for the existence of MBD as an entity is (1) the similarity between its symptoms and the symptoms of children with proven organic brain disease and (2) the remarkable response to certain medications, *a response not found in non-MBD children* [Gross and Wilson, 1974, p. 6, emphasis added].

It should be obvious that the logic of the type of evidence given under (1) is not compelling. Whether or not the evidence listed under (2) is compelling is discussed below as a means of illustrating the variable relationships that exist between treatments and causes.

Relation of Treatment to Causes

It is often assumed that the effectiveness of a treatment in alleviating a behavioral problem reveals, if not the cause of the problem, at least something about what is maintaining it. The error in such logic should be obvious, but it may be helpful to illustrate the fallacy by continuing the discussion of the hyperkinetic-minimal brain dysfunction (MBD) labels. As already noted, it is often stated that MBD is a disease entity in part because of the presumed *uniqueness* of the response of children with this disease to amphetamine-like drugs. A closer examination of this statement leads to serious reservations about both its validity and the logic that leads from it to the conclusion that these hyperkinetic-MBD children have some brain dysfunction.

It has been frequently reported that hyperkinetic-MBD children given amphetamine-like drugs display a reduction in motor activity and an increase in attention span. These changes, which apparently are reliable, often lead to a reduction in their troublesome behavior and a consequent improvement in school performance. These responses of hyperkinetic-MBD children to a drug considered to be a stimulant have been called "paradoxical" and therefore considered indicative of a biochemical abnormality in the brain.

It should be noted that statements implying that the response of hyperkinetic-MBD children to amphetamine-like drugs is unique are not supported by any evidence. It was not thought possible to study a population of normal prepubertal children taking comparable doses of such drugs because of the clear ethical restraints on experimentation in this area. Recently, however, the results of an experiment with normal children were reported (Rapoport et al.,

1978). The subjects were fourteen children of "parents from the biomedical and mental health community,"[4] who had superior school performance and no behavioral indices associated with the "hyperkinetic-MBD syndrome." The children were given dextroamphetamine within the dose range normally prescribed for hyperkinetic children. The children's general behavior and performance on a battery of tests were recorded before the administration of the drug, while under the influence of the drug, and following the administration of a placebo. The results indicated that under the influence of dextroamphetamine the children showed decreased motor activity and generally improved attention, including superior memory. The authors conclude:

> The major finding is that children with no behavioral or learning difficulties, and in fact superior intellectual performance, showed behavioral and cognitive responses, that is, motor calming and improved performance, and some electrophysiological changes following amphetamine administration similar to those of hyperactive-MBD children. These results indicate that models of MBD which assume that patients have an altered behavioral response to stimulants compared to normal children are not appropriate for the hyperactive child syndrome. Conversely, hypotheses of biological abnormalities in MBD, such as dopamine depletion or low arousal, are not necessary to explain the effects of stimulants in hyperkinetic children. It is important that no diagnostic significance be inferred from a beneficial drug effect: diagnostic labels in themselves, when incorrectly applied, may have deleterious effects upon children's behavior and achievement [Rapoport et al., 1978, p. 562].

Some of the children diagnosed as MBD may indeed have some demonstrable brain dysfunction. It should be clear, however, that drugs, psychotherapy, behavior therapy, psychosurgery, and in fact any treatment, may alleviate symptoms for reasons that have nothing to do with the cause of the symptoms. A biological treatment can bring about improvements in a behavior problem produced primarily by environmental circumstances. Tranquilizing drugs, for example, may be effective in reducing environmentally induced tension.[5] Similarly, nonbiological therapies may be beneficial even

---

[4] There are clearly ethical questions raised by parents (even those in the mental health community) "volunteering" their own children for a drug experiment, but this is not the place to discuss these issues.

[5] It may also be recalled that Egas Moniz, the "father of psychosurgery," postulated (with evidence) that as a result of Pavlovian conditioning the morbid ideas of "people who suffer from melancholia and are tormented by unhappy compulsive ideas . . . become deeply rooted in the synaptic complex." Moniz decided, therefore, "to sever the connecting fibers of the neurons in question" [from Moniz' Nobel Prize acceptance speech].

where constitutional factors are involved. Thus, psychotherapy might help a person adjust by encouraging insight into a genetically determined predisposition, and behavior therapies may achieve some success in teaching brain-injured patients methods of coping with their deficits. Moreover, there are any number of examples of alleviating symptoms of a "physical disorder" with "physical" treatments that are not directly related to the primary cause. Prior to the discovery of a deficiency in dopamine in the brains of Parkinson patients, for example, it was common practice to administer drugs such as scopolamine, which blocked the action of brain acetylcholine rather than addressing the dopamine deficiency. Although we now believe we have some understanding of why anti-acetylcholine drugs were sometimes helpful, it is clear the medication is not always targeted specifically (and probably never exclusively) to the cause of the problem.

The complexity of the relationship between "causes" and "treatments" is further illuminated by considering the often tenuous relationship between "causes" and "diseases." A single "cause" may produce different diseases, and a disease such as diabetes, for example, may have many different causes. It is rare indeed even in cases of a "biological disease" to find all patients with the same underlying impairment. Not all diabetics, to continue using this example, have low insulin responses. In mental disorders, it is rare even to find any general consensus on what underlying impairment or life experience to search for. When a biological factor (usually a biochemical measure) is postulated as a contributory cause of a mental disorder, the supporting data are inevitably presented as average figures; there are always individuals with the disorder who are well within the range of a normal population.

Moreover, the evidence that people with a particular disease tend on the average to differ from others on some biological measure does not establish the direction of the relationship. Any particular biochemical or structural factor that is reported to be characteristic of a given diagnostic group may have little to do with the cause of the troublesome symptoms. An unusual biochemical measure may be produced by the behavioral problem rather than being the cause. Similarly, it has become increasingly clear in this pharmacological age that very long-lasting biochemical or structural changes, such as alteration in the number of biochemical receptors on nerve cell membranes, may be iatrogenic—that is, induced by the drug treatment—rather than causal.

The fact that the connections between treatments and causes of mental disorders are often very indirect and sometimes nonexistent may underlie many of the undesirable "side effects" of treatment. "Side effects" have been commonly described as concomitants of drug treatments and surgery, but they may occur with any type of treatment, including psychotherapy (although by convention we do not refer to the adverse consequences of psychotherapy as "side effects"). The point here is that where treatment is not directed both accurately and selectively to the cause of a disorder, the possibility of "side effects" is greater. (See the discussion of the relation between animal experiments and psychosurgery in Part II.)

Dangers of a Strong Conceptual Bias

Almost by definition, a bias tends to create conditions for selective perception and overemphasis that may induce serious errors in judgment. Preconceptions of the causes of behavior disorders are impossible to avoid entirely, but where there is little attempt to question premature conclusions, tragic consequences can result.

An example of the tragic consequences of a strong bias has recently been published in two separate accounts of the common misdiagnoses of dystonias. Dystonia is the name given to a group of movement disorders that are characterized by spasticity (sustained muscular contractions) and sometimes also by twisting movements. Patients with this disorder sometimes are forced to assume unusual postures because of muscle dysfunctions. Most dystonias are believed to result from abnormalities in the basal ganglia of the brain. Some of these are caused by encephalitis, but most cannot be traced to any infectious process. A significant proportion of dystonias have been shown to be of genetic origin, following an autosomal recessive pattern of inheritance.

In a recent report by Lesser and Fahn (1978), the results of a survey of the history of 84 patients with confirmed dystonia were described. In 44 percent (37 of 84 patients) of the cases, the patients' movement disorders were considered to be due to emotional disorders. Lesser and Fahn report that "These patients had received without benefit a variety of psychiatric therapies including psychoanalysis for up to 2 years, psychoanalytic psychotherapy, behavioral therapy, hypnosis, and pharmacotherapy."

Cooper (1973) in his book *The Victim Is Always the Same* describes in detail several cases in which dystonia was treated as a psychological problem, with tragic results. The patients described by Cooper underwent several types of therapy because the symptoms were considered to be evidence of either conversion hysteria or learned behaviors used to get attention. In the latter instances, the patient often received behavior therapy consisting of the use of rewards (and in a few instances, punishment) designed to extinguish what were assumed to be learned patterns. Parents were inevitably made to feel guilty for having somehow rewarded these "attention getting behaviors" in the past. In one case, where the conversion hysteria hypothesis was being pursued, a psychiatrist offered the following "explanation" of the patient's various postures.

> He [a 17-year-old] learned in good time a good deal about the meaning of his symptoms, how his sticking his stomach out was, on the one hand, imitating his mother's pregnancy with his younger sister, whereas on the other hand, it was putting his penis forward and asserting himself as a man. Inevitably, whenever he sticks his stomach out, he withdraws it rapidly and sticks his buttocks out. He could see in time how this was, in part, related to his fear that harm would be done to his penis, when it is stuck out, and sticking out his anus prominently was an invitation for sexual attack from the rear [cited by Cooper, 1973, p. 52].

Tragic consequences can result from any kind of theoretical orientation, but obviously the danger is greater when the treatment must proceed for a long time before any judgment of effectiveness can be made, where the dangers of adverse side effects are significant, and where a better alternative exists.

Summary

It was not possible to describe all the "explanatory models" of mental disorders, nor to describe any of them fully. The intent was to illustrate some of the major types of models that have been proposed. These models vary in many ways, but particularly in respect to their reliance on explanatory factors outside or inside a person. Thus, sociological and biological theories are located at opposite ends of the continuum, with various psychological theories being distributed over the middle range. It was stressed that probably all mental disorders have multiple contributory causes and that a very doctrinaire approach almost always produces distortions (sometimes having dangerous consequences) and often a closed-minded attitude toward new ideas and evidence.

Also discussed was the complexity of the relationship between causes and treatments. It was argued that this relationship is much less restraining than often assumed. Thus, biological interventions may be effective treatment for disorders primarily caused by environmental factors, and the converse may also be true. It follows that the cause of a disorder can not be assumed from the efficacy of the treatment. Moreover, it may be dangerous to make this assumption.

In essence, the purpose of this chapter was to illustrate some of the sources of confusion about causes and treatments of mental disorders. No attempt was made to restrict the discussion to psychosurgery. Unquestionably, some of the issues raised do not apply to either the patients of psychosurgery or their circumstances. However, it may be true that more of the issues apply to psychosurgery than some people appear to realize.

CHAPTER 16

Violence: A Localizable Problem?

Stephan L. Chorover

"Human violence is the most threatening problem in our world today." With this presumably unarguable assertion, Vernon Mark and Frank Ervin introduced their 1970 monograph *Violence and the Brain* (Mark and Ervin, 1970, p. 1). As no reader of this volume need be told, their analyses of, and proposed solutions for, the formidable and complex problem of human violence have been the focus of much controversy ever since. In retrospect, it is perhaps not surprising that proposals, like theirs, to use brain surgery as a means of dealing with the problem of violence received an attentive hearing at the time. But, as the war in Indochina, the unrest on college campuses, and the strife on inner-city streets began to subside, the psychosurgery debate began to take on a slightly less intense, yet perhaps a more deeply serious scientific and social character.

Today, thanks largely to growing public awareness of the relevant scientific and ethical issues, we are beset by fewer proposals to cre-

---

This chapter is dedicated to the memory of Hans-Lukas Teuber—mentor, colleague, friend.

ate a "psychocivilized society" through the use of electrical brain stimulation (Delgado, 1969). We no longer find psychosurgeons promoting brain operations as an allegedly simple, humane, and cost-effective means of transforming "the violent young criminal . . . into a responsible, well-adjusted citizen."[1] And it is almost impossible to imagine reading a letter in a current issue of the *Journal of the American Medical Association* from three Boston physicians who would like to see mass neurological screening programs established to locate people with "low violence thresholds," allegedly traceable to "episodic dyscontrol syndromes" or some epileptiform variety of "limbic brain disease" (Mark, Sweet, and Ervin, 1967). Which is only to say that it is no longer as easy as it once was for psychosurgeons (and other psychotechnologists) to promote brain manipulation as a means of social control.

From my particular vantage point—as a neuropsychologist and an observer of developments in various fields of psychotechnology—there has been some substantial progress in "the psychosurgery debate." That the employment of brain surgery as an instrument of social control is now generally regarded as unwarranted is shown, for example, by the National Commission's statement that *"the use of psychosurgery for any purpose other than to provide treatment to individual patients would be inappropriate and should be prohibited."* (National Commission, 1977, p. 58, emphasis in original.) But appearances are sometimes deceptive, and distinctions between "control" and "treatment" are often far from clear-cut. One characteristic of this situation is the ease with which medical jargon can be used to camouflage otherwise obvious exercises in behavior control (Chorover, 1974; Chorover, 1976b, pp. 730–767; Chorover, 1979, chap. 7). Psychotechnologists who are in a position to define and deal with socially problematical behavior, including "abnormal aggressive behavior" (Mark and Ordia, 1976), apparently would like to have it both ways. Thus, by conflating terminology from different realms of discourse, psychosurgeons sometimes make it appear that psychosurgery is being done *to* a person, primarily in the interests of others, and, sometimes, that it is being done *for* the person, primarily in his or her own interests. As a result, it may be difficult or impossible to determine just whose interests the psychosurgeon in a given instance actually represents. Consider, as a case in point, the following passage from a recent

---

[1] M. H. Brown, quoted in I. Calder, "Noted surgeon claims . . . brain surgery could transform the most violent murderer into a normal citizen," *National Enquirer*, July 9, 1972, p. 3.

article advocating hypothalamotomy as a form of "sedative neuro-surgery" in the treatment (or management) of aggressive behavior:

> Sedative neurosurgery is used to manage assaultive and aggressive patients who are very difficult to manage either at home or in special institutions. They are always on the rampage and often break out into catastrophic violence. Apart from the medical problems of their management, they are a great nuisance and danger to members of their families and their neighbors. Treatment to keep them quiet is necessary to maintain peace inside the family and to protect the safety of neighbors. . . . A well-performed operation of sedative neurosurgery does not make a patient worse or inert; the only change is quieting of behavior [Balasubramaniam and Kanaka, 1976, p. 775].

As it happens, the authors of the foregoing passage do not practice psychosurgery in the United States. It might be objected, therefore, that they are not subject to prevailing domestic standards of psycho-surgical practice and ought not necessarily be expected to conform with the injunction against the use of brain surgery for explicit behavior control purposes. But the deeper question to consider is whether prevailing domestic standards of psychosurgical practice (as represented, for example, by the National Commission's statement quoted earlier) effectively preclude the use of brain surgery for explicit purposes of behavior control. I believe that they do not. My purpose in this paper is to argue that, moral and technical and political considerations aside, it is logically incorrect and scientifically unwarranted to treat individual patients with psychosurgery in cases involving violence and other socially problematical forms of human behavior.

Clarification of Terms

In order to make the grounds for my argument explicit, it is first of all necessary to clarify the meaning of certain terms. By *psychosurgery*, I mean what the National Commission's report on the subject describes as "brain surgery performed either (1) on normal brain tissue of a person, for the purpose of changing or controlling the behavior or emotions of such person, or (2) on diseased brain tissue of a person, if the primary purpose of performing the procedure is to control, change or affect any behavioral or emotional disturbance of such person" (National Commission, 1977, p. 57).

It may seem altogether obvious, but it needs to be pointed out here, that the main (indeed, the *only*) logical justification for psycho-surgical intervention in any case derives from the proposition that there is a relationship between the brain and behavior. Taken by itself, this proposition can hardly be considered controversial. On the contrary, it is simply the basic tenet of the entire field of neuropsychology. As I have stated elsewhere, "one thing is clear: the coherence, continuity, and complexity of our conscious experience depend upon the organization and integrity of our brains" (Chorover, 1976b, p. 731). This is not to say, however, that anyone really understands *how* our brains work, or *what*, precisely, the nature of the relationship is between the neural organization of the brain, on the one hand, and the psychological organization of experience, on the other. I stress the uncertainty that prevails in such matters, not to disparage the enormously exciting progress that is being made by researchers in diverse fields of neuroscience, but merely to caution against the uncritical acceptance of a further proposition that is commonly advanced in defense of psychosurgical intervention. As put by a contemporary psychosurgeon, the latter proposition is "that human behavior, including violent assaultive action, *is an expression of* the functioning brain" (Sweet, 1970, p. vii, emphasis added).

What, precisely, does this mean? If we understand it to mean that a person must have a functioning brain in order to engage in a violent assaultive action, then the proposition is obviously unarguable. But in order to serve as a logical justification for psychosurgery, it must *also* mean that violent assaultive action results primarily from (i.e., is *caused by*) something taking place in the brain of the person who engages in the action. In fact, Sweet, in a defense of the idea that all human behavior, including violence "is an expression of the functioning brain," has added: "It follows that one way to understand and control the current colossal problem of violence is to increase our knowledge of those brain mechanisms relating to emotion in general and to dangerous aggression in particular" (see Mark and Ervin, 1970, in Foreword). This is a very dubious proposition indeed.

The notion that violence springs primarily from the individual's brain becomes even more dubious when we recognize the essentially social (or antisocial) nature of violent assaultive actions. The term *violence* generally refers to a behavioral *transaction* in which one person exerts upon another person (or thing) an action considered (by the recipient or others) to be injurious and unwarranted. In other words, a violent assaultive action is an action that occurs in a social context of which the actor is only one—albeit an essential—*part*. Thus, unless one wishes to assert that the context (including the person or thing toward which the assaultive action is directed) is *also* an expression of the functioning brain of the person who commits the action, it necessarily follows that the action in question, whatever it may be, involves more (perhaps much more) than the "expression" of a particular brain. Indeed, if there is no *logical* basis for considering violence as reducible to a property or process located in a particular individual, then there is no *a priori* basis for believing that the causes of violent behavior can be localized or treated within the brain of the person who is identified (by someone) as expressing "abnormal aggressive behavior" (Mark and Ordia, 1976, pp. 722–729).

Yet, according to Mark and Ordia (1976, p. 722), the phrase "abnormal aggressive behavior" refers to something that can be located and treated within the brains of certain patients. Their argument is typical of the ones that many psychosurgeons are now finding it necessary to fashion in order to justify their practices in the light of growing skepticism. For that reason alone, what they have to say on the subject is worth examining closely. They write:

> There are two kinds of patients with abnormal aggressive behavior who have been treated by brain surgery. The first group has structural or functional brain abnormalities related to the aggressive behavior. Surgery in these patients is primarily an attempt to treat their brain abnormalities. The second group has abnormal aggression without detectable structural or functional brain defects. Brain surgery in these patients is used only to modify behavior [Mark and Ordia, 1976, p. 722].

Mark and Ordia criticize "some of the critics of the surgery of aggression" for failing "to differentiate between these two groups of patients." Moreover, after asserting (without the benefit of argument) that fear of the potential abuses of psychosurgery is based partly "on a misinterpretation of the words 'aggression' and 'violence'," they go on to stipulate "the kind of violent behavior for which neurological treatment might be legitimate" (Mark and Ordia, 1976, p. 722). It is, they say, "personal violent behavior, unwarranted and usually unprovoked [including] acts that directly attempt to, or actually do, injure or destroy another person or thing" (Mark and Ordia, 1976, pp. 722–723; Mark and Neville, 1973).

Mark and Ordia explicitly disavow any intention to apply this definition to violence in general, and they purport to exclude "aggressive behavior consistently organized for a political motive." But this disavowal, however well intended, overlooks the fact that judgments about motives underlying personal behavior are inevitably made from perspectives influenced by the observer's presuppositions and beliefs about the propriety or justifiability of certain forms of behavior. What this means is *not* that it is necessary for observers (in this case, psychosurgeons) to "be more objective" or to withhold their judgments about the justifiability of particular acts of "personal violent behavior." But it does mean that it is incumbent upon those who take it upon themselves to evaluate behavior as "unwarranted" or "unprovoked" to make their own perspectives explicit. In other words, it takes a *normative* point of view to perceive a particular act (or set of acts) as abnormal, and the failure to acknowledge the existence of a socially defined frame of reference only serves to create the false and misleading impression that standards for judging the propriety of behavior exist independently of the observer's point of view. There is, I believe, a great deal of social bias inherent in all efforts ostensibly intended to define controversial human problems (such as violence) in an essentially "value-free," "morally and ethically neutral," and "strictly objective" way. Moreover, concealment of those biases is itself a practical necessity for purposes of definition and control. But bias is not my main focus here. Suffice it only to repeat, in this context, that the power to diagnose—that is, to give names to—problematical behavior is one aspect of the power to define the limits of allowable behavioral diversity in a society. And, in any society, the power to give names and to enforce definitions is a touchstone of social control (Chorover, 1979).

Attempts to Localize Behavior

If we assume that Mark and Ordia, together with others who share their view of violence, are intent upon treating "abnormal aggressive behavior" by means of psychosurgery, it becomes necessary to ask what criteria they propose to use to identify individuals for whom "neurological treatment may be legitimate." Here is their answer:

> Of course, we would not approve neurosurgical treatment, unless the abnormally aggressive act or violent behavior could be traced to a recognized neurological or psychiatric disease state, a disease that could not be treated by non-surgical methods, i.e., medical or psychiatric management (Mark and Ordia, 1976, p. 723].

This presumably means that a necessary (albeit perhaps not sufficient) precondition for the neurosurgical treatment of abnormal aggressive behavior is that the behavior in question be traceable to an otherwise untreatable "neurological or psychiatric disease state." It may be noted, at once, that this ostensible justification is a slightly adumbrated version of the idea that "human behavior, including violent assaultive action, is an expression of the functioning brain."

In this case, however, we are faced with the additional proposition that certain violent assaultive actions are "expressions" of a localizable neurological or psychiatric derangement. This, then, is the proposition that we must carefully consider, for it comprises, at the present time, the only available rationale for psychosurgery that appears consonant both with traditionally accepted concepts of medical diagnosis and treatment, and with proscriptions against the use of such surgery for any purpose other than to provide treatment to individual patients. But, as I said earlier, appearances may be deceptive.

Reduced to essentials, this rationale implies that the legitimacy of "the surgery of violence or aggression" ultimately rests upon the traceability of certain abnormal behavioral acts to certain correspondingly abnormal conditions within the brain of the particular actor. Evidently, any serious effort to evaluate this rationale must begin by addressing the meaning of the term "disease state" and by clarifying the notion that "violent behavior could be traced" to some such process or thing. Bearing in mind what has already been said about the logical problems inherent in attempts to reduce violence to the status of a personal problem, let us consider the term "disease state" and the notion of "traceability" a bit more closely.

According to generally accepted technical and popular usage, a *disease* is a "definite morbid process having a characteristic train of symptoms; it may affect the whole body or any of its parts, and its etiology, pathology, and prognosis may be known or unknown" (*Dorland's Illustrated Medical Dictionary*, 23rd ed., Phil.: Saunders, 1957). One thing that this definition makes plain is that the term "disease" properly refers to a state of affairs that (if it exists at all) must exist somewhere within the physical boundaries of a particular person. More to the point, it is "a situation or condition (one might well call it both a *state* and a *process*) of an organ, part, structure, or system of the body in which there is an incorrect function resulting from the effect of heredity, infection, diet, or environment" (*Random House Dictionary of the English Language*, 1967). Of course, the word "disease" has sometimes been used in a broad metaphorical sense to refer to a wide variety of other situations (including allegedly "unhealthy" states of affairs that may prevail within certain societies at particular times). Implicit in such usage is the idea that the locus of the disordered function lies somewhere within the material or conceptual domain of the supposedly deranged *system*. It is accordingly necessary to reemphasize that in order to serve as a logically or scientifically plausible justification for a particular form of intervention (e.g., psychosurgery), the "disease state" in question must be presumed to be localizable—that is, to have a tangible existence within the boundaries of the identified system (e.g., the person). Hence, the proposition that an abnormally aggressive act (or acts) of violence may be traceable to a particular disease state asserts, in effect, that the behavior in question is logically or scientifically attributable to a definite morbid process located (or at least in principle localizable) within the *identified patient.*

The "localization" problem under discussion here bears a close resemblance to the more general age-old question of brain–behavior relationships. More specifically, it recalls the kinds of questions that arise whenever a neuropsychologist is inclined to ascribe a specific aspect of behavior to events taking place within a particular brain locus. Since most readers are presumably familiar with the "localization of function" controversy, I think that a brief reference to it may shed some light on the psychosurgical inclination to ascribe violent behavior to definite processes taking place within a particular person.

As I have previously argued elsewhere (Chorover, 1966; Chorover, 1974; Chorover, 1976a; Chorover, 1976b; Chorover, 1979), most neuropsychologists no longer consider it tenable to maintain the existence of a strict dichotomy between the traditionally antithetical doctrines of "localization" and "mass action," which dominated discussions about the relationships between brain function and behavior in an earlier day. It is today quite evident that the more complex and subtle neurobehavioral characteristics of individual organisms—that is, those internal states and processes that constitute *a necessary but not a sufficient basis* for the interpersonal and social activities of human beings (and other "higher organisms")—ultimately do not lend themselves to simple dichotomous ascription. In other words, everything that we know about the subject today seems to deny the simplistic presumption that neuropsychological processes are comprehensible in *either* strict "localizationist" *or* diffuse "mass actionist" terms. It is becoming increasingly clear that in most—if not all—cases where something significant is known about brain–behavior relationships, it is to *neither* discretely localized *nor* extensively interconnected neural subsystems, but to *both*—and especially to their mutual and reciprocal interaction—that characteristics like the aforementioned ones are most readily ascribable. The point is worth pursuing.

In stressing—as I have just done—that the problem of localization of function is concerned with the neural organization of brain systems whose integrity is a necessary but not sufficient basis for interpersonal and social behavior, it is my intention to point out that it is meaningless to talk about such activities as if they are merely (or even mainly) something "expressed" (literally "pressed out" or manifested) by an individual brain existing in a material, conceptual, or social vacuum. By insisting that violence is *essentially* a transaction and hence a problem that needs to be addressed in interpersonal or social terms, I mean to suggest that it is simply not reducible to a personal attribute. I mean to assert, further, that it is simply not meaningful—in any scientific sense—to define or deal with violence as if it exists or could exist independently of the specific material, conceptual, and social context of which it is a part.

Let me be yet more specific. Even in those rare cases where a definite morbid process is shown by tangible physical evidence to exist in the brain of a particular individual who has been observed, coincidentally, to exhibit abnormal aggressive behavior, it is not logically (or psychologically) justifiable to simply attribute the latter facts to the former. Why not? Because social behavior is comprehensible only in terms of reciprocal causal processes; I know of no aspect of it (including violent assaultive action) that is intelligibly "traceable" in a linear fashion to events in a single person or brain. Of course, if all that one ultimately aspires to do is to lend a semblance of legitimacy to the psychosurgical taming of "aggressive patients who are very difficult to manage," then a linear causal argument may suffice for expediency. But to assert that the causes of a human problem (whether violence or any other) are traceable to some process or state within allegedly malfunctioning individual brains is in no sense scientifically or logically credible. On the contrary, if one aspires to lend any scientific substance to the solution of human problems (including the problems raised by the existence of violence), it becomes necessary to reject the linear causal model and to identify this one-sided localizationist doctrine as a false and misleading species of "biological determinism" (Lewontin, 1977). I suspect that much of the frustration engendered by "the psychosurgery debate" may be due, at least in part, to the inherent epistemological inadequacies of the biological determinist doctrines that pervade prevailing concepts of brain–behavior relationships. Current conditions, however, seem propitious for the rejection of such doctrines, and some of them have lately been effectively debunked (Sociobiology Study Group, 1977; Chorover, 1979, chap. 7).

My central argument here has been that complex human problems are not, in any meaningful sense, reducible to either personal disorders or localizable brain states or processes. To understand them, we must look beyond specific acts to the overall neuropsychological and social context of which both brain and behavior are a part. I have come to this view partly on the basis of my experience as a participant in "the psychosurgery debate," where the conceptual frameworks of the biological, behavioral, and social sciences are so tightly interwoven. From my own vantage point I am beginning to glimpse what seems to me to be a somewhat more unified picture of brain–behavior relationships and the nature of human problems—a view that may be capable, moreover, of encompassing or integrating the complementary and overlapping aspects of existence represented by the organization of the brain, the individual, and the society. While much still remains obscure, it is now more evident than ever to me that psychosurgery is controversial precisely because it is a combined biological-psychological and social enterprise. It is destined to remain the focus of debate, moreover, unless or until we devise a more unified conceptual framework capable of accounting harmoniously for the multiple and reciprocal patterns among the organization of the brain, and behavior of the individual, and the dynamics of the larger social context.

As I have argued more extensively elsewhere (Chorover, 1979, chap. 7), psychosurgery and other forms of psychotechnology generally take the individual person as the main locus for intervention. But so long as we pursue this approach, we will never even come close to solving the problems of violence and aggression or any other serious human problems that threaten our survival. If it is the case, as I believe it is, that the most pressing human problems are essentially interpersonal and transactional, then all efforts to define and deal with them in terms of a particular individual's actions— ignoring other demonstrable dimensions of such problems—must be rejected as reflecting a fundamentally biased (and unscientific) approach. The individual "localizationist" perspective is thus more than merely mistaken. It is also a barrier to meaningful social change. Whether by intention or otherwise, it reflects and reinforces an unwillingness to undertake the social, political, and economic steps that must be taken in order to transform our violent and problem-ridden society into one that is more peaceful and more responsive to fundamental human needs. My point is not that serious human problems are amenable to quick and easy social solutions, but rather that the pursuit of psychosurgical and other psychotechnological "remedies" tends to serve as an excuse for not pursuing more rational alternative or complementary approaches.

An Interactional Model

It is becoming increasingly clear that those who would make a serious contribution to the solution of urgent human problems must first abandon the tendency to define and deal with them in traditional either–or (social or personal) terms. What I have tried to show in this article is that the ostensibly scientific rationale for psychosurgery rests upon a grossly simplistic and untenable notion of brain –behavior and personal–social relationships. I would like to conclude by making a few hopefully constructive remarks about the prospects for progressing beyond crude neuropsychological reductionism in both scientific and social affairs.

By the term *neuropsychological reductionism*, I mean, in the present context, an epistemological position from which behavior is seen as an "expression of" or as "traceable to" particular or localizable brain states (or processes). This perspective is prevalent among contemporary neuropsychologists and evidently derives from a more general principle of reductionism that has its counterpart (or, more precisely, its prototype) in the domain of classical physics. There, until fairly recently, it was a generally accepted and largely unexamined assumption that the world and its contents were ultimately comprehensible through a process of analysis in which relatively large and evidently complex entities or events were effectively "disassembled" or "reduced" to reveal their constituents. The latter were then regarded as separate, relatively smaller, and ostensibly simpler "elementary parts."

The idea that behavior is traceable to particular brain processes is thus analogous to the idea that the structure of the material universe is, as a whole, traceable through successively more minute stages, down to the level of some simple, unchanging, independently existing and fundamentally unanalyzable elementary constituents. Both viewpoints are deeply ingrained in our way of thinking (Weisskopf, 1972). Nonetheless, around the beginning of this century, a series of developments in the field of high-energy physics began to challenge the basic tenets of this approach.

The first step in this process was the revision of Newton's original concept of the atom as the "solid, massy, hard, impenetrable" fundamental building block of the material universe. Just before World War I, it was shown that atoms—far from being solid and impenetrable—were actually composite entities encompassing relatively vast regions of "empty" space in which virtually massless particles (electrons) orbited around a relatively tiny "massy" nucleus to which they were bound by intra-atomic forces. Soon thereafter, it was discovered that the nucleus was itself neither impenetrable nor unanalyzable but rather a composite structure consisting of other particles (protons and neutrons). At that point it was generally believed by physicists that the three "basic building blocks" of matter had finally been uncovered. But this view did not prevail for long. As experimental techniques were progressively improved and as new, more sensitive, higher-energy methods of particle detection came into existence, more and more "elementary" constituent particles were discovered. The number increased from three to six by 1935 and then to eighteen by 1955. Today, more than two hundred "elementary" particles have been identified, and investigations at the present technological limits of experimental physics are mainly focused upon the search for still more infinitesimal particles (quarks), which, according to some physicists, form the general class of elementary entities that finally will be shown to include *the* "fundamental building block."

But the point of all this—especially as it relates to the matter at hand—is that the physicists' present inability to find an elementary particle that is not itself a composite entity may not be a temporary state of affairs. On the contrary, it may have a deeper meaning. At very least, it has led *some* physicists (admittedly only a small minority at present) to raise some fundamental questions about the validity of the entire "elementary particle" view. Some of them, recognizing that the technological limits of observation have changed continuously and that increasing powers of observation have engendered the discovery of newer and previously unsuspected particles, have come to regard it as probable that a truly fundamental elementary particle (that is, an entity of essentially "impenetrable hardness," in the Newtonian sense) does not exist, and will therefore never be found. This conjecture, however unsettling it may at first appear, has opened up the search for alternative ways of comprehending the structure and behavior of the material world. One alternative that has emerged, and that stands in direct opposition to the basic tenets of reductionism, may be particularly pertinent to the present discussion. To be more specific, it may help us to go beyond the generally unsatisfactory ideas (1) that the social behavior of particular persons is in some meaningful sense "traceable to" (or an "expression of") localizable brain states or processes, and (2) that human problems of social interaction (including violence) are reducible to specific acts expressed by particular persons. The physicist David Bohm is one of the leading proponents of a viewpoint which denies the classical reductionist idea that the world must be (or can be) analyzed into separately and independently existing "elementary" parts. Here is how he puts his alternative conception:

> We have reversed the usual classical notion that the "elementary parts" of the world are the fundamental reality, and that the various systems are merely particular contingent forms and arrangements of these parts. Rather, we say that inseparable quantum interconnectedness of the whole universe is the fundamental reality, and that relatively independently behaving parts are merely particular and contingent forms within this whole [Bohm and Hiley, 1975, p. 102].

If it is assumed, however provisionally, that this is a reasonable view of the matter and if one agrees, further, that the various systems that we call brains, individuals, and social organizations can only exist within the material and conceptual boundaries of "the whole universe" to which this principle of inseparable interconnectedness applies, certain conclusions appear to follow. For one thing, it becomes reasonable to stop treating human problems as if they were essentially reducible to individual behavioral acts, and to stop regarding the social actions of individuals as reducible, in turn, to localizable brain processes. At very least, it becomes reasonable to insist that proposals to treat human problems reductionistically must be carefully considered and—when possible—counterposed by the conscious realization that neither individual persons nor specific brain states are separately or independently existing "elementary parts." On the contrary, they are composite entities which happen to be found at a particular level of organization and whose mode of organization—like that of the so-called elementary particles—is manifested by "a set of relationships that reach outward and inward to other things" (Stapp, 1971, p. 1310). What emerges from this perspective is a view of the brain, of human behavior, and of human problems that is consonant with a scientifically sophisticated view of the world as a whole. Such a view reveals *not* a set of phenomena comprehensible in *either* reductionistic *or* holistic terms, but rather a complex, interpenetrating, and ultimately irreducible web of relationships among events taking place at many levels simultaneously. As one famous physicist put it, "the world thus appears as a complicated tissue of events, in which connections of different kinds alternate or overlap or combine and thereby determine the texture of the whole" (Heisenberg, 1958, p. 107).

Does this view offer a scientifically and socially meaningful alternative to the naive reductionistic, linear causal doctrines of biological determinism? Does it provide a more intellectually, emotionally and practically satisfying conceptual framework for understanding violence? Does it shed any real light on the age-old riddle of relationships between brain and mind or between individual and society? Perhaps it is too soon to tell. But it is not premature to insist that this alternative perspective exists and that it deserves to be taken seriously. At very least, those who choose to take it seriously may with reason expect that anyone who purports to be following a scientific approach to social violence and other human problems will be able to present a reasonable rationale for so doing. But, in the last analysis, all of us who aim to contribute to the rational solution of threatening human problems must heed a demand that is implied in the nature and organization of human social existence itself. And human social existence demands to be recognized as a complicated tissue of interpenetrating and mutually interdependent events in which multifarious reciprocal causal connections among neurobiological, individual, and social processes alternate, overlap, and combine, thereby determining the texture of the whole.

CHAPTER 17

The Meaning of "Experimental"

Gerald T. Perkoff

It is abundantly clear that it is difficult to discuss psychosurgery—or for that matter any other controversial medical intervention—without raising complex questions about its medical and ethical justifiability. Many participants in such discussions simply assert that a disputed medical intervention is "acceptable treatment" or "experimentation," but rarely is there any discussion of the criteria used for assigning these labels.

The word "experimental" has, of course, been used many times to describe psychosurgery, most frequently in a pejorative sense designed to rally opposition to such procedures—for many people the label "experimental" implies the use of humans as guinea pigs. The appropriateness of the label is usually assumed however, and not discussed. But what is an experiment in medicine, and how are experiments and therapy related? What guidelines can be identified that allow us to characterize a procedure or action as "experimental" or "therapeutic"? In this chapter, I will review concepts that have been proposed to help establish criteria for characterizing a medical procedure as "experimental" and will try to develop them further. Sparse though it is, the literature contains enough information to allow identification of several common threads, which can be woven into a general approach to this problem that may be useful in making decisions in the future.

Review of the Arguments

It may be helpful to use as a point of departure the assertion by many highly respected physician/investigators that "human experimentation is a daily occurrence in the practice of medicine because of the uniqueness of the individual" (F. O. Moore, 1975, p. 15). This position reflects the view, held by many, that every therapeutic encounter is an experiment inasmuch as even the outcome of known therapy is unknown for any particular patient. In essence, it begs the question by maintaining that everything a physician does is an experiment. But every physician–patient relationship is not an experiment. For most proposed treatments, considerable information is available on which to base a reasonable judgment of the likelihood of success or failure. Although the physician is not absolved of the responsibility of making careful observations and learning from every patient, this does not make every therapeutic encounter an experiment.

The clearest and most complete early discussion of this problem was offered by Claude Bernard, who devoted an entire section of his *Introduction to the Study of Experimental Medicine* (1865) to the definition of an experiment and the criteria for distinguishing experimentation from simple observation as well as from a "novel" or innovative therapeutic action. Bernard covered almost every point made later by others and distinguished between observation and experimentation quite simply. He said that observations "show" facts, while experiments "teach" about facts by a "sequence of reasoning." He argued persuasively that a major characteristic identifying something as experimental is the careful, sequential reasoning process that has its formal expression in the design of the data-collecting process. It was Bernard's view that we should classify a procedure as experimental not only on the bases of the reasoning behind it and the design, but also on the attempt to place the information obtained into some explanatory scheme built upon pre-existing knowledge. Bernard used the same criteria to distinguish experimentation from a "novelty" or from innovative therapy. Experimentation is characterized by reasoning and design, while novel manipulation or even innovative therapy is not primarily intended to yield knowledge.

Bernard also quoted Zimmerman, who carried this thought further by stating that knowledge gained in an experiment is "the fruit of an effort we make"—that is, a purposeful seeking of knowledge (cited in Bernard, 1865). This definition adds an additional theme, the "motive" or intent of the physician/investigator. Evidence of a physician's motive is derived from the specific effort expended to make it possible to draw conclusions and to obtain new knowledge. However, even Bernard departed from his own criteria when he stated that "physicians make therapeutic experiments daily on their patients" (Bernard, 1865).

This confusion continues into the modern literature. Schwitalla (1929), emphasized the importance of clinical research, arguing that such research was often for the patient's benefit, but he maintained that "the term research is stretched too far in its meaning" when applied to the individual patient. Schwitalla restated one of Bernard's keystones when he distinguished "applied" from "pure" research, defining the latter as "formal, experimental, creative" research. In the terms "formal" and "creative" we again encounter the ideas of design and the sequence of reasoning that separate things "experimental" from things "observational" or "novel." McCance (1951) tried to clarify this confusion but instead contributed to it when he stated that an attempt to cure an individual patient generally is not regarded as an experiment, but added, "yet it undoubtedly may be, if the results are observed and followed up, for the essence of treatment is to do some things positive to a patient, i.e., alter his condition, in the hope that the effect will be of benefit to him" (p. 189). Nevertheless, he too returned to the importance of motive by emphasizing that things that are done to patients that are not directly related to their benefit are experimental, and by stating that it is the "mental approach"—that is, the "motive"—of the person performing the procedure that helps determine whether it is innovative therapy or experimentation.

This was the state of thinking until recently, when Jonas (1970) commented that when a new therapy—either one still under investigation or one devised by the physician for a particular patient—is used when there is no known therapy for that patient's disorder, it is therapy rather than experimentation. This is so because the purpose is to discharge the physician's responsibility to treat the patient. Thus, even though the treatment is new and its use might therefore yield knowledge, it is different in its motivation from an experiment in which something is done to a patient for the express purpose of learning. More recently, in a discussion of psychosurgery and experimentation, Mark and Neville said that procedures done to determine the outcome, with no expectation of direct benefit to the particular patient being operated upon, had to be classified as experimental (Mark and Neville, 1973). And finally, Veatch has identified the degree of organization of procedures as important in their characterization as experiments; that is, the "design" for the obtaining of new knowledge is what makes procedures "experimental" (Veatch, 1977). This important point tells us that a high degree of novelty of a procedure is not sufficient to justify the label "experimental."

Four themes are common to this earlier literature and must be included in any model designed to help determine whether a medical procedure is experimental or therapeutic: (1) The importance of the knowledge or lack of knowledge of the outcome of the intervention planned. If the outcome is known, the procedure is not experimental. (2) The motive of the physician/investigator. If the purpose of intervention is solely to help the patient, it is treatment; if it is planned solely for the purpose of and with the express design of gaining new knowledge, it is experimental. The common problem of mixed motives will be discussed later. (3) The presence or absence of a specific design to obtain reliable data and to reach valid conclusions. (4) Whether or not there exists a known therapy for the condition in question. From a legal point of view, this is especially important for determining whether physicians are only discharging their responsibility to treat a patient by urging a new and untried treatment. In this case, the use of a new therapy does not constitute an experiment, even if the physician learns something in the process. Of course, in specific instances, the claim that there is "no other known treatment" for the condition can be disputed. It is important to consider the different models that have been used to define situations as "experimental" and to see whether any of them contain all four necessary elements.

Three different models have been presented to deal with these issues. One is a practical bureaucratic model now in use, which makes simple and absolute determinations based upon outcome as the only acceptable discriminant between experimental and therapeutic actions or materials. I call this the Practical Governmental Model, best illustrated by the procedures the Food and Drug Administration (FDA) uses to develop information about safety and efficacy of new drugs before approving them for marketing to the general public (Levine, 1975). The second is a Medical Investigative Model, specifically relating to clinical studies on human subjects (Levine,

1975). The third and most complete is a Legal Model, which includes a "decision tree" by means of which individual cases may be described and classified (Dickens, 1975).

Practical Governmental Model

The FDA takes a simple approach to these issues for the purposes of drug evaluation. It arbitrarily defines all drugs as "experimental" until both their safety and efficacy have been demonstrated. This method begins with evidence from animal studies and proceeds in a stepwise manner through a series of human studies until specific evidence is obtained that leads to acceptance or rejection of a drug for marketing. This is an outcome model in its purest form and takes no account of any of the other factors mentioned. The "motive" of the physician or investigator does not enter into the final determination, although a physician who tests a new drug for safety or efficacy clearly is experimenting when he does the work that leads to this determination. Further, the availability or lack of availability of any other efficacious therapy is not taken into account when a new drug is tested. This is done only later when a drug newly determined to be efficacious is tested against earlier forms of treatment. And the only design that is important in the efficacy determination is that of the particular studies required to provide the results (outcome) upon which the FDA can base its final decision. Nevertheless, this model has wide potential applicability, being suitable for evaluation of new surgical procedures, marketing and deployment of new and expensive technological advances, prostheses and the like. However, it avoids the real issue of what is "experimental," since it uses an arbitrary, predetermined classification based only on the availability of knowledge of outcomes. This model could be applied only with great difficulty to more complicated problems such as the identification of the specific characteristics of parts of randomized clinical trials (RCT),[1] to operations that may affect symptoms but not longevity, or to many other complex clinical and investigative situations.

---

[1] For the purposes of this discussion, a *randomized clinical* (or *controlled*) *trial* is defined as a study in which patients with a particular illness or problem are distributed randomly by some specific statistical design among two groups, the members of which thereby have similar characteristics. Following randomization, one form of treatment is given to patients in one group and a second to patients in the other. Measurements are made during treatment that yield data upon which a decision is based about the advantage or lack of advantage of one treatment over the other (after Cochrane, 1972).

Medical Investigative Model

The Medical Investigative Model is a much more complete and clinically applicable model than the one just described. It deals specifically with the knotty problem of clinical research and the relationship of experimentation to therapy in the same patient. Levine defines research as:

> any manipulation of a human being—or of anything related to that human being that might subsequently result in manipulation of that human being—which is done with the intent of developing new knowledge and which differs in any way from customary medical or other professional practice [Levine, 1975].

According to this definition, if the physician/investigator's only motive is to help his patient, then what he does is treatment and not research or experimentation. Conversely, if the only motive is to acquire new knowledge, then what is done is experimental and not treatment. Recognizing that the situation rarely is this pure in clinical investigation or medical practice, Levine describes a series of interreactions between research and treatment that define boundaries and overlaps from different points of view. The simplest boundaries are between physician and investigator, at least when their motives are single-purposed and obvious. Any clear motive to pursue either treatment or research effectively differentiates these roles. A second set of interactions exists between any given action in research or medical practice and its review by peer groups or regulatory bodies. For example, study sections of the National Institutes of Health, composed of investigators' peers, review research proposals believed by the investigators to be experimental. The members of those groups explicitly or implicitly help decide whether or not a procedure is experimental, according to their estimates of the state of knowledge, the perceived motive of the investigator, and the quality of the design. The FDA, as already noted, classifies procedures as experimental or nonexperimental according to the outcomes of studies of efficacy and safety. By fitting the physician/investigator and the practice/peer review interactions into a graphic model, Levine identifies nineteen overlap areas to help define the boundaries between research and treatment, public and private interest, acceptable and nonacceptable treatment, and so on. Unfortunately, except in his clear definition of research, Levine does not provide us with any system of reasoning by which we can resolve the overlap problems he so systematically enumerates. Nor does he help us with problems that contain elements of both research and treatment.

It should be noted that the theme of motive recurs repeatedly in this model, and that the importance of a known or unknown outcome also is emphasized in the discussion of overlaps and boundaries between the physician's actions and the actions of regulatory agencies. Like Jonas, Levine makes the important point that the existence or lack of existence of orthodox therapy for a given condition is a major determinant in classifying a procedure as research —research being, in Levine's words, something that "differs in any way from customary medical practice."

The Medical Investigative Model also emphasizes that the experimental/therapeutic relationships are the same, from an ethical point of view, in some kinds of social science research (for example, educational research or health services research) as in medical investigation, and apply as well to nonphysician researcher/providers as to medical doctors. Levine thus carries us well along the way to the development of a general model that might be used for decision making related to the complex interaction which is the topic of this chapter.

The concept of "orthodox therapy" for given conditions leads us directly to the Legal Model, which depends heavily on the presence or absence of such therapy for certain critical decisions.

Legal Model

Decision Criteria

With law and medicine intertwined in so many ways today—and especially with respect to psychosurgery—it is interesting that the most detailed model of the factors, methods, and concepts that can be used to decide whether a procedure is experimental or therapeutic comes from legal exposition (Dickens, 1975). Bernard Dickens reviewed the Canadian legal literature and pulled together various important issues into a decision tree that advances our thinking in this area and at the same time provides a practical tool for making decisions in specific cases. All of the factors already identified are specifically codified in this model—motive, knowledge of outcome, design, and availability of orthodox therapy—giving us some confidence that this legal approach takes advantage of prior philosophical, ethical, investigative, and medical thought, as well as of prior legal decisions.

Dickens discusses the problem from several perspectives. He reminds us that from the patient's perspective, unless he is simply a volunteer for an experiment, he has come to a physician with a problem and expects that physician to make an informed effort to correct the problem. In other words, he expects treatment—and views the physician's procedures as such, even if they have other characteristics typical of experimentation. Since the patient seeks therapy, what is done must be therapy unless it is explained otherwise and the patient's own motivation changed. In the legal sense, then, the patient's motive becomes as important a determining factor from his own point of view as does the professional's from his. This view may seem to confuse the issue, since the question can be fairly asked, What if the treatment is part of a direct experimental trial, or of a clinical comparison, with clear design, investigative motivation, and unknown outcome? Consideration of the physician's point of view helps clarify these points.

A professional's motivation can be quite direct, even in the management of a sick patient with a new treatment, according to Dickens. Even though the new therapeutic procedure may be intended to yield knowledge, if this knowledge is obtained in an effort that is undertaken solely for the patient's benefit, the process in which physician and patient are involved is therapeutic. The doctor-patient relationship implies a responsibility on the physician's part to help the patient who comes to him with a problem. The acceptance of this responsibility makes the relationship a therapeutic one even though the motivations of the physician may be mixed—that is, a helping motive plus an interest in new knowledge. As we shall see in the discussion of randomized clinical trials, experimental studies may be designed to yield knowledge as their primary goal but at the same time include therapies that have known benefit for the patient. Likewise, in a therapeutic relationship some aspects of the helping process can be experimental and designed to yield new knowledge.

An additional point is worth making here, because the question often has come up in relation to psychosurgery. What if there is no orthodox therapy for the condition in question? Even in the absence of an orthodox therapy—a decision that is made by legal precedent, peer opinion, and search of medical literature—it is the physician's responsibility to help or to try to help a patient who comes to him for help. In this situation, the use of a new, unorthodox, untried therapy, even one that might be considered novel, is a therapeutic use—even though new knowledge may accrue—because the physician's motive is determined by his direct responsibility to help the patient. This argument is carried further in the Legal Model, which states that if there *is* an orthodox therapy available, then a new therapy must be considered experimental and its use designed to yield knowledge, and this must be explained to the patient. Otherwise, the use of a new therapy constitutes negligence on the part of the doctor, who is expected to use accepted, orthodox treatment. If the physician has mixed motives, any sign of investigational motive may render at least part of the situation experimental. Obviously, in some situations, both therapeutic and experimental motives are present.

Resolution of this conflict is partially accomplished by the example of the RCT, in which two therapies known to be at least partially effective are compared with one another to determine which is better and should become (or remain) the orthodox therapy. In this situation, if both treatments are known to be effective, then neither is experimental, as the outcome of their use is known. Likewise, if the patient sought out the doctor for help, his treatment is considered therapeutic. But the *process of comparison* of the two treatments may be considered experimental if the physician, through his mixed motives, designs the process to yield new information. As defined, therefore, an RCT can have both therapeutic and experimental aspects. It is the design to provide new knowledge that is the experiment in this case, not the treatments.

No matter which model is being considered, the question of knowledge of the outcome seems to be paramount. Inherent in the questions about the existence of an orthodox therapy, about safety and efficacy, and about the presence or absence of a design for obtaining new knowledge, and even in the belief expressed by some that every therapeutic encounter is an experiment, is the stated or implied rule: If what we do has a known outcome, then it is not experimental. If what we do has an unknown outcome, it is either experimental, in which case we must design its use to gain the required knowledge, or else it is merely negligent. This outcome determinent is of course modified in the many ways discussed previously, but in all of them is the principle first enunciated by Bernard and later cited and expanded upon by every other medical, legal, or philosophical authority. That principle is that ignorance is remedied by the seeking of knowledge and that this seeking is best done by purposeful manipulation. The design of that manipulation, which is evidence of a sequence of reasoning, makes the seeking experimental. These principles are laid out graphically in Figure 17.1.

In this diagram, medical actions are divided into three categories: diagnostic, therapeutic, and nontherapeutic. The principles followed throughout are set forth most simply in relation to diagnostic proce-

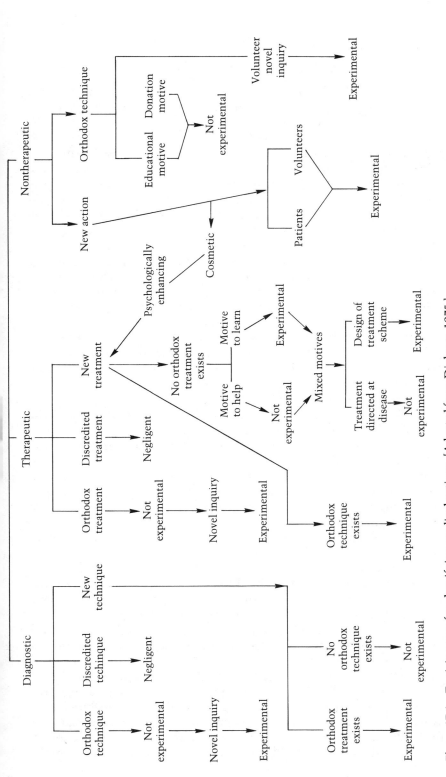

Figure 17.1 Decision tree for classifying medical actions. [Adapted from Dickens, 1975.]

dures. When the diagnostic technique being used is an orthodox technique, its use is not experimental. If a discredited procedure is used, this would be considered negligent. If a new, untested technique is used and an orthodox technique exists, then the use of the former is considered experimental, provided the experimental requirements of design, reasoning, and consent are met. Exactly the same process of reasoning is applied to therapeutic actions, with the same decision results. In considering therapeutic decisions, however, we now must add an additional branch point to account for the additional factor to be considered in the therapeutic situation— physician's motive. Where no orthodox therapy exists and the motive of the physician is purely to help the patient, he is discharging his responsibility to help the patient by his actions. These actions, therefore, are considered therapeutic, not experimental. If, on the other hand, his motive is purely to learn and no helping is involved, his action must be classified as experimental.

If the physician's motives are mixed, then his actions are experimental insofar as they are designed to yield information—and it would be considered negligent for the physician not to design them so—even if the treatment is carried out for the patient's benefit. The clearest example of this situation is the new treatment for an incurable disease or the randomized clinical trial, both of which have the special features already described.

Dickens considers "cosmetic" procedures as nontherapeutic. However, since they may result in psychological benefit to the patient they also fit into the therapeutic scheme as actions performed to correct a patient's problem. The classification of their use as therapeutic or experimental then follows the same outline as do other treatments.

In nontherapeutic situations, the study of a new treatment or technique in volunteers clearly is experimental and subject to all the qualifications about design and reasoning already alluded to. In patients, this decision may be modified by motivation, and by other factors already described, but the very fact of study conducted in a nontherapeutic situation implies that the motive is to learn and that knowledge is lacking. This fulfills the main characteristics of experimental situations. The decision tree also allows for nontherapeutic actions in three additional situations. The first is the performance of orthodox procedures for the education or training of health professionals. The informed participation by a patient in the teaching of physical diagnosis and the use of patient specimens for repeated laboratory analyses by technicians in training are examples of this kind. A more complex situation, but one that fits the line of reasoning already developed, has to do with donations, for example, of blood or of an organ for transplantation. If one donates blood or submits to removal, say, of a kidney for purposes of donation to a patient in need, the clinical situation is dominated by the gift relationship (Titmus, 1971). The physician may use the blood or organ in a patient whose treatment is part of an experiment (as in a randomized clinical trial), but the actual donation is not experimental if an orthodox procedure is used to accomplish the donation. If a new procedure is used, then its use is subject to the same reasoning as is any other such new procedure, already described. This third situation is the now familiar one of study of an orthodox procedure by means of a novel inquiry or comparison, and is considered experimental under these terms.

Applications

Although psychosurgery has occupied a special position in the public eye and in the ethical literature, the same considerations apply to it as to any other procedure or treatment. The additional complexities of informed consent and the other ethical issues that are especially difficult for psychosurgery do not change this. If the outcome of a psychosurgical procedure is known—that is, if there is agreement among a significant sample of experts about the clinical situations in which its use is or is not effective—then the procedure is not experimental. If the outcome with a particular use is known to be bad, that use represents negligence. If the outcome is unknown, the psychosurgical procedure is experimental, and its use requires a design for obtaining information, the evidence of a sequence of reasoning, and a clear recognition by the patient (or his surrogates) and the physician of the motives of the physician in prescribing the procedure. If no orthodox procedure exists, then the psychosurgical procedures can be considered therapeutic, provided the physician's motives are *purely* therapeutic. Otherwise, the situation almost certainly will contain mixed motives and should be considered experimental to the extent and in the manner outlined above. This carries us into the more traditional areas of informed consent and the many difficulties associated with informed consent from a patient who has a condition that might be treated by a psychosurgical procedure. But those considerations are subsequent to the recognition of the conditions that make the procedure experimental or not experimental, and do not enter into that determination.

Especially in the case of psychosurgery, the application of the principles just developed would be clearer if we had specific procedures for determining whether an outcome is known or unknown.

This remains most difficult to do, since a physicians' beliefs about outcome may be influenced by his motives in suggesting any given therapeutic procedure in the first place. Moreover, such influences may not be wholly conscious.

How can we resolve this difficult problem? Dickens says that lawyers arrive at a determination by a combination of legal precedent, literature search, and the opinions of peers. In medicine we do the same. Experts (specialists) organize into committees or are asked to serve in the public interest for just such judgments. Two recent examples concern the treatment of hypertension (Moser et al., 1977) and the prevention of bacterial endocarditis in various clinical situations (Kaplan et al., 1977); there are many others that could be cited. And medical literature does reflect significant agreement or disagreement about treatment outcomes. Thus, while an exact set of guidelines is difficult to specify, a generally applicable method has precedent in medical as well as in legal circles. However, challenges to opinions developed by this method can be expected to occur periodically until majority opinion becomes overwhelming.

Two additional examples can be cited to help clarify how our principles may be applied to complex clinical and research situations. The first is the current, rapidly growing practice of treating coronary heart disease by means of coronary artery bypass graft surgery (CABG). Medical therapy is an old and established means of treatment for patients with angina pectoris, the chest pain associated with coronary atherosclerosis and believed to be related in some as yet undetermined way to restriction of coronary blood flow by the atherosclerotic process (Murphy et al., 1977). Such therapy relieves pain in most patients but requires constant medical supervision and the use of either regular or intermittent medication, or both. CABG now has been shown to relieve the symptoms of angina pectoris in the large majority of patients, perhaps more often than, but certainly as well as, medical treatment, and it does so in a short period of time as a direct result of the operation. Is the use of CABG for angina pectoris experimental because the procedure still is relatively new, controversial, and costly—or is it therapeutic? By all the criteria enumerated during the present discussion, the use of CABG for *angina pectoris* can only be considered therapeutic, since the outcome is known. However, if one used a new technique for the surgery, that new technique would be experimental and would have to be compared with orthodox techniques for the treatment. This would call for a design and the other stated characteristics required for experimental procedures. The use of a surgical approach itself would not be experimental, and the clinical situation would contain mixed motives with the characteristics associated with action in such a setting.

However, many believe that CABG may prolong life as well as relieve symptoms. Indeed, for one form of coronary heart disease, left main coronary artery disease, this seems well demonstrated (Braunwald, 1977). In this latter circumstance, CABG surely is not experimental. However, in other forms of coronary heart disease, the effect of CABG on prolongation of life is hotly disputed (Hiatt, 1977, DeBakey and Lawrie, 1978). In this situation, by the criteria enunciated, use of CABG would be experimental and should be carried out only with attention to design, informed consent, and all the other characteristics of experiments. Thus, a single procedure used in one set of circumstances and with one type of information provided the patient would be considered therapeutic, while the *same procedure* in the *same patient*, done for another purpose would require a different designation, a different set of information for and consents from the patient. Any other approach could be considered negligent according to the reasoning we have developed here. Even in this complex situation, then, our model holds.

A final example indicates other complexities and shows how this decision problem spills over into another area of major medical and ethical concern—responsibility for payment for care and procedures. Let us take again the example of the randomized clinical trial of two forms of treatment, which are not experimental in themselves, inasmuch as each may have some known effectiveness, but which are being compared in a design purposely conceived to establish which is the more effective treatment. The comparison of the two, therefore, constitutes an experiment, while their actual use is therapeutic. Let us also assume that the condition being treated is metastatic cancer of a type for which there is no known cure, and of which the outcome would be death unless successful treatment could be found. In this instance, the motivation of the patient surely is to be helped—a prime characteristic of the therapeutic relationship. Since there is no effective orthodox treatment, the physician is required by his responsibility to the patient to use any new therapy available to try to help his patient. The motives of the physician, however, are mixed, since he is comparing two treatments of known partial effectiveness and has set up a design that he believes will yield that information to him, so he will do better with the next patient he cares for. This makes the situation experimental. In the course of the treatments, certain diagnostic procedures are used. They are believed necessary, at least in part, to follow the results of treatment and to monitor for toxicity of therapy. To some additional extent, they also are part of the design to give information about comparative effectiveness of the two treatments being used. Some of these procedures are done on a regular timed basis, with the times decided upon in advance and the procedures performed whether or not there are immediate clinical indications for them. These procedures may be the same kind as those used to follow the results of therapy. According to our model, unless the procedures are used solely for therapeutic purposes—and they can hardly be in the posited situation of mixed motivation on the part of the physician—they are part of the experiment. In today's complex medical world, then, these should be paid for by research funds, and not be charged to the patient. Those that are used for therapeutic purposes alone, however, would be legitimate charges to treatment and should be paid for by the patient or his third party carrier. Solomon himself would be sorely tried to unravel the various motivations and outcomes in such a situation, one that comes up every day in any major medical center. The same considerations would apply equally well to any study of the relative outcomes of psychosurgical procedures, in which two procedures were compared and in which mixed therapeutic and "knowledge-gaining" motives existed.

Monitoring Procedures

As we consider possible ways such decisions might be monitored and applied to the real world of medical and surgical treatment, it is well to remember again that only four principles have been identified throughout the literature and this discussion. They must be kept in mind, since any system devised to deal with such complex and emotional issues must address all of them. These issues are: (1) Is the outcome of the act to be initiated known or unknown? (2) Is the motivation of the physician/investigator purely to help the patient or purely to gain new knowledge, or is it mixed? (3) Is there evidence in the way in which the action is taken that there was a design that would yield information and that a sequence of reasoning went into that design or will go into the analysis of the results? (4) Is there an orthodox therapy for the condition being treated? Other modifying factors are important, especially those legal considerations that raise the issue of negligence. But in the main, these four principles are the ones to consider for the purposes of monitoring.

One way to monitor the development and implementation of new treatments and procedures, including surgical procedures and technological innovations, would be to follow the FDA model strictly and insist that the outcome always is "unknown" until satisfactory evidence of safety and efficacy is available and ruled upon. This could be applied in most of the straightforward instances we have cited but, as a pure outcome model, would give us little help with the frequent complex situations where the motivations of the physician and patient are mixed and where knowledge of outcome is known for one aspect of the problem but not the other. The CABG example cited above would not fit well into this model, for example, nor would randomized clinical trials carried out in patients with serious or incurable diseases. The complicated bureaucratic process required to provide information to the regulatory agency would itself discourage investigators from making the kinds of comparisons needed when a new and untried therapy carried out. This would likely be so unless such work could be done only in research centers. Even then, the stepwise, rule-following procedures would be cumbersome, and the delays now known in drug development, implementation, and acceptance would be compounded many-fold in more controversial treatments such as those for cancer, heart disease, or indeed, psychosurgery.

A more practical way to pursue such monitoring information—an experimental procedure itself by the principles outlined here—would be to expand and assign increased responsibility to the Human Experimentation Committees of all institutions. Such groups could take an active role in the evaluation of therapeutic/experimental procedures not usually submitted to them for ruling under the present practices. To do so, they would have to be expanded into Bioethics and Experimentation Committees, would have to follow some defined model or decision tree like, but not necessarily the same as, that discussed here. They would study a statistically derived, prospective sample of the practice in their institution or area to identify the motivations of the physicians, the level of knowledge of outcome of the procedures used and how that level changes, the degree to which orthodox therapy does or does not exist, the presence or absence of research design, and the presence or absence of a process of reasoning to yield information. This effort could be carried out initially and then on an ongoing basis as a means for continued monitoring of practice in the local institution or region under jurisdiction. Defined procedures for gathering information and hearing appeals would be needed, and the committees would be expanded to include people with medical, ethical, consumer, economic, and social skills of a wide variety. Such an approach would permit the development of local procedures, practices and decision rules that would reflect the characteristics of the particular area, making them more likely to be accepted and participated in by the physicians and patients whose care they would most directly affect. Such an idea presented here, in a most limited form, would have to be developed further in each area and institution, but seems preferable to a centralized bureau that would make rulings on a national basis without knowledge of individual circumstances and modifying factors.

Perhaps the best way to close this discussion is to say, as Dickens did, that what I have said here cannot be considered a complete analysis of this complicated and important subject: no one exposition could be. But perhaps these considerations have organized and advanced existing thought in a way that might serve as a basis for future discussions of this important, interesting, and perplexing problem—what is the meaning of the word "experimental"?

PART V

Legal Issues

CHAPTER 18

Psychosurgery Legislation and Case Law

Francis C. Pizzulli

Various models for regulating psychosurgery have been legislated, adjudicated, or recommended by advisory commissions. The models give us a picture of the various approaches to regulating innovative surgery, biomedical research, and mental health therapies generally in a context of uncertainty as to the patient's capacity for informed consent and the efficacy and safety of the proposed procedures. Thus, the controversy over psychosurgery has provided the impetus for the articulation of these models, but the approaches taken toward the issues of committee review, proxy consent, and the like have important implications outside the psychosurgery debate.

Regulatory models may operate on an ad hoc basis, through the imposition of uniform standards, or, most typically, through a combination of the two methods. For example, by means of the common law of malpractice—that is, negligence by a medical professional —courts may regulate the practice of psychosurgery, on a post hoc basis, by applying general rules on informed consent and standard of care to particular cases. Regulation via the tort of negligence is discussed by Morse in this book.

Legislation may regulate psychosurgery by setting out hard-and-fast rules concerning what types of procedures may or may not be performed, and upon what category of patients. Alternatively, or in combination with such per se rule making, legislation may provide for decision-making machinery on certain issues and relegate to the chosen decision-making body—whether a court, executive agency, advisory commission, or ad hoc committee—the tasks of identifying substantive principles and applying principles to specific cases. Grimm reviews legislative efforts in this book.

Constitutional principles may also serve as a regulatory force. Constitutional issues may arise when there is "state action," as when patients institutionalized in state-sponsored facilities are subjected to treatment without their consent. (In a related vein, Delgado discusses the role of due process principles when a prisoner requests release on the grounds that he has been "cured" by psychosurgery or other organic therapies.) Moreover, legislation that controls access to psychosurgery is subject to review to ensure the protection of constitutionally guaranteed freedoms that may be embodied in the free choice of or access to mental health therapies.

This paper will focus on the regulatory models set forth in Oregon and California legislation. The state legislation will then be examined in light of two judicial decisions concerning restraints on the use of psychosurgery. Emphasis will be placed on constitutional "freedom of choice and thought" limitations upon the regulation of mental health therapies. The provocative First Amendment "freedom of mentation" argument endorsed in the two court decisions is analyzed, and the criticisms of it are evaluated.

Legislative Models

Oregon and California have statutes that regulate the practice of psychosurgery in a comprehensive manner. The Oregon Act is noteworthy for its reliance upon multidisciplinary review and its provision for proxy (that is, guardian) consent to psychosurgery in those cases where the patient lacks the capacity for informed consent.[1] California has two acts that regulate psychosurgery, one for those confined pursuant to the criminal laws (the Penal Code Act)[2] and another act that regulates all other situations in which psycho-

---

[1] 35 Ore. Rev. Stat. § 426.700 *et seq.*
[2] Cal. Penal Code § 2670 *et seq.* (West Supp. 1978).

surgery may be proposed (the Civil Law Act).[3] (The predecessor of the Civil Law Act[4] was struck down as unconstitutional in a court decision discussed later.) The Penal Code Act provides for judicial review of proposed psychosurgery, while the Civil Law Act requires peer review by certain medical specialists. The California Acts are also distinguished by their prohibition of proxy consent in the case of incompetents and minors.

Oregon

Oregon passed its Act in 1973. The Act covers psychosurgery (and intracranial brain stimulation by means of implantation of electrodes) intended to be performed on a prisoner, inmate of a mental health institution, or private patient. Any physician intending to perform psychosurgery must file a petition with the Psychosurgery Review Board alleging (1) that a patient is in need of such treatment, (2) that the patient or legal guardian has consented, and (3) that the proposed operation has legitimate clinical value.

The Review Board must hold a "consent hearing" within a month after the filing of such petition. The Act sets out various points that must be put to the patient or legal guardian. They include a fair explanation of the procedures, including identification of those that are experimental; a description of benefits and risks; disclosure of appropriate alternative treatments; disclosure of the right to consult with legal counsel and to revoke the consent at any time. The patient or guardian may be represented by legal counsel at the consent hearing.

If a patient appears to be incapable of giving informed consent, the necessary consent shall be given or withheld by the legal guardian of the patient. Thus, the Act permits psychosurgery upon those lacking the capacity for informed consent, and, apparently, even if the incompetent patient indicates an unwillingness to undergo the psychosurgical operation.

If a patient or guardian gives an informed consent, the Review Board next engages in a substantive review of the proposed operation. It must determine whether the operation has clinical merit and is an appropriate treatment for the specific patient. This determination calls for both a general and specific inquiry: not only must the

---

[3] Cal. Welf. and Inst. Code § 5325 *et seq.* (West Supp. 1978).
[4] Cal. Welf. and Inst. Code § 5325 *et seq.* (West Supp. 1976).

proposed operation have legitimate clinical value, it must also be determined to be appropriate for the specific patient in question. Such a determination requires that (1) all conventional therapies have been attempted, (2) the criteria for selection of the patient have been met, (3) the operation offers hope of saving life, reestablishing health, or alleviating suffering, and (4) all other viable alternative methods of treatment have been tried and have failed to produce satisfactory results. The requirement of exhaustion of viable alternative methods of treatment in addition to exhaustion of conventional therapies indicates a legislative presumption that such other treatments, even when experimental, are less intrusive than psychosurgery.

The Oregon Act highlights several issues that must be addressed in a regulatory model. Perhaps the most critical decision made by the Oregon Legislature is the authorization of psychosurgery upon those incompetent to consent. Thus, Oregon permits proxy consent by the legal guardian to psychosurgery. Moreover, the Act does not preclude the performance of psychosurgery on members of special populations, such as prisoners and children. The Act does not require judicial review, nor does it flatly prohibit any particular procedure. It does require, however, approval by the Review Board, which entails slightly more than peer review by other neurosurgeons or related professionals. The Review Board is composed of nine persons appointed by the governor. Membership of the board is specified as follows: one board-certified neurologist; two board-certified neurosurgeons; two board-certified psychiatrists; one clinical psychologist; one neuroscientist actively engaged in research on the nervous system; and two members of the public, one of whom shall be a lawyer. No individual directly involved on conducting psychosurgery shall be a member of the Review Board, and a majority of six is required to effect decisions of the Review Board.

Thus, the Oregon model is distinguished by its provision for multidisciplinary review and proxy consent, and its requirement of exhaustion of viable alternative therapies. To date, there has been no reported case of psychosurgery having been performed under the Act (but see Grimm's chapter in this book).

California

The California Penal Code and Civil Law Acts have in common a prohibition of proxy consent to psychosurgery. The California Acts differ, however, with respect to the means of reviewing decisions to undergo psychosurgery and to the requirement of exhaustion of alternative therapies.

Penal Code Act   The Penal Code Act was legislated in 1974 and received its impetus from an article by Michael Shapiro published that year in the Southern California Law Review (Shapiro, 1974). The Penal Code Act regulates the use of organic therapies (for example, psychosurgery, electrical stimulation of the brain, drugs used in programs of aversive conditioning) upon prisoners confined in public or private hospitals, sanitariums, and the like. The preamble or declaration of policy of the Penal Code Act states in part:

> It is hereby recognized and declared that all persons, including all persons involuntarily confined, have a fundamental right against enforced interference with their thought processes, states of mind, and patterns of mentation through the use of organic therapies. . . .

The Penal Code Act protects against enforced interference by requiring an informed consent, in writing, from a psychosurgery patient. The test for informed consent is carefully defined so that a person confined shall not be deemed incapable of informed consent solely by virtue of being diagnosed as a mentally ill, disordered, abnormal, or mentally defective person. By implication, someone who has not been adjudged legally incompetent for purposes of appointment of a guardian or conservator may still be considered to lack the specific capacity for informed consent to psychosurgery. This fine discrimination between states of mental illness reflects the increasing recognition by legislatures and courts of the various capacities that may be affected by mental illness. For example, civil commitment statutes should pertain to the capacity of a person to decide whether he or she is in need of hospitalization. At times this may be a different capacity from that of consent to psychosurgery.

In order to be found capable of informed consent a person must be provided with, and able to understand and act upon, various items of information, which may be described as follows:

1. The nature and seriousness of the person's illness or defect.

2. The nature of the proposed psychosurgery.

3. The likelihood of improvement or deterioration with and without the psychosurgery.

4. The nature, likelihood, and extent of changes in behavior or mentation and of side effects caused by the surgery.

5. The uncertainty of the cost–benefit equation of the particular psychosurgery and the degree to which it is considered experimental.

6. The reasonable alternative organic therapy or "psychotherapeutic modality of therapy," or "nonorganic behavior modification program."

Once a written informed consent is obtained, the decision of the patient and attending physician must be reviewed by a court. The superintendent of the confining institution must petition a local court of general jurisdiction for an order authorizing the psychosurgery. (Conversely, such courts have jurisdiction over petitions for orders to prohibit unauthorized organic therapies.) In the case of an indigent patient, the court will appoint counsel (similar to the Oregon Review Board) and an independent medical expert in the patient's behalf. Speedy resolution of the issues is provided for by requiring that the hearing on the petition be held within ten to twenty days after the filing of the petition.

The reviewing court must evaluate both the sufficiency of the informed consent and the substantive merits of the proposed psychosurgery, and must find the superintendent's petition supported by "clear and convincing evidence"—a standard calling for a greater degree of certitude than the "preponderance of the evidence" standard usually employed in civil adjudications. In order to pass the substantive review, the superintendent must show that (1) the psychosurgery would be beneficial; (2) there is a "compelling interest"—a concept derived from the constitutional law of fundamental rights—justifying the psychosurgery; (3) there are no "less onerous alternatives" (a similarly derived concept) to the psychosurgery; and (4) the psychosurgery is in accordance with sound medical-psychiatric practice.

The requirement that there be no less onerous alternatives to psychosurgery should be distinguished from a requirement of exhaustion of all other viable alternative therapies. The no-less-onerous-alternative test does not conclusively presume that psychosurgery is the most onerous alternative. It thereby allows room for development in validation of psychosurgical procedures so that, for example, a patient does not necessarily have to undergo a long period of potentially debilitating shock therapy before psychosurgery can be performed.

Because the patient must both have the capacity for informed consent and have been shown to have granted it, the court may not approve psychosurgery on the basis of proxy consent. In this regard, the Penal Code Act treats psychosurgery differently from other organic therapies, which may be administered upon one found incompetent to give informed consent.

Civil Law Act   The Civil Law Act, which applies to all psychosurgery performed in the state not covered by the Penal Code Act, was passed in 1974 and was reenacted with substantial modifications in 1976 in the wake of a court decision striking it down. The declaration of policy of the Civil Law Act reflects the Legislature's awareness that regulation of mental health therapies implicates constitutional values:

> Recognizing the danger of a violation of a mental patient's constitutional right to privacy, the Legislature intends by this enactment to assure that the integrity and free choice of every such patient is fully recognized and protected. Because those who are emotionally disturbed are vulnerable to being unduly influenced, the Legislature believes the protection of their rights requires a careful process of informing and consenting in order to assure the protection and vindication of their rights.

The Civil Law Act has a number of provisions substantially similar to those of the Penal Code Act. For example, the elements of informed consent are similar, and a person is not precluded from having the capacity to give consent solely because of a diagnosis of mental illness. Likewise, proxy consent to psychosurgery is prohibited. The ban on proxy consent is elaborated upon by a prohibition of any psychosurgery upon minors—those under the age of eighteen years.

The Civil Law Act nevertheless deviates from the Penal Code Act in a few notable ways. The Penal Code Act appears to have a broader definition of psychosurgery in that it includes destruction of brain tissues by electronic or chemical means and also includes implantation of electrodes. Moreover, the Civil Law Act incorporates two "cooling-off periods"—a concept perhaps borrowed from consumer protection law—into the consent process for psychosurgery. A written consent may be given only after twenty-four hours have expired from the time the required information is presented orally to the patient. Then there must be a delay of at least seventy-two hours following the written consent before the psychosurgery may be performed.

There are, moreover, two major distinctions between the Acts. Under the Civil Law Act the substantive standard for evaluating the proposed psychosurgery is that "all other appropriate treatment modalities have been exhausted" and that the psychosurgery is "definitely indicated" and is "the least drastic alternative available for the treatment of the patient at the time." The requirement of exhaustion of alternative therapies is similar to the Oregon Act rule. Unfortunately, the requirement reflects what may occur when there is a lack of a unified legislative approach. In an area where one would suppose that greater safeguards on the use of psychosurgery are desired—the special population composed of prisoners—there is no exhaustion requirement, whereas an indisputably voluntary and competent noninstitutionalized patient is burdened with the requirement. The Civil Law Act is also a bit curious in its rule that psychosurgery must be the least drastic alternative available (that is, that there be no less onerous alternative). The rule is somewhat obscure in light of the exhaustion-of-therapies requirement; once all other therapies are exhausted, the only alternative to psychosurgery to be balanced on the least-drastic-alternative scale is no treatment at all.

The second major difference between the California Acts lies in the provision for review of the psychosurgery decision. The Civil Law Act relies on peer review rather than judicial review—a distinction that does make sense in light of the lesser need for special safeguards when not dealing with prisoners. The pure peer review approach differs from the multidisciplinary review tack taken by the Oregon Act. A review committee composed of three physicians not otherwise involved in the treatment of the patient must personally examine the patient and unanimously concur in the treating physician's determinations under the substantive standard and in the conclusion that the patient has the capacity for consent. The review committee members must be either board-certified or eligible psychiatrists or neurosurgeons; two must be appointed by the county mental health director, and one must be appointed by the facility. (In the case of a noninstitutionalized patient, presumably "facility" refers to the institution in which the psychosurgery is to be performed, although the Act is unclear on this point.) The Civil Law Act does not identify the party or entity financially responsible for the work of a review committee.

It may be said that, in a sense, the review procedure takes the form of an expansion of the patient–physician relationship to include additional physicians. There are no lay members on the review committee. Because the physician members are reviewing not only the capacity for informed consent but also the issue of whether the psychosurgery is medically indicated, it is reasonable to say that they are acting *qua* physician, and given the fact that they personally examine the patient, the statement could be expanded to the form "*qua* physician in a patient–physician relationship." Under the Civil Law Act, there should then be no question involving application of the patient–physician privilege to refuse to disclose confidential communications in a judicial proceeding, leaving aside the issue of whether the privilege is a meaningful one in light of several exceptions to the privilege and the already existing ethical obligation of confidentiality.

Experience Under the California Acts   Several years have elapsed since the California Acts went into effect. It is reported that only two psychosurgical operations have been performed pursuant to the 1976 Civil Law Act. The costly and time-consuming review procedures are often blamed for discouraging psychosurgery. Indeed, somewhat similar review procedures for shock therapy, described later in this chapter, are blamed by some physicians for a reputedly drastic reduction in the number of shock treatments and the outright discontinuance of shock therapy in a number of major state and private hospitals. Shock therapy patients have been required to pay the fees of the review committee, which are not insignificant.

The reason for the absence of psychosurgery under the Penal Code Act is all too clear (Kelley, 1978). The State Department of Corrections has promulgated regulations that flatly forbid psychosurgery on prisoners—and, for that matter, all other organic therapies except shock therapy (which has a requirement of committee review in addition to the statutorily prescribed judicial review).[5] Yet the regulations seem to be wrongheaded. The Legislature could have chosen to prohibit psychosurgery if it so desired. It declined to do so and instead set up a judicial review procedure for approving decisions to undergo organic therapy. The Department's paternalistic per se prohibition is thus neither within the letter nor the spirit of the Penal Code Act.

The Edmund Kemper case illustrates the impact the Department's regulations may have. Kemper has committed some dozen brutal mutilation murders of hitchhikers and of close family members. Most of the murders were committed after Kemper had undergone every accepted form of therapy and had been released. He is now serving a life sentence. He has made persistent, educated, and poignant requests that he be permitted to undergo psychosurgery to ameliorate his uncontrollable rages, with the knowledge that in any

---

[5] 15 Cal. Admin. Code § 3343 *et seq.* (1977).

event parole, even in the distant future, is improbable. Kemper's attempts to bypass the regulations have been judicially rebuffed. This is but one unfortunate result of a paternalistic policy.

We should digress momentarily to note the parole factor in this equation. In an intriguing and provocative article, Richard Delgado (1977a) has argued that if, as a result of organic therapy, a prisoner's psyche is sufficiently reconstructed to constitute a "new person," continued confinement would be unconstitutional. (A request for release of a prisoner who has undergone brain surgery has in fact been made in England; the outcome is unknown.) Delgado's argument with respect to the deterrence and rehabilitation rationales of punishment and the criminal justice system may well be persuasive, but his analysis of the retribution function is not the only reasonable one. Delgado himself concedes that retribution is past-looking— that is, looks to the "old person." Moreover, atonement cannot be achieved by a technological fix, but only by a long, arduous, and painful process of conscious contrition—as any novena attendant in the dead of winter could testify to. Further, acceptance of Delgado's "new person" argument, even if factually supportable, is at odds with our democratic notions of free will, which are implicitly anchored to the belief that the citizen's character and behavior are not predictable events of bioelectrochemical processes. Thus, Kemper's request for psychosurgery should not be denied because of the fear that he will then have to be released.

Case Law

Two courts have analyzed in depth issues surrounding the regulation of psychosurgery. These two cases will be reviewed with an eye toward the constitutional issues they raise and their applicability to other organic therapies.

Aden v. Younger

Aden v. Younger[6] is the leading case on the issues concerning the regulation of psychosurgery and organic therapies generally. In Aden, a California appellate court reviewed the 1974 Civil Law Act on psychosurgery and shock therapy. The Act was struck down because of the invalidity of certain provisions without which the Act could not stand.

---

[6] 57 Cal. App. 3d 662 (1976).

Petitioners in *Aden* were patients and their attending physicians who requested a judicial declaration of the constitutionality of the 1974 Act, without reference to any particular factual situation. The 1974 Act had a peer review committee requirement similar to that of its successor Civil Law Act, for both psychosurgery and shock therapy. Proxy consent to psychosurgery was prohibited, though proxy consent to shock therapy was (and is now) permitted. In addition, the attending physician and the committee members were required to find that the mode of treatment was "critically needed for the welfare of the patient." These provisions, and others, were attacked on various grounds, including due process, equal protection, and right of privacy—all issues of constitutional stature.

The critical argument before the court was that due process was violated by the state's action limiting the patient's right to select and consent to medical procedures. The court did find a fundamental constitutional right to decide whether one should undergo psychosurgery. But the court did not base such a right upon a constitutional right of privacy broad enough to cover decision-making with respect to all medical procedures. Instead, the court found freedom of thought values implicit in the First Amendment protection of speech to be highly relevant in broadening the constitutional right of privacy to include privacy of the mind.

The *Aden* court explored the nexus between the First Amendment and the right of privacy as follows:

> The right to be free in the exercise of one's thoughts is essential to the exercise of other constitutionally guaranteed rights. First Amendment rights of free speech would mean little if the state were to control thought. . . . Here the state has sought to control neither what is thought by mental patients, nor how they think. Rather, the state is attempting to regulate the use of procedures which touch upon thought processes in significant ways, with neither the intention nor the effect of regulating thought processes, per se. Yet despite the lack of any showing the state has attempted to regulate freedom of thought, this legislation may diminish this right. If so, the legislation can only be sustained by showing (1) it is necessary to further a "compelling state interest" and (2) the least drastic means has been employed to further those interests. . . .

The court was perceptive in noting that the interest in protecting freedom of thought and privacy of the mind is not unidimensional, but is at stake where there is a denial of access to mental health therapy as well as where there is coercive use of such therapy:

> Freedom of thought is intimately touched upon by any regulation of procedures affecting thought and feelings. In an effort to protect freedom of thought, the state has put procedural and substantive obstacles in the path of those who both need and desire certain forms of treat-

ment, and in that way their freedom of thought remains impaired because they cannot get treatment. . . . Some patients will be denied treatment as a natural and intended result of this legislation.

Thus, because of the possible denial of access to mental health therapy, the court invoked the standard of judicial review of legislation known as the *standard of strict scrutiny* to determine whether the 1974 Act was constitutional under the federal Constitution. The choice of a standard of review is very important. It is far more difficult to show that legislation serves a compelling state interest and employs the least drastic means than to show that legislation merely has a "rational basis"—the usual standard of review when no fundamental constitutional rights are at stake. Moreover, under the standard of strict scrutiny the state has the burden of proof in justifying the legislation, whereas under the rational basis standard, doubts and uncertainties regarding the validity of the legislation are resolved in favor of the state.

Under the standard of strict scrutiny, the *Aden* court found the requirement of committee review to be the most difficult aspect of the 1974 Act to evaluate. (Compulsory notification of next of kin of a proposed psychosurgery patient was more readily struck down.) The state's interests in enacting the 1974 Act—identified generally as protection of the right to refuse treatment and the avoidance of "unnecessary administration of hazardous and intrusive treatments"—would have to be balanced against the First Amendment and privacy values infringed upon by a denial of therapy. The court's analysis separated out two issues: (1) committee review of consent and (2) committee review of the merits of a proposed therapy.

The *Aden* opionion had little problem in upholding the requirement of committee review of the capacity for informed consent to psychosurgery (and shock therapy) in light of the state's interest in protecting patients from unconsented-to and unnecessary treatment. The class of patients sought to be protected by the 1974 Act included those who had guardians or conservators, those who were involuntarily admitted to state and private mental institutions, and those who were voluntarily admitted to such institutions. Because there is reason to suspect incompetence on the part of such patients, the court reasoned that their privacy may be uniformly invaded to the extent of requiring third party review of the informed consent process.

The issue of substantive review of the merits of the therapy chosen by the attending physician and patient, however, could not be resolved on a uniform basis. The court found a need to distinguish between involuntarily and voluntarily admitted patients. (Those who were incompetent to consent to psychosurgery were excluded from the analysis because the Act prohibited proxy consent, and therefore committee review, in their behalf.)

The *Aden* court upheld the requirement of substantive committee review in regard to voluntary patients found competent to consent, on the grounds that the hazardous and experimental nature of psychosurgery is a sound reason for its regulation as a treatment of last resort. While the record before the court reflected a more pessimistic view of psychosurgical procedures than that found, say, in the report of the National Commission for the Protection of Human Subjects of Biomedical and Behavioral Research (National Commission, 1977), the court's analysis is instructive:

> There are sound reasons why the treating physician's assessment of his patient's competency and voluntariness may not always be objective, and he may not necessarily be the best or most objective judge of how appropriate an experimental procedure would be. Because the consequences to the patient of such a procedure are so serious, and the effects he may suffer are so intrusive and irreversible, tort damages are totally inadequate. The need for some form of restraint is a sufficiently compelling state interest to justify the attendant invasion of the patient's right to privacy.

Given the sound analysis of substantive committee review of psychosurgery in the voluntary patient context, the court could have easily disposed of the involuntary patient situation on the same grounds: the hazardous and experimental nature of psychosurgery. Unfortunately, however, a different approach was ostensibly borrowed from the *Kaimowitz*[7] case (discussed subsequently), which only served to muddle the opinion.

The *Aden* opinion viewed the involuntary patient situation as posing the dilemma of either withholding psychosurgery from such a patient, on the grounds that the duress of detainment made adequate confirmation of the voluntariness of an informed consent impossible, or providing a substitute decision maker for the patient. The court then upheld the substantive review requirement as a substitute decision-making process, justified by the compelling interest in preventing involuntary use of psychosurgery.

But there is no such dilemma. The distinguishing premise, that informed consent of an involuntary patient can never be adequately confirmed, simply cannot bear the weight of the argument. The voluntariness of a consent by a psychotic patient with manic-

---

[7] *Kaimowitz* v. *Department of Mental Health*, Civil No. 73-19434-AW (Cir. Ct., Wayne Co., Mich., July 10, 1973).

depression is a difficult to ascertain if the patient is involuntarily admitted at the behest of an impatient stepparent or if the patient decides to be voluntarily admitted via the compassionate and persistent entreaties of a trusted friend. Indeed, the *Aden* opinion itself mentions elsewhere that voluntary patients are susceptible to many of the pressures exerted upon involuntary patients, and that "the 'voluntary' label is a creation of the legislature, and often only means the patient did not formally protest hospitalization." And even if there are differences between voluntary and involuntary patients, as respective classes, they must be truly significant to justify placing different barriers to access to constitutionally protected interests.

The dilemma is unwittingly unraveled by the court's own conclusion that a substitute decision-making process is justified by the interest in preventing involuntary treatment, which is a *non sequitur*. In the first place, it is inaccurate to describe committee review as making the treatment decision. The committee review is not a true substantive decision-making process. Because of the statutory requirement of informed consent, the review process can only substitute a "no" decision for an "action-X" proposal. It may not propose action-X where a patient has not given informed consent.

Crucially, then, the court's errant approach to a perceived problem in diagnosis of voluntariness can be viewed as the introduction of a partial-proxy consent concept. That is, where capacity is attenuated but not negated, the composite consent of the patient and the review committee shall constitute a unitary informed consent. But, the locus of personal autonomy cannot easily be circumscribed so as to encompass a three-person peer review committee.

If the *Aden* court were truly impressed with the involuntariness argument of the *Kaimowitz* decision, it could have announced a rule uniformly prohibiting psychosurgery on involuntary patients, as did *Kaimowitz*. But in wisely rejecting that result it made a similar error of paternalism in referring to a substitute decision-making process. The *Aden* court would have done better to modify its paternalistic approach by stating that where capacity to consent is questionable, it is not unconstitutional for a review committee to err on the side of withholding psychosurgery. But a problem remains with even this modified approach. It fails to take into account that constitutional rights are at stake, and thus a particular involuntary patient's capacity to consent should be decided on an individual rather than on a class basis.

The fact that *Aden* upheld substantive committee review of psychosurgery does not mean that its constitutional analysis is without bite. The court's analysis of the shock therapy provisions of the 1974 Act illustrates this point. In the case of voluntary patients found competent to consent to shock therapy, the court held the requirement of substantive review to be unconstitutional as an impermissible invasion of the patient's right to privacy. The court reached its conclusion upon a careful review of shock therapy procedures, which it did not find to be experimental or as hazardous as psychosurgery. In relying upon a United States Supreme Court decision striking down a committee review requirement for obtaining abortions, the *Aden* court explained:

> Where informed consent is adequately insured, there is no justification for infringing upon the patient's right to privacy in selecting and consenting to the treatment. The state has varied interests which are served by the regulation of ECT, but these interests are not served where the patient and his physician are the best judges of the patient's health, safety and welfare.

In addition to its analysis of committee review, the *Aden* opinion is also noteworthy for its handling of two other issues that are bound to surface repeatedly in efforts at regulating mental health therapies. One is a requirement of demonstrating some sort of qualitatively special need for a particular therapy. The 1974 Act required a showing that psychosurgery or shock therapy was "critically needed for the welfare of the patient" before such therapies would be utilized. The requirement was held to violate due process because it was impermissibly "vague": that is, so vague that persons of common intelligence must necessarily guess at its meaning and differ as to its application.

The court's conclusion appears reasonable. How could the "critically needed" criterion answer such questions as whether certain treatments are indicated where: (1) there is a stable condition of severe psychosis, as opposed to a danger of deterioration, (2) there is complete psychological dysfunction, but no self-destructive tendencies, or (3) there is an inability to remain employed or married. The problem is exacerbated by the recognized lack of certainty in psychiatric diagnoses and prognoses. Moreover, it would appear difficult enough to compare various therapies in order to determine which is the "least onerous alternative," without requiring an evaluation in the abstract, so to speak, of a single therapy's need vis-à-vis critical need.

The *Aden* court's difficulty in infusing the "critically needed" criterion with meaning may indicate that where strict regulation of a therapy is desired, it would be advisable to have the regulation depend less upon noncomparative, qualitative assessments to be made by individual physicians, and more upon standards or assessments to be set forth by means of administrative regulations, review committees, and the like.

Another issue of import treated in the *Aden* opinion involves what is known as the "therapeutic privilege" to avoid application of the informed consent doctrine. The therapeutic privilege provides the physician, in a malpractice suit, with the defense that nondisclosure of risks was justified on the grounds that disclosure would have so seriously disturbed the patient that the patient would not have been able to dispassionately weigh the risks of refusing to undergo the recommended treatment. The patient's waiver of the disclosure requirement is implied and constitutes a defense to malpractice, just as an express request to be left uninformed would be a defense. The petitioners in *Aden* challenged the statutory requirement of compulsory disclosure of risks on the ground that it conflicted with the common law therapeutic privilege. But the court correctly stated that the statutory requirement may be superimposed upon the common law matrix of rights and duties because the Act is designed to protect the patient's rights and is not in derogation of them.

While statutes regulating therapies may require full explication of material risks as a means of bypassing the therapeutic privilege exception to the informed consent doctrine, the better approach would be to have the courts reexamine the therapeutic privilege exception itself. The exception appears to be at odds with the underlying theory of the informed consent doctrine. If the patient is unable to act upon all of the pertinent information on a proposed therapy because disclosure of some information would cause an emotional disturbance, then it is problematic whether the patient can give an informed consent. The therapeutic privilege should not be used as a means of creating informed consent. Moreover, it is difficult to put practical bounds on the scope of the therapeutic privilege: how does one decide what is unnecessarily disturbing?

Kaimowitz v. Department of Mental Health

Kaimowitz v. *Department of Mental Health*, alluded to above, was a well-publicized case involving the proposed use of psychosurgery upon a patient charged with murder and rape/necrophilia and committed pursuant to a criminal sexual psychopath statute. The patient obtained release by means of a writ of habeas corpus, successfully arguing that the criminal sexual psychopath law was unconstitutional. The writ was granted by a three-judge Michigan state trial court, which was specially convened because of the controversial nature of the case. The court also went on to rule on the proposed psychosurgery, to which the patient had withdrawn his consent, on the debatable grounds that the psychosurgery issue would likely recur and thus was not mooted by the patient's release and withdrawal of consent.

Kaimowitz served as a landmark case for at least two reasons: (1) it was viewed as holding that involuntarily detained patients could never give truly informed consent to a psychosurgical procedure, and (2) it was the first court to consider in depth constitutional First Amendment and privacy issues of mental health therapy or behavior control. (As a trial court opinion, it is not binding legal precedent for any other court.)

Because the *Kaimowitz* court reached some controversial conclusions and developed the constitutional arguments in questionable ways, it is tempting to wish that various counsel before it had not argued that the case was ripe for judgment rather than moot. The court, however, did push the psychosurgery debate forward by introducing key pertinent legal concepts. On the other hand, the *Kaimowitz* opinion is not likely to be a persuasive precedent in many courts because it was not published in an official or substitute case report system. Court rules usually require that an opinion be published before it may be cited and relied upon.

The patient in *Kaimowitz*, and his parents, had signed consent forms for participation in a study comparing the effects of amygdalotomy with a certain chemotherapy (cyproterone acetate) on uncontrollable aggression. The court was concerned about both the effect of institutionalization upon the patient's ability to give informed consent and the allegations that the proposed amygdalotomy entailed hazardous and unknown effects. Underlying the court's unease was the recognition that there is no medically recognized syndrome for aggression and undesirable behavior associated with nonorganic brain abnormality.

The court analyzed the doctrine of informed consent as containing three criteria: competency, voluntariness, and knowledge. Competency to consent was found diminished by the fact of involuntary commitment and the effects of institutionalization. The court also found the voluntariness requirement wanting in light of the inherently coercive environment of a total institution. Moreover, the consent was ruled to be unknowledgeable because the proposed procedure was deemed to lack a sound scientific basis for predicting risks and benefits. The parents' consent was also considered to be inadequate, although the reasoning for such a conclusion is far from clear. The nub of the argument is that a parent or guardian "cannot do that which the patient, absent a guardian, would be legally unable to do." The argument is circular in nature, and would lead to the invalidation of proxy consent to any therapy.

Indeed, on a closer examination, the *Kaimowitz* court's analysis of the patient's consent is similarly confusing, if not confused. The court's analysis appeared to conclude that the patient's consent was defective on each of the three independent and sufficient grounds for invalidation: incompetency, involuntariness, and lack of knowledge. Some have seized upon this ostensible analysis to conclude that *Kaimowitz* precludes any person's valid consent to psychosurgery on the grounds that the experimental nature of psychosurgery would make knowledgeable consent thereto impossible. But it must be noted that the record before the court was based on evidence adduced in 1973 and was focused upon a particular psychosurgical procedure—amygdalotomy for treatment of uncontrollable aggression—and upon a specific context—the involuntarily detained patient. Thus, the court stated that its holding did not prevent involuntarily confined patients from consenting to all neurological procedures; and, if amygdalotomy were to become an accepted, nonexperimental procedure, the court indicated that the involuntarily detained patient might be able to consent to it. This reasoning indicates that the court's tripartite analysis of informed consent must be viewed as three interrelated and mutually dependent conclusions on the criteria of competence, voluntariness, and knowledge.

It is apparent that under the *Kaimowitz* analysis, a court would strike down substantial portions of the Oregon and California legislative models—for example, those provisions permitting proxy consent and psychosurgery on prisoners and involuntary patients. But the *Kaimowitz* court's ostensible flat ban on psychosurgery upon those involuntarily confined has been criticized severely and has not been followed by other courts (to wit, *Aden*). Moreover, while the decision has been used by some advocates to suggest a broader prohibition that would include not only all psychosurgical procedures but other organic therapies as well, it could easily be distinguished on the basis of the narrowly focused procedure and facts before it.

The *Kaimowitz* analysis of the constitutional issues at stake, while on the right track, also suffered from a failure to carefully develop and explain the logical sequence of the arguments. As an alternative means to the tripartite analysis of informed consent for invalidating the patient's consent, the court stated that the constitutional protections afforded by First Amendment freedom of expression and the right of privacy prevented the state from accepting the patient's consent to the proposed amygdalotomy. It appears that the court was concluding either: (1) that an involuntarily confined patient's constitutional right to freedom of expression—and, by implication, mentation—and privacy prevented the patient, regardless of capacity for informed consent, from giving a valid consent; or (2) that the constitutional protections require an irrebuttable presumption that all such patients be deemed incompetent to consent.

Both conclusions, however, are wrongheaded, principally for the reason that they ignore the fact that such constitutional protections are based upon an interest in individual autonomy. If a person decided to permit an intrusion into his or her privacy, or to undergo a mental health therapy that affects mentation, then such an exercise of individual autonomy should be honored. At least that is the case where a person is otherwise competent to consent. The defect in the *Kaimowitz* analysis is that it used the constitutional arguments to leap to an across-the-board conclusion of incompetence, thereby disrespecting the potential for exercising individual autonomy. (Mason, 1974; Shapiro, 1975)

But surely the Constitution can no more completely preclude competent consent to psychosurgery than it can forbid consent to psychotherapy, or consent to alter one's mentation by reading in the privacy of one's home. Indeed, application of the *Kaimowitz* analysis to the question of access to other mentation-altering materials —for example, books—would result in a conclusion that state censorship was justified because it protected the citizen's First Amendment rights! Thus, while the *Kaimowitz* court might have been the first to address the legal issues of psychosurgery, it is unlikely to be a persuasive opinion because of its highly paternalistic bent.

The First Amendment Theory

The *Aden* and *Kaimowitz* courts relied heavily on the First Amendment theory of protection of mentation. They are not the only courts to discern a constitutional freedom of expression issue in the context of mental health therapies. The United States Court of Appeals for the Ninth Circuit has indicated that the use of succinylcholine upon a prisoner without his consent, as part of an aversive conditioning program, raises "serious constitutional questions respecting . . . impermissible tinkering with the mental processes"[8]

---

[8] *Mackey v. Procunier*, 447 F.2d 877 (9th Cir. 1973).

(Leinwand, 1976). The court cited First Amendment and privacy cases in support of its position. The United States Court of Appeals for the Third Circuit has seized upon this statement, and the *Kaimowitz* opinion, in holding that involuntary administration of drugs such as Thorazine and Mellaril upon an involuntarily detained patient may constitute an infringement of First Amendment rights.[9] Recently, a federal district court has enjoined, absent patient consent, guardian consent, or well-defined emergency conditions, medication of inpatients at the May and Austin units of Boston State Hospital, based on the First Amendment and privacy arguments.[10] (The First Amendment is also being relied upon in a suit brought by an inmate of a Veterans Administration hospital over a bilateral prefrontal lobotomy allegedly performed without his consent a number of years ago.)[11]

The invocation of constitutional doctrines in cases in which psychosurgery and other mental health therapies are performed in the context of state action warrants careful analysis. The emergence of a powerful, fundamental constitutional right analysis regarding rights of access to such therapies and rights against their involuntary administration is especially important because of its potential for materially restructuring rights and obligations in the psychiatric ward. A legal analysis of a psychosurgery regulation is therefore necessarily contingent upon a constitutional analysis focusing on First Amendment and privacy considerations (Spece, 1972). It can safely be said that any legal analysis of psychosurgery and organic therapies that does not take the constitutional arguments into account (for example, Annas, 1977) is seriously deficient. Because of the amorphous nature of the right of privacy, and its common application to matters affecting the family and procreation, the First Amendment argument is of primary importance.

The First Amendment argument is at once both novel and creative and yet so commonsensical that one wonders why it had not surfaced previously. Perhaps the advent of intrusive organic therapies, which have the capacity for significantly altering mental processes, has inevitably led to the elucidation of such an argument. The argument that the First Amendment protects, as a fundamental right, a person's ability to generate ideas, thoughts, moods, emotions, and mental activity generally—that is, freedom of mentation—has been

---

[9] *Scott* v. *Plante,* 532 F.2d 939 (3rd Cir. 1976); see *Rennie* v. *Klein,* 462 F. Supp. 1131 (D. N.J. 1978); see also *State* v. *Maryott,* 6 Wash. App. 96, 492 P.2d 239 (1971).

[10] *Rogers* v. *Okin,* Civil No. 75-1610-T (D. Mass., Oct. 29, 1979).

[11] *Cofer* v. *U.S.,* Civil No. C75-169T (W.D. Wash.) (filed 1975).

formulated by Shapiro (1974, pp. 256–257) in the context of organic therapy essentially as follows:

1. The First Amendment protects communication of virtually all kinds, whether written, verbal, pictorial or in symbolic form and whether cognitive or emotive in nature;

2. Communication entails the transmission and reception of whatever is communicated;

3. Transmission and reception necessarily involve mentation on the part of both the person transmitting and the person receiving;

4. It is in fact impossible to distinguish in advance mentation which will be involved in or necessary to transmission and reception from mentation which will not;

5. If communication is to be protected, *all* mentation (regardless of its potential involvement in transmission or reception) must therefore be protected;

6. Coerced use and regulation of therapies (and other agents and procedures) which alter or interfere with mentation raises a First Amendment issue; and

7. Coerced use of, or denial of access to, such therapies which "intrusively" alter or interfere with mentation is a "direct" abridgment of a First Amendment right and must be justified by the government under the standard of strict scrutiny; that is, the government must show a compelling state interest in such coercion or denial which cannot be implemented in a less drastic/onerous/intrusive manner.

The difficulty of some commentators in accepting Shapiro's argument lies principally with Steps 3 and 7.

The Connection Between Mentation and Communication

It is important to point out that the connection between mentation and communication in Step 3 of the First Amendment argument is not merely an empirical connection such as that between printing presses or auditory canals and communication. Mentation is not simply a means of or aid to communication; mentation is a *logically prior antecedent* of any communication. Thus, the connection is different from an empirical deduction such as "reading requires eating, since one must eat to live, and live to read"; one can posit thinking without positing eating.

Given this background, Step 5 of the First Amendment argument then becomes more readily acceptable. One may argue that if communication is to be protected, all mentation must therefore be protected, because it is impossible as a practical matter, given the current state of behavioral science, to determine which induced mentational changes will have an impact upon expression and which will not. In the First Amendment area of protected freedoms, overinclusiveness should be preferred to underinclusiveness.

Samuel Shuman, in an otherwise sensitive discussion of the issues surrounding the use of psychosurgery, criticizes the First Amendment argument's premise regarding the mentation–communication connection (Shuman, 1977). He contends that Step 3 is not a statement regarding a necessary antecedent, but rather a conclusion based on "definitional fiat." The contention is based on his argument that there is "no axiom or linguistic inference rule [which] posits that mentation is a necessary antecedent of communication" (p. 119); the connection between mentation and communication is an empirical one. Shuman's argument is ingenuous, at best. Whether or not the connection between mentation and communication can be derived from linguistic rules, the fact is that people do regard the connection as a necessary one. If Shuman were correct, it should be possible to hypothesize a system of human "communication"—as we commonly refer to that term—without mentation. Such a hypothesization is awaited.

Shuman's confusion is illustrated by his counter-argument that many things are logically prior antecedents to communication—one example being a language system—and that, despite this relationship, "no legal consequences follow either possibly or necessarily" (Shuman, 1977, p. 120). If Shuman is maintaining that there would be no First Amendment issues if the government were to prohibit all communication in Indo-European languages, then I suppose he can just as easily say that coerced interference with mentation does not possibly or necessarily raise a First Amendment issue.

The Role, and Criteria, of Intrusiveness

It is perhaps because of the potentially broad scope of the First Amendment argument (Step 6) that some commentators have been unable to accept it (Edgar, 1975). Obviously, a legal doctrine that construed any mentation-altering activity—for example, public school education—as unconstitutional mind control would be frivolous. But the critical issue to be considered here is whether a significant First Amendment issue is raised in the case of mental health therapy, which would invoke the standard of strict scrutiny—that is, whether the governmental regulation of mentation-altering therapy can be considered as "directly abridging the freedom of mentation" (Step 7). Here, "directly" is used in the legal sense. There is clearly a direct abridgement if an "intrusive" therapy is administered upon a person without that person's informed consent, or if the state denies access to such a therapy. (This is true regardless of whether a therapy alters mentation directly or indirectly, in the empirical sense—for example, chemotherapy vis-à-vis conditioning.) While there can be little dispute that psychosurgery is an intrusive therapy, the role, and criteria, of intrusiveness have engendered considerable confusion for some commentators (Shuman, 1977).

Several points regarding the concept of intrusiveness should be made. First, there are two roles for the concept of intrusiveness. One role is to serve as an *empirical* litmus test for determining whether a governmental regulation raises a significant First Amendment claim. For example, involuntary administration of psychosurgery directly abridges a First Amendment right; governmental pamphleting does not. Another role is to determine, once there is found a direct abridgment of a right and the government has demonstrated a compelling state interest in support thereof, whether there are less "intrusive" (that is, less drastic or onerous) alternative means of regulation that would implement the compelling state interest. This is the legal sense of intrusiveness, which may incorporate, at times, the empirical sense; for example, it may well be a less intrusive (legal) alternative to have proxy consent to chemotherapy rather than to psychosurgery, which generally is more intrusive (empirical).

For purposes of understanding the First Amendment argument, it is the empirical sense of the concept of intrusiveness that is relevant. It should be clear, then, that describing a therapy as intrusive in this empirical sense does not necessarily denote that the government has "intruded" upon one's liberty. Liberty and autonomy are infringed when one's competent consent is overridden by imposing, or denying access to, mentation-affecting therapies. But not all such infringements invoke the standard of strict scrutiny of governmental action. It is the role of intrusiveness to provide an empirical touchstone for determining when strict scrutiny is required. Shuman's inability to recognize this role of intrusiveness vitiates the merits of his critique of the First Amendment argument.

Perhaps distinguishing between the two senses of autonomy at stake will serve to place the primary role of intrusiveness in perspective. Personal autonomy has both an internal and an external facet. Governmental coercion or denial infringes autonomy from an external point of view; let us call this "autonomy$_1$." A therapy such as psychosurgery effects a massive change in one's mentation and thus alters one's internal autonomy or native capacities: "autonomy$_2$" (Shapiro, 1975). It is this latter facet of autonomy, autonomy$_2$, with which the primary role of intrusiveness is concerned.

It should be pointed out that an intrusive alteration of mentation can constitute either an improvement or deterioration in one's health and behavior. Indeed, successful psychosurgery would be a clear case of an intrusive, as well as effective, alteration of mentation. (The distinction between effectiveness and intrusiveness of therapies is discussed by Shapiro in this book.) For legal purposes, the negative connotation of intrusiveness is brought into play by governmental imposition or denial. In sum, for a significant First Amendment issue to arise, both external autonomy$_1$ and internal autonomy$_2$ must be at stake; for example, the government must infringe autonomy$_1$ by imposing psychosurgery—which intrusively alters autonomy$_2$—upon someone who lacks the capacity to consent.

What, then, are the criteria of intrusiveness by which we can determine what other therapies are intrusive? Shapiro (1974, p. 262) sets out a quorum of interdependent criteria:

1. The extent to which the effects of the therapy upon mentation are reversible.

2. The extent to which the resulting psychic state is "foreign," "abnormal" or "unnatural" for the person in question, rather than simply a restoration of his or her prior psychic state (this is closely related to the "magnitude" or "intensity" of the change).

3. The rapidity with which the effects occur.

4. The scope of the change in the total "ecology" of the mind's functions.

5. The extent to which one can resist *acting* in ways impelled by the psychic effects of the therapy.

6. The duration of the change.

As is evident by the above criteria, the intrusiveness of a particular therapy is an empirical question. Thus, the First Amendment argument is fully attentive to individual conditions and responsive to refinements of particular therapies.

Reevaluation of Legislative Models and Committee Review

Given the willingness of courts to embrace the First Amendment argument for protection of mentation, several features of the legislative models described here should bear careful examination as psychosurgery, as well as the First Amendment argument, is continually refined. In particular, policy makers should be keenly aware of the role of committee review, whether in regulating psychosurgery or other therapies. When well-defined psychosurgical procedures become validated and on a par with, say, shock therapy, with respect to risks, several legislative provisions will have to be reexamined—for example, the mandatory substantive committee review of the Oregon Act and the California Civil Law Act. The California Department of Corrections' flat ban on psychosurgery on prisoners is even less likely to survive.

The prohibition in California of proxy consent to psychosurgery should also be rethought as procedures become validated. It may be difficult, however, to argue that such a prohibition is unconstitutional, because there is less of an infringement of autonomy when an incompetent's desire for therapy is not honored. On the other hand, it seems wise, as a policy matter, not to deny those otherwise destined to institutionalization with physical and pharmacological restraints some possible relief from suffering. If there is a strong concern about undue manipulation in the proxy consent area, even with committee review mechanisms, giving the incompetent patient the power to "dissent" or "assent" to therapy may be a useful compromise; this is the approach taken by the National Commission (National Commission, 1977).

Policy issues will no doubt revolve primarily around the uses and abuses of committee review. It is quite likely that difficult issues concerning the use of risky or experimental therapies will increasingly be dealt with by the utilization of committee review. Several extant examples of committee review should be reviewed to identify the proper uses and formats of committee review, and, as a corollary, to distinguish between consent review and substantive review.

One example is the California Civil Law Act requirement that a competent patient's consent to shock therapy in a private physician's office, a clinic, or at home, must be reviewed by a board-certified or eligible psychiatrist or neurologist other than the patient's attending physician (that is, a committee of one). Upon personal examination of the patient, the reviewer must concur that the patient has manifested competent consent. Presumably, it is open for the attending physician merely to obtain the gratis consultation of a partner, although such a route is arguably outside the spirit of the requirement. Whether most physicians who administer shock therapy have a readily accessible partner is questionable. (The petitioners in *Aden* sought, unsuccessfully, to raise the factual issue of whether there are a sufficient number of psychiatrists available for review committees.)

This consent review should be recognized, as it was by the *Aden* court, as posing the genuine risk of preventing a suitable patient from obtaining needed therapy. This risk is independent of the risk that the second physician may simply err in concluding there is no informed consent. To the patient, the time and emotional expense of obtaining another consultation may seem to be too much trouble, particularly when the patient must bear the financial cost of the second set of consultations. The patient's choice of a physician is entitled to respect, and the requirement of a personal examination by another physician is an invasion, in a very real sense, of the patient's privacy and his or her confidential relationship with the physician of choice.

The role of an attorney in consent review is another troubling issue. The California Civil Law Act permits a patient's attorney, after committee review and approval, to initiate court review of a patient/physician decision to use shock therapy if the attorney suspects the patient to be incompetent. What additional expertise the attorney brings to bear on the competency issue is unclear. Nevertheless, the Legislature, in recognition of the economic incentive for an attorney to err on the side of suggesting incompetency, has indicated that a second attorney would be more appropriate as counsel in the court proceeding. The patient may thus have to foot two legal bills.

There will be increasing pressure to make committee review mandatory for various mental health therapies with strong behavior modification potential, even if they are "accepted" medical treatment (Annas, 1977). Perhaps use of a new genre of major tranquilizers may move committee review out of the psychosurgery/shock therapy area. The rationales for compulsory use of such review committees should be carefully set out. It may well be that the use of institutional review boards (IRBs) to review experimentation protocols can be grounded primarily upon the need to balance the public's interest in obtaining knowledge against the risk to the patient, and the need to ensure that an appropriate cross section of people is subject to the protocol. Those considerations may not be appropriate for requiring review of a validated therapy in, say, a private setting. In the latter situation, there is a severely attenuated need to determine whether there is an appropriate cross section of patients. Moreover, there is less need to balance public versus private interests because it is less likely that the treatment is intended to lead to generalizable knowledge, and whatever risks there are to the patient are probably outweighed by the therapeutic benefits to be obtained. Thus, other considerations may be of primary importance for justifying review of mental health therapy; for example, the factors identified by the *Aden* court, of suspicion of incompetency to consent and of potential hazard.

That the concept of multidisciplinary committee review needs to be defined is evidenced by the makeup of the short-lived multidisciplinary committee to review consent to surgery for temporal lobe epilepsy at Boston City Hospital. There were eleven people on the committee, only two of whom were physicians. They included one physician, one psychiatrist, two lawyers, a political scientist, a minister, a sociologist, a research biogeneticist, a medical student, and "two representatives from the local community" (Annas, Glantz, and Katz, 1977). Apparently, no politicians or cultists were available.

Annas urged the use of such layperson committees after reviewing the Boston City Hospital committee's work in the two cases it handled. In one case, the consent of a minor and her parents to surgery was approved after the eleven-person committee had met with the patient and parents three times over a two-week period, with the final session being videotaped. In the second case, the patient was not so resilient and strong-willed. The committee met with a patient and his family "a number of times" over some eight months before determining that it was really the adult patient's parents who wanted the operation—a determination allegedly "confirmed" by the patient. When the patient returned six months later demanding that he be relieved from his seizures and suffering, the eleven committee members again engaged in "extended discussions" with the patient and his family, and again decided that surgery could not be done because their gut reaction was that "the patient did not want surgery" (Annas, Glantz, and Katz, 1977). Annas' only hedge on the use of such consent committees is that they may have to be strengthened in order to fully "protect" patients' rights. Such a scenario is pathetic. With the exception of the psychiatrist, none of the committee members was particularly qualified to adjudge capacity for informed consent. If what is truly desired is a grueling test of the patient's resolve, more efficient devices could certainly be concocted.

Annas' criticism of the National Commission's concern with the patient's privacy and confidentiality in the context of committee review is also without support (see Annas, 1977; Annas, Glantz, and Katz, 1977). The National Commission recommended that personal interviewing of a psychosurgery patient by a multidisciplinary IRB be optional for the patient, having implicitly noted in its Report the California Civil Law Act procedure of consent review by specialist physicians, which is covered by the patient–physician privilege to refuse to testify. Annas argues that, under the California Act, the communications expressed in the personal examination by three psychiatrists and neurosurgeons do not come within the patient–physician testimonial privilege. The argument is unsupportable, as explained above. At any rate, the dispute over testimonial privilege is already marked by a number of exceptions and does not guarantee as much confidentiality as it connotes. While Annas is correct in suggesting that the legislature could require that confidentiality be maintained by nonphysicians, there is obviously a great distinction between a physician maintaining a confidence pursuant to a long professional tradition, and the state requiring a patient to confess his or her innermost thoughts to "community representatives." If nonmedical review is deemed necessary, a court hearing (National Commission, 1977), closed to all but patient, examining physicians, and counsel, would be quite preferable to such multidisciplinary committee review.

Even though Annas' legal arguments lack merit, his concern with the potential for undue social control through the guise of therapy should not be passed over lightly. Despite the extreme view in some quarters that mental illness is a convenient myth for legitimizing the control of aberrant behavior, the trend is to find biological causes, and thus biological "fixes," for such behavior. Nor is the concern with medical expansionism relevant only in the context of coerced treatment. As Willard Gaylin points out, "the universal terror of illness, operating under the imprimatur of the medical establishment, will then make coercion in the traditional sense unnecessary" (Gaylin, 1975).

But the strident protests by critics of psychosurgery are not nearly discriminating enough. Psychosurgery is not the only therapy that may be founded in part on value-laden conclusions about behavior (Neville, 1975). "Behavioral and emotional disorders always constitute an inextricable mixture of biological and psychosocial factors so that the notion of a purely biological approach to the treatment of mental illness is illusory" (Vaughan, 1975). Criticism of psycho-surgery for its focus on behavior rather than on biological causes fails to appreciate that most somatic treatment in psychiatry is based upon a trial-and-error modification of behavior (for example, depression) rather than upon any etiology or pathophysiology (Vaughan, 1975). Indeed, if social engineering is what is feared by the anti-psychosurgery critics, they might be advised to explore the be-havior control issues raised by institutional sponsorship of neonatal conditioning and preschool education, or for that matter, television programming and advertising. As well as being capable of im-plementation on a mass scale, such powerful sensory inputs, parti-cularly if introduced at a youthful age, can carry the fixity of organic change (Gaylin, 1975).

Does this relativism leave us analytically impotent to distinguish between implanting an electrode and implanting an idea? I submit it does not. Faithful adherence to the criteria of intrusiveness as set forth above, and as amplified upon in the future, should enable us to distinguish, say, psychosurgery from adult education, pursuant to a unified legal theory. Obviously, a "conditioning" program that is reversible (at least, in its early stage), directed at a narrow range of behavior, requiring a great deal of ongoing, conscious cooperation to succeed, and intended to reinstate the subject's previous normal behavior, is not, by itself, as grave a threat to liberty as coerced psychosurgery.

Extensions of the First Amendment Argument

The First Amendment argument, and perhaps also the privacy argument, developed in regard to psychosurgery has implica-tions in other areas as well. Regulations of various psychoactive agents—for example, marijuana—are intended to control the ways in which the mind processes sensory inputs and to preempt the choices that together comprise a person's psyche (Tribe, 1978), and thus are subject to the First Amendment analysis.

The marijuana laws present the other side of the tension in dis-tinguishing therapy from social control. Obviously, consent capac-ity of adult marijuana users cannot be disputed, and a candid defense of the law on the grounds of control of behavior or life style is unlikely. Thus, in the marijuana cases the state has usually de-fended its statute on grounds that marijuana is harmful to health —that is, "bad" therapy. With the exception of at least one state court,[12] the state has won, needing only to show a "rational basis" for the legislation.

It will not be surprising if marijuana laws are challenged under the *Aden* court and Shapiro First Amendment analyses. What standard of review is applicable will be an important factor. It can be argued that people are denied access to a mentation-affecting agent; the fact that emotive-oriented mentation is predominantly influenced by marijuana appears consistent with established case law that protects both cognitive and emotive functions of communication. On the other hand, whether there are alternative means of attaining the mental states induced by marijuana is also relevant. The availability to the state of recent studies indicating the harmful effects of marijuana may well serve to uphold the laws.

Conclusion

The need to regulate innovative surgery as well as innovative drugs is recognized. Inflexible legislative rules and paternalistic denials of access are undesirable and at times unconstitutional. Regulation of mental health therapies generally will remain uncertain as developing constitutional concepts and theories of proxy consent remain in flux.

Proper functions of committee review should be identified. The patient's privacy should not be invaded by a consent review committee composed of nonprofessional advocates. Involvement of family members or friends chosen at the discretion of the patient is less burdensome; cooling-off periods might also be utilized.

Where there is proxy consent to intrusive therapies, process values militate for third party substantive review, whether by committee or court. If review is by committee, some nonexpert involvement may be appropriate (for example, IRBs where therapy is part of a research program).

Acceptance of the First Amendment argument may stimulate reexamination of regulations of low-risk psychoactive agents in private, nontherapeutic contexts.

---

[12] *Ravin* v. *State*, 537 P.2d 494 (Alas. 1975); see also *People* v. *Sinclair*, 387 Mich. 91, 194 N.W.2d 878 (1972) (Kavanagh, J., concurring); *State* v. *Kantner*, 53 Haw. 327, 493 P.2d 306, *cert. denied*, 409 U.S. 218 (1972) (dissenting and concurring opinions).

CHAPTER 19

Malpractice Liability for Psychosurgery

Stephen J. Morse

Previous chapters in this book have offered a theoretical scheme for analyzing legal regulation of psychosurgery (see Shapiro's chapter) and an overview of current legal regulation (see Pizzulli's chapter). (See also Annas and Glantz, 1974; Edgar, 1975; Shuman, 1977.) This chapter will attempt the narrower task of identifying and analyzing malpractice issues that are peculiar to psychosurgery. There is little specific material to work with, however, because no appellate case involving modern psychosurgical techniques has been discovered. General malpractice law will therefore be relied on to develop issues germane to psychosurgery, but no overview of malpractice will be presented.

I shall first present a brief statement of malpractice law. Next, I shall review the practice of psychosurgery and its psychiatric and psychological rationale and then shall analyze the standard of care that should be applicable to psychiatrists and neurosurgeons who engage in psychosurgery. Then a comparative analysis of the liability of psychiatrists and neurosurgeons will be presented. Following that, I shall examine the relevance to malpractice liability of violations of statutes, regulations, and institutional and professional guidelines. Next, experimentation and damage issues will be touched upon briefly, and finally the adequacy of tort law as a tool to regulate psychosurgery will be examined.

I shall argue throughout that psychosurgery is an extraordinary treatment and that a high standard of care should be imposed on its practitioners. Very little is known about why it is efficacious, and the extant efficacy data are rather scanty and of low scientific quality. Further, psychosurgery irreversibly destroys healthy brain tissue, with little knowledge of the possible long-term effects of doing so. There is simply not very much scientific or clinical consensus among psychiatrists, psychologists, and neurosurgerons about the indications, contraindications, and efficacy of psychosurgery. Indeed, some believe that it is never indicated.

For purposes of this discussion, however, I shall treat psychosurgery as a minimally acceptable, proven treatment. If psychosurgery is not an accepted treatment, then performing it is malpractice and the discussion need not go further. Others in this volume have already debated the validity of psychosurgery, and I shall not add another chapter to that debate. Here I shall simply accept, only for the purpose of discussion, that although psychosurgery is an extraordinary procedure, there is enough evidence of its beneficial effects to consider psychosurgery a nonexperimental, appropriate treatment for some psychiatric conditions. This does not mean that it is not necessary to learn much more about it. It does mean, however, that psychosurgery may sometimes be indicated and that the risks and benefits of the treatment can be explained to a patient with reasonable medical precision and certainty.

Medical Malpractice[1]

Recovery for medical malpractice aims to compensate an injured patient for physical and emotional injury resulting from the physician's failure to treat the patient with reasonable skill or to obtain the patient's informed consent to the treatment. A failure in either

---

[1] There is no one law of malpractice because each state develops its own law. Throughout this paper, therefore, most statements about malpractice will necessarily be generalizations based on current, dominant trends in the United States. Interested readers can refer to the following standard works on which I have heavily relied for general statements about malpractice: Dawidoff, 1973; Holder, 1978; King, 1977; Louisell and Williams, 1970/1977; Waltz and Inbau, 1971; see also, Annas and Glantz, 1974, pp. 251–258.

case is said to violate the physician's duty to apply the required *standard of care,* and the physician will be liable for damages proximately caused by the failure. In traditional legal language, malpractice actions are tort claims based on negligence. A minority of jurisdictions still treat an operation performed without proper consent as a battery, but the majority view is to treat the failure to obtain informed consent as a malpractice action based on negligence (King, 1977; Waltz and Inbau, 1971).

The Practice of Psychosurgery

The problems treated by psychosurgery are psychiatric or psychological in nature (Laitinen, 1977). Psychosurgery patients usually begin treatment with psychiatrists, and when a psychiatric proponent of psychosurgery believes that other techniques are unlikely ever to prove effective with certain patients, he or she will refer the patient to one of the relatively small number of neurosurgeons who perform psychosurgery. Of course, neurosurgeons are not psychiatrists, but those who perform psychosurgery certainly have some familiarity with psychiatry. In any case, it should be recognized that the primary indications for psychosurgery and the primary alternative treatments are psychiatric or psychological.

It should also be recognized that psychiatry and related disciplines are comparatively undeveloped. Professionals daily face clinical phenomena about which little is known and about which little can be done except in the most rudimentary sense. At all stages of the clinical mental health process—diagnosis, prognosis, and treatment —there is insufficient adequate theory or scientific data and few objective criteria to guide decision making. Thus, psychosurgery is a treatment that is part of a quite rudimentary science.

Psychosurgery has been employed vastly less often than other psychiatric treatments that are considered standard.[2] This has been especially true in the last decade or two. Moreover, there has been less scientific study of the efficacy of psychosurgery, and the efficacy studies performed to date have largely been of very poor scientific quality. Despite the lack of experience and high-quality data,

---

[2] Throughout this paper, unless otherwise noted, all statements about psychosurgery will be based on two reviews of the literature: Valenstein's excellent, comprehensive 1977 review, and the 1977 paper by Bridges and Bartlett. I should say, however, that the conclusions reached by both these papers concerning the efficacy of psychosurgery seem to me to be overly optimistic in light of the scientific quality of the studies relied on.

however, there is some weak evidence that psychosurgery may change certain behaviors. Nevertheless, some responsible commentators believe that there is no adequate scientific evidence for the efficacy of psychosurgery. As noted, however, this paper will accept for the purpose of discussion the proposition that in some cases psychosurgery may be more efficacious and less dangerous than other treatments for changing some abnormal behavior.

Psychosurgery seems most useful for ameliorating persistent, severe abnormalities of mood and emotion, such as depression, anxiety, phobias, obsessions, and compulsions. (It is also evidently useful for decreasing persistent pain, but psychosurgery for pain is not for a primarily psychiatric condition.) There is vast disagreement, however, concerning whether psychosurgery is useful for other disordered behaviors, such as schizophrenic behavior, sexual misconduct, assaultiveness, and others.

It is also generally believed that for the following reasons psychosurgery should be a treatment of "last resort": it causes irreversible brain damage; surgery is always risky to some degree; efficacy data are limited; and the possible side effects, such as convulsions, intellectual deficits, emotional flattening, or impulsivity, may be serious (although newer, precise procedures produce serious side effects far less often than older, cruder procedures). Further, the brain is an infinitely complex organ, and psychosurgery may cause less measurable or long-term effects that are not yet known. Thus, psychosurgery is considered appropriate mainly for patients whose chronic disorders have proved refractory to other treatments. The desire to consider psychosurgery a last resort for intractable conditions is understandable, but doing so may pose a paradox because some claim that intractable conditions with poor prognoses are least likely to be ameliorated by psychosurgery (see Rachman's chapter in this volume).

Although much theoretical speculation has attempted to account for the seeming efficacy of psychosurgery, its therapeutic mechanism is unknown. There is even some reason to believe that destruction of brain tissue may not be the primary therapeutic agent. The lack of understanding of the therapeutic mechanism is not terribly surprising, however, given the difficulty of establishing precise correlations between the functions of various areas of the brain and most social and intellectual behavior. Indeed, most psychosurgeons tend to employ the same techniques for all patients, and all techniques seem to work about equally well on similar patients. Thus, for unknown reasons a number of different procedures for destroying brain tissue seem to have equally efficacious effects in changing different behaviors.

The Standard of Skill

The standard of skill required of physicians, under the general standard of care, is usually either *customary practice* (often restricted to the locale in which the physician practices) or the often higher and preferred standard of *reasonable competence*. In the case of a specialist, the standard of skill is determined by reference to other specialists in the same field. In all jurisdictions, the legal standard of medical skill required is considered to be primarily a matter of expert knowledge, proof of which requires expert opinion. Sometimes a judge or jury can decide if this aspect of the standard of care has been violated without hearing expert evidence, but such cases are rare.

Defining an appropriate standard of skill for psychosurgery is a substantial problem because so little is performed and so little is known about it. It seems proper, therefore, that the reference group for deriving the standard of skill ought to be those surgeons and psychiatrists *nationwide* who have considerable experience performing psychosurgery and are highly skilled at doing so. Customary practice or reasonable competence based on locale is not an appropriate standard because for this extraordinary treatment there are too few qualified practitioners in any locale to derive a reasonable standard; a larger reference group is needed. The legally required standard of skill is meant to protect the public, and it is suggested here that because psychosurgery is an extraordinary treatment, the standard of reasonable competence should be high. Thus, neurosurgeons who perform only two or three operations per year or psychiatrists who have little experience with psychosurgery should be held to the standard of their more experienced colleages.

The small number of psychiatrists and neurosurgeons who engage in psychosurgery raises the question of whether the recommendation or performance of psychosurgery is ever reasonable medical practice. Indeed, among neurosurgeons and psychiatrists there is strong disagreement over whether psychosurgery is ever indicated in the absence of brain pathology, and probably the vast majority of both groups believe that recommending or performing psychosurgery is a professional error. To deal with such intraprofessional disputes, the law of malpractice has developed what is called the *respectable minority* doctrine. According to this doctrine, if a procedure is accepted by a respectable minority of practitioners in the field, recommendation or performance of the procedure will not be considered negligent even if an untoward result occurs and, in hindsight, the recommendation or treatment does not seem to have been a wise choice.

The question is whether psychosurgery commands a respectable minority. On the one hand, the minority of psychiatrists and neurosurgeons who approve of psychosurgery is quite tiny and the efficacy evidence is equivocal. On the other hand, there is some evidence for the efficacy of psychosurgery, and it is probably only somewhat less convincing than the evidence adduced for other intrusive treatments that are more commonly in use (for example, ECT, about which there is considerably more literature, but which is also of generally poor scientific quality; see Costello, 1976; Turek and Hanlon, 1977; but see American Psychiatric Association, 1978; Royal College of Psychiatrists, 1977).

Much of the vehement opposition to psychosurgery stems from the fact that it irreversibly destroys healthy brain tissue, the supposed source of personality and identity, without any real understanding of why destruction ameliorates certain disordered behavior. Still, there is some evidence of efficacy, and those neurosurgeons and psychiatrists who believe psychosurgery is sometimes indicated are not an evil or lunatic fringe. Future scientific discoveries may prove that the present advocates of psychosurgery were misguided, but given the general state of brain science and psychiatric art, it is reasonable to argue that a treatment that may restore some chronic patients to more normal functioning with few serious side effects is minimally acceptable.

A perhaps analogous case drawn from physical medicine is the jejunoileal bypass, an infrequently performed operation wherein a substantial portion of the small intestine of severely obese patients is surgically rendered nonfunctional in order to control their obesity. There is great controversy about this procedure, which renders healthy tissue nonfunctional and has serious side effects. But the treatment is efficacious and accepted by a respectable minority of practitioners; performing it under the appropriate conditions therefore would not constitute malpractice per se. Likewise, the respectable minority doctrine may reasonably apply to the practice of psychosurgery.

In malpractice actions, the standard of skill required in a particular case and whether it was met are matters of proof. With the help of expert testimony provided by the litigants, each case is decided on its own facts. It will be useful here, however, to explore the substantive standard of skill and to suggest what it should be. The crucial issues are ensuring that an accurate determination is made that the patient suffers from a condition for which psychosurgery is appropriate, and that all other, less intrusive appropriate treatments have been reasonably tried without success or hope of future success. I shall assume for purposes of discussion that the neurosurgeon and attending team skillfully perform the physical operation and provide proper postoperative care.

Diagnostic and Related Problems

Accurate diagnosis of mental disorders poses numerous theoretical and practical difficulties. To begin with, the disorders defined by the currently predominant diagnostic scheme are not highly valid; that is, the allegedly discrete disorders designated by particular diagnostic labels often do not seem to exist in reality as they are defined by the most widely used diagnostic scheme (Ennis and Litwack, 1974; Frank, 1975; Zigler and Phillips, 1961). In other words, a diagnosis often does not convey specific, accurate information about how the patient is presently behaving, why he is behaving that way, how he is likely to behave in the future, or what is the best treatment for him. Further, most diagnoses are rather vague, and the same behavioral manifestations may be indicative of many disorders. In sum, the value of present diagnoses for clinical or research purposes is problematic, albeit improving as mental health scientists increasingly employ operationalized and validated diagnostic criteria.

In addition to being of questionable validity, present diagnoses are often quite unreliable, even when made by highly qualified practitioners—an outcome partially produced by their invalidity (Spitzer, Endicott, and Robins, 1975; Helzer et al., 1977a). By and large, diagnostic reliability in mental health refers to the degree of agreement about diagnosis reached, preferably independently, by diagnosticians (Kendell, 1975). Empirical studies demonstrate that diagnostic agreement, although definitely improving, rarely rises much over 50 percent, even for the most severe and well-known mental disorders such as schizophrenia or severe affective disorder (Helzer et al., 1977b; Spitzer and Fleiss, 1974). There tends to be much greater agreement among diagnosticians, however, if they limit themselves to observations of behavior, without special regard to what may be rather artificial diagnostic categories (Overall et al., 1977; Luria and Berry, 1979). Thus, a diagnosis of delusion is more likely to be reliable than a diagnosis of schizophrenia. And, in the most general sense, all observers will agree that there is something wrong with the person who behaves extremely abnormally (Morse, 1978).

Even if referral for psychosurgery is made on the basis of pure behavioral phenomenology, reliability will still be a problem. For instance, there is little agreement, except at the extremes, about whether depression or anxiety is severe. For another example, the differential diagnosis of schizophrenia and depressive disorders is often difficult (Taylor, Gaztanaga, and Abrams, 1974). If psychosurgery is based on behavioral signs and is limited to severe cases, however, diagnostic reliability may not be as great a problem as critics of psychiatric diagnosis might fear. Still there will be room for disagreement because there are few well-operationalized and scientifically agreed upon criteria for the conditions for which psychosurgery is indicated, or for deciding when a condition is severely or truly chronic. Determining whether skillful diagnosis was made will be difficult for the courts, but reasonable operationalization of criteria and consultation with other professionals (which will be discussed later in the chapter) ought to rationalize the diagnostic process to a reasonable degree.

Another question related to diagnosis is whether it is a professional error to perform psychosurgery on a patient who suffers from a condition other than the persistent states of mood or emotion that are generally recognized to be the primary indications for psychosurgery. For other conditions, such as thought disorder or sexual deviation, there is much disagreement about efficacy among the small number of psychiatrists and neurosurgeons who advocate psychosurgery, and the evidence is highly equivocal.

Two approaches to this question might be adopted. Psychosurgery for other than the generally agreed upon indications might be considered negligent per se because arguably there is no respectable medical minority that supports its use in these cases. In view of the lack of knowledge about efficacy for these other conditions and the large general opposition to psychosurgery, the negligence per se approach has much to commend it because it would allow patients to recover damages when a treatment of unproven efficacy is performed upon them and injures them. On the other hand, there is some, albeit very weak, evidence for the efficacy of psychosurgery for these other conditions, and it might be considered an undue restriction effectively to ban it entirely because of the negligence per se rule. After all, some chronically disabled persons might be benefited, and it would be unreasonable to deny this possibility to them.

Courts might ultimately decide this issue either way. Psychiatrists and neurosurgeons who recommend and perform psychosurgery in such cases should recognize that a court might find that psychosurgery is simply not indicated for these conditions in light of present scientific and clinical knowledge. At the very least, psychosurgery for these other conditions should be accompanied by full disclosure to the patient of the risks involved. But even such full disclosure might not insulate the participating professionals from liability if the patient is harmed (Waltz and Scheuneman, 1970).

Exhaustion of Treatment Alternatives

Malpractice liability for psychosurgery might also depend on whether psychosurgery should always be a treatment of last resort and, if so, how the question of whether all appropriate treatment alternatives have been exhausted should be determined. These issues raise some questions about psychiatric treatment in general. Unfortunately, *knowledge* of how to treat psychiatric disorders is most incomplete. Many biological, psychological, and social treatment methods of varying efficacy have been discovered, but for the most part the therapeutic mechanisms of these treatments are unknown and it is rarely claimed that the treatments cure the alleged underlying illnesses that produce disordered behavior. Psychiatric treatments primarily change the behaviors that are the indicators of psychiatric illness. In nearly all instances there is considerable dispute about which treatment is the most appropriate for the disordered behavior in question (see generally, Group for the Advancement of Psychiatry, 1975) or about which specific treatment within a class of treatments is appropriate (for example, Goldberg et al., 1972). Finally, many of the standard treatments used for the most severe disorders (for example, psychotropic medications, electroconvulsive therapy, and certain forms of behavior therapy) are quite intrusive (see Shapiro, 1974) or have serious side effects that may be irreversible (see, for example, Special Report, 1973).

Ironically, the long-term failure of other treatments before resort to psychosurgery may lead to increasing severity and chronicity of the patient's condition, decreasing the expectation of a favorable outcome for psychosurgery. Such a situation calls for a cost–benefit analysis: The risks and benefits of possibly premature psychosurgery must be balanced against the risks and benefits of performing the surgery too late. Still, it is submitted that for a variety of reasons the appropriate standard of care is to treat psychosurgery as a treatment of true last resort, thus "favoring" the error of waiting too long. As noted repeatedly, psychosurgery produces irreversible brain damage with uncertain effects; the efficacy data are equivocal; and psychiatric conditions, even chronic ones, can sometimes be surprisingly labile and show spontaneous remissions. Prudence dictates, therefore, that psychosurgery should not be performed until all other customary, reasonable alternative forms of treatment have been exhausted and a substantial period of time has elapsed during which the person has remained chronically, severely disordered.

There are two major counter-arguments to the position that all other customary treatments should be exhausted before attempting psychosurgery. The first is that some identifiable patients clearly will not improve with other treatments and might regress unless some heroic intervention stems their potential deterioration. This is certainly true of some individuals, but, unfortunately, clinicians have no highly valid prediction tools to identify such persons—and there is little guarantee that psychosurgery will provide a cure. Further, as noted, psychiatric conditions are labile, and, contrary to expectations, even some hopelessly chronic patients seem to improve.

The second counter-argument is that many of the supposedly less-intrusive treatments also have serious risks, especially if they are used intensively or over a long term. For instance, long-term use of antipsychotic medication carries with it the risk of irreversible neurological damage, for example, tardive dyskinesia (Special Report, 1973); and heavy use of electroconvulsive therapy might cause serious and perhaps permanent memory deficits (Freidberg, 1977; but see Fink, 1978). There is some force to the second counter-argument, but it fails for a number of reasons. The risks of antipsychotic medications are not large in this context because most of the conditions for which psychosurgery is arguably indicated are not treated by antipsychotic medication. The major exception, of course, is chronic, severe anxiety, for which antipsychotic medication may be the treatment of choice in some instances. In any case, even if drugs and ECT have risks, these risks are more clearly delineated and are not more serious than the risks of psychosurgery. Finally, the seriously risky side effects of drugs and ECT typically have a gradual onset that can be monitored, and these treatments can therefore be discontinued before serious, irreversible damage occurs.

If the principle that psychosurgery should be a treatment of last resort is accepted, it still remains to operationalize the principle so that courts may determine if it has been adhered to. Although much homage is paid to this principle, few writers have attempted to operationalize the criteria for exhaustion of other remedies (Valenstein, 1977). The difficulty here, of course, is the general lack of agreement in mental health science about which treatments are appropriate for which conditions and how long they must be employed at what intensity before the professional can reasonably conclude that the alternative customary treatments have failed. This problem is especially acute in psychiatry because of the plethora of treatment modalities now available. Few mental health clinicians are highly trained in more than a small number of the available techniques, especially the many psychotherapies (see Morse and Watson, 1977), and it is probable that many professionals are not knowledgeable about (or even aware of) large numbers of alternative treatments. Thus, in addition to disagreement over what constitutes exhaustion of alternatives, few clinicians will be competent to exhaust them alone or to conclude reasonably without consultation that they have been exhausted. A further consequence of the enormous number of reasonable treatments is that exhaustion of all alternatives might be prohibitively expensive and time-consuming.

Given the problems outlined, it is fair to predict that no uniform set of criteria for the exhaustion of alternatives is likely to be agreed upon by professionals. Confronted by such ambiguity, as always the courts will have to apply a standard of reasonableness based on the evidence given by expert witnesses. I suggest, however, that the sole opinion of the primary treating psychiatrist that all reasonable alternatives have been exhausted should be per se insufficient. There should be consultation with at least one other psychiatrist who has a different viewpoint about the appropriateness of various treatments for different conditions. Such consultation would give the primary psychiatrist further information and a check on his or her decisions, decisions which might be biased by a set of personal treatment preferences, and at the same time would provide a check on diagnostic reliability. If the primary psychiatrist is not competent to employ all these treatment modalities, referral to another clinician should be made. At the least, however, the courts should require that all reasonable alternative chemotherapies should be employed, as well as various forms of psychotherapy and behavior therapy (see Older, 1974). For persistent depression, some would argue that ECT should also be tried if chemotherapy and psychological therapies fail. And all these treatments should be performed by clinicians who are highly skilled in their use.

Thus, the standard for assessing that psychosurgery has been employed only as a treatment of last resort should be (1) that a reasonable number of alternative treatments have been attempted by clinicians clearly skilled in those treatments, (2) that each has been attempted for a reasonable period of time at the appropriate intensity, but without reasonable success or likelihood of future success, and (3) that reasonable consultation has been sought before concluding that a recommendation of psychosurgery is appropriate. If it is argued that the standard suggested is too high and too costly, the most persuasive answer is that psychosurgery is a purely empirical treatment of dubious efficacy that produces irreversible brain damage with uncertain effects. Before such a treatment is attempted, reasonable, customary alternatives with equal or higher expectations of efficacy should be exhausted. Sound professional practice should demand no less, and the law should require that this standard be applied.

If practitioners generally treated psychosurgery as a treatment of last resort, then arguably a *prima facie* case of negligence would be established if psychosurgery were performed earlier than usual in a course of treatment. The defendants would then have the burden of demonstrating that in this particular case there was sufficient scientific and clinical justification for earlier surgery. Given the present state of the evidence concerning psychosurgery, I estimate that it would be extremely difficult for psychosurgery malpractice defendants to rebut the *prima facie* case of negligence arising from unusually early surgery.

The Standard of Informed Consent

Adults have a near absolute right to control their bodies. Unauthorized intrusions are a source of liability in tort and under some conditions may be constitutional violations as well. Persons can refuse clearly warranted medical treatment, even if it may be lifesaving and quite riskless. In order to respect the patient's right to self-determination and bodily privacy, and thus to meet the required standard of care, the physician must obtain the patient's informed consent to the proposed course of treatment. Informed consent authorizes the physician's intrusion into the patient's body and avoids possible liability so long as the treatment is performed with reasonable skill.

Although the standard of care is usually proven by expert testimony, according to modern cases,[3] the standard of care for informed consent should be decided largely by lay persons. Lay persons are not competent to judge medical questions without expert assistance, but they are competent to judge the social question of how much information a patient must have in order to uphold the patient's right to self-determination.

The standard criteria for informed consent are that it should be competent, knowledgeable, and voluntary[4] (see generally Barnhart,

---

[3] *Canterbury* v. *Spence*, 464 F.2d. 772 (D.C. Cir. 1972).
[4] *Kaimowitz* v. *Department of Mental Health*, Civil No. 73-19434-AW (Cir. Ct., Wayne Co., Mich., July 10, 1973), *1 Mental Disability Law Reporter 147* (Sept./Oct. 1976).

Pinkerton, and Roth, 1977; Myers, 1967; Waltz and Scheuneman, 1970).

Competence

A person is considered legally competent to give consent if he or she is capable of rationally deciding whether to accept or reject the proffered treatment (see Meisel, Roth, and Lidz, 1977; Note, 1974). Note that the standard focuses on the person's decision-making competence, not on the decision finally reached. Focusing on capacity rather than on outcome preserves the patient's autonomy and dignity because it respects the patient's decision, if he or she is capable of choosing rationally, even if the decision reached appears irrational in a particular case. Unfortunately, there is no legal operational definition of the required degree of decision-making capacity. It has been suggested, however, that the criteria for competence should be that the patient ought to be able to attend to and weigh the data relevant to the decision at hand within reasonable, broad, culturally determined limits (Morse, 1978).

It should be recognized that the legal criteria for competence are social and legal and not medical. Medical or psychiatric data may help inform a legal decision maker, but deciding who is legally capable of exercising the right to self-determination is an issue the law must ultimately decide for itself. There are no scientific tests that can determine with any degree of certainty whether a person is capable of attending to and weighing the data relevant to the decision. Making this determination requires a common-sense judgment about the person in light of all relevant medical and nonmedical information (including his or her reasoning concerning the decision in question).

The difficult issue in the context of psychosurgery, of course, is that the proposed patients are presumably severely and chronically mentally ill—a condition that usually presupposes some deficit in the capacity for rational behavior, at least in certain areas of one's life (M. S. Moore, 1975). Indeed, for many decades the law treated persons adjudicated mentally ill (for example, involuntarily committed patients) as incompetent. More recently, however, the law has recognized that mentally disordered persons, including those who are severely disordered, are not necessarily legally incompetent for most, if not all, purposes[5] (Brakel and Rock, 1971). Simply be-

---

[5] *Vecchione* v. *Wohlgemuth*, 377 F. Supp. 1361 (E.D. Pa. 1974).

cause a person suffers from a persistent disorder of mood or emotion does not mean, therefore, that the person is necessarily incapable of making a rational treatment decision. Most prime candidates for psychosurgery do not suffer from severe thought disorders and should be presumed competent to decide for themselves whether to undergo psychosurgery (see Goldstein, 1978). Thus, the emerging and better view is that competence should be decided on a case-by-case basis, with particular reference in each case to the specific capacity that is in question (for example, ability to make a rational treatment decision, ability to manage one's financial affairs, and so on).

A consent given by an incompetent person is not legally sufficient authorization for a medical procedure. Consequently, if the psychiatrist and surgeon fear that a particular patient is incapable of attending to and weighing data relevant to the decision, a court order for the appointment of a legal guardian must be obtained. There are limits, however, to the ability of a guardian to give proxy consent; courts will not allow guardians to consent to treatments that are not sufficiently beneficial to the ward.[6] Nevertheless, it is likely that if psychosurgery is a reasonably acceptable treatment, a court would authorize its performance on an incompetent patient where the medical evidence clearly demonstrated that it was indicated.[7]

If a competent *or* an incompetent patient refuses psychosurgery, however, the National Commission for the Protection of Human Subjects of Biomedical and Behavioral Research (1977) suggests that surgery should not be performed. It is submitted that this is a wise recommendation because, in the face of an uncertain and risky treatment, it maximizes respect for the patient. Of course, if a court sanctions the performance of psychosurgery contrary to the objection of the patient, the treatment will be validly performed despite the lack of consent by the patient.

Knowledge About the Treatment

Informed consent must be knowledgeable. Even if treatment is medically indicated, the decision to accept it must be made by the patient. Therefore, the patient must have sufficient information about the treatment to allow him or her to decide intelligently

---

[6] *In re Richardson,* 284 So.2d 185 La. App. 173.

[7] Compare *Kaimowitz, op. cit.*

whether or not to undergo the treatment. All *material* facts concerning the benefits and risks of the proposed treatment and its alternatives (such as no treatment or continuation of alternative treatments) must be disclosed in nontechnical language that is comprehensible to the patient.[8]

The legal definition of materiality is not clear, but not every risk, no matter how unlikely, must be explained to the patient; only significant information that would be likely to affect the patient's decision to undergo the treatment must be disclosed. The physician's fear that the customary disclosure of material facts might deter the patient from undergoing the treatment is clearly *not* the type of consideration that should excuse the usual disclosure requirement.[9] If disclosure of certain facts would be likely to harm the patient or to interfere with the success of the treatment, those facts need not be disclosed. But when the extraordinary treatment of psychosurgery is contemplated, the physicians should bear a heavy burden of proof when trying to justify less disclosure than usual.

It is suggested that particularly full disclosure of behavioral effects ought to be given to prospective psychosurgery patients. After all, behavioral changes do affect one's basic personality and identity. The behavioral and social ramifications of psychosurgery are so controversial that it seems reasonable to claim that all behavioral risks should be considered material. Further, because psychosurgery is of dubious efficacy, it is reasonable to require unusually full disclosure of the physical risks as well. After all, if the psychiatric benefits are problematical, the physical risks become more material to the patient's personal cost–benefit analysis. But there is no duty to disclose unknown risks, and the materialization of such a risk should not lead to liability so long as psychosurgery was a reasonable treatment for the patient in question and was performed skillfully (Waltz and Scheuneman, 1970). On the other hand, if the surgery is performed on the basis of a misdiagnosis or prematurely, then informed consent should not insulate the psychiatrist and neurosurgeon from liability (Waltz and Scheuneman, 1970).

I also suggest that patients should be told about the intense controversy concerning the value of psychosurgery. The psychiatrist and surgeon should be able to state their opinion that the treatment is indicated, but it seems wiser for the patient to know that only a small minority of experts believe that psychosurgery is appropriate.

---

[8] *Cobbs* v. *Grant*, 8 Cal.3d 229, 104 Cal. Rptr. 505, 502 P.2d 1 (1972).
[9] *Canterbury, op. cit.*

Compared with the ordinary course of medical practice, the suggestions made here would require unusually heavy disclosure. It is submitted, however, that psychosurgery is an extraordinary and controversial procedure that should be undergone only by patients who are completely aware of the likely outcomes of the treatment. I recognize that other medical treatments may be equally extraordinary and controversial—for example, the jejunoileal bypass—but I would suggest that extraordinary disclosure should be made in those cases as well. The result of extraordinary disclosure may be that some patients will refuse the treatment who might otherwise have accepted psychosurgery and benefited from it if the more usual, less cumbersome disclosure requirements were followed. This risk appears justified, however, in view of the weak efficacy data and the extraordinary nature of the treatment.

Voluntary Consent

The third criterion for an informed consent is that it must be voluntary; if the consent is the product of coercion, the treatment infringes the patient's right to self-determination. For purposes of discussing voluntariness, it is useful to distinguish between voluntary patients and patients who are under involuntary restraint—for example, patients who are civilly committed or prisoners. We shall discuss these separately, but it should be remembered that nearly all psychosurgery on restrained persons is now or is likely to be regulated by legislation (National Commission, 1977).

Voluntary patients who are candidates for psychosurgery typically will have been severely and chronically disabled for quite some time, a condition that will tend to make them emotionally vulnerable to various pressures. The pressures from the entreaties of families and friends (who will have been frustrated, angered, and saddened by the patient's condition) and the forceful, authoritative recommendations from medical professionals will arguably be more coercive on psychosurgery candidates than on candidates for other medical treatments. Despite this, it would be an infringement on the autonomy of the potential psychosurgery patient to assume that he or she is incapable of consenting freely to the procedure. In the absence of judicial or administrative review, the patient's primary protection must therefore be his or her own autonomy and the ethical, restrained conduct of the physicians or other mental health professionals involved with the case. If a jurisdiction requires some form of judicial or administrative review of all psychosurgery decisions, a finding that the consent was voluntary would insulate the participating professionals from liability in this regard.

In addition to the pressures that might induce a chronically disabled mental patient to undergo psychosurgery, the involuntarily institutionalized patient faces other, more coercive pressures. The patient may rightly or wrongly believe that a penalty, such as loss of privileges or the opportunity to be released, will flow from refusal to accept treatment. A more subtle factor might be the conscious or unconscious desire to please the institutional staff, which exerts considerable control over the inmate's life. Finally, the additional attention a psychosurgery patient is likely to receive may itself induce the inmate to accept psychosurgery.[10]

Factors like those just adduced have led some to claim that obtaining truly voluntary consent from an involuntarily institutionalized person is impossible and that psychosurgery should never be performed in such cases[11] (Mark, 1973). Others argue that although there are greater pressures on inmates, a total ban on psychosurgery would deny some needy patients the benefits of psychosurgery—a result that should be avoided if possible (Shapiro, 1974). Those who do not wish a complete ban usually propose the promulgation of legislative or institutional guidelines to ensure that no undue pressure is brought to bear. If such guidelines were instituted, scrupulous compliance with them would surely insulate the participating professionals from liability.

Having examined the standard of care for skill and informed consent, we shall now turn briefly to an examination of the comparative liability of the various professionals for violation of the standard.

Responsibility for Violations of the Standard of Care

Primary responsibility for diagnosis, exhaustion of alternative treatments, and the initial recommendation of psychosurgery must rest with the psychiatrist. Some might argue, however, that once the psychiatrist refers the patient to a neurosurgeon, responsibility for the psychosurgery shifts to the surgeon, insulating the psychiatrist from possible liability for his or her previous lack of skill. While a court might accept this argument, I submit that it would be unwise to do so. The primary psychiatrist and the neurosurgeon should be

---

[10] *Kaimowitz, op. cit.*
[11] *Kaimowitz, op. cit.*

jointly liable for injuries resulting from improper diagnosis and failure to exhaust alternative treatments. The primary indications for psychosurgery are psychiatric, and the participating neurosurgeon is unlikely also to be a psychiatrist. The neurosurgeon must therefore rely heavily on the opinions and recommendations of the psychiatrist, and the psychiatrist should be liable.

In the same way that referral to a neurosurgeon should not insulate the psychiatrist from liability, reasonable reliance by the surgeon on the psychiatrist should not insulate the former from all responsibility for psychiatric aspects of the case. The surgeon is operating on the basis of mainly psychiatric indications and therefore should be responsible for proper treatment in regard to the psychiatric factors. In addition to interviewing the patient, the neurosurgeon therefore ought to review thoroughly the psychiatric recommendations. Ideally, the psychiatrist should provide extensive written documentation of diagnosis, treatment decisions, and referrals for treatment and consultation. It is suggested that the neurosurgeon consult an independent psychiatrist in order to evaluate the psychiatric recommendations. In an area of great clinical and scientific uncertainty, such a further general check on the adequacy of the psychiatric referral would help protect the patient and the primary psychiatrist and neurosurgeon.

After reviewing the case and deciding that psychosurgery is indicated, the surgeon must decide which operation to perform. As we have seen, most psychosurgeons use the same operation on all patients, and for the most part there is not convincing evidence that any one operation is most appropriate for particular conditions. Until such data are collected, the only reasonable course is to hold that the requisite standard of care is met if the psychosurgeon competently performs an operation that experienced psychosurgeons consider one of the reasonably acceptable alternatives. Failure to meet this standard of care would constitute a *prima facie* case of negligence. Thus, for example, if a neurosurgeon who rarely performs psychosurgery attempted a prefrontal lobotomy, a heavy burden would fall on the surgeon to justify the treatment if the patient suffered harm.

Although the choice of a surgical technique seems to be a decision that is uniquely a surgeon's, a strong argument can be made that the psychiatrist should also be liable if an improper technique is chosen. First, the psychiatrist should only refer patients to experienced, skilled psychosurgeons. Moreover, the psychiatrist should be aware of the efficacy and risk data, and should have a duty to ensure that the surgeon uses one of the reasonable techniques for the patient in question. Again, the surgery is meant to alleviate a psychiatric condition, and its success or failure will be measured largely by psychiatric criteria. The psychiatrist should therefore consult with the surgeon about the choice of technique and should bear responsibility for the untoward results of an improper choice to which he or she assents.

Since malpractice law is in part a regulatory tool that aims to ensure proper medical care, the joint liability of psychiatrists and neurosurgeons suggested here would lead to a greater number of scientific and clinical checks on the decision to recommend and perform psychosurgery than if liability were not joint. The checks suggested would be something of a burden on psychiatrists and neurosurgeons, but it is likely that much greater care would be exercised before this extraordinary treatment was employed.

The psychiatrist and neurosurgeon should also be jointly responsible for disclosing the psychiatric and neurological benefits and risks of psychosurgery and for assessing the competence and consent of the patient. The psychiatrist will generally have more complete information about the psychiatric aspects, but the surgeon should also be aware of them because he is performing the surgery for psychiatric reasons. The psychiatrist and the neurosurgeon are equally well situated to assess competence and consent (see Morse, 1978). Moreover, joint liability will encourage both the psychiatrist and the neurosurgeon to ensure that the full, necessary disclosures are made.

In sum, for nearly all aspects of psychosurgery, public policy will be served better if the psychiatrist and neurosurgeon are held jointly liable for injuries resulting from failure to exercise due care.

The Effect of Statutory Administrative, Institutional, or Professional Regulations

Because psychosurgery is such an extraordinary treatment, it is likely that there will be growing regulation of it at various levels. In the previous chapter of this volume, Pizzulli pointed out that some states have already passed statutes regulating the practice of psychosurgery, and the National Commission (1977) has promulgated a series of guidelines that include the establishment of institutional review boards and a national psychosurgery advisory board. The question raised is what effect such guidelines will have on psychosurgery malpractice liability.

The usual rule in the law of malpractice is that violation of a statute or administrative regulation will constitute either weighty evidence of negligence or negligence per se if an injury is caused that is proximately related to said violation. Violation of institutional or professional guidelines is typically treated simply as evidence of negligence. For an extraordinary treatment like psychosurgery, there is a powerful argument that violation of a statute or regulation that results in injury should lead to liability per se and that violation of institutional or professional guidelines should constitute very powerful evidence of negligence. (It should be mentioned in passing that a hospital or review board might be liable if a patient is injured by negligent psychosurgery that has not been performed or reviewed in conformity with the hospital or review board's applicable guidelines.)[12]

Because of the lack of consensus concerning psychosurgery and the intense opposition to it, specific guidelines would reduce the uncertainties that face professionals who participate in psychosurgery. More important, such regulations would protect patients by announcing a uniform and relatively unambiguous set of standards for various aspects of the practice of psychosurgery. The argument against such regulation is that the state or other outsiders have no business interfering in the practice of medicine. The noninterventionist argument carries some weight, but the state, professional organizations, and institutions like hospitals can argue reasonably that they have a compelling interest in ensuring that an extraordinary treatment like psychosurgery is performed only under the proper conditions.

Powerful new technologies that have so much potential for altering behavior and personality cannot be considered simply medical procedures. They raise social and moral issues far wider than their medical implications. Consequently, regulation of these technologies is entirely appropriate and probably will benefit professionals and patients. Assuming the regulations are reasonable, they should not constitute an undue limitation on the appropriate and effective practice of psychosurgery. Such regulations might lead to a delay or lack of proper treatment in some cases, but these few unfortunate cases are a necessary cost of the proper limitation of psychosurgery.

Experimentation

For our purposes, three types of experimentation may be delineated. First, a new, untested psychosurgical technique may be attempted by an individual surgeon for clinical purposes. Second, a new tech-

---

[12] *Darling* v. *Charlestown Comm. Mem. Hosp.*, 33 Ill.2d 326, 211 N.E.2d 253 (1965), *cert. denied* 383 U.S. 946 (1966).

nique may be attempted for both clinical and scientific purposes as part of a consciously designed study. Third, scientists may attempt various experiments (for example, examining the effects of brain stimulation) during the course of a standard psychosurgical procedure ("adjunctive experimentation").

Physicians who attempt new techniques for primarily clinical purposes run a great risk of liability unless there is quite substantial scientific and clinical evidence pointing to the likely clinical usefulness of the treatment. If such evidence is insufficient or the technique is unreasonably risky and the patient is harmed, even "complete" disclosure will not insulate the physicians from liability (Waltz and Scheuneman, 1970). Where performance of a technique is per se wrongful (for example, attempting a technique without sufficient basis), consent becomes irrelevant. Similarly, if the treatment or adjunctive experimentation is performed as part of a study, all concerned (that is, the physicians and the sponsoring organization) will be liable if there are insufficient data reasonably to risk performing the study. However, if there are sufficient background data, treatment is not unreasonably risky, the risks and benefits of the experimental procedure are fully disclosed, and applicable regulatory guidelines for the performance of experimentation on human subjects are conformed to, there will be no liability for the individual surgeon and the other participants in a study if the operation is performed skillfully.

One can estimate that because of the extreme controversy concerning "standard" psychosurgery, individual surgeons and study participants should be very careful about proceeding with experimental psychosurgery, especially with involuntary patients. Courts may very likely view experimental psychosurgery or adjunctive experimentation with extreme skepticism. Individual surgeons who are not "protected" by participation in a study and compliance with research regulations will be especially exposed to liability. A final point is that all psychosurgery on children, which is rare in any case, is likely to be considered experimental because of the utter paucity of high-quality data concerning its indications and efficacy for this patient group.

Damages

If a medical procedure is performed properly and with the patient's informed consent, the physician will not be liable for untoward results, including side effects, complications, or simply unbeneficial outcomes. Thus, the participating professionals will not be liable for such sequelae of psychosurgery (for example, no change, seizures, deficits in abstract reasoning) if the patient was fully informed and if an appropriate operation for his accurately diagnosed condition was skillfully performed after reasonable exhaustion of more conservative and customary psychiatric therapies. The psychiatrist and neurosurgeon who treat the patient negligently or do not obtain the patient's informed consent will be liable in malpractice for injuries that result proximately from the physicians' failures.

Some possible harms, such as loss of employment resulting from untoward impairment—for example, from seizures—will lead to typical recovery claims and should present no particular difficulty. A more complex issue would be presented by deficits in abstract reasoning capacity or personality changes such as increased emotional lability. Unless these results are tied to loss of earning capacity or the like, calculating damages based on them would be very speculative. Further, it is conceivable that psychosurgery might blunt the emotional distress that would typically flow from untoward results. Such cases would present an interesting paradox. The patient has suffered injury, and in addition, has suffered a further injury, blunting of the usual and normal reaction to distress, that decreases the patient's distress from the injuries suffered. Thus, the patient has suffered multiple injuries but feels less distressed than he or she would normally feel. Whether this patient should recover more or less than the "normally" distressed patient is a matter the courts will have to decide as the issue arises.

Another issue worth mentioning in passing is the measure of damages for failure to obtain informed consent. As always, the cause of action in malpractice requires injury to the patient that is proximately caused by the physician's failure to exercise due care. Recovery will be possible for failure to obtain informed consent only if the undisclosed risk materializes and the physician's disclosure of the significant risk would have led the patient to reject the treatment.[13]

Assuming that the physician is liable, should the measure of damages be the loss from the undisclosed but now materialized risk, or should it be the *difference* between the patient's condition as it would have been with no treatment and the patient's condition after the surgery and the materialization of the undisclosed risk? Provided that the surgery was performed skillfully, the latter measure seems fairer because the patient recovers only for the actual loss occa-

---

[13] *Canterbury, op. cit.*

sioned by the surgery (Waltz and Inbau, 1971), but proper calculation requires an estimate of the probable course of the patient's condition in the absence of treatment. This requires psychiatric prognostication, an area in which knowledge is severely limited. Still, the latter standard is fairer and courts should attempt to apply it. (If the failure to obtain informed consent is treated as a battery, then the physician will be liable for every injury that is proximately caused by the touching. A battery action is the minority position, however.)

A final damage issue is whether physicians ought to be "strictly liable" for any injuries that result from psychosurgery; that is, should recovery be allowed for injuries caused by psychosurgery even if it is performed properly and with informed consent? The argument in favor of strict liability is that psychosurgery is such an innovative and "minority" treatment that physicians should bear the costs of all injuries that are occasioned by it. It is argued further that strict liability will appropriately cause physicians to be extremely cautious before recommending or performing psychosurgery. There is some precedent in Anglo-American law for applying strict liability to innovative treatments (Waltz and Inbau, 1971), but this does not seem the wisest course.

As a general matter, strict liability will impede medical progress and needed treatment in some cases. Further, if the patient is fully informed and there is scientific and clinical basis for the treatment, then there seems little reason to hold a physician liable for untoward results if the treatment is performed satisfactorily. I have assumed throughout this paper that psychosurgery does meet a minimal level of scientific and clinical acceptability. Little if any psychosurgery would be performed if strict liability were applied. Some would argue that this is the best outcome, but if so, it should be achieved directly by legislative restriction or banning of psychosurgery, and not indirectly by means of an unduly harsh tort remedy.

Conclusion: Tort Law as a Regulatory Tool

Tort law is a customary means of regulating medical practice and compensating patients for injuries caused by negligence. It is therefore extendable to the performance of psychosurgery as well as to the performance of any other medical treatment. But, as so many commentators have noted, psychosurgery raises vast ethical, social, and political as well as medico-psychiatric issues. How society should respond to a medical technique that changes behavior by destroying healthy brain tissue is a much broader question than a decision about treatment for a disease.

In an area so controversial and lacking in hard data, judge-made tort law is not an adequate regulatory tool. Tort remedies lead to piecemeal regulation because the development of coherent doctrine depends on the existence of sufficient numbers of plaintiffs and defendants who are prepared to litigate. Even then the courts will only decide the questions brought before them; other equally important questions may not be raised and decided because of the vagaries of the litigation process.

If psychosurgery requires extraordinary regulation because it is an extraordinary treatment, then the legislature or an administrative agency is the appropriate institution to give full consideration to the issues and to promulgate comprehensive regulations. If legislative or administrative regulation is accomplished, malpractice law will remain as a secondary mechanism for ensuring that physicians obey the regulations and perform psychosurgery properly, and a primary mechanism for compensating patients. But tort law alone cannot be successful as the sole regulatory tool if psychosurgery is as extraordinary as it seems to be.

CHAPTER 20

Regulation of Psychosurgery

Robert J. Grimm

Oregon and California now have statutes regulating psychosurgical practice, and such regulation is being considered elsewhere. The Oregon psychosurgery bill[1] became law on July 1, 1973, and the California legislation[2] on psychosurgery and electroconsulsive therapy (ECT) became effective on January 1, 1977. Later, in March of 1977, a National Commission task force report (National Commission, 1977) was sent to the White House, Congress, and the Secretary of the Department of Health, Education and Welfare (DHEW) spelling out the circumstances under which psychosurgery could be performed where federal money is involved. These efforts bespeak the extraordinary concern that has arisen over brain surgery for psychiatric problems. As a coauthor of the Oregon bill, I witnessed its origin, design, and consequences, and in this chapter I shall discuss the Oregon legislation and then compare it with the California

---

[1] Senate Bill (SB) 298, Oregon Legislative Assembly, 1973; 10 pages.
[2] Assembly Bill (AB) No. 1032, California Legislative Assembly, 1976. Reprinted as Chapter 1109 of California Welfare Institutional code; 10 pages.

legislation and the National Commission's recommendations to show the advantages and disadvantages of such efforts.

1973 Oregon Bill (SB 298)

In the fall of 1972, Senator Hallock of the Oregon legislature introduced a bill (SB 298) to restrict the use of psychosurgery and ECT on state institution patients. At that time, a number of bills were introduced in the Oregon legislature with the intent of subjecting to review all treatments of the mentally disturbed. These bills made "the unspoken allegation that those who performed organic therapies, including psychosurgery and brain stimulation, would use their skills in the service of political and social ambitions or as a final weapon in the closed closets of the penal system and back wards of the state hospital."[3] Stevie Remington of the Oregon branch of the American Civil Liberties Union (ACLU) asked that I review the medical and technical content of SB 298 as it pertained to civil liberties matters. As I was ignorant of the issues involved, I consulted thirty or so acquaintances in neurology, psychiatry, neurosurgery, and the basic neurosciences in Oregon to obtain their views about psychosurgery. I also talked to members of the clergy, friends in the arts, and lawyers, since psychosurgery raised a number of complicated issues other than those strictly medical.

From these discussions and a review of psychosurgery literature, I concluded that such operations were at best empirical and at worse experimental. Rather than engaging in prolonged debate over a subject for which decisive clinical data were lacking, I raised the point that there were enough significant questions about psychosurgery to preclude informed consent. Colleagues did not disagree, but they were divided about what should be done. Some opposed any effort to restrict psychosurgery, not because of the merits of the case, but because of a general concern over further government involvement in medical practice. The few neurosurgeons doing cingulotomies or other psychosurgical procedures in Oregon at the time were not enthusiastic about regulatory control. One, however, conceded that a formal review process for selecting patients would relieve him of the burden of making such decisions alone. Additional material summarizing the concern and discussion over psychosurgery in Ore-

---

[3] Rushmer, D. S., Chairman, Oregon Psychosurgery Board (Personal communication to the National Commission for the Protection of Human Subjects of Biomedical and Behavioral Research, November 3, 1976).

gon at the time has been published (Dow, Grimm, and Rushmer, 1975).

I subsequently drafted a position statement for the Oregon branch of the ACLU[4] in opposition to psychosurgery and critical of certain features of the Hallock bill. Following this testimony, and that of my colleagues Donald Rushmer and Curtis Bell, Senator Hallock requested that I, Rushmer, and Henry Crawford, legislative assistant of the Oregon Medical Association (OMA) rewrite the bill. With the aid of Robert Simpson, a hospital lawyer, we completely overhauled SB 298 and dropped its ECT section. ECT was a separate and controversial issue whose inclusion would have jeopardized the bill's passage.

The revised bill was designed to amend existing Oregon mental health statutes (ORS 426-700, 426-755, 677-190). It opens with a preamble (unusual for legislation) of four paragraphs. The first acknowledges that the brain is the source of an individual's identity; the second, that the free and full use of the brain is an inalienable right and a prerequisite for human life; and the third, that any deliberate irreversible alteration of brain to change behavior shall not be considered except in the most extraordinary situations and only as a last resort. The final paragraph of the preamble makes it clear that the Act's intent is to provide the strictest possible control over the advocacy and practice of psychosurgery.

The Oregon bill (act) has sixteen sections. The first (S,1) defines the terms of psychosurgery, experimental, and other key terms. The second (S,2) stipulates that all physicians must comply with the Act. A nine-member Review Board is established, with six appointments by the governor and three by the OMA for specific terms. The makeup of the Board is prescribed: one neurologist, two neurosurgeons, two psychiatrists, one clinical psychologist, one neuroscientist, one lawyer, and one lay member of the public. Appointments are for four years (S,3,4). Any institution or physician can petition (S,6) the Board for psychosurgery or intracranial brain stimulation[5] by arguing three points: (1) that the patient needs psychosurgery; (2) that informed consent has been obtained, and (3) that the proposed surgery has legitimate clinical value. The rest of

---

[4]Grimm, R. J. *Advocacy of psychosurgery and intracranial brain stimulation in the voluntarily committed: medical, legal, and ethical objections.* Oregon district branch, American Civil Liberties Union statement to Senate Human Resources Committee Hearing on SB 298, Oregon Legislature, March 20, 1973.

[5]I shall comment only on psychosurgery in the Oregon bill. Provisions for regulating intracranial brain stimulation (IBS) are identical.

S,6 provides for a Board hearing within twenty days to ascertain that a proper consent has been obtained. The work of the hearing (S,7) is to decide whether consent was voluntary and informed. If the patient is incompetent or a juvenile, a legal guardian decides whether or not to grant consent.

The Psychosurgery Board is entitled to review the clinical and research literature pertaining to psychosurgery, to conduct consultations with knowledgeable persons regarding the efficacy of proposed techniques, to assess fully the clinical data of the patient proposed for surgery, and, after deciding whether or not conventional therapies have been exhausted, either permit or reject the petition (S,8). The Board is empowered (S,9) to take depositions, issue subpoenas, and gather information about the efficacy of specific psychosurgical procedures. Steps for providing a legal guardian are outlined (S,10). Patients have a right to be represented by counsel at the consent hearing (S,11). The petitioners and/or surgeon must report the clinical results of the psychosurgical operation (S,12). The Psychosurgical Board is shielded from invalid or criminal liability (S,13), as are surgeons (S,14). Physicians or institutions doing psychosurgery without Board permission are liable for civil damages (S,15); in the case of a surgeon, the Act specifies revocation of medical license. The date scheduled for the Act to become law was July 1, 1973 (S,16).

SB 298 was guided through amending sessions of both the Senate (May 10, 1973) and the House (June 18, 1973) by Donald Rushmer. It was unanimously passed on June 18, 1973, was signed by Governor Tom McCall, and became effective on July 1, 1973.

Consequences

A Psychosurgery Board was convened by December 1973. It immediately saw that verifying informed consent, determining that all conventional therapies had been exhausted, and establishing that a particular psychosurgical operation actually worked were formidable, if not impossible, tasks. Informed consent was not the problem; there were sufficient models available for determining this. Rather, how was it to be determined that *all* conventional therapies had been exhausted, or that any specific psychosurgical procedure actually worked?

Within one class of therapies—for example, drugs—the Board agreed that only one member of the class need to have been tried and proved ineffective. Documentation was required that a therapeutic end point had not been reached in a patient. It was suggested that an adequate period of trial and failure with a full range of conventional therapies would probably require one to two years. The Board also requested an accurate diagnosis and psychiatric evaluation of the patient's disorder to permit it to determine the patient's need for psychosurgery. With regard to the requirement that a proposed psychosurgical procedure be demonstrated to be valid, the Board decided to adopt a wait-and-see attitude as to what would be needed.

An instructive letter to physicians[6] was prepared by George Kjaera, a psychiatrist on the Board. Using depression as a model, the letter showed what the Board needed in order to decide the merits of each petition for psychosurgery. The letter was sent to the Oregon physicians in September of 1974. Between July 1, 1973, and January 1, 1980 the Board received six cases for consideration. They are highly instructive:

Case 1 was a 22-year-old housewife with a normal IQ and neuropsychological function but with psychological test findings compatible with a diagnosis of psychosis. The petitioner had met none of the Board requirements. There was no adequate history, no documentation of therapies used without success, and no evidence for an informed consent. The petition was eventually abandoned because of the patient's ambivalence.

Case 2 was a 34-year-old obsessive accountant whose work had decompensated intermittently over a period of three years. He had been treated with various tranquilizers, antidepressants, ECT, and insight therapy, all without benefit. While the Board awaited documentation of these therapies, the petition was withdrawn, as the patient was reported to have recovered.

Case 3 was a middle-aged woman who had been treated for twenty-five years by her family practitioner. Past diagnoses included agitated depression, chronic anxiety with hypochondriasis, acute anxiety, menopausal depression, and pseudoneurotic schizophrenia. One Board member commented that from the data presented he could not tell whether the patient suffered from multiple pulmonary emboli or an anxiety reaction. Drug therapy included major tranquilizers and antidepressants. At the time of the hearing the patient was on thioridazine (Mellaril), a major tranquilizer. She had seen several psychiatrists but had usually left hospitals against their advice. Quite commonly, after arriving home she would call the psychiatrist repeatedly and demand that something be done. Commitment to a state hospital was formally recommended. This terminated the psychiatrist's in-

---

[6] Psychosurgery Review Board letter, Donald S. Rushmer, Board Chairman, to Oregon physicians, September 1974, outlining requirements to comply with SB 298 and including sample consent forms and letters of petition.

volvement with her case. It was reported that she had been treated with ECT, but the dates of such therapy were not in her physician's record.

During the hearing, the patient was ambivalent and withdrew her consent at several points during the proceedings. When reassured that she could withdraw her consent at any time, she tentatively consented to the psychosurgical operation. Since her clinical data were vague and uncertain, the Board requested a psychiatric evaluation and treatment history. Her petition was withdrawn as she died of a pulmonary embolus several months later.

Case 4 was a 30-year-old inmate in a state hospital. He had been in and out of correction institutions since the age of nine. He was Court-committed for murder but judged not guilty of murder by reason of insanity. He was clearly dangerous, but he was never considered mentally incompetent. Because of his violent nature and repeated assaults on guards (including the killing of a prison guard) and patients, many therapies had been tried. Although the petitioners declined to document all these therapies, the Board heard testimony that all major tranquilizers and anticonvulsants had individually and in combinations been tried on the patient and had failed to control him. Fluphenazine (Prolixin), a long-acting injectible tranquilizer, had been tried in large, frequent dosage (4cc. per week), as had other drugs. Finally, weekly "maintenance" ECT proved successful. During the first Board hearing, the patient sat with his face on the table drooling and oblivious to the proceedings. He was disoriented and completely unable to understand what was going on.

At a second hearing several weeks later, the patient was more alert. He responded to questions in a childlike fashion but could not recall whether or not the operation had been performed. The diagnosis offered at the time was an antisocial, explosive passive-aggressive personality. The Board requested that the petitioners appoint a competent and neutral guardian, who would be provided with legal counsel to effect a valid consent. The director of the petitioning institution had himself appointed guardian until the Board convinced a judge that it would be contrary to the spirit of the Act to allow the petitioner to be also the legal guardian. Thereafter, the case lapsed, as no guardian was appointed. To complicate matters further, the petitioners had recommended a radio frequency (RF) lesion cingulotomy to treat the patient's aggressiveness. Neither the Board nor outside reviewers could establish, on the basis of their knowledge or the literature, that the cingulate gyrus was a conventional or useful target for aggression control. The neurosurgeon petitioner was experienced with this lesion site and was not interested in changing it.

This case eventually resulted in the resignation of two Psychosurgery Board members. All Board members were reportedly moved by this patient's plight and wanted something better done. But they possessed no power to practice medicine—that is, to refer the patient to a more knowledgeable neurosurgeon or to prescribe alternative therapies—and hence the resignations.

Case 5 was a 41-year-old man who had suffered from manic-depression for eleven years and had responded poorly to conventional therapy. The petition was the first of the five to provide an adequate documentation of all therapies and their failure and the first to be presented to the Board as a case of last resort. Psychotherapy had been attempted over the course of several years without success. ECT yielded only temporary improvement. Drug therapy included tranquilizers, antidepressants (including monoamine oxidase inhibitors), hypnotics, minor tranquilizers, anticonvulsants, and thyroid hormone, all carried to the limits of toxicity with no effect on the patient's mood swings. The patient was considered a high risk for suicide. At the consent hearing, the Board was impressed that the patient was quite capable of giving an informed consent. The Board asked that the patient receive a battery of psychological tests, skull films, and isotope and computer tomogram (CT) brain scans before a final decision. The required tests were completed. During this preparation, the patient contacted friends in the medical profession for papers on psychosurgery for his own review. As a result of all this and the information received at the consent hearing, the patient asked that his application be suspended. Also, he had gotten better. As stated by the referring psychiatrist, "The patient has maintained excellent progress with the combination of medication and psychotherapy. For the first time in almost ten years he's had relative stability, has begun working consistently again and has improved family relationships. It is understandable that he wishes the application for psychosurgery to be suspended at this time."[7]

Case 6 was a 23-year-old unmarried man with a seven-year history of a severe obsessive-compulsive disorder dominated by phobias, ruminations, withdrawal, and isolation. The number 21, blue trucks, certain hyphenated words, and particular noises that occurred by chance while he was swallowing, walking on his left foot, or exhaling all triggered fear responses and heightened his apprehension. School and work environments were impossible places, as he could not protect himself from the unscheduled occurrence of these aforementioned events. He gradually spent more time alone in his acoustically-tiled room, listening to selective music by earphone.

A well-documented record existed for innumerable medical and nonmedical therapies between 1972 and 1979 without evidence that any had worked. They included single and combination drug programs of phenothiazines, butyrophenones, tricyclic antidepressants, MAO inhibitors, anticonvulsants (phenytoin), minor tranquilizers, L-tryptophan, and megavitamins. No fewer than six different mental health facilities had been involved. Treatments included behavioral modification and desensitization, psychotherapy, and various types of counseling in both inpatient and outpatient settings, all without any significant effect. Seventeen multiple-monitored ECT sessions similarly failed.

---

[7] Rushmer, *op. cit.*

With this documented record of treatment failure, the patient's knowledgeable consent, and literature presented supporting the efficacy of psychosurgery for this disorder, the Board approved the patient for psychosurgery on December 15, 1978. Bilateral lesions were placed in the cingulate gyrus in January 1979 at a Portland hospital by an experienced neurosurgeon. The procedure was without success, according to the patient's psychiatrist.

The Psychosurgery Board has no data on the number of cases that psychiatrists have sent elsewhere for surgery. Some Oregon psychiatrists have informally threatened to do so. If cases have been sent out of Oregon, observers agree that the number would be few.

In the first year of the statute's existence, there was no money for legal consultation, secretarial help, xeroxing, library services, mailings, and so on. The State's Attorney General's office supplied legal help and the State's Mental Health Division gave secretarial assistance. In 1974–1975, the Psychosurgery Board's chairman petitioned the Oregon legislature's interim (between sessions) governing body, the Emergency Board, for $10,000. This was granted. In subsequent years the administrative budget has been $5,000–6,000 each year.

Proper funding, legal assistance, a heterogeneous group of professionals obliged to judge each case on its own merits, and requirement of informed consent, the exhaustion of conventional therapies, and scientific proof that a given operative procedure works have been the major elements of the Oregon experience in regulating psychosurgery. The Oregon statute has been in effect now for over seven years, and in my view the Psychosurgery Board has worked well, administering a rigorous statute that makes it reasonably difficult to perform psychosurgery in all but well-conceived clinical situations.

1977 California Bill (AB 1032)

On January 1, 1977, revised legislation for the control of psychosurgery and ECT (AB 1032), sponsored by California Assemblyman John Vascancellos, became law. It passed by a 72–2 Assembly and 23–1 Senate vote and was signed by Governor Brown on September 20, 1976. Vascancellos' original 1974 bill (AB 4481)[8] had been de-

---

[8] California Assembly Bill (AB) No. 4481, 1974, to amend California Welfare and Institutional Code, Chapter 1534, was signed by Governor Ronald Reagan on September 27, 1974. The test case, *Doe, Roe et al.* v. *Younger and Mayer,* 4 Civil 14407, was eventually argued before California's Fourth District Appellate Court, Division One, on June 11, 1975.

clared unconstitutional by the California Court of Appeals in April 1976 because of vague language, invasion of privacy (the bill required responsible relatives of the patients be notified), failure to provide for an adequate competency hearing, and invalid sanctions.

AB 1032 redefined informed consent, clarifying requirements for informing patients about proposed treatments and their options. It provided distinctions between voluntary and involuntary patients with respect to obtaining consent to ECT. Safeguards were added to protect confidentiality. Although much of the controversy over the eventual passage of AB 1032 concerned ECT regulations, I shall focus only on its psychosurgery provisions.

AB 1032 has fifteen sections; it amended certain parts of the existing California Welfare Institutional Code relating to mental health (sections 5325 through 5326,95 and 5715,3, and it repealed 5325,5). The first section (S,1) identifies the legislative intent to ensure the integrity and free choice of mental patients, recognizes their vulnerability, and itemizes their rights, including the right to refuse psychosurgery. It also specifies that such rights should be posted in English and Spanish.

Professionals in charge of a treatment facility can waive certain patients' rights (S,2) but not the right to refuse ECT or psychosurgery. Physicians in facilities administering ECT or psychosurgery (S,3) must report the numbers of treatments, the patients receiving the treatments, and any side effects and consequences. This information must be presented annually to the California legislature. Voluntary informed consent is stipulated, and it is expressly stated what information must be given to a patient (S,3,5) and what constitutes an informed consent (S,4,5, and 6).

The heart of the psychosurgery provisions of the California bill is S,7, which states that psychosurgery can be performed only if there is a written consent. Optimally, a close relative or guardian of the patient will be involved in the consent procedure. The attending physician must document the reasons for the procedure and demonstrate that all other appropriate therapies have been tried without success and that psychosurgery is needed. Three physicians other than the treating or petitioning physician must examine the patient and unanimously agree with the petitioner's views. They must also agree that the patient has the capacity to give an informed consent. Psychosurgery cannot be performed for at least seventy-two hours following a patient's written consent. Under no circumstances can it be performed on minors. Formal consent, once given, can be withdrawn at any time.

Sections 8, 8.5, 9, and 9.5 deal essentially with ECT. Sections 10 through 15 deal with administrative and legal aspects including sanctions.

Consequences

The passage of AB 1032 is instructive in light of the opposition and criticism to the original Vascancellos bill. In 1974, AB 4481, regulating ECT and psychosurgery, was passed by a vote of 72–0 in the California Assembly and 30–1 in the Senate and signed by Governor Reagan on September 27, 1974. Five public hearings and two meetings had been held involving psychiatrists, mental health directors, hospital spokesmen, and private citizens. The original bill's intent was to recognize and protect the free choice of therapy by mental patients. AB 4481 was scheduled to become law on January 1, 1975. In the meantime, some physicians refused to perform shock therapy on the grounds that provisions of AB 4481 were vague and that violation of its provisions subjected a physician to severe penalties. A temporary restraining order was issued on December 30, 1974, blocking California's Attorney General and the Director of Health from enforcing the bill. The case went to the California Fourth District Court of Appeals on a writ of mandate (*Doe, Roe et al.* v. *Younger and Mayer*, 4 Civil 14407) and was argued on June 11, 1975.

The court's decision declaring AB 4481 unconstitutional, on the basis of four counts noted earlier, was handed down on April 23, 1976.[9] The court largely upheld the basic thrust and intent of the legislation, and acknowledged that both psychosurgery and ECT were not fully understood, that the risks of psychosurgery were disputed, and, that adverse effects of ECT were not fully known or agreed upon. Regulation of intrusive and possibly hazardous forms of medical treatment was held to be a proper exercise of the state's police power, and public health and safety protection in the field of medical practice was deemed a legitimate function of the police power of the state. Importantly, the court held that mental patients should be distinguished from other patients because of the questions about their competency to give consent and, thus, their ability to voluntarily accept treatment. It therefore held: "These circumstances make the separate treatment of mental patients clearly rational related to the objective of ensuring their rights to refuse treatment. The special regulation of psychosurgery and ECT is also a

---

[9] District Court Appeal, Fourth Appellate District, Division One, State of California, April 23, 1976; 32 pages.

reasonable classification because these procedures, associated with mental illness, present a great danger of violating the patient's rights."

During the California hearings in April of 1975 on AB 1032, opposition was voiced by the California Medical Association, the local branch of the American Psychiatric Association, the Board of Medical Examiners, the Sacramento Director of Mental Health, and other local mental health unit directors. Support for AB 1032 came from the California Mental Health Association, the Association of Humanistic Psychology, the Youth Law Study, the Institute for the Study of Medical Ethics, the Friends Committee, the California Democratic Council, the ACLU, and the Libertarian Party. Additional support for AB 1032 came from the Department of Health, the Association for Humanistic Psychology, the Network Against Psychiatric Abuse (NAPA), the Citizens Commission for Human Rights, the San Francisco Mental Health Advisory Board, the California Democratic Council, the National Organization of Women (NOW), the Los Angeles County Mental Health Service, and the Youth Law Center of San Francisco. The California Hospital Association remained neutral.

AB 1032 subsequently passed. There were more than fifty changes from the original Vascancellos bill, most of which dealt with ECT, the center of controversy over AB 4481. Persons on both sides of the issues were unhappy with the final product. Former mental patients and others who favored the bill believed it gave too much power to physicians. Physicians, on the other hand, wanted no statutory regulations at all and opposed the civil penalty provision of the bill. Since passage of AB 1032 in 1977, California's Department of Mental Health records no reported psychosurgery cases through November 1, 1979, the date of the author's inquiry.

The National Commission's Recommendations

On March 14, 1977, a congressionally mandated report by the National Commission for the Protection of Human Subjects of Biomedical and Behavioral Research (National Commission, 1977) was completed and forwarded to DHEW Secretary Joseph Califano to be published by mid-May of that year for public comment. This publication, the product of two years' work, has two sections: an appendix and a report with recommendations. The appendix consists of three contract studies prepared especially for the Commission: a survey of the psychosurgical literature (1971–1976) by Elliot S.

Valenstein and two clinical studies, one conducted by Allan Mirsky and Maressa Orzack and the other by Hans-Lukas Teuber, Suzanne Corkin, and Thomas E. Twitchell. Valenstein's study contains a review of 629 articles dealing with psychosurgery and an appendix of clinical material, letters, and a review of postoperative complications after 1970. The two clinical studies (61 operated patients) document detailed efforts to assess the postoperative and, where possible, preoperative neuropsychological status of patients subjected to different psychosurgical operations.

The second part of the Commission's work is a seventy-six-page document entitled *Report and Recommendations: Psychosurgery*, which is divided into an introduction defining the Commission's work and seven chapters: a background review of the psychosurgery controversy; specific issues; legal considerations; commentary on the Commission studies (Appendix); minority conferences and public hearings material; recommendations (Chapter 6); and a dissenting statement by Commission member Patricia A. King.

The Commission affirmed that the use of psychosurgery for any purpose other than to provide treatment to psychiatrically impaired persons would and should be prohibited. Safeguards were recommended to prevent use of psychosurgery for purposes of social or institutional control. Eight recommendations were made.

Recommendation 1: Until the safety and usefulness of a psychosurgical operation has been shown, such operations should only be performed after a decision by an Institutional Review Board (IRB) approved by DHEW for the special purpose of reviewing psychosurgery, and only after such an IRB has determined: (1) that the surgeon is competent to perform the operation, (2) that the proposed surgery is appropriate, (3) that adequate pre- and postoperative evaluations will be performed, and (4) that the patient is informed and has consented.

Recommendation 2: Psychosurgery can be performed on adults voluntarily residing in mental hospitals with IRBs provided that a National Psychosurgery Advisory Board (a second proposed board) has determined that a specific psychosurgical operation works for a particular psychiatric disorder. Where such patients are research subjects, previously established Commission guidelines for the study of institutionalized mental patients obtain. As institutionalized people may be exceptionally vulnerable to suggestion as a consequence of their disability, dependent status, or depersonalization resulting from confinement, the designated IRB is admonished to scrutinize the adequacy and integrity of consent by such persons.

Recommendation 3: Ordinarily, psychosurgery should not be performed on prisoners, involuntarily committed patients, or incompetents unless certain conditions are met. If an individual cannot give an informed consent, Recommendation 3 suggests a mechanism whereby guarantees protecting a patient's right can be given by another. The Commission held that no individual should be denied a potentially beneficial psychosurgical operation simply because he or she was involuntarily confined or unable to understand what was at stake. However, the Commission advised that psychosurgery should not be performed over a patient's objection, even if the patient is incompetent and a guardian has given consent.

Recommendation 4: Psychosurgery was not ruled out for children, but it was not to be recommended unless passed on by a national psychosurgery advisory board, and met other tests. The Commission did not categorically wish to deny children the possible advantages of a new therapy that might be safer than, for example, long-term drug use.

Recommendation 5: DHEW should establish a mechanism for compiling and assessing information about psychosurgery, its occurrence in the United States, indications for its use, and the patients who receive it.

Recommendation 6: DHEW should evaluate psychosurgical operations and their efficacy, and also document that such surgery, where performed, was in compliance with adopted regulations.

Recommendation 7: Sanctions up to and including the withholding of federal funds should be provided to ensure compliance with adopted regulations.

Recommendation 8: Congress should take appropriate action to assure that psychosurgery is performed in compliance with DHEW regulations.

Table 20.1 summarizes some of the major similarities and differences in the current statutes regulating psychosurgery and the DHEW-contracted task force proposals for federal legislation.

Consequences

The Commission report was completed by DHEW on May 2, 1977, approved for public notice by Secretary Califano on May 13, 1977, and subsequently published in the *Federal Register* on May 23, 1977 (42: 26318–26332), seeking public comment by November 21, 1977.

Table 20.1 Comparison of Major Features of Current State Statutes and HEW Task Force Proposals for Federal Psychosurgery Regulations

	Oregon	California	HEW
Defines terms	Yes	Yes	Yes
Requires informed consent	Yes	Yes	Yes
Requires competency determination	Yes	Yes	Yes
Permits guardian consent for incompetents	Yes	No	Yes
Permits individual to refuse surgery	Yes	Yes	Yes
Permits incompetent to refuse surgery	No	Yes	Yes
Permits psychosurgery on children	Yes	No	Yes
Subjects psychosurgery procedures to review	Yes	Yes	Yes
Requires documentation of prior treatment failure	Yes	No	Yes
Requires documentation of psychiatric diagnosis	Yes	No	No
Requires specification of need	Yes	Yes	Yes
Requires documentation that specific operations work for designated disorders	Yes	No	Yes
Limits psychosurgery to specific institutions	No	No	Yes
Provides sanctions	Yes	Yes	Yes

Califano, reviewing the Commission's work and public comment, concluded his own efforts on November 6, 1978, and published his determination (in accordance with P.L. 93-348: National Research Act) in the *Federal Register* on November 15, 1978 (*43*: 53242–53243). It is not generally appreciated that the Secretary's final recommendations for a federal policy on psychosurgery essentially overruled the recommendations of the National Commission and outlawed for the time being psychosurgery on children, prisoners, incompetents, and the involuntarily committed.

Basically, the 1978 DHEW recommendations proposed the establishment of a Joint Commission on Psychosurgery (JCP) to voluntarily regulate psychosurgery through the issuance of guidelines and the formation of local psychosurgery review panels. Additionally, Califano promised the eventual publication of DHEW regulations for Public Health Service (PHS) hospitals or institutions with either PHS or DHEW support, and for patients funded by Medicaid or Medicare. A national registry of psychosurgery procedures would be set up by the JCP.

After Califano's November 15, 1978, determination, the work of the proposals was divided between the office of the General Council to the Secretary (regulations) and the Alcohol, Drug Abuse, and Mental Health Administration of DHEW (establishment of a JCP and a psychosurgery case registry). As of November 1, 1979, DHEW regulations had not been drafted, and two contract announcements in 1979 searching for an organization to develop a JCP and a psychosurgery registry produced no acceptable responses.

Comment

Through January 1, 1980, one psychosurgical procedure has been performed in Oregon since 1973 and none (reported) in California since 1977. It is rumored that a few patients from Oregon have been sent elsewhere for such operations, but no documentation has been presented. The Oregon and California bills effectively killed psychosurgery, but the reasons are by no means clear. One hears grumblings from private practice and academic circles in Oregon that the red tape involved in getting a patient through a Board review requires an inordinate amount of time and "hassle" for petitioners. There is some truth in this. To obtain approval for psychosurgery in Oregon, you have to demonstrate that a proper diagnosis has been made, that conventional therapies have been exhausted, that the procedure is needed, that your patient understands the risks and accepts them, and finally, that the treatment you seek, works. If the request for psychosurgery is for a minor, a prisoner, or an incompetent, procedural matters are even more difficult.

Practically speaking, obtaining Board approval in Oregon for psychosurgery requires perseverance, a belief in what you are doing, good clinical records, and some knowledge of the relevant literature. As a number of practitioners meet these requirements—especially where convictions about therapy are strong and a specific patient's welfare is at stake—the "hassle factor" argument would appear to be specious. Cases 5 and 6, reviewed earlier, shows that it is possible in Oregon to comply with regulations and obtain Board approval. Case 5 also illustrates an unexpected outcome of the Oregon legislation: When a delay is interposed between a psychosurgery petition and its final approval, for one reason or another the informed patient may drop out.

As no one has denied the logic or reasonableness of the legal, ethical, or medical steps pursuant to obtaining Board approval in Oregon, the decline in psychosurgery should be examined on other grounds. (In the two-year period prior to passage of the Oregon legislation, I estimated, from conversations with Portland neurosurgeons, that between 30 and 40 operations per year—mostly cingulotomies—being done in the state, exclusive of operations for pain. It is my contention that psychosurgery came to an end in Oregon simply because a careful look at the data on its efficacy, the multiplicity of brain targets for a diverse number of conditions, the selection of patients, the murkiness of psychiatric systematics and theory, and the diverse opinions on the management of disturbed patients argued against the practice of what appeared to some to be high-level phrenology. Where bureaucratic and legislative intrusion into a specific medical practice is successful, the practice is already moribund.

The experience with the Vascancellos bill in California has been more contentious because of its ECT sections, but the outcome on psychosurgery is essentially the same as in Oregon. There have been a few court challenges to the psychosurgery portion of the bill, but all failed. The office in the California Mental Health Division responsible for the psychosurgery registry in that state has no record of any procedure since the 1977 bill became law. Thus, for all intents and purposes, regulatory legislation in Oregon in 1973 and in California in 1977 effectively ended psychosurgery in these states with only one reported case (Oregon) in the period from 1973 to 1980.

As of late 1979, the consequence of the National Commission's efforts on psychosurgery has yet to generate specific federal guidelines on the subject or any enthusiasm in the federal or private sector for the establishment of a national review board. The National Commission's efforts should be viewed as a "consciousness raising" in the latter part of the 1970s of the complex issues surrounding psychosurgery at a national level. In my view, this effort contributed to the further decline of psychosurgery in the United States; by 1979, there were perhaps no more than 150–200 cases per year being done in the United States.

The Commission focused a great deal of their time on the general question of consent. They left open the possibility of psychosurgery on children, prisoners, incompetents, and the involuntarily committed. For critics, this reflected a too-heavy weighting of traditional scientific and clinical prerogatives against public sensitivities, available data, and the view that persons of limited capacity or persons involuntarily incarcerated were in no position to give knowledgeable and uncoerced consent to a damaging procedure on their own brain.

The promised DHEW regulations, banning psychosurgery on certain classes of subjects and strictly proscribing the direct or indirect role of federal funding in institutions performing psychosurgery, can only be expected to further inhibit psychosurgery practice in the United States. Finally, given the nonresponse to the DHEW contract proposals for the establishment of a JCP and registry, psychosurgery in the United States seems to be dying a natural or unnatural death, depending upon one's point of view.

It is of interest that Secretary Califano's belief that psychosurgery could be regulated on a voluntary basis by local psychosurgery boards is becoming a reality. Recently, a psychosurgery bill proposed by Representative Janet Clark of the Minnesota House of Representatives was countered by guidelines drafted by the Minnesota Medical Association that followed Califano on the matter of children, incompetents, prisoners, and the involuntarily confined, established a local review board, and recognized the issues listed in Table 20.1.

In summary, legislative regulation of psychosurgery in two Western states effectively ended the practice by 1980. Additionally, the spilling-over of the debate on psychosurgery out of traditional psychiatric and neurosurgical circles and into the public forum has had a complex but generally inhibiting effect on its continuation. Since the early 1970s, the number of procedures has continued to diminish. Failure of psychosurgeons and psychiatrists to obtain support from colleagues in the clinical and basic neurosciences rests, in my judgment, not on fears of lawsuits, radical voices, and misguided thinking, but on knowledgeable reflection that such procedures were essentially prescientific and phrenological in concept without sound theoretical or clinical foundation and contrary to current thinking on the biology of the mind–behavior transaction. In the last analysis, regulation of psychosurgery came about because of its inadequate scientific base, which weakened the argument of noninterference in clinical judgment prerogatives by its physician supporters. Such arguments were no match for intelligent inquiry, critical data, and the application of humanistic precepts as knowledgeable, informed, and uncoerced consent. The real significance of the psychosurgery regulation in the 1970s lies, not with the merits of scientific or clinical arguments, but in the legacy of a serious and applied concern for the adequacy of legal, ethical, and scientific issues where treatment of the mentally disturbed is concerned.

Medical controversies are difficult to resolve in public arenas.

Anyone familiar with legislative hearing rooms knows the impossibility of providing legislators with adequate clinical and scientific information on the questions involved, let alone on more difficult social and ethical issues, which are often partisan, impassioned, and divisive. Legislative forums may be good for the "emotional juices," but they produce a winners-versus-losers division, with chronic disgruntlement in its wake.

What is needed in each state are small, dedicated standing councils that would update for the legislatures (and the public) the salient features of controversial medical and scientific practice with respect to treatment outcomes and the ethical, legal, religious, and political questions sometimes raised. Such councils, formulated from the best talent locally available, should be provided with special core libraries where students of these issues could study. The purpose of such councils would be to crystallize issues at local levels for public discussion and to provide elected representatives with an authoritative local resource. Where elected representatives are treated to reliable information translated into plain English, and from persons they know or who are locally based, their decisions about medical issues would be greatly improved and all of us would be the better for it.

CHAPTER 21

The Concept of Informed Consent

Samuel I. Shuman

Judicial Precedents

Precedents Prior to the Kaimowitz Case

Probably the single most frequently quoted statement about informed consent is that of Justice Cardozo, made while he was still on the bench in New York: "Every human being of adult years, with sound mind, has a right to determine what shall be done with his own body."[1] As is so often the case, the problem comes, not in understanding the thrust of the general principle, but in articulating general rules for advancing the policies behind the principle. Nowhere is this difficult development from general principles to rules better illustrated than in the development of the concept of informed consent. The problem has been especially difficult in the context of experimental medicine because there have been so few significant judicial pronouncements about informed consent as ap-

---

[1] *Schloendorff* v. *Society of N.Y. Hosp.*, 211 N.Y. 125, 105 N.E. 92, 93 (1914).

plicable to experimental medicine. The decision of the Michigan court in the *Kaimowitz*[2] case is a dramatic exception. Perhaps the most significant earlier precedent was another Michigan case, *Fortner* v. *Koch*, in which the court said, "we recognize the fact that, if the general practice of medicine and surgery is to progress, there must be a certain amount of experimentation carried on; but such experiments must be done with the knowledge and consent of the patient, or those responsible for him, and must not vary too radically from the accepted method of procedure."[3]

Before turning to the *Kaimowitz* decision, which speaks directly to the issue of informed consent in experimental medicine, let us briefly consider a modern precedent that has had a far-reaching effect on the general concept of informed consent. That precedent is the decision in the 1972 case of *Canterbury* v. *Spence*,[4] in which the court declined to follow the prevailing view that informed consent requires only that the physician disclose risks normally disclosed by other physicians in the community. This so-called objective community standard, which relied upon expert testimony to establish the prevailing standard, was dropped in *Canterbury*. Instead, it was held that the jury must decide "(1) whether a reasonable patient would have deemed undisclosed information 'significant' in deciding whether to submit to a course of treatment (materiality); and (2) whether a reasonable patient would have foregone that treatment had the information been disclosed (approximate cause)."[5] This modification of the previously prevailing standard has been followed in a number of recent informed consent cases.

The net result of this development is to compel the physician to make those disclosures that the so-called reasonable or prudent patient would expect were he asked to grant consent. Consequently, if the physician fails to make those disclosures, which if made would cause a reasonable patient to withhold consent, then the physician may be liable for damages. In substituting the "prudent patient" test for the "objective standard," the court in *Canterbury* added that a risk would be deemed material and therefore subject to disclosure "when a reasonable person, in what the physician knows, or should know, to be the patient's position, would be likely to attach signifi-

---

[2] *Kaimowitz* v. *Department of Mental Health*, Civil No. 73-19434-AW (Cir. Ct., Wayne Co., Mich., July 10, 1973). Summarized at 42 U.S.L.W. 2063 (July 31, 1973). References are to the slip opinion.
[3] 272 Mich. 373, 261 N.W. 762 (1935).
[4] *Canterbury* v. *Spence*, 464 F.2d 772 (D.C. Cir. 1972), *cert. denied* 409 U.S. 1064 (1972).
[5] Id. at 783.

cance to the risk or cluster of risks in deciding."[6] While the *Canterbury* test was not developed in the context of experimental medicine, it is interesting to note that the informed consent requirements for experimentation with human subjects laid down by HEW, FDA, and the VA are operationally very close, if not identical, to the *Canterbury* requirements. The net effect is that, for treatment or experiment, disclosures must be sufficient to enable a reasonably prudent person, be he patient, subject, or one legally empowered to grant permission on behalf of a patient or subject, to make an informed decision; this means a decision where the knowledge requirements have been satisfied.

Kaimowitz v. *Department of Mental Health*

In this leading case, the Michigan circuit court, a court of original jurisdiction and not an appellate court, confronted directly the specific issue of consent for a procedure that was deemed to be experimental and that was being considered for someone already institutionalized on the grounds of mental disability. The prospective subject in that case had for some seventeen years been institutionalized as a criminal sexual psychopath.

Before proceeding to trial on the issue of consent with an involuntarily committed subject, the court considered the constitutionality of the criminal sexual psychopath provision, pursuant to which the prospective subject had been detained for all those years. The court found the statute to be unconstitutional and ordered the subject released from the institution. Despite the release of the subject, it was urged that the trial proceed on the consent issues, and the several counsel, although representing different interests in the case, agreed that the following two questions should be considered by the court:

1. After failure of established therapies, may an adult or the legally appointed guardian, if the adult is involuntarily detained at a facility within the State Department of Mental Health, give legally adequate consent to an innovative or experimental surgical procedure on the brain, if there is demonstrable physical abnormality of the brain and the procedure is designed to ameliorate behavior which is either personally tormenting to the patient or so profoundly disruptive that the patient cannot safely live or live with others?

[6]Id. at 783.

2. If the answer to the above question is yes, then is it legal in the state to undertake an innovative or experimental surgical procedure on the brain of an adult involuntarily detained at a facility within the jurisdiction of the State Department of Mental Health, if there is demonstrable physical abnormality of the brain and the procedure is designed to ameliorate behavior which is personally tormenting to the patient or so profoundly disruptive that the patient cannot safely live or live with others?

After hearing argument to the contrary, the court held that the issues raised by these two questions were not moot since the state might find another subject for the proposed experimental procedure. The court heard complex testimony about the particular procedure involved, a procedure denominated as psychosurgery, and made the following major findings:

1. Psychosurgery should never be undertaken upon involuntarily committed populations, when there is a high-risk, low-benefit ratio as demonstrated in this case. This is because of the impossibility of obtaining truly informed consent from such populations.

2. Generally, individuals are allowed free choice about whether to undergo experimental medical procedures. But the State has the power to modify this free choice concerning the experimental medical procedures when it cannot be freely given, or when the result would be contrary to public policy. For example, it is obvious that a person may not consent to acts that will constitute murder, manslaughter, or mayhem upon himself. In short, there are times when the State, for good reason, should withhold a person's ability to consent to certain medical procedures.

3. We do not agree that a truly informed consent cannot be given for a regular surgical procedure by a patient, institutionalized or not. The law has long recognized that such valid consent can be given. But we do hold that informed consent cannot be given by an involuntarily detained mental patient for experimental psychosurgery. . . .

4. To be legally adequate, a subject's informed consent must be competent, knowing, and voluntary.

5. Involuntarily confined mental patients live in an inherently coercive institutional environment. Indirect and subtle psychological coercion has profound effect upon the patient population. Involuntarily confined patients cannot reason as equals with the doctors and administrators over whether they should undergo psychosurgery. They are not able to voluntarily give informed consent because of the inherent inequality of their position.

6. The keystone to any intrusion upon the body of a person must be full, adequate, and informed consent. The integrity of the individual must be protected from invasion into his body and personality not voluntarily agreed to. Consent is not an idle or symbolic art; it is a fundamental requirement for the protection of the individual's integrity.

We, therefore, conclude that involuntarily detained mental patients cannot give informed and adequate consent to experimental psychosurgical procedures on the brain.

7. The State's interest in performing psychosurgery and the legal ability of the involuntarily detained mental patient to give consent must bow to the First Amendment, which protects the generation and free flow of ideas from unwarranted interference with one's mental processes.

To allow an involuntarily detained mental patient to consent to the type of psychosurgery proposed in this case, and to permit the State to perform it, would be to condone State action in violation of basic First Amendment rights of such patients, because impairing the power to generate ideas inhibits the full dissemination of ideas.

Federal Agency Regulations

Pursuant to regulations that became effective in July of 1974,[7] and applicable to any HEW research involving human subjects, informed consent was defined as follows:

"Informed consent" means the knowing consent of an individual or his legally authorized representative, so situated as to be able to exercise free power of choice without undue inducement or any element of force, fraud, deceit, duress, or other form of constraint or coercion. The basic elements of information necessary to such consent include:

1. A fair explanation of the procedures to be followed, and their purposes, including identification of any procedures which are experimental;

2. A description of any attendant discomforts and risks reasonably to be expected;

3. A description of any benefits reasonably to be expected;

4. A disclosure of any appropriate alternative procedures that might be advantageous for the subject;

5. An offer to answer any inquiries concerning the procedures; and

6. An instruction that the person is free to withdraw his consent and to discontinue participation in the project or activity at any time without prejudice to the subject.

The Energy Research and Development Administration's proposed regulations for research involving human subjects contain the same definitional standards for informed consent.

The 1977 Institutional Guide to Consumer Product Safety Commission Policy (on protection of human subjects)[8] contains the following provisions on informed consent:

---

[7] 39 Fed. Reg. 18913 (May 30, 1974).
[8] CPSC Publication, May 1977, U.S. Gov't Printing Office: 1977-720-000/8853.

Informed consent is the agreement obtained from a subject, or from his authorized representative, to the subject's participation in an activity.

The basic elements of informed consent are: [the same as those promulgated by HEW].

In addition, the agreement, written or oral, entered into by the subject, should include no exculpatory language through which the subject is made to waive, or to appear to waive, any of his or her legal rights, or to release the institution or its agents from liability for negligence.

Consent should be obtained, whenever practicable, from the subjects themselves. When the subject group will include individuals who are not legally or physically capable of giving informed consent, because of age, mental incapacity, or inability to communicate, the review committee should consider the validity of consent by next of kin, legal guardians, or by other qualified third parties representative of the subject's interest. In such instances, careful consideration should be given by the committee not only to whether these third parties can be presumed to have the necessary depth of interest and concern with the subjects' rights and welfare, but also to whether these third parties will be legally authorized to expose the subjects to the risks involved.

The review committee will determine if the consent required, whether to be secured before the fact, in writing or orally, or after the fact following debriefing, or whether implicit in voluntary participation in an adequately advertised activity, is appropriate in light of the risks to the subject, and the circumstances of the project.

The review committee will also determine if the information to be given to the subject, or to qualified third parties, in writing or orally, is a fair explanation of the project or activity, of its possible benefits, and of its attendant hazards.

Where an activity involves therapy, diagnosis, or management, and a professional/patient relationship exists, it is necessary "to recognize that each patient's mental and emotional condition is important. . . . and that in discussing the element of risk, a certain amount of discretion must be employed consistent with full disclosure of fact necessary to any informed consent". [Salgo vs. Leland Stanford Jr. University Board of Trustees (154 C.A. 2nd 560; 317 P. 2d 1701).]

Where an activity does not involve therapy, diagnosis, or management, and a professional/subject, rather than a professional/patient, relationship exists, "the subject is entitled to a full and frank disclosure of all the facts, probabilities, and opinions which a reasonable man might be expected to consider before giving his consent". [Halushka vs. University of Saskatchewan (1965) 53 D.L.R. (2d).]

When debriefing procedures are considered as a necessary part of the plan, the committee should ascertain that these will be complete and prompt.

The Public Health Service rules for programs in which sterilization is available provide that:[9]

---

[9] 38 Fed. Reg. 26459 (Sept. 21, 1973).

§ 50.302 Definitions

A person "legally incapable of giving consent" includes any person who (1) under State law, is a minor whose consent to the sterilization would not be legally effective, (2) has been adjudicated incompetent by a court of competent jurisdiction, or (3) in the judgment of a responsible program or project official, appears to be incapable of giving informed consent because of a mental condition or lack of mental capacity.

§ 50.303 General policy

(1) A Review Committee, as described in § 50.304, has reviewed and approved the sterilization, and

(2) In the case of an individual who is legally incapable of giving consent, a court of competent jurisdiction has determined that the proposed sterilization is in the best interests of the patient.

In no case shall sterilization be performed on a legally competent individual, irrespective of age, unless that individual has given written informed consent to the sterilization.

The National Commission's Recommendations

Pursuant to the National Research Service Award Act, enacted by Congress in 1974,[10] there has been established a commission, known as the National Commission for the Protection of Human Subjects of Biomedical and Behavioral Research. As regards such research, this eleven-member Commission has made the most important current contributions to the development of the issues surrounding the problem of informed consent.

Research with Prisoners

In the Report and Recommendations on Research Involving Prisoners,[11] the Commission prefaced its recommendations with a section titled "Deliberations and Conclusions." In this section, the Commission states:

> To respect a person is to allow that person to live in accord with his or her deliberate choices. Since the choices of prisoners in all matters except those explicitly withdrawn by law should be respected, as courts increasingly affirm, it seems at first glance that the principle of respect for persons requires that prisoners not be deprived of the opportunity to volunteer for research. Indeed, systematic deprivation of this freedom would also violate the principle of justice, since it

---

[10] Public Law 93-348; 88 Stat. 342; M.R. 7724.
[11] DHEW Publication No. (OS) 76-131.

would arbitrarily deprive one class of person of benefits available to others—namely, the benefits of participation in research.

However, the application of the principles of respect and justice allows another interpretation, which the Commission favors. When persons seem regularly to engage in activities which, were they stronger or in better circumstances, they would avoid, respect dictates that they be protected against those forces that appear to compel their choices. It has become evident to the Commission that, although prisoners who participate in research affirm that they do so freely, the conditions of social and economic deprivation in which they live compromise their freedom. The Commission believes, therefore, that the appropriate expression of respect consists in protection from exploitation. . . .

Reflection upon these principles and upon the actual conditions of imprisonment in our society has led the Commission to believe that prisoners are, as a consequence of being prisoners, more subject to coerced choice and more readily available for the imposition of burdens which others will not willingly bear. Thus, it has inclined towards protections as the most appropriate expression of respect for prisoners as persons and toward redistribution of those burdens of risk and inconvenience which are presently concentrated upon prisoners.

While these recommendations do not specifically develop criteria for informed consent with an institutionalized population, the material is relevant because it does concern such a population. Recommendation 3 requires that there be "a high degree of voluntariness on the part of the prospective participants and of openness on the part of the institution(s)" and further provides that minimum requirements for such voluntariness and openness "include adequate living conditions, provisions for effective redress of grievances, separation of research participation from parole considerations, and public scrutiny." In the comment following this recommendation, the Commission specifies some seventeen quite precise living standards, which are deemed relevant in determining whether or not the institution can even be considered as one within which research might be conducted with an institutionalized population.

Recommendation 4 provides that, in reviewing research proposals, at least the following should be considered: "the risks involved, provisions for obtaining informed consent, safeguards to protect individual dignity and confidentiality, procedures for the selection of subjects, and provisions for providing compensation for research-related injury." In the comment following this recommendation, the Commission states: "In negotiations regarding consent, it should be determined that the written or verbal comprehensibility of the information presented is appropriate to the subject population." The comment also contains the statement that "prisoners who are minors, mentally disabled or retarded should not be included as subjects unless the research is related to their particular condition, and complies with the standards for research involving those groups as well as those for prisoners."

Research with Children

In September 1977, the Commission issued its final recommendations on research with children.[12] As regards informed consent, the most relevant material is contained in Recommendation 7, where the Commission provides:

> The Institutional Review Board should determine that adequate provisions are made for: (A) soliciting the assent of the children (when capable) and the permission of their parents or guardians; and, when appropriate, (B) monitoring the solicitation of assent and permission, and involving at least one parent or guardian in the conduct of the research. A child's objection to participation in research should be binding unless the intervention holds out a prospect of direct benefit that is important to the health or well-being of the child and is available only in the context of the research.

Commenting upon this recommendation, the Commission further develops the problem of consent and lack of competence.

> The Commission uses the term parental or guardian "permission," rather than "consent," in order to distinguish what a person may do autonomously (consent) from what one may do on behalf of another (grant permission). Parental permission normally will be required for the participation of children in research. In addition, assent of the children should be required when they are seven years of age or older. The Commission uses the term "assent" rather than "consent" in this context, to distinguish a child's agreement from a legally valid consent. . . .
> Parental or guardian permission should reflect the collective judgment of the family that an infant or child may participate in research. . . . The IRB [Institutional Review Board] should determine for each project whether permission of one or both parents should be required, a substitute mechanism may be used, or the provision may be waived. In making such determination, the IRB should consider the nature of the activities described in the research protocol and the age, status and condition of the subjects. . . .
> The Commission believes that children who are seven years of age or older are generally capable of understanding the procedures and general purpose of research and of indicating their wishes regarding participation. Their assent should be required in addition to parental permission. However, if any child over six years of age is incapacitated

---

[12] DHEW Publication No. (OS) 77-0004.

so that he or she cannot reasonably be consulted, then parental permission should be sufficient, as it is for infants. The objection of a child of any age to participation in research should be binding except as noted below.

If the research protocol includes an intervention from which the subjects might derive significant benefit to their health or welfare, and that intervention is available only in a research context, the objection of a small child may be overridden. . . . As children mature, their ability to perceive and act in their own best interest increases; thus, their wishes with respect to such research should carry increasingly more weight. When school age children disagree with their parents regarding participation in such research, the IRB may wish to have a third party discuss the matter with all concerned and be present during the consent process. Although parents may legally override the objections of school age children in such cases, the burden of that decision becomes heavier in relation to the maturity of the particular child.

Disclosure requirements for assent and permission are the same as those for legally valid informed consent. Similarly, children and parents or guardians should be free from duress. In order to assure full understanding and freedom of choice, the IRB may determine that there is a need for an advocate to be present during the decision-making process. The need for third-party involvement in this process will vary according to the risk presented by the research, and the autonomy of the subjects. The advocate should be an individual who has the experience and perceptiveness to fulfill such a role and who is not related in any way (except in the role as advocate or member of the IRB) to the research or the investigators.

Finally, the IRB should pay particular attention to the explanation and consent form, if any, to assure that appropriate language is used.

Recommendation 10 provides that children who are institutionalized as mentally infirm may participate in research only if the further conditions regarding research with the institutionalized mentally infirm are fulfilled.

Commission Regulations on Psychosurgery

On March 14, 1977, the Commission submitted its recommendations and report on psychosurgery to the President, Congress, and HEW.[13] In a chapter preceding the actual recommendations, the Commission dealt with "legal considerations" and there considered the *Kaimowitz* case. I quote from the Commission report.

---

[13] DHEW Publication No. (OS) 77-0001.

The informed consent and constitutional rulings of *Kaimowitz* have not been universally accepted. *Kaimowitz'* argument that involuntarily detained persons do not have the capacity for informed consent to psychosurgery has been criticized by commentators. Moreover, the California penal legislation, enacted after the *Kaimowitz* decision, rejected the theory that involuntary confinement by itself precluded capacity for consent to risky experimental therapy. The constitutional barriers to valid consent set up by *Kaimowitz* have been greeted even more skeptically. It is not clear whether the court was concluding that (1) an involuntarily confined patient's free speech and privacy rights prevented the patient, regardless of his or her capacity for informed consent, from giving a valid consent, or (2) the constitutional protections required a conclusive presumption that all such patients be considered incompetent to consent. The first interpretation is severely questioned when applied to patients who would otherwise have the capacity for informed consent. Commentators have argued that the Constitution can no more preclude consent to psychosurgery than it can forbid consent to standard psychotherapy. In both cases, the Constitution protects the competent individual's right to choose whether or not to permit interference with his or her mental activity. The second interpretation has also been criticized harshly. A "conclusive or irrebuttable presumption" of incompetency would appear to conflict with First Amendment and privacy cases which require that individuated rulings must be made on claims which involve infringement of fundamental rights. . . .

Aside from *Kaimowitz*, which refused to recognize proxy consent to amygdalotomy, there have been no cases that have decided the difficult issues raised by third-party consent to psychosurgery. A complete prohibition of psychosurgery upon patients lacking the capacity for consent, however, may not be a permissible approach. . . .

Conclusion—The *Kaimowitz* approach might not prevail today. With new data indicating that certain psychosurgical procedures are less hazardous than previously thought and potentially of significant therapeutic value, the Oregon model (requiring committee review of both consent and the merits of the therapy, as well as a reporting system recognizing proxy consent, and permitting psychosurgery on involuntarily detained patients) should be secure from constitutional or informed consent doctrine challenges.

As regards the use of psychosurgery with institutionalized populations, the Commission states:

> Because institutionalized persons may be vulnerable as a consequence of their disability or the dependence and depersonalization which often result from confinement, the IRB should scrutinize with care the consent of such persons to determine whether it is adequate. If the IRB has good reason to believe a patient is unable to give informed consent to psychosurgery, the provisions of Recommendation (3) will apply.

Recommendation (3) A psychosurgical procedure should not be performed on an adult patient who (i) is a prisoner, (ii) is involuntarily committed to a mental institution, (iii) has a legal guardian of the person, or (iv) is believed by the Institutional Review Board (IRB) to be incapable of giving informed consent to such procedure, unless all of the following conditions are satisfied: (A) A national psychosurgery advisory board has determined that the specific psychosurgical procedure has demonstrable benefit for the treatment of an individual with the psychiatric symptom or disorder of the patient; (B) If the operation is to be performed as part of a research project, the conditions set forth in the Commission's report on research involving prisoners or report on research involving the institutionalized mentally infirm, as applicable, are fulfilled; (C) The conditions of recommendation (1) are fulfilled at the institution where the operation is to be performed, and such institution is separate from any prison or institution where the patient is regularly confined; (D) The patient has given informed consent or, if the patient is believed by the IRB to be incapable of giving informed consent, the patient's guardian of the person has given informed consent and the patient does not object; and (E) A court in which the patient had legal representation has approved the performance of the operation. (One Commission member dissented.)

Comment: Fairness requires that individuals should not be denied access to potentially beneficial therapy simply because they are involuntarily confined or unable to give informed consent. The Commission recognizes, however, that such individuals are vulnerable to coercion and that psychosurgery may be proposed in attempts to modify behavior for social or institutional purposes not coinciding with the patients' own interests or desires. Accordingly, the Commission recommends court review and, in some instances, appointment of a legal guardian in addition to the required determinations by an IRB and the national Psychosurgery Advisory Board. The Commission also recommends that the IRB review and the surgery itself be performed at a facility that is administratively independent of any facility in which the patient is regularly confined. . . .

The IRB and court should ascertain that a prisoner or other person involuntarily confined is never compelled to undergo psychosurgery or unduly influenced to consent to psychosurgery by the promise of probation, parole, reduction of sentence, release or otherwise.

Consent given on behalf of mental patients who are unable to give legally valid consent themselves should be reviewed with an awareness of the potential for conflict of interest inherent in such third-party consent. The consenting guardian should not be affiliated with the institution where the patient is confined or where the psychosurgery is to be performed. Consent given by the legal guardian of a patient who is not institutionalized should also be scrutinized to take into account the potential conflicts of interest that may be associated with the responsibility of providing care for such persons.

If the IRB has good reason to believe that a patient, lacking a legal guardian, is incapable of giving informed consent for psychosurgery, the IRB should withhold approval of the operation pending authorization by a court and consent of a legal guardian, if one is appointed. If no court accepts jurisdiction, however, the operation should not be performed on such a patient. Similarly, in states that do not accept third-party consent for psychosurgery, a psychosurgical procedure should not be performed on a patient believed by the IRB to be unable to give informed consent for such an operation. *In no case should a psychosurgical procedure be performed over the objection of an adult patient, even following adjudication of incompetence and with the consent of a legal guardian.*

The Commission recognizes that portions of the recommendation are at variance with the opinion of the Michigan court in *Kaimowitz* v. *Department of Mental Health* (1973). The Commission agrees with the *Kaimowitz* opinion that institutionalization may diminish the ability of prisoners and mental patients to make free choices by removing opportunities for asserting or exercising self-determination. On the other hand, it seems unfair to exclude prisoners or involuntarily confined patients from the opportunity to seek benefit from the new therapies on the basis of an unrebuttable presumption of diminished capacity or by prohibiting third-party consent. Therefore, the Commission recommends that such persons be permitted to obtain psychosurgery, subject to the extensive review requirements described above, and the expressed willingness of the patient to undergo the surgery.

Research with Institutionalized Mentally Infirm

At the last meeting of the Commission for which I have summary minutes available, November 11 and 12, 1977, the Commission did consider again the subject of research with institutionalized mentally infirm, and what follows is taken from what appear to be the final recommendations (with minor word changes still possible).[14] I quote here only from the provisions most directly concerned with the consent issue.

> *Recommendation (2)* Research that does not present more than minimal risk to subjects who are institutionalized as mentally infirm may be conducted or supported provided an Institutional Review Board has determined that. . . .
>
> (B) Adequate provisions are made to assure that no subject will participate in the research unless (i) the subject has assented or (ii) if the research is relevant to the subject's condition and the subject is incapable of assenting in a meaningful way, the subject does not object to such participation.
>
> *Recommendation (3)* Research in which more than minimal risk to subjects is presented by an intervention that holds out the prospect

---

[14] Summary Minutes, National Commission for the Protection of Human Subjects, Nov. 11–12, 1977.

of direct benefit for the individual subjects, or by a monitoring procedure required for the well-being of the subjects, may involve those institutionalized as mentally infirm provided. . . .

(B) If the subject is an adult, the subject has assented or does not object and, where appropriate, a third party has consented on behalf of the subject, under the following conditions: (i) the consent process should be observed by an adviser appointed for this purpose by the Institutional Review Board; (ii) if the consent auditor determines that the subject has the ability to understand the nature of the procedures to be used in the proposed research and the attendant risk and anticipated benefit, and can communicate his or her choice in a meaningful manner, the assent of the subject should be deemed sufficient (if there has been an adjudication of incompetency, the consent of a guardian may also be required by state law); (iii) if the consent auditor determines that assent cannot be given (under the standard described in paragraph (B)(ii), above), a guardian of the person may consent on behalf of the subject (if a guardian of the person has not been appointed, such appointment should be requested at a court of competent jurisdiction); and (iv) the subject should not be involved in research over his or her objection unless such participation has been specifically authorized by a court of competent jurisdiction; and

(C) If the subject is a child, the subject has assented (if capable) and the subject's parent(s) or guardian have consented; a child who is institutionalized as mentally infirm should not be involved in research over his or her objection unless such participation has been specifically authorized by a court of competent jurisdiction.

Recommendation (4) Research in which more than minimal risk to subjects is presented by an intervention that does not hold out the prospect of direct benefit for the individual subjects, or by a monitoring procedure that is not required for the well-being of the subjects, may involve those institutionalized as mentally infirm, provided. . . .

(B) If the subject is an adult, the subject has assented or does not object and, where appropriate, a third party has consented on behalf of the subject, under the following conditions: (i) the consent process should be observed by an adviser appointed for this purpose by the Institutional Review Board; (ii) if the consent auditor determines that the subject has the ability to understand the nature of the procedures to be used in the proposed research and the attendant risk and anticipated benefit, and can communicate his or her choice in a meaningful manner, the assent of the subject should be deemed sufficient (if there has been an adjudication of incompetency, the consent of a guardian may also be required by state law); (iii) if the consent auditor determines that assent cannot be given (under the standard described in paragraph (B)(ii), above) a guardian of the person may consent on behalf of the subject (if a guardian of the person has not been appointed, such appointment should be requested at a court of competent jurisdiction); and (iv) the subject should not be involved in research over his or her objection; and

(C) If the subject is a child, the requirements of the commission's recommendation (5) on research involving children are satisfied.

AAMD "Consent Handbook"

In 1977 the American Association on Mental Deficiency published an eighty-page "Consent Handbook."[15] The handbook represents one of the first efforts to deal systematically with the problems of consent across the broad spectrum of issues and thus represents one of the first consent "codes." Hence, despite what may be the special interests and biases of the AAMD, the handbook deserves careful consideration, even if it lacks the status of a judicial precedent, a federal agency rule, or a recommendation promulgated by a commission created pursuant to an act of Congress.

The following is taken from the discussion on experimentation:

> Proposals recently have been made to exclude from research projects at least institutionalized mentally retarded persons. But this development is alarming. It threatens an abrupt decline in research: the major hope for new knowledge that could benefit mentally retarded people.
>
> By now, it is apparent that principles of normalization require that retarded persons not be excluded automatically from participation in research projects. However, their own inherent mental limitations and, at times, the potentially coercive elements of the environments in which they find themselves or in which the research will be conducted must be recognized and reflected in consent procedures.
>
> MINIMUM REQUIREMENTS OF ALL RESEARCH PROPOSALS. A retarded person should NOT be asked to participate in a proposed project if the research objectives can be met, within reason, by the use of nonretarded subjects. Further, the study must have a significant potential for directly benefiting a given participant or for contributing new knowledge that might benefit other retarded individuals or their families or prevent mental retardation. (Note that the "direct benefit rule" is only one criterion for participation in research; there is another criterion.)
>
> If the proposed project meets these conditions, then it must be reviewed and endorsed as scientifically sound. Moreover, the plans and procedures for securing consent also must be reviewed and endorsed as adequate. Two types of review, then, are required: one as to scientific methodology, and another as to the adequacy of consent. . . .
>
> Mentally retarded people must not be exploited as research subjects. They should not be used merely for the investigator's convenience. To put it another way, non-retarded people should not be used when the research objectives can be met equally by them [*sic*]. This is so because they are more likely to comprehend explanations regarding conditions of participation, risk, intrusiveness, and reversibility. Yet, under some circumstances, it is wholly appropriate for retarded people

---

[15] Turnbull, H. R., Ed., *Consent Handbook*, Am. Assoc. on Mental Deficiency, Inc. Special Publication No. 3 (1977).

to be included in a project. This may occur, for example, when institutionalized mentally retarded people furnish the only subjects for research, such as research on the effects on the retarded of institutionalization or de-institutionalization.

Conclusion

It should be clear from what has been presented above as "the existing state of the art," that the trend is toward maximizing individual autonomy, even where the price paid for such autonomy may
be some significant diminution in the *medical* good health of the
autonomous patient or subject. The one apparent deviation from
this trend, back toward "the doctor knows best" tradition, is where
children or mentally disabled persons may have their desires overridden when the intervention is experimental, but therapeutic. The
generalized principle that would appear to accommodate both the
trend and the seeming deviation is that the autonomy of individuals
should be respected so long as the individual is competent enough
to be treated as autonomous. To this principle must be added the
standard for determining who should be considered competent—
namely, those who have not been judicially declared to be incompetent and children who are "capable of understanding the procedures
and general purpose of research and of indicating their wishes."

The long and short of all these rules and judicial precedents is that
if courts, parents, and doctors concur in the judgment that one deserves to be respected as a competent human being, then there is
some reasonable chance that one may be able to decide for oneself
about participation in biomedical experimentation. As offensive as
this may seem to some, the relevant question is not whether the test
is objectionable, but rather whether there is some better way to
achieve the presumably shared objectives of maximization of autonomy, prevention of exploitation, and fairness in the distribution of
unavoidable burdens. Hence the question becomes not whether the
Commission rules and court decisions frustrate any of these shared
goals, but rather whether there is a better way to prevent exploitation while properly respecting autonomy and principles of distribu-
tive justice.

In a post-trial brief submitted to the court in the *Kaimowitz* case, I
presented arguments contrary to the conclusions reached by that
court and much closer to the recommendations ultimately promulgated by the National Commission. The portion of that brief dealing with informed consent appears as an appendix in my recently

published *Psychosurgery and the Medical Control of Violence* (Shuman, 1977). In addition, there is some further discussion on the informed consent issue in that book.

Since my own views on the relevant issues are thus already readily accessible, perhaps it will suffice if I here conclude by suggesting that, on balance, the Commission's recommendations do strike me as generally reasonable and fair in that they do effect an acceptable adjustment of the shared objectives. There is a rather clear preference for mechanisms that should prevent exploitation, even when the price paid for the preference is a diminution in autonomy. I prefer the opposite risk and would generally aim at the maximization of autonomy, even when doing so might create greater risks of possible exploitation. But the Commission recommendations are so clearly within the domain "where reasonable men may differ," that it would be a disservice to try to pick them apart. Instead, it is to be hoped that HEW will soon issue the final rules that it was supposed to formulate after receiving Commission recommendations, and that the relevant professions can then see what the actual consequences are of working, for the first time, under reasonably explicit rules designed to cover biomedical research with human subjects. (It is interesting to note the following item in the Summary Minutes for the Commission meeting in November: "Commission members agreed to write a letter to HEW Secretary Califano, calling his attention to the fact that departmental action on the Commission's report and recommendations regarding research involving prisoners is several months overdue.")

CHAPTER 22

Legal and Ethical Reflections on Neurosurgical Intervention

William A. Carnahan and Vernon H. Mark

When considering neurosurgical intervention, the general reader is deluged by arguments calling for judicial, legislative, and administrative involvement in the clinical practice of neurosurgery. In our view, these arguments are both quite unconvincing and essentially without merit.

Anti-Neurosurgical Arguments

The arguments for some type of governmental involvement cluster into six groupings. First, the brain is considered to be a unique bodily organ and thus deserving of governmental protection. Second, the neurosurgeon cannot be considered an impartial decision maker. Due to the fee-for-service nature of his profession, he has an economic incentive to invade the cranial vault. Third, neurosurgical intervention is often in aid of experimental goals rather than patient care. Fourth, the irreversibility of the procedure distinguishes neurosurgery from other forms of surgical intervention. Fifth, the

risks so outweigh the benefits to the patient that public policy requires governmental regulation of the nature and scope of permissible neurosurgical practice. Sixth, the consent of the patient, which
is the legally required touchstone for neurosurgical intervention,
cannot be assured.

Brain Ideology

Perhaps the most frenetic argument advanced for governmental involvement is that of the uniqueness of the brain. But why, one may
ask, is the brain unique? Not so, according to the ancient Greeks
who espoused a "radiator" theory of the brain according to which
the sole function of the brain was to cool one's blood. Quite so,
according to the judicial panel in the *Kaimowitz* decision, which
opted for a "generator" theory according to which a major function
of the brain is to generate ideas.[1] Just as history has proven the
ancient Greeks to have erred, neurophysiology may yet prove the
court in *Kaimowitz* to be in error. As the neurosurgeon Wilder Penfield has noted:

> In the end I conclude that there is no good evidence, in spite of new
> methods, such as the employment of stimulating electrodes, the study
> of conscious patients and the analysis of epileptic attacks, that the
> brain alone can carry out the work that the mind does. I conclude that
> it is easier to rationalize man's being on the basis of two elements
> than on the basis of one. But I believe that one should not pretend to
> draw a final scientific conclusion, in man's study of man, until the
> nature of the energy responsible for mind-action is discovered as, in
> my own opinion, it will be. [Penfield, 1978, p. 114]

In short, the evidence for the brain as the bastion of free will and
thus of its preferred organ status does not presently exist. Eccles, a
neurophysiologist, and Popper, a philosopher, have recently come to
this view after an exhaustive and critical appraisal of the world
literature (Popper and Eccles, 1977). Eccles has coined the phrase
"self-conscious mind" to describe the vehicle of human thought and
ideas. It is clear, however, that even this Nobel laureate is not able to
give this concept a substance that is independent of the brain.

Of more practical import than whether the brain is or is not the
"seat of the soul" is whether there is any evidence that modern
neurosurgical intervention deprives a particular patient of his or her

---

[1] *Kaimowitz* v. *Department of Mental Health*, Civil No. 73-19434-AW (Cir. Ct.,
Wayne Co., Mich., July 10, 1973), 1 MLRP 147, 152 (1976).

"unique" qualities as a side effect of attempting to relieve symptomatology. In reviewing the results of both frontal and temporal surgery, a recent National Commission (1977) as well as Andersen (1972), a neuropsychologist, and Vaernet (Vaernet and Madsen, 1970), a neurosurgeon, found no evidence of major cognitive and personality changes occurring. Prescinding from presently unanswerable ontological arguments, no adverse impact from limited neurosurgical intervention on one's "soul" or "mind" is either detectable or demonstrable.

Economic Incentives

The argument that a neurosurgeon might have an economic incentive to enthusiastically embrace neurosurgery where clinically unnecessary has plausible appeal. However, the argument is not new and certainly not applicable only to the neurosurgeon.[2] In 1906, the English surgical profession bore the brunt of George Bernard Shaw's scathing wit as he remarked:

> That any sane nation, having observed that you could provide for the supply of bread by giving bakers a pecuniary interest in baking for you, should go on to give a surgeon a pecuniary interest in cutting off your leg, is enough to make one despair of political humanity. . . .
> Scandalized voices murmur that these operations are necessary. They may be. It may also be necessary to hang a man or pull down a house. But we take good care not to make the hangman and the housebreaker the judges of that. If we did, no man's neck would be safe and no man's house stable [Shaw, 1963, p. 1].

The correctives for unnecessary surgery lie not in governmental involvement in clinical decision making, but rather in efforts to affect financial incentives. One promising approach is that of a mandatory second opinion where such procedures are reimbursed either by government or by regulated third-party payers.

Experimentation

The argument here suggests that the clinical ethos favors advancing the goals of medical science rather than responding prudently to the patient's condition. Again, this argument is not new and certainly

---

[2] Psychiatric neurosurgery is only a small part of neurosurgical practice, and only a handful of neurosurgeons are interested in this field. Even during the "frontal lobotomy fad" of the forties, the most frequently performed procedure, transorbital leucotomy, was done by psychiatrists, not neurosurgeons. In practical terms, unnecessary disc surgery or carotid angiography is much more likely to occur than psychiatric neurosurgery.

not idiosyncratic to neurosurgery. In the mid-fifteenth century, the philosopher Lorenzo Valla wrote:

> It seems to me that the doctor who experiments with new and still untried medication, instead of curing his patient with medicines already proved by experience, is odious and execrable. I should judge him the same way as the helmsman who favors an uncharted course to that long used by others to save their ships and merchandise [Valla, 1967, p. 42].

No one could or would wish to disagree. Medical history has shown, however, that when conventional treatment proves fruitless, originality and innovation, grounded on reasonable clinical hypotheses, should be encouraged. There are countless examples of "conventional treatment," such as bloodletting and purging, which were accepted for centuries without question by patient and physician alike—even though needless suffering or death were the all too frequent results. On the other hand, almost every advance and improvement in medical diagnosis and treatment, including the antibiotic treatment of infectious disease and open heart surgery for "blue babies," have resulted from innovation or frank experimentation. Conformity to the tried and true in any art guarantees mediocrity. Medicine is no exception.

Irreversibility

The argument here focuses on the fact that destroyed brain tissue does not regenerate itself. Thus a mistake—should there be one —cannot be remedied. But irreversibility characterizes many surgical procedures, and no evidence can be adduced to single out neurosurgery for paternalistic surveillance.

Moreover, the fact that brain tissue is nonregenerative does not mean that brain function is nontransferable. One of the major problems of modern limited frontal lobe and limbic surgery for psychiatric symptoms is, not that too much tissue will be destroyed, producing irreversible intellectual deficits, but that too little will be inactivated, allowing the return of disabling symptoms (Sweet, 1973).

Risk–Benefit

The argument that risk–benefit ratios are so weighted against the patient that public policy requires governmental regulation of neurosurgical procedures can be refuted by the one example of the amygdalotomy—surgery on the amygdaloid portion of the limbic brain. In 1973, the *Kaimowitz* decision denounced amygdalotomy in general as being of high risk and of no known benefit. Four years later, the National Commission for the Protection of Human Subjects of Biomedical and Behavioral Research felt far from confident of this judicial finding:

> With respect to the questions of safety and efficacy, it is clear that the information presented to the Michigan court in 1973 regarding amygdalotomy differs significantly from that which has been presented to the Commission regarding four other psychosurgical procedures. The Commission believes that the information presented on its record justifies its recommendation, for at least some psychosurgical procedures have been shown to present a potential for significant benefit, and the risks of such surgery do not appear to be nearly as great as previously supposed [National Commission, 1977, p. 67].

In fact, the evidence adduced by Andersen (1972) and Vaernet (Vaernet and Madsen, 1972) in their neurological and psychometric evaluation of amygdalotomized patients showed minimal deficits in the face of genuine relief of clinical symptoms.[3]

Informed Consent

The patient has a legal right to decline neurosurgical intervention. This right was succinctly phrased by the late Judge Cardozo when he wrote:

> Every human being of adult years and sound mind has a right to determine what shall be done with his own body; and a surgeon who performs an operation without his patient's consent, commits [a battery] . . . for which he is liable in damages. . . . This is true except in cases of emergency where the patient is unconscious and where it is necessary to operate before consent can be obtained.[4]

Moreover, for consent to be legally sufficient, it must be "informed":

> Indeed the very nature of "consent" implies the added notion of "informed" because consent, in itself, includes the notion of freedom. It is

---

[3] Andersen did not report any differences in psychometric testing in 2 patients with bilateral amygdalotomies as compared with 11 patients with unilateral operations. Olsenes et al. (1976) could find no significant psychometric deficits in 40 psychomotor epileptic patients who underwent amygdalotomy, 25 of whom had a bilateral operation. Heimburger et al. (1978) reported on the results of amygdalotomy in 58 patients who have had long-term follow-ups with thorough psychiatric and psychometric examinations before and many years after surgery. Fifteen of these patients had a bilateral operation. No significant deficits were produced by the operations.
[4] *Schloendorff* v. *Society of N.Y. Hosp.*, 211 N.Y. 125, 129–130, 105 N.E. 92, 93 (1914) (Cardozo, J.).

obvious that one who is not free to refuse is neither free to consent. [O'Donnell, 1974, p. 1]

Minimally, informed consent requires that the patient has the mental capacity to rationally understand the procedures involved, realistically assess the benefit-risk ratios, and voluntarily accept or decline the treatment. The duty of disclosing therapeutic risks devolves upon the physician.

> Physicians are now expected to make a professional judgment as to whether or not a patient is capable of informed consent. The determination of informed consent is based on a clinical judgment of whether or not the patient understands his need for treatment and the alternative risks, his level of competence to make a decision regarding treatment and voluntariness of his decision. [Peszke, 1975, p. 828]

When the patient possesses consentual capacity and declines treatment, the matter should end. Where, however, the patient lacks consentual capacity, the question of surrogate decision making arises. In this instance, the surrogate decision maker does well to be guided by Professor Rawls' "theory of primary goods":

> Others are authorized and sometimes required to act on our behalf to do what we would do for ourselves if we were rational, this authorization coming into effect only when we cannot look after our own good. Paternalistic decisions are to be guided by the individual's own subtle preferences and interests insofar as they are not irrational, or failing a knowledge of these, by the theory of primary goods. . . . We try to get for him the things he presumably wants whatever else he wants. [Rawls, 1971, p. 249]

In our view, these legal doctrines are sufficient to protect patients' freedom of choice where neurosurgical intervention is sought to correct or modify brain dysfunction and behavioral symptoms resulting from a clinically recognized disease entity. Where, however, behavioral symptoms are not associated with clinically recognizable brain pathophysiology, the issue becomes one of whether the procedure has been shown to be clearly efficacious and safe. In this situation, the neurosurgeon is not trying to modify and control brain dysfunction but rather to alter the behavior of the patient. If demonstrable clinical efficacy and safety are absent, a series of constraints such as the following, recommended by the National Commission for the Protection of Human Subjects of Biomedical and Behavioral Research, are worthy of consideration:

> Until the safety and efficacy of any psychosurgical procedure have been demonstrated, such procedure should be performed only at an institution with an institutional review board (IRB) approved by DHEW specifically for reviewing proposed psychosurgery, and only after such IRB has determined that: (A) the surgeon has the compe-

tence to perform the procedure; (B) It is appropriate, based upon sufficient assessment of the patient, to perform the procedure on that
patient; (C) Adequate pre- and post-operative evaluations will be performed; and (D) The patient has given informed consent. . . . [National
Commission, 1977, p. 57].

When the safety and efficacy of such procedures have been demonstrated, they should be treated no differently than any other surgical
procedure.

Innovative Neurosurgery

With the exception of the now controversial decision by the *Kaimowitz* court,[5] the law has not precluded a patient from consenting to
and the neurosurgeon from performing innovative surgery.[6] The
problem here is not so much one of legal constraint as it is one of
medical ethics. In our view, the solution depends upon the presence
of clinically recognizable brain pathophysiology. If present, the decision should rest with the patient. If absent, the procedure should be
treated as surgical intervention on normal brain tissue with peer
review required prior to demonstration of safety and efficacy.

Thus, we would suggest that a requirement of peer review pending
a demonstration of safety and efficacy depends not on whether one
wishes to characterize a particular procedure as innovative, but
rather on the presence or absence of pathological brain tissue or
pathophysiological brain processes. Where either is present, there
are no compelling arguments to persuade one that decision making
should not rest between patient and physician.

Electrical or Chemical Stimulation of the Brain

Electrical stimulation of the brain (ESB) or chemical brain stimulation seeks by implantations of electrodes and the use of electric
voltages or by the deposition of chemicals to activate or inhibit
rather than eliminate brain tissue. Legally, the ground rules for pa-

---

[5] See generally R. Singer, Consent of the unfree. In B. D. Sales (Ed.), *Law and human
behavior* I (New York: Plenum Press, 1977), pp. 1–43.

"The opinion was badly muddled. Although the court unmistakably held that
consent to this operation was invalid, it went out of its way in dictum to declare that
consent to 'normal' operations would not be invalid but failed to explain why. It did
not address the question of whether confined persons could consent to experimental
but not clearly irreversible procedures. Indeed, even the basis of its specific holding
was opaque" (p. 2, footnotes omitted).

[6] See *Carpenter* v. *Blake*, 60 Barb. 488 (N.Y. App. Div. 1871), reversed on other
grounds, 50 N.Y. 696 (1872), affirmed 75 N.Y. 12 (1878).

tient consent are the same as those for other forms of neurosurgical intervention.[7] It should be borne in mind, however, that the effects of stimulation are reversible and that arguments relating to procedures that inactivate or remove brain tissue are not pertinent to brain stimulation (Ervin, Brown, and Mark, 1966; Mark et al., 1969).

Conclusion

For the most part, the psychiatric neurosurgical debate rests upon an Orwellian hysteria which portends thought control to be just around the neurosurgical corner.[8] As the philosopher Robert Neville has written:

> The philosophic perspective on psychosurgery views it as a microcosmic example of the macrocosmic problem of social control in the hands of professional groups. The cacophony of opinions and accusations reflect not so much direct interests in psychosurgery as the diverse feelings that psychosurgery represents those larger and more important problems. Thus, if we could but find a way to limit the application of psychosurgery to cases of scientifically demonstrated mental illness—narrowing the class of mental illness to those conditions whose designation as such is genuinely scientific—and to clarify and establish adequate procedures of due process by which to declare a person mentally ill and thereby a candidate for powerful treatments, we would have solved more than the problems of psychosurgery. [Neville, 1974, pp. 352–353]

We think that a patient fares better under a system of care that may be prone to occasional excess under the banner of scientific progress than under a system of care that becomes captive to the law of bureaucratic inertia. In one, the patient may choose to raise or lower the banner for his own perceived good. In the other, the expected result could be flying the banner continually at half-mast.

---

[7] See R. Singer, Consent of the unfree. In B. D. Sales (Ed.), *Law and human behavior* I (New York: Plenum Press, 1977), pp. 1–43.

"Still other methods, such as electrical stimulation of the brain (ESB), are potentially usable for behavior control but seem to involve enormous difficulties for the controller; at least at the moment. Thus, for purposes of the discussion of consent, psychosurgery can remain the paradigmatic method; if one can consent to this operation, it could be argued, one could consent to all the rest." (pp. 30–32, footnotes omitted)

[8] See, e.g., S. Knowles, Beyond the "Cuckoo's Nest": A proposal for federal regulation of psychosurgery. *Harvard Journal of Legislation*, 1975, *12*, 610–667.

"Psychosurgery is also a potential tool of those who would control behavior. . . . While such fears of psychotechnological control of society are often exaggerated, certainly those uses already proposed have far reaching and enormous consequences. . . . *Whether or not such fears are justified*, the potential medical and social dangers warrant federal legislative action." (pp. 626–627, emphasis added, footnotes omitted)

PART VI

Ethical Issues

CHAPTER 23

Brain-Disabling Therapies

Peter R. Breggin

Psychosurgery is an apt choice as a model for ethical and scientific issues in psychiatry because it in many ways epitomizes *all* somatic psychiatric treatment. As a therapy, psychosurgery displays in the extreme the contradictions and problems inherent in modern psychiatric treatment—especially the most commonly used hospital treatments, electroshock and the major tranquilizers (Breggin, 1975b). I have recently proposed and elaborated in detail upon what I call the brain-disabling hypothesis to explain the shared effects of these major somatic therapies (Breggin, 1979).

In the early 1970s, I originated the controversy over psychosurgery and carried it to both the public and the profession in an effort to stem the "second wave" predicted by the psychosurgeons. I presented my views in the *Congressional Record* (Breggin, 1972a), before the United States Senate (Breggin, 1973e), through radio and TV (Breggin, 1972e), in lay articles (Breggin, 1973b and c; Breggin and Greenberg, 1972), in court (Breggin, 1973d), in a law review article (Breggin, 1975a), in letters to medical and scientific publications (Breggin, 1972d, 1972f, 1973e) and in reports in medical sources

(Breggin, 1972b, 1973e, 1975b, 1977b). Perhaps most important in regard to the controversy, these efforts resulted in extensive newspaper and magazine coverage of the issue by many outstanding journalists, including Dietz (1972, 1973a, 1973b), D'Arazien (1972), Brownfeld (1973), Mason (1970), Parachini (1973), Hampton (1972), Trotter (1973a, 1956b) and von Hoffman (1971), who were deeply concerned about the dangers of psychosurgery.

The motivating force behind this activity was not merely my concern with psychosurgery as it was being utilized at the moment. My original estimate of only 500–1,000 operations a year in the United States has been confirmed. I was concerned with both the political motives of the psychosurgeons and with the brain-disabling psychiatric model that is carried to its extreme in psychosurgery. The public and the psychiatric community quickly became aware that the issues were broader than the immediate practice of psychosurgery. The psychosurgery controversy rallied many community and political leaders, eventuating in my founding the Center for the Study of Psychiatry, an organization concerned with the overall impact of psychiatry upon individual well-being, humanistic values, and civil and political liberties (Trotter, 1973b). At the same time, many psychiatrists who personally opposed psychosurgery nonetheless hesitated to raise their voices in criticism. Part of the reason was that they had only heard reports of my concerns about the political implications of psychosurgery without actually reading the data with which I backed up these concerns (Breggin, 1973a and b, 1975a). But more important, they were also aware of the larger principles at stake. While they might oppose psychosurgery as a dangerous, radical, and experimental extension of psychiatric principles, they did not wish to support a general criticism that might equally undermine the use of other brain-disabling therapies, such as electroshock and the major tranquilizers.

Human Values in Psychiatry

In the field of medicine, the object of the treatment is indeed "an object"—the body of the person. But even in this relatively objective arena, first principles and humanistic values have become increasingly important. How much more important they must be within psychiatry, where the object of the treatment is not an "object" at all, but a *person*. The arena of medicine, in its narrowest definition, is bodily dysfunction. The arena of psychiatry is the activity of persons—their thoughts and feelings, and their actions. As I have analyzed in *The Psychology of Freedom* (Breggin, in press), it is impossible to make any safe or sensible progress in this field without giving primary consideration to such broad philosophical considerations as "the nature of the human being" or "the purpose of human life."

Even experimental data concerning the effects and efficacy of a psychiatric treatment cannot be properly interpreted without giving consideration to such fundamental questions as "What are the highest human functions?" and "What are the ethical and philosophical implications of impairing or sacrificing any one of these functions?" Who determines the effect or efficacy of the treatment—the allegedly objective physician or the more personally affected patient? Is it relevant if a patient believes that he has lost his ability to recall certain past events, even though so-called objective tests can demonstrate no loss? Does it matter than the patient complains of difficulty thinking, even though the surgeon or psychiatrist can find no clinical evidence for this impairment? How does anyone, physician or patient, weigh a person's loss of emotional spontaneity against the presumed gain of leaving the hospital or returning to work?

These issues are as large as human life itself, for it is human life that psychosurgery and psychiatric treatment attempt to modify. I have wrestled with these issues in my novels (Breggin, 1971a), essays (Breggin, 1971b, 1972c, 1974, 1975c and d, 1977a), and most extensively in *The Psychology of Freedom* (Breggin, in press). They have also been explored by Szasz, especially in *The Myth of Mental Illness* (1974) and *The Myth of Psychotherapy* (1978). Szasz has challenged the core concepts of "mental illness" and "psychotherapy" as attempts to corrupt philosophical, political, and religious questions with medical and scientific language. He has argued cogently that psychiatrists in particular have attempted to gain a monopoly over larger human concerns by capturing them with medical and scientific terminology.

The meaning, purpose, and value of life itself lie at the heart of any serious inquiry concerning the effects or efficacy of psychosurgery and the somatic treatments in psychiatry. Need I say that such a subject can only be approached cautiously and with full recognition of the limits of any individual critic? Need I say that any one essay on the subject can at best focus upon a small piece of the problem? My own intention is to present a few of the more important principles involved in my criticism of psychosurgery and the somatic treatments, and to illustrate them with historical and experimental data. My larger hope is to stimulate a more profound concern for the implications of these interventions into the human brain and into the lives of individual human beings.

Reasoning Capacity

Reason, which enables the scientist and philosopher—and, indeed, all capable men and women—to evaluate facts and theories, also plays a crucial role in our daily lives. The most complex form of reason—abstract thinking and the manipulation of symbols—is required for the simplest daily tasks, such as communicating with others, taking care of bills, making a grocery list, following a recipe, or understanding directions to a friend's home. Nearly all the activities that distinguish human beings from lower animals require the use of abstract thinking. Thus, many philosophers have agreed with Aristotle in labeling reason the highest and most characteristic human function.

Irrationality itself presumes the existence of reason and can be looked upon as abused or faulty reasoning. A lower animal cannot become "irrational" because it lacks the fundamental capacity. The animal cannot imagine that it is Jesus or that it is controlled by radio waves. It cannot grow to hate itself or to wish itself dead. These are self-destructive *uses* of abstract, symbolic reason (Breggin, in press).

What is *reason?* Here the inquiry could grow endlessly in complexity. For my purposes, I shall select one aspect of reason that is especially pertinent to the somatic treatments in psychiatry. Reason is *systematic choice making*. The person who reasons is making decisions or choices between various real or imagined alternatives. He is choosing among, comparing, or evaluating various potential actions. If my reader changes his mind after studying my viewpoint, or even if my reader holds on to his original position, he has made a *systematic choice* between alternatives.

Reason thus presupposes and contains within it the concept of *free will* or *volition*. By free will or volition I mean the inner experience of choosing, deciding, and ultimately making up one's own mind (Breggin, in press). It is an *action*—albeit a private one. When these private actions seek expression in the world, they become a more objectively observable phenomenon—*human conduct*. It is the hypothesis of this study that the somatic therapies—psychosurgery, electroshock, and the major tranquilizers—bring the conduct of the patient under the control of the psychiatrist by rendering the patient less able to think, to choose, and to act.

Emotional Capacity

As reason contains within it the idea of volition or choice, emotion suggests the idea of involuntary reactivity. While these are subtle and difficult distinctions, no one believes that the emotions are wholly subject to reason or to the will of the individual. Most definitions of emotion recognize its reactive, reflexive nature and link emotion to bodily processes that lie somewhat or wholly beyond individual control. Emotions are nonetheless extremely important, even indispensable, as signals concerning our state of well-being (Breggin, in press).

The capacity to feel and to recognize various emotions is central to the proper function of reason. Emotions, such as pain or pleasure, sexual desire or hunger, are *signals* conveying information about the well-being, needs, and desires of the individual. The individual must learn what is making him miserable in order to alleviate it, and he must learn what makes him happy in order to pursue it. Even if he decides to pursue what makes him miserable, and to ignore what makes him happy, as so many people do, he must feel and recognize his emotional signals in order to guide his decision making and his conduct. Anything that dulls or impairs emotional responsiveness will, therefore, compromise the ability of the individual to choose among the various alternatives in life.

Beyond giving relevant information about health, well-being, and appetites, emotions play a crucial role in the individual's ability to think and to exert his will. The overall emotional state of the individual has a great deal to do with how much effort, concentration, or willpower he will exert in thinking or acting. It is well known that fatigue, chronic illness, and other bodily impairments can vastly reduce these emotional reserves. Any somatic treatment that produces a similar apathy, dulling, or fatigue would similarly render the individual less able or willing to reason and to carry out his decisions, especially in the face of adversity or restraint.

Knowing the importance of emotional signals, the wise man who steps upon a tack does not choose to cut the pain fibers from his foot to his brain. Nor does he decide to blunt the pain perception in his brain in order to deal with the tack. He may not like the pain he feels when stepping upon the tack, but he nonetheless welcomes it as a signal that his health or well-being has been threatened. He could dull his awareness or concern about pain to enable himself more easily to go through life walking upon tacks. But he would fear the consequences of multiple tack wounds; and he would fear the consequences of impairing pain perception in general, knowing how it signals him of other more serious dangers to his health and well-being. He would also be repelled at the thought of reducing his overall capacity to think and feel about himself and life. He would not wish to simplify or to impair his human function by disabling his brain.

Personal Sovereignty and Personal Freedom

Personal sovereignty is the concept I use to summarize and to name the inner experience of free will, reason, and emotion (Breggin, 1975d, 1977a, in press). A person who is "personally sovereign" can *choose to experience his emotional signals and to reason systematically.* Personal sovereignty is *inner freedom.* It is wholly subjective, and no one knows its limits. It can be viewed as both a right and as a capacity.

Personal freedom is the external or public expression of personal sovereignty. It is the right and the capacity of the individual to express his thoughts and feelings through actions. Unlike personal sovereignty, personal freedom can be directly examined by others. It also has known limits. Some of the limits are ethical, and may be set by the individual himself. Thus the individual may choose not to steal or to murder. Personal freedom also has many objective limits —everything from the inherent mortality of the body to the competing and conflicting desires of various individuals.

The high value I place upon personal sovereignty and personal freedom provides the *philosophical basis* for my criticism of psychosurgery, electroshock, the major tranquilizers, and most other somatic therapies in psychiatry. Factual evidence that these therapies disable the brain and compromise personal sovereignty and personal freedom provides the *scientific basis* of my criticism.

Effects of Brain-Disabling Therapies

My hypothesis is that the primary somatic therapies—psychosurgery, electroshock, and the major tranquilizers—disrupt normal brain function and thereby compromise the individual's personal sovereignty and personal freedom. Disabling the brain is the most important, overriding effect of these treatments.

The *psychological effects* of these treatments are of course far more complex and subtle than indicated by the hypothesis, which deals exclusively with the specific effect of producing brain damage or dysfunction. Psychologically, some people may seek out brain dysfunction as a method of avoiding themselves and their problems, or as an attempt to achieve a "high" or euphoria. Sniffing glue or inhaling nitrous oxide are typical nonpsychiatric methods of achieving such a state. Electroshock, psychosurgery, and some medications can provide a medically sanctioned method of achieving the same impaired state, including an irrational sense of well-being (euphoria). Nonetheless, the individual compromises his personal sovereignty and personal freedom, even though he does it voluntarily. Various placebo effects may also result from the positive expectations of the person submitting to one or another somatic therapy. Still more important, in my experience, is the effectiveness of these treatments as intimidators and enforcers on hospital wards. As I first wrote in "Coercion of Voluntary Patients in an Open Hospital" (Breggin, 1964), the major tranquilizers and electroshock loom as important threats in controlling the conduct of hospital inmates. In this study, however, I wish to focus on the single most important effects of these somatic interventions—the production of brain disability in the interest of controlling the patient.

Each of these suppressive interventions—psychosurgery, electroshock, and the major tranquilizers—produces a different form of brain damage or dysfunction. Furthermore, different psychosurgical operations can produce somewhat different results. The discarded technique of removing a large portion of the cerebral cortex had a more obvious effect upon intelligence than a deeper lesion in the limbic system, which suppresses emotional responsiveness. But *all* the somatic therapies affect important aspects of personal sovereignty and personal freedom.

Obviously, not all possible interventions in the brain disrupt personal sovereignty or personal freedom. Some interventions may cure or ameliorate a disease process. Neurosurgery may remove a scar, relieving pressure in the cranium. Sometimes as a side effect in neurosurgery there is some loss of personal sovereignty if damage is done to the limbic system in the process of treating the disease. Sometimes there may be a more direct loss of personal freedom if, for example, the motor area of the cortex is damaged during surgery, causing the paralysis of a limb. But these are untoward or unwanted consequences of neurosurgical interventions. Psychosurgery, by contrast, is psychiatric surgery. Its *aim* is to modify thoughts, feelings, or conduct, and it accomplishes this by compromising the brain functions required for personal sovereignty or personal freedom (Breggin, 1972a, 1975b, in press).

Psychosurgery, electroshock, or the major tranquilizers *always compromise normal brain function.* In those few uses in which abnormal tissue is indeed treated, the psychiatric effect is nonetheless achieved by further compromising whatever *normal function* remains in the tissue. Thus, a surgical intervention or a drug may be used to control aggressive responses in a child who has physiological retardation of the brain or epilepsy. But the effect of the psychosurgical lesion will not be produced specifically by destruction of the malfunctioning tissue. The "taming" effect will be produced in a wide variety of areas in the limbic system, and it will be produced in exactly the same fashion as it is produced in humans and animals with normal brains—by causing further brain damage and dysfunction. To repeat, the commonly used psychiatric interventions act by compromising normal brain function.

While these principles are easiest to explain in regard to psychosurgery, they are equally true for electroshock and the major tranquilizers. Furthermore, they are true regardless of the mental or physical state of the person to whom the treatments are administered. Even if so-called mental illness is biological in origin (I do not believe that it is), this would have no effect whatsoever upon the hypothesis that the somatic interventions achieve their effect by disrupting normal brain function.

Consider a person who has a verifiable brain disease, such as a tumor or a more generalized drug intoxication or atherosclerosis. This person will be subdued by electroshock or a major tranquilizer in exactly the same fashion as a person with a normal brain. There may be a difference of degree, however, which is wholly accounted for by the hypothesis that the intervention disrupts normal brain function. The person with a brain disease may require a smaller surgical lesion, fewer shock treatments or a lesser drug dose in order to achieve the anticipated effect. This is because the person's brain function has already been disrupted by a disease process, and is therefore more easily compromised by a lesser psychiatric intervention.

This is a crucial and easily misunderstood point: The hypothesis that the somatic therapies are suppressive of normal brain function is wholly independent of the controversy concerning the biological nature of mental illness. Put most baldly, a blow on the head is a blow on the head, regardless of the thoughts, feelings, convictions, or physical state of the recipient. The only exception has already been examined. The blow may have a more severe effect if the person already has brain damage or dysfunction.

In *Electroshock: Its Brain-Disabling Effects* (1979), I examine in more detail the unproven assumption that a particular abnormal chemical reaction, for example, a dopamine abnormality, is corrected by the somatic interventions. This position is untenable for several reasons that I can only summarize here. First, even if a subtle biochemical abnormality exists, the various somatic interventions produce generalized, widespread changes throughout the brain. Electroshock, for example, significantly disrupts nearly every measurable biological function in the brain. Second, the disruption in these biochemical systems, including dopamine metabolism, is comparable to that following any form of severe trauma, hardly supporting a "therapeutic" specificity for any of the treatments. Third, the overall organic and psychological dysfunctions produced by the somatic treatments, including apathy, euphoria, and increased tractability or docility, are gross and overwhelming. It makes no sense to disconnect the "therapeutic effect" from the obvious, disabling effects that dominate the thoughts, feelings, and conduct of the patient.

The brain-disabling hypothesis is independent of the differences in effect found among the various somatic interventions. Even though various somatic interventions differ in their specific effects, each produces an overall or *generalized* brain dysfunction. A major tranquilizer cannot suppress a person's "delusions of grandeur" without equally suppressing the person's overall capacity to reason, to feel, and to make decisions. A surgical disruption in the limbic system cannot remove "aggression" without disrupting widespread mental functions. One could deduce this from an understanding of mental function itself. Delusions of grandeur, aggression, and other categories of human thought or action, such as depression or anxiety, relate to the overall experience of the individual as a thinking, feeling, willing human being (Breggin, in press).

If observations on the subjective experience of humans were not enough to verify the integration of thoughts, feelings, and decision making, physiological and anatomical studies of the brain confirm the integrated nature of brain function. One cannot pluck a "thought" or a "feeling" out of the brain as one might pluck an olive from a tree. Any primer on functional neuroanatomy demonstrates the naiveté inherent in attempting to isolate brain function in such a specific manner. Within this book, the issue is examined in greater depth by Chorover.

In summary, the somatic therapies produce brain damage and dysfunction and thereby compromise the personal sovereignty and personal freedom of the individual. This effect is not accidental, and it is not secondary to some other effect: it is not a side effect. It is the specific effect of the treatment.

Motivation for Somatic Psychiatric Interventions

What purpose, we may ask, does it serve the psychiatrist to reduce the personal sovereignty and personal freedom of the patient? The answer is not hard to find: the psychiatrist (or psychosurgeon) gains *control* over the patient. More specifically, the psychiatrist or psychosurgeon may render the person less troublesome to himself or to others by rendering him less able to think, to feel, to choose, and to act.

As I review the effects of the somatic therapies in more specific detail in the following sections, it will become apparent that the psychiatrists who pioneered these treatments knew exactly what they were doing. They describe in vivid detail the reduction of the patient to a more robot-like, less troublesome, and less vital status with psychosurgery, electroshock, and the major tranquilizers. When it is understood that each of these interventions had its origins in the custodial state mental hospital, it becomes more obvious why even well-meaning physicians might turn to extreme methods to subdue the difficult, unruly, and anguished populations of these institutions.

Each major somatic therapy originated as part of psychiatry's efforts to control the massive numbers of inmates under its charge, and, if possible, to render them malleable enough for useful work in the hospital or for discharge into the community (Breggin, 1974, 1975c, 1975d, 1979). Psychosurgery, ECT, and the major tranquilizers share a common origin with the vast majority of other psychiatric interventions over the years—from castration and whipping to arsenic poisoning and forced submersion in bathtubs (Breggin, 1979). The power of the newer interventions derives from their direct assault upon the brain rather than upon the body, and specifically, their ability to tame patients without too frequently killing them.

The extension of these treatments from the involuntary mental patient population to the outpatient and even the private office patient is another and more complex matter. Historically, this transition has always come after the wide-scale application of these treatments to the involuntary state mental hospital patient, and *none* of these treatments has been widely accepted by the voluntary private patient. Few people willingly submit to psychosurgery, electroshock, or the major tranquilizers when they have been informed about their effects, and fewer still willingly submit a second or third time. Of those who do actively seek these treatments, many undoubtedly do so very self-destructively.

The Major Tranquilizers: Pharmacological Lobotomy

From 1954 through 1958 I helped develop the first large mental hospital volunteer program using college students (Umbarger et al., 1962) and personally witnessed the "miracle" wrought by the introduction of the major tranquilizers into the state mental hospitals of the Boston area during that period of time. During two summers I was also an investigator in related research projects. There can be no doubt about the effect of the medications. Prior to their introduction, electroshock treatment and insulin coma therapy were the mainstays of patient control. When an individual was difficult to manage within the confines of these foul-smelling, dilapidated, overcrowded concentration camps, he was involuntarily subjected to a brutal series of shocks or comas, often rendering him more tractable and more willing to hide his craziness or rebellion (Breggin, 1979). Nonetheless, the wards remained very unruly, and for the hospital staff they were often dangerous. But with the advent of the major tranquilizers a dramatic change took place. Instead of the traditional disorderly madhouse filled with upset, outraged inmates, we now had a storehouse filled with apathetic, robot-like nonpersons. This was my personal introduction to the miracle of modern psychiatry.

It is generally accepted that at least two-thirds of hospitalized psychiatric patients receive no other treatment than drugs, usually a phenothiazine. I have investigated a number of mental hospitals, state and private, and have frequently found this figure too conservative. Even in hospitals in which the director or his staff have estimated that two-thirds of the patients receive major tranquilizers, an actual count of medication cards on the wards has sometimes yielded a figure nearer to 95 percent. To the hundreds of thousands of patients subjected to these drugs in hospitals on any given day must be added another substantial number receiving them in outpatient clinics. Literally tens of millions of people have been administered these drugs over the past twenty-five years (Crane, 1973).

The phenothiazines vary among themselves with respect to side effects and duration of action, but nonetheless present a remarkably consistent pattern. Chlorpromazine was the first of this group introduced into North America in 1953, and it remains the prototype. Its brand name in the United States is Thorazine, and in Canada and England, Largactil. Other brand names of related phenothiazines are Mellaril, Stelazine, Sparine, Compazine, Trilafon, Prolixin, Permitil, Serentil, Tindal, Quide and Vesprin. The butyrophenones (brand name Haldol) and the thioxanthenes (brand name Taractan) may also be included among the "major tranquilizers." While these differ from the phenothiazines, their effects and side effects are very similar. On the other hand, the "minor tranquilizers" vary widely among themselves and differ vastly from the phenothiazines in their actions and side effects. My analysis of the major tranquilizers should not be applied to them.

The first report on the psychiatric effects of the phenothiazines was published in France in 1952 by Delay and Deniker (Jarvick, 1970).

With doses in the low range of modern clinical usage, they achieved the following effect:

> Sitting or lying, the patient is motionless in his bed, often pale with eyelids lowered. He remains silent most of the time. If he is questioned, he answers slowly and deliberately in a monotonous, indifferent voice; he expresses himself in a few words and becomes silent.

They consider the patient's behavior to be "fairly appropriate and adaptable," "But he rarely initiates a question and he does not express his anxiety, desires or preferences." There is an "apparent indifference or the slowing of responses to external stimuli" and a "diminution of initiative and anxiety."

The first report on the first major tranquilizer clearly describes its total assault on personal sovereignty and personal freedom. The patient is rendered "adaptable," and this is accomplished by suppressing his spontaneity, his responsiveness, his desires and preferences, and his communications. It is no exaggeration to describe this as the making of a tractable inmate in a suppressive state mental hospital.

Heinz Lehmann's first English-language article promoting the same medication, published from Canada, gives substantially the same description of its effects (Lehmann and Hanrahan, 1954). Again employing doses in the low range of current clinical use, Lehmann remarks that the patients continue to suffer from "retardation," "emotional indifference," and "lethargy," even after the initial drowsiness has worn off. He compares the drug experience to that of "an exhausting illness" with fatigue and malaise. This frank description of a generalized assault on the patient's personal sovereignty and personal freedom is reinforced by Lehmann's conclusion that "We have not observed a direct influence of the drug on delusional systems or hallucinatory phenomena." Despite this admission, he highly promotes the drug, clearly demonstrating that his enthusiasm for it is based on its suppressor effects.

In later years, Lehmann would change his viewpoint and take the position that the major tranquilizers are antipsychotic agents with specific effects upon delusions and hallucinations. But his fundamental observations would remain the same (Lehmann, 1955):

> Many patients dislike the "empty feeling" resulting from the reduction of drive and spontaneity which is apparently *one of the most characteristic effects of this substance* [emphasis added].

In this publication, Lehmann becomes perhaps the first observer to speak of the major tranquilizers as "a pharmacological substitute for lobotomy."

Over the following years, a most remarkable transformation would take place in the psychiatric literature. Though the dosage of the drugs would increase, the reports on its overall suppressive effects would be gradually eradicated from clinical and research reports. Instead of the submissive, apathetic, and robot-like conduct reported by the original investigators and still obvious today on any mental hospital ward, the clinical and research literature would tout specific antipsychotic effects. Instead of reporting how all spontaneous conduct and all spontaneous communications are reduced by the pharmacological agent, investigators would select a few limited "symptoms" and report their diminution.

In 1958 and 1959, the arbitrary transformation from suppressor agent to "antipsychotic" agent was graphically displayed in a comparison of two of the most widely read resources in psychiatry. Noyes and Kolb (1958) in *Modern Clinical Psychiatry*, perhaps the single most influential textbook of psychiatry, continued to describe how the typical patient receiving maximum benefit from his treatment would become robot-like with "indifference both to his surroundings and to his symptoms."

> Even though not somnolent, the patient may lie quietly in bed, unoccupied and staring ahead. He may answer questions readily and to the point but offer little or no spontaneous conversation; however, questioning shows that he is fully aware of his circumstances.

But one year later, a lengthy chapter on the phenothiazines by Paul Hoch (1959) in the *American Handbook of Psychiatry* contained no word about the overall apathy, lassitude, and indifference produced by these agents. Instead, the focus was on "the reduction of symptomatology in a schizophrenic patient" and the alleviation of "the emotional push behind the delusional ideas." No one reading the analysis would know that *all* thoughts, feelings, communications, and actions had been leveled.

After the late 1950s, one must generally go to sources outside psychiatry, such as *Drill's Pharmacology in Medicine* (DiPalma, 1971), to find frank descriptions of the phenothiazones as agents that suppress the central nervous system, especially the reticular activating system, producing apathy and indifference in human beings. Even the early objectivity of Goodman and Gillman's famous *The Pharmacological Basis of Therapeutics* (1956) gives way to psychiatric propaganda in the 1970 edition. The author Jarvick (1970) does recognize the actual facts when he states:

> All the phenothiazines used in psychiatry diminish spontaneous motor activity in every species of animal studied, including man. . . .

Indifference to environmental stimuli and consequent taming are easily seen in naturally aggressive wild animals such as monkeys.

He also acknowledges the "emotional quieting and affective indifference" as well as the impaired attention in intellectual tasks that characterizes the drug response in humans. But he nonetheless repeats the unsubstantiated claim that phenothiazines have a specific antipsychotic effect.

Similarly, a 1968 National Institute of Mental Health report by the experienced researcher Albert DiMascio cites massive evidence that the phenothiazines produce a decline in perception, memory, reasoning, mental speed, libido, and just about every measurable human function, but nonetheless concludes that these effects "have not been reported in psychiatric patients undergoing pharmacotherapy." True, findings of apathy and globally depressed activity were not being reported very frequently after the 1950s; but they remained obvious to the most casual visitor on any mental hospital ward.

Later research purporting to demonstrate the "antipsychotic" effects of the phenothiazines has, in reality, confirmed the overall suppressive effects. In the *Clinical Handbook of Psychopharmacology*, Gerald Klerman (1970), one of the nation's leading exponents of psychopharmacology, reviewed the research literature and renewed the claim that the phenothiazines are antipsychotic agents. Gone are the original picturesque descriptions of patients suffering from apathy, lassitude, and chronic exhaustion, much as persons with debilitating illnesses. There is no mention whatsoever of these phenomena. Instead, the patients are rated on a variety of arbitrarily selected "symptoms" before and after the treatment. Even so, the four most "improved" behaviors turn out to be "combativeness, hyperactivity, tension, and hostility," in descending order. This is the "taming effect" seen in animals and humans alike, and it has nothing to do with any "antipsychotic" effect. The ratings of symptom reduction show that "delusions" and "hallucinations" are reduced hardly at all. Since the patients must have become relatively inactive and noncommunicative after being medicated, it is surprising that there is so little reduction in these "symptoms." It is as if the patient's psychotic manifestations are *more* resistant to the drugs than other aspects of conduct. Nonetheless, Klerman concludes that there is an antipsychotic effect.

In the same symposium in which Klerman argues for the antipsychotic effect of the drugs, Allan Mirsky (1970) shows that these substances make normal monkeys "drowsy," "indifferent," and generally inattentive. The dose, pound for pound, is in the low range of starter doses for humans.

I need not go through the embarrassing task of citing psychiatric expert after psychiatric expert who claims a specific antipsychotic effect for the major tranquilizers wholly without evidence and wholly in the face of overwhelming proof that these drugs produce a reduction in *all spontaneous activity* in humans and animals alike, regardless of the presence or absence of any psychiatric problems. Research evidence indicates that the major tranquilizers suppress function throughout the brain, but that they especially disrupt brain functions associated with arousal, activation, or overall drive state. They "de-fuse" the individual. In so doing, the phenothiazines cut at the heart of personal sovereignty and personal freedom, rendering the individual less able to generate *any* thoughts, feelings, or actions.

What remains open to question is the *permanency* of these suppressive effects following the termination of treatment. It is now known that permanent brain damage manifested as tardive dyskinesia can frequently be found following long-term, and sometimes short-term, administration of the major tranquilizers (American College of Neuropsychopharmacology, 1973; Crane, 1973). The afflicted individual is left with a variety of permanent and disfiguring tics and spasms. The damage is irreversible even after the discontinuation of medication. Are patients with tardive dyskinesia also afflicted with permanent apathy? No one has as yet taken the problem seriously under investigation. I harbor a fear that we are producing a permanent "deep lobotomy" in tens of thousands of psychiatric patients by permanently impairing the arousal center of the brain.

Whether the object is to tame a captured animal for transportation to a zoo or to subdue a psychiatric patient, the major tranquilizers render the individual less able to think, to feel, to choose, and to act on his own initiative. Because these drugs strike deeply into the arousal centers of the brain, emotional drive seems more obviously impaired than reasoning or thinking. But all mental functions are depressed, and the de-fused individual remains relatively unable to exercise personal sovereignty or personal freedom. He is much more easily controlled.

Brain Damage and Dysfunction from Electroconvulsive Treatment

Electroconvulsive treatment (ECT) is far more widely used than most psychiatrists and the public realize. Estimates from a variety of sources place the number of ECT patients at fifty thousand to one hundred thousand each year in the United States (Breggin, 1979; Grosser, 1974). Most of these patients are treated in private psychiatric hospitals, where shock treatment is often the main form of therapy administered to 50 percent or more of routine admissions. General hospitals also use the treatment frequently. However, the large state hospitals, which have no financial gain from using the therapy, have often discontinued it entirely. The decline of its use in state hospitals, and its widespread use among a limited number of practitioners, account for the fact that few people realize how frequent its use remains (Breggin, 1979).

The number of treatments administered to individual patients varies widely. I have personally known patients who have received 50, 100, and 150 treatments over a period of months or a few years in modern private psychiatric hospitals. Even the number given at any one session varies from 1 to 10 or more. The average range, however, appears to be 8–12 treatments administered once every other day.

The range of patients given electroshock also varies far more than the average practitioner realizes. The Massachusetts study indicated that depression, as anticipated, characterized the majority of patients, but large numbers of individuals with diagnoses of schizophrenia, neuroses, and personality disorders were also treated with ECT (Breggin, 1979).

In short, many psychiatrists and hospitals appear to consider electroshock the treatment of choice for most patients, while other psychiatrists and hospitals rarely, if ever, use it.

That shock is utterly harmless and that no evidence supports any other contention is the standard view in authoritative textbooks and review articles, all of which are written by advocates of the treatment. I was therefore astonished when I began to review the psychiatric literature concerning ECT and found many dozens of articles indicating permanent brain damage and dysfunction following one or more ECTs in animals or humans. Even those articles cited as proof of the harmlessness of ECT on actual inspection frequently indicate the occurrence of severe brain damage. After years of research I have recently completed a book in which I present six clinical cases of my own and review several hundred articles pertinent to the subject (Breggin, 1979).

Both the older methods of ECT and the newer modified ECT (using artificial respiration and oxygenation combined with muscle "relaxants" to produce paralysis during the electrically induced convulsion) cause an acute brain syndrome largely indistinguishable from that produced by any other severe trauma to the brain. The individual after one to three or four treatments becomes grossly disoriented to time, place, and person; loses his capacity to reason abstractly; becomes apathetic, or perhaps euphoric, with an unstable, abnormal mood; and is impaired in insight and judgment. The person always requires supervision and in many cases becomes extremely helpless.

As in the phenothiazine literature, the first clinical reports concerning ECT are the most graphic, but the same data can be gleaned from more modern aseptic studies or from observing modified ECT in a psychiatric hospital. In 1942, in the first detailed clinical report, Lowenbach and Stainbrook opened with the following remark:

> A generalized convulsion leaves a human being in a state in which all that is called the personality has been extinguished.

The authors describe the stupor and incoherency that follows the very first convulsion, as well as the frank terror:

> But the patient is not yet talking and does not follow simple commands. It becomes, however, increasingly easier to control his restlessness and to calm what appears to the observer to be terror-manifesting reactions. . . . The first sentences uttered are also usually incomprehensible. But as time goes on it is possible to establish question and answer sequences. From now on, the perplexity of the patient arising from his inability to grasp the situation pervades his statements.

They go on to note that it takes the patient twenty to thirty minutes to be able to write his name after the first shock, and that during this period of time, the brain wave patterns are abnormal. Lowenbach and Stainbrook (1942) directly connect the therapeutic effect to the brain dysfunction, observing that "if the patient becomes almost immediately his pre-shock self, then the therapeutic procedure has been in vain." They advocate using the period of confusion as a time for conditioning the patient to new ways of thinking and acting. This is a graphic illustration of the hypothesis that the somatic therapies act by producing brain dysfunction and by compromising personal sovereignty and personal freedom.

The modern literature amply shows that multiple electroshock treatments produce an escalation of mental and physical deterioration with a correspondingly longer recovery time. That this deterioration is the sought-after effect is demonstrated by the fact that electroshock courses almost always exceed three or four treatments, when gross deterioration first becomes apparent, and by the fact that many therapists use the severity of the organic brain syndrome as the "titration point" for concluding treatment. Some proponents of shock have observed that to the degree that recent modifications may ameliorate some of the effects of the treatment, the modified shock treatment course must be prolonged. Many clinical groups are now using more than one modified shock in a session, which produces more rapid organic and mental deterioration.

Does shock treatment, especially modified shock treatment, produce brain damage? Certainly no one can doubt that an individual with a florid acute organic brain syndrome has received a devastating insult to brain tissue and brain function, however temporary. If the destructive effects of shock treatment are not always permanent, then the cure is not always permanent either. Indeed, the treatment is notorious for its stopgap effects. It is entirely possible that some patients largely recover from the effects of the treatment, for many patients obviously return to their former mental states, with all their old problems, often complicated by a fear and distrust of the doctors who administered the treatment. But beyond the basic hypothesis that treatment result is related to brain dysfunction and the loss of mental capacities, it is important to establish that the damaging effects of this treatment can be permanent. In this regard I want to summarize the findings I have published in detail in my recent book (Breggin, 1979).

The six clinical cases, three men and three women, ranged in age from eighteen to fifty at the time of treatment. Three received short courses (eight or fewer treatments) and three received long courses (fifty or more). Each person was followed up for more than four years after treatment, most for many years. Each person received modified electroshock without known untoward reactions, and at least four of six were considered treatment successes by the treating doctors. Each person had had a responsible job or educational status shortly prior to treatment, and none had any previous history of complaints referable to brain function or to memory. Only one person had an extensive neurological work-up including an EEG both before and after treatment, and in this case there were major brain wave changes consistent with those reported in the literature following ECT. A brain scan and other tests showed significant loss of brain tissue, and there were positive neurological signs. A battery of standard psychological tests also demonstrated brain damage. This person had received a short course of ECT.

The most significant complaints of the patients centered around retrograde memory loss. The period of days during which the shock was administered was entirely blanked out for some of the patients, but fragments could be recalled by others. For people receiving long courses lasting over a year or more, this constituted a significant loss of personal memories and personal identity. Each person also lost most, if not all, memory of a period of a few months leading up to the treatment. Only one person's losses were limited to that few months, however, and in both the short- and long-course groups, all but one person had significant memory losses reaching back several years, and in two or three instances, even into childhood. This pattern of memory loss was identical to that reported by I. L. Janis in a series of before and after studies of personal memories following routine ECT (Janis, 1948, 1950; Janis and Astrachan, 1951).

Two of the six people reported losing a significant, incapacitating degree of current mental functioning, especially the ability to concentrate, to persist, to memorize, and to learn new material. Of the four others, who claimed to have no significant degree of impairment in ongoing function, two appeared to function normally and two definitely did not. Despite claims of no impairment, one case displayed frank signs of a chronic organic brain syndrome, including inappropriate affect (euphoria), perseveration, and irrelevance in speech, and the other demonstrated organic brain damage and deficits on psychological testing.

These six people are not a representative sample and cannot be taken as illustrative of what typically happens to ECT patients. However, my own experience indicates that *most patients* continue to complain of memory loss following ECT—a finding that is confirmed in the literature when series of patients are interviewed long after the treatment. The literature is also replete with reports of people who have lost recall for many years of their lives in part or *in toto*. The problem is sufficiently great that many authorities have warned against giving ECT to people whose jobs require memory work and mental agility (Breggin, 1979).

Probably the most convincing part of the literature is experimental rather than clinical. A variety of animal studies indicate that ECT given in clinical doses produces diffuse brain damage characterized by damage to small blood vessels, petechial hemorrhage, glial proliferation, and sometimes cell death. In the best controlled study by Hans Hartelius (1952), the pathologist was able to select out the treated animals from the control animals in every case by examining their brains after a few ECTs, and several animals showed cell death as well as the typical hemorrhagic picture.

Significantly, dozens of autopsies reported in the literature show an identical picture of frequent widespread petechial hemorrhage, occasional massive hemorrhage, many cellular changes, and occasional cell death. There are also many reports of central nervous system death following one or more treatments. Also of great weight, many brain wave studies of modified and unmodified ECT show permanent slow wave changes roughly proportional to the number of treatments administered (Breggin, 1979).

The mechanism of cell damage has been explored in a variety of interesting ways. Most conclusively it has been shown that small amounts of electric current even without convulsion produce severe spasm of the small blood vessels. Since modern ECT uses at least as much current as the older methods, and often much more, little amelioration can be expected from modifications of oxygenation and respiration alone. The current breaks through the skull at many places and travels down the vascular tree, causing diffuse damage; but the largest intensity of current strikes the anterior temporal lobe, accounting for the severe memory loss, and the frontal lobe, accounting for lobotomy-like effects (Breggin, 1979).

ECT, like the phenothiazines, had its origin in the attempt to control large state hospital populations. Nowadays it is more frequently administered to patients in private hospitals. As the literature repeatedly observes, these patients may initially volunteer for the treatment under the impression that it is harmless, but after one or two treatments they become terrified and almost universally ask to have it ended. In my own clinical and forensic experience, I have *never* seen a course of ECT terminated because the patient becomes terrified of his mental losses and begs to have it terminated. The treatment is invariably continued until the patient is no longer able to protest or to resist, or even to recall or to understand what is happening. Nowhere in the Western world today do we find such a gross, obvious, and frequent assault upon personal sovereignty and personal freedom. Given such an obvious devastating impact on the patient, the burden must rest upon those who promote the treatment to explain how its major effect could be anything other than mental dysfunction, with its associated euphoria or submissive helplessness.

From Lobotomy to Stereotaxic Surgery

Exactly like the phenothiazine tranquilizers and electroshock, lobotomy was invented as a technology to control the overcrowded madhouses, and like electroshock and the phenothiazines its primary result was the transformation of madhouses into storehouses. By 1954, when the phenothiazine tranquilizers were introduced into North American state mental hospitals, lobotomy had already run its course. It was on the way out not because of the phenothiazines, but because of its damaging effects upon the individual. A high percentage of patients were so mentally incapacitated that they died from self-neglect (Vosburg, 1962).

If electroshock has remained alive and well largely through the efforts of a limited number of proponents who perform the great majority of treatments, psychosurgery has been kept barely alive by a *handful* of proponents, perhaps no more than five or six major figures, who perform most of the operations in the country (Breggin, 1972a). If the public was largely unaware of a resurgent interest in electroshock, it was totally unaware of a resurgence in psycho-surgery. In 1971, when I first alerted the profession and the public to the reality of a growing second wave of psychosurgery, I had to provide massive documentation before reasonable people would be-lieve that anyone was performing the operation. That I did convince the public is probably the major reason that the operation did not enjoy the second wave so enthusiastically predicted by its leading proponents in the early 1970s.

Why the public furor about an operation performed on less than 1,000 patients a year in the United States? Why was I so intent upon drawing its dangers to public attention? First and foremost, there was the operation itself. Regardless of the limited number of people subjected to the surgery, I have considered it a very harmful and irrational intervention. Second, there is the ever-present danger of a much more wide-scale application of the surgery if and when the psychosurgeons find access to the large state mental hospitals, the prisons (Aarons, 1972; Breggin, 1975a, 1975b), or the institutions for the retarded (Andy, 1966, 1970; P. L. Breggin, 1974), each of which was targeted as containing potential patient populations. Third, there was blatant political rhetoric by a limited number of psychiatrists and psychosurgeons who were explicitly advocating the surgery for the control of black violence in the ghetto—a subject I have researched and examined in great detail (Breggin, 1975a). That these psychosurgeons had federal support, including Justice Depart-ment and National Institute of Mental Health grants, added fuel to the fire of public concern (Breggin, 1973a and b, 1975 a and b; Brown-feld, 1973; Parachini, 1973; Trotter, 1973a).

The Political Threat

The point that psychiatrists and psychosurgeons were openly and in print advocating psychosurgery for the control of racial violence is of extreme importance. With the exception of a number of black chil-dren operated on in Mississippi (Andy, 1966, 1970; Breggin, 1972a;

P. L. Breggin, 1974; Mason, 1973) and a still smaller group of black prisoners operated on in California (Aarons, 1972), significant numbers of black people had not been operated on during the initial phase of the second wave of psychosurgery. Most modern psychosurgery, like most electroshock, is carried out on people who are covered by insurance programs. However, somewhat of a precedent had been set during the first wave when the dean of lobotomy, Walter Freeman, claimed that psychosurgery was especially effective on poor people, people with simpler occupations, and black people (Freeman and Watts, 1950). More frightening, prominent figures in the resurgence of psychosurgery in the late 1960s made strong, published claims connecting brain disease and urban rioting and disorder, and suggested psychosurgery as a possible solution to the political violence sweeping the American cities (Breggin, 1975a; Mark et al., 1967; Mark and Ervin, 1960; Mason, 1970; Rodin, 1973; Rosenfeld, 1968). One of the nation's best-known neurosurgeons advocated before a legislative body that the leaders of urban uprisings might make suitable candidates for psychosurgery, and the story was carried without criticism in the *New York Times* (Bird, 1968).

Given the political campaign being mounted by the psychosurgeons, I was not reassured by later claims that the surgery was too difficult to apply on a mass basis. First, the *threat* of its use against black urban leaders seemed a serious intimidating force in itself. Second, the surgery need not be used widely to have a vast effect, not only as an intimidator and as a method of neutralizing leadership, but as a technique for redefining political problems as medical ones. By proposing psychosurgery as a "cure" for urban violence, the psychosurgeons further distracted the nation from the *political* issues. Third, the mass application of any technique is largely an engineering problem. Where there is a will, there is a way to mass produce almost any technology. Perhaps the initial stereotaxic experiments would have led to a simpler technology, much as Walter Freeman reduced a major operation, prefrontal lobotomy, into a simple five-minute office procedure involving an ice pick around the eyeballs. All in all, it was the psychosurgeons themselves who were raising the political issue with enthusiasm, and I took them at their word. That we no longer hear the psychosurgeons making claims to save America from violence is strictly a product of the massive effort to alert the public and the Congress to this threat.

The proposed use of psychosurgery as a method of political control in an extreme way illustrates my basic hypothesis that the somatic interventions serve the purpose of compromising *personal sover-*

eignty and *personal freedom*. The hypothesis is nowhere better illustrated than in the clinical effects of psychosurgery, past and present.

The Threat to Personal Sovereignty

The most complete experimental study of lobotomy effects is a little-known book, *Personality Changes Following Frontal Leucotomy*, by P. MacDonald Tow, published in 1955. More than twenty years ago it should have laid to rest the myth that lobotomy effects are difficult to document, define, or demonstrate. Using a multiplicity of tests aimed at a variety of human mental functions, Tow came to the following conclusions:

> Tests of some intellectual functions show very significant change. There seems to be impairment of the powers of abstraction and synthesis; of perception of relations and differences; of the ability to deal with complex situations, planning, and thinking out of the next action and its consequences; and appreciation of one's own mistakes. These are, of course, not several discrete functions, but they are several closely related aspects of intellectual activity, which the tests show to be impaired. There is also impairment of the power of sustained attention and of the capacity for fine discrimination; and a dulled appreciation of the subject's own level of success or failure.

Because they most closely approximated the inner experience of the patient, the before and after autobiographies were the most poignant and sensitive indicators of the effect of lobotomy on the patients. Post-surgery autobiographies showed a difficulty producing anything creative or self-aware, sometimes mixed with a terrible fear of being harmed and controlled by scientific and psychiatric technology. Tow believed these patients to be more "schizophrenic" after their lobotomies, a phenomenon recently reported following cingulotomy (Escobar and Shandel, 1977). I have observed a florid paranoid schizophrenia with terror of being controlled by psychiatric technology following amygdalotomy (Breggin, 1973a, 1973b, 1973c).

Overall, Tow described the patients as "more simple" and as reduced in their "humanity":

> Possibly the truest and most accurate way of describing the net effect on the total personality is to say that he is more simple; and being more simple he has rather less insight into his own performance. . . . The higher mental processes suffer most; and one might say that it is the upper limit or the discriminative aspect of psychological function which is blunted. The conclusion would be that after loss of the pre-

frontal area there is a generalized impairment of mental activity, and that this impairment is greater in the higher and more peculiarly human functions than in others.

Tow's analysis fits well into my own, for the functions he is describing can easily be understood as personal sovereignty—the capacity and willingness to think, to feel, and to act on the highest human level. The resultant loss of personal freedom is also obvious.

Tow was no anti-lobotomist. On the contrary, he was a staunch defender of lobotomizing chronic state mental hospital patients on the grounds that the lobotomy would make them less morally sensitive to their awful condition and plight (Tow, 1952). Nor was Tow the only lobotomist to understand that lobotomy worked precisely because it made "good inmates." Some of the best-known lobotomists and lobotomy studies during the first wave advocated lobotomy because it helped adjust the patients to the "mundane realities" of state hospital life (Freeman and Watts, 1950; Freeman, 1959; Greenblatt, Arnot, and Solomon, 1950).

Studies of modern psychosurgical techniques in animals and humans alike show that they reduce the highest human faculties, making the individual less able to think abstractly, to experience his emotions, and to act decisively. The effect, as in electroshock or in phenothiazine medication, is a generalized one, and it depends upon damaging normal brain function. The effect is independent of any psychiatric disorder, and works alike in monkeys and in people. It can be achieved by destroying tissue in almost any part of the normal brain required for the proper function of volition, thought, or feeling.

Unfortunately, modern psychosurgeons have *never* exposed their patients to independent analysis by individuals who are critical of psychosurgery. Nor have critics of psychosurgery been consulted in developing objective standards for evaluating psychosurgery. My personal observations are based on patients who have come to me on their own for help following psychosurgery (Breggin, 1973a, b, and c). In several instances, patients of well-known surgeons who claim *never* to have had bad outcomes have contacted me for interviews and have displayed a post-lobotomy syndrome as well as other mental and physical side effects.

The recent studies by the National Commission on Psychosurgery (1977) illustrate the reluctance of the psychosurgeons to subject their patients to independent analysis. Although the Commission was established specifically at my request in an amendment through the office of Senator J. Glenn Beall, Jr., all critics of psychosurgery were systematically excluded from participating at any point in the studies. As a result, no attempts were made to measure the crucial functions of autonomy or personal sovereignty, and obvious signs of organic brain damage, such as euphoria and denial, were consistently interpreted as improvements. The results of these studies are critically examined elsewhere in this volume.

One need not have firsthand personal experience to discover the reality that the newer forms of surgery provide the same old service. First we have animal studies showing, for example, that amygdalotomized monkeys become helpless and unable to survive in their natural habitats (Breggin, 1975b). Some psychosurgeons, especially those operating outside the United States, have also stated their intent to "sedate" and "control" patients by means of modern stereotaxic surgery (Balasubramaniam et al., 1969, 1970). The "blunting" of emotions has also been cited as the major and desired outcome of *all* psychosurgical methods by the neurosurgeon William Scoville (1972).

One of the few in-depth psychological evaluations of modern-day psychosurgery patients also demonstrates the hypothesis that psychosurgery produces brain damage and dysfunction, impairing personal sovereignty and rendering the patient more helpless and manageable. The author is Ruth Andersen (1972), who works with Kjeld Vaernet, a Danish psychosurgeon and co-editor of *Psychosurgery*, the compendium in which the study appears. Andersen found a classic post-lobotomy syndrome typically following amygdalotomy:

> Typically the patient tends to become more inert, and shows less zest and intensity of emotions. His spontaneous activity tends to be reduced, and he becomes less capable of creative productivity, which is independent of the intelligence level. . . . With these changes in initiative and control of behavior, our patients resemble those with frontal lobe lesions.

Andersen claims that this constitutes no "serious disturbances in the establishment and execution of their major life plans," and then, contrary to her own assertions, goes on to declare that after surgery the patient has "become more dependent on the circumstances in the outer world" and "will make the most of this gain in well-structured situations of a somewhat monotonous and simple character." That statement—the last in the paper—brings me to the conclusion of my own study as well. Psychosurgery, like electroshock and the major tranquilizers, produces brain damage and dysfunction, rendering the patient less able to exercise personal sovereignty and personal freedom. He becomes a less able and less complete person, but a person easier to control and to manipulate. When euphoria appears as a reaction to the brain damage, the patient may deny any harmful effects and praise the treatment in an irrational manner (Breggin, 1979).

Summary

The major somatic therapies—phenothiazine tranquilizers, electroshock, and psychosurgery—share many common characteristics as brain-disabling interventions. Each originated as a technique for the control of inmates in oppressive overcrowded state mental hospitals. Each helped turn the "madhouse" into a "storehouse" by reducing the capacity and the willingness of the inmates to make trouble for themselves or for others. Each was openly described as a suppressive agent in the original research literature, and then became sanitized in subsequent generations of promotional publications. Each has been refined over the years without modifying its essentially destructive purpose and effect.

Despite a variety of differences, each of the major somatic therapies achieves its primary effect through the same mechanism—the production of brain damage and brain dysfunction causing a reduction in the capacity to exercise personal sovereignty and personal freedom. By disrupting normal brain function, the somatic therapies render the person less able, "more simple," or more childlike, ultimately making the person more susceptible to manipulation and control.

CHAPTER 24

Informed Consent and Review Committees

George J. Annas

The Doctrine of Informed Consent

The legal doctrine of informed consent has been developed for two primary purposes: the promotion of self-determination and the enhancement of rational decision making (Annas, Glantz, and Katz, 1977, pp. 33–38). The first is promoted by leaving the ultimate decision concerning treatment in the patient's hands, the second by providing the patient with a specified amount of information before he is asked to make a decision. The informational component of the informed consent doctrine in psychosurgery has been best described by the Massachusetts Department of Mental Health Psychosurgery Task Force, all fourteen members of which agreed that the following elements should be set forth in a written document signed by the patient before any psychosurgical procedure was performed.

> *How the procedure is performed.* It is the duty of the physician responsible for performing the procedure to explain to the subject, in lay terms, how the procedure is performed. The physician must also make himself available to answer any questions that the subject may have.

The risks involved in the procedure. Risks of death or serious disability (e.g., paralysis, blindness, deafness, impotence, etc.) must be disclosed even if the probability of their occurring is minimal. Any risk that is expected to occur with more than 1% frequency must be disclosed even though it may not be considered serious (e.g., headache, temporary loss of memory, etc.). Any probability of the procedure making the problem for which surgery is being recommended worse, must also be fully disclosed.

The benefits to be derived from the procedure. The subject must be told how successful or unsuccessful this particular procedure has been in the past with other patients as well as the probability for a successful outcome in his particular case. The subject must understand that success is not guaranteed, and what success means to the physician.

Available alternative modes of treatment. The subject must understand what, if any, alternative modes of treatment are available. The risks, benefits, and probabilities of success of these treatments must be explained to the subject.

An understanding that a procedure is experimental or investigational, if it is, and what these terms mean. This should include the number of times the procedure has been performed and the outcomes.

The ability to rescind his consent at any time. The subject must understand that he will not suffer in any way by withdrawing his consent and that alternative modes of therapy will be made available. The subject should also understand that if he decides not to undergo the procedure at this time, he may change his mind at a later date and the procedure will be performed at that time [Stone, 1975].[1]

While the disclosure of such information is a necessary means for protecting the rights of patients, it is not sufficient when psychosurgery is contemplated. The quest for additional safeguards has led many to turn to review committees of various sorts to help ensure both that the patient is fully informed and understands the proposed treatment, and that his or her consent is voluntary. These review committees have been used in a variety of situations.

Review Committees

In the *Kaimowitz* case,[2] discussed elsewhere in this volume, a three-person "human rights committee" was designated to ensure that Louis Smith's rights were protected. At least one member of this

---

[1] The Task Force was split 8–6 on the issue of individual patient interviews with a multidisciplinary review committee, the majority favoring such a procedure.

[2] *Kaimowitz v. Department of Mental Health,* Civil No. 73-19434-AW (Cir. Ct., Wayne Co., Mich., July 10, 1973) [slip opinion].

committee personally interviewed Smith to determine the voluntariness and competence of his consent. Although Smith convinced him of his willingness to participate in the experiment, he later withdrew his consent after he was released from custody. This raises some real questions as to the voluntary nature of the original consent and the quality of the review committee's determination, and about review committees in general (Annas, 1976).

A multidisciplinary review committee, consisting of a physician, a psychiatrist, two lawyers, a political scientist, a medical student, a sociologist, a research biochemist, and two representatives from the local community, was established at the Boston City Hospital in 1972 (Annas, Glantz, and Katz, 1977, pp. 232–233). The Committee reviewed two cases in depth. Although both involved temporal lobe epilepsy, and thus not the type of psychosurgery usually subject to either controversy or regulations, review if appropriate for epilepsy is *a fortiori* appropriate for other modes of psychosurgery (except for intractable pain). In one case, the Committee met with the patient, who was suffering from temporal lobe epilepsy, and his family a number of times over a period of approximately eight months. The Committee determined, and the patient confirmed, that it was the adult patient's parents who were desirous of the operation and not the patient. Six months after this decision, the patient returned to the surgeon and the Committee with another request for "something to be done" about his seizures. Meetings were held with both the surgeon and the Committee. After extended discussion with both the patient and his parents, the Committee again concluded that the patient did not want surgery, and surgery was not performed.

In another case, involving a minor who was suffering from severe temporal lobe epilepsy, the Committee met with the patient and her parents approximately three times over a two-week period. The final session was videotaped. Consent to an experimental psychosurgical procedure was obtained and approved by the Committee. Weeks after the procedure was performed, the father of the patient contacted the Committee chairman to express his appreciation for the thoughtfulness and completeness that characterized the Committee's work. He concluded that he, his child, and his wife all felt they understood the alternatives, the risks, and the possibilities of success of the surgery in a way they could not have if the Committee had not discussed these issues with them.

The experiences with patients at the Boston City Hospital, while limited, were all positive, and no patient or family member interviewed ever objected to the procedure or raised the issue of "breach of privacy" or confidentiality.

Similar experiences have been reported in Oregon, where state law mandates committee review prior to psychosurgery. As of mid-1977, the Committee had reviewed five cases, all involving considerably different circumstances (Annas, Glantz, and Katz, 1977, pp. 230–231). Of the five, three patients withdrew their consent shortly after the petitions for review were filed. Final decisions were not reached by the time of this writing on the others, but much valuable information was obtained about each of these cases by the review panel, which personally interviewed the patient-applicants (see Grimm, this volume). The Oregon experience suggests that a consent committee that personally interviews the patient can be a powerful tool both in determining the competency and knowledgeability of the patient, and in helping the patient to make an informed decision. It performs this latter function by acting as a neutral and authoritative entity to which the patient can communicate his or her questions and concerns and from which unbiased and knowledgeable answers can be obtained.

In this regard, the recommendations of the National Commission for the Protection of Human Subjects of Biomedical and Behavioral Research are disappointing. While endorsing the idea of review boards in general, the Commission has recommended drastically limiting their access to the patient himself. The Commission specifically recommends that psychosurgery research only be done in institutions that have an Institutional Review Board (IRB) formed and approved specifically to review proposed psychosurgery, and then only after the IRB has made a determination that:

a. the surgeon has the competence to perform the procedure;
b. it is appropriate, based upon sufficient assessment of the patient, to perform the procedure on that patient;
c. adequate pre- and post-operative evaluations will be performed; and
d. the patient has given informed consent.[3]

In its commentary to this recommendation, the Commission states, regarding informed consent:

> The consent by each patient should be reviewed by the IRB as a whole to assure that the patient's rights are protected. This review should focus on procedures or forms employed in the *consent process*, as well as the *circumstances of the actual consent* given by each patient. The IRB *may* require that a *third person*, unaffiliated with the surgical team or the patient's referring physician, observe or participate in the consent process. The IRB may also require that an examination by

---

[3] "Report and Recommendations on Psychosurgery," 42 *Fed. Reg.* 263329 (May 23, 1977).

appropriate consultants or a hearing before the IRB be conducted to determine the patient's ability to give informed consent to psychosurgery [emphasis added].[4]

This paragraph is followed by language that makes it clear that this "third person" participation is optional with the IRB, and is to be preferred to interviewing the patient before the entire IRB. Such "third person" participation in the consent process is grossly inferior to complete IRB participation, and is likely to place the IRB in the position of being a rubber stamp. If the IRB is to take into account the actual consent process, as the Commission suggested, the whole board must be personally involved in it and must discuss it with the patient. This is especially vital in psychosurgery, where many other treatments have been tried unsuccessfully, surgery looks like an "easy" out for the patient, and the surgeon involved is generally a "true believer."

Indeed, even mandatory appearances before review committees have won court approval. In reviewing the California statute that requires review of patient consent by a committee composed of three physicians who personally interview the patient, the court notes that such a review is justified for incompetent patients or patients whose competence is suspect in order to promote "the state's interest in protecting patients from unconsented-to and unnecessary psychosurgery"—and that such a review can ensure that the patient is competent and the consent voluntary. The court further approves such review for involuntarily committed patients whose voluntary consent can "never be adequately confirmed," as the only alternative to an outright prohibition of psychosurgery on this population. The court finds the most difficulty with requiring the review procedure for competent and voluntary patients, but approves it, explaining:

There are sound reasons why the treating physician's assessment of his patient's competency and voluntariness may not always be objective, and he may not necessarily be the best or most objective judge of how appropriate an experimental procedure would be. Because the consequences to the patient are so serious, and the effects he may suffer are so intrusive and irreversible, tort damages are totally inadequate. The need for some form of restraint is a sufficiently compelling state interest to justify the attendant invasion of the patient's right to privacy. The right is not absolute and must give way to appropriate regulation.[5]

---

[4] "Report and Recommendations on Psychosurgery," *op cit.*
[5] *Aden* v. *Younger*, 129 Cal. Rptr. 535, 549 (Ct. App. 4th Dist., Div. 1, 1976).

The court also and significantly approved the requirement that the three physicians be unanimous in their decision, saying, "Requiring unanimity by the review committee ensures each approved treatment is an appropriate use of an experimental procedure."

Additional Safeguards

Franz Ingelfinger has argued that informed consent is not meaningful in the hospital setting because of the control doctors exercise over their patients. In his view, "the subject's only real protection . . . depends on the conscience and compassion of the investigator and his peers" (Ingelfinger, 1972). Although our society has been willing to rely on this form of protection in the past, recent developments in medical technology and an increasing awareness of past abuses have made the establishment of more stringent safeguards imperative. Community sensibilities will no longer allow, for example, the unregulated research of scientists who respond to arguments affirming the special nature of the human brain as opposed to other organs with the contention that "[t]he inviolability of the brain is only a social construct, like nudity" (Delgado, 1973).

Because of the limitations of informed consent, especially with regard to experimental procedures on potentially incompetent or involuntary subjects, more protections are called for. One such protection that merits additional experimentation itself is the involvement of community representatives and nonmedical professionals in the decision-making process. The problems posed by psychosurgery and many other medical procedures are not capable of resolution merely on the basis of medical considerations. It is for this reason, and because of the tendency of peer review committees to act as rubber stamps for the research protocols of members of their own profession, that significant nonmedical representation on review committees should be assured.

Our experience with multidisciplinary committees, however, is so limited that we must guard against their becoming a mechanism that merely serves a legitimizing function on the basis of inadequate consideration. The criteria they employ and the decisions they reach should receive constant scrutiny to assure that the rights of patients are being protected. IRBs should probably not interview individual patients, since this has never been their function and there is no indication that they can do it well. A multidisciplinary committee should, however, be specially formed for this purpose. In addition, certain procedural safeguards should be built into the review process. First, a prospective patient should always be represented by legal counsel during committee proceedings, and should have the right to cross-examine witnesses and challenge documents presented. Second, the committees should follow written standards for review of voluntariness, competency, information, knowledgeability of the patient, and appropriateness of the procedure; keep minutes of their meetings; and record individual votes for every decision. The keeping of detailed minutes and the recording of votes should act as a safeguard against the diffusion of personal responsibility (Milgram, 1973; Milgram, 1974).[6] If the research proposal and the consent of the patient are reviewed and approved according to such procedures, individuals legally competent to give their informed consent should be allowed to undergo psychosurgical operations.

Certain classes of prospective patients, however, require more stringent protection. The confinement or status of prisoners, institutionalized mental patients, and children makes them especially vulnerable. Thus, in addition to committee review and approval, there should be established a presumption, rebuttable only in a court of law, that psychosurgery cannot be performed on them. To rebut this presumption, the proponent of psychosurgery should be required to demonstrate beyond a reasonable doubt that the patient's consent is both voluntary and knowledgeable, and that there is a reasonable probability that the procedure will produce the desired effect. Although this proposal may amount to a *de facto* ban on the performance of psychosurgery on members of these groups, it would permit such operations under extremely compelling circumstances.

It is much too early in our experience with the mechanism of multidisciplinary review to reach any final conclusions with respect to its ability to regulate potentially abusive medical procedures. It is clear, however, that the current system of regulation is not only woefully inadequate, but almost nonexistent. For the present, the establishment of review committees along the lines suggested offers a regulatory approach that permits the medical community to proceed with research on the human brain without sacrificing the individual rights of patients.

Finally, I would urge the creation of some federal agency to begin to examine the question of which technologies or surgical procedures *should* be developed. At some point, procedures, like drugs

---

[6] Stanley Milgram's experiments have demonstrated that the fragmentation of responsibility may lead average individuals to commit inhuman acts. Thus, the proliferation of committees proposed by NIH may prove self-defeating.

and devices, assume a life of their own, and regulation becomes difficult, if not impossible. The question of whether or not we should control human behavior by brain manipulation should be answered before the question of how we should conduct research in this area comes to be viewed as the only relevant question (Casper, 1976; Task Force of the Presidential Advisory Group on Anticipated Advances in Science and Technology, 1976).[7]

---

[7] The entire question of psychosurgery regulation and research may be an appropriate one to use in a pilot study on the concept of a "Science Court."

CHAPTER 25

Effective Psychosurgery: The Greater Danger?

George J. Annas

Dangers of Current Psychosurgery

Psychosurgery of established effectiveness may pose a greater danger to society than current experimental psychosurgery. It could pose a danger to individual patients because less emphasis would be placed on the need to obtain voluntary, competent, informed and understanding consent; and it could pose a danger to society in that its use could be broadened to include "treatment" of certain behaviors deemed undesirable by the majority. While psychosurgery may never become "standard medical procedure," it is worth spending at least some time speculating about the implications of such a possibility.

While a landmark case in many respects, the *Kaimowitz* decision (discussed elsewhere in this volume) has major drawbacks. Its holding, for example, that Louis Smith could not give his informed consent to psychosurgery was based primarily on the finding that psychosurgery was "experimental." The court went on to emphasize that it believed a different situation would present itself if the proposed surgery were an "accepted" treatment:

When the state of medical knowledge develops to the extent that the type of psychosurgical intervention proposed here becomes an accepted neurosurgical procedure and is no longer experimental, it is possible, with appropriate review mechanisms, that involuntarily detained mental patients could consent to such an operation.

This qualification of the court's opinion, of course, flies in the face of its finding that an involuntarily committed mental patient cannot give adequate consent because the phenomenon of institutionalization diminishes the capacity to consent, rendering the patient in effect "incompetent." In the court's words, "Institutionalization tends to strip the individual of the support which permits him to maintain his sense of self-worth and the value of his own physical and mental integrity." Likewise, the court found that no such consent could be voluntary since a closed institution has "an inherently coercive atmosphere even though no direct pressures may be placed upon him. . . . Involuntarily confined patients cannot reason as equals with the doctors . . . and are unable to give informed consent because of the inherent inequality in their position."

Neither the coercive atmosphere of the mental institution nor the phenomenon of institutionalization would change if psychosurgery became standard medical procedure. What could change, however, is our current belief that only the patient himself should be permitted to consent to such a procedure. The result might be the use of psychosurgery on significant numbers of institutionalized patients against their wills.

The problem is one of treating all prospective patients as if they were identical, and all prospective medical treatments as if they were fungible. The fact is, as is well-recognized in experimental settings, that very different factors are relevant in obtaining the consent of a child, a prisoner, a mental patient, or an outpatient to be used as an experimental subject. The law also recognizes that procedures with varying degrees of risk require varying degrees of disclosure. No disclosures concerning risks of donating blood need be made, since these are minimal and generally known. However, all risks of death and serious disability must be disclosed, as well as alternatives and problems of recuperation, before a patient is asked to consent to surgery under general anesthesia. The greater the risks and the wider the alternatives, the more disclosures required.

Technology has a momentum of its own, and a technology that has been recognized as effective will bring into play a whole host of pressures to put it to use. Use on violent prisoners, for example, will be proposed both as a method of "rehabilitation" and as a cost-savings mechanism. As has been recognized by a few writers, including Kittrie (1971) and Shuman (1977), what is at stake once deviance has been defined as illness and a medical solution advanced is "the right to be unhealthy." While this right has always been circumscribed by society, the recent increase in medicine's turf has caused it to become more and more constricted. For example, drug addiction and public drunkenness, once universally considered crimes, are now generally dealt with as illnesses for which the appropriate remedy is enforced medical treatment. Since the "indications" for psychosurgery are virtually limitless, and have at the extreme even included such things as drug addiction and homosexuality, its potential as a medical intervention to "cure" social deviance is also virtually limitless.

Regulatory Options

There are a number of options. The first is to hold that the potential abuses of effective psychosurgery are so menacing that only an immediate ban on psychosurgery experimentation can prevent them. Such an argument could draw some strength from historical precedent, such as the highly regulated use of drugs in so-called hyperactive children. Another option is to require the types of review safeguards recommended for experimental psychosurgery by the National Commission even after psychosurgery becomes "accepted" medical procedure. A third is to dispense with the Commission's recommendations that pertain to the scientific rationale and review, but continue the requirements for informed consent and review of the consent process. A modification of this third position would be to retain the informed consent review process for all patients capable of giving consent themselves, but to eliminate from consideration for the procedure all patients incapable of so consenting. A fourth approach would be to develop some general set of criteria that define when procedures like psychosurgery can be performed on individuals without their informed consent.

My own bias is to favor the modified third approach, since it is the only one that promotes and protects the individual's right of self-determination and ensures that his brain will not be violated and altered without his own agreement and cooperation. Physicians might argue that this would eliminate a major group of patients —those who need the operation but are too "sick" to know that they do, and so will not consent to it. The response is that this is a risk well worth running, since the benefit is speculative but the harm produced by involuntary major surgery is not.

Efforts to produce a set of compromise principles also merit further exploration. Shuman (1977), for example, has suggested that there might be a limitation on the "right to be unhealthy" when five conditions are met:

1. The unhealthy condition is corrigible.

2. The evidence for the condition is regarded as biological by the relevant scientific community.

3. The curative therapy is not experimental.

4. The therapy carries no unreasonable risk of organic or psychological harm.

5. The condition has previously imposed, and would continue to impose, significant social cost to the community (Shuman, 1977, p. 205).

While this list is acknowledged as tentative and subject to many varying interpretations, it is a potentially fruitful avenue that should be pursued by those who would propose psychosurgery on anyone without the patient's own informed consent.

Limiting access to certain things (like accepted medical treatments) on the basis of danger or inability to consent is not without legal precedent. A number of states, including Massachusetts, have recently passed statutes making it a crime to sterilize anyone without his or her "knowledgeable" consent. While sterilization is not deemed experimental by anyone, the experimental standard of "knowledgeable" consent has been applied to this procedure by the legislature because of past abuses involving children and the mentally retarded. There is little doubt that a similar approach, applied to nonexperimental psychosurgery, would survive constitutional challenge (Annas, Glantz, and Katz, 1977, pp. 51–53).

Indeed, the state could probably ban experimental psychosurgery altogether if it found that the prospect of effective psychosurgery posed unjustifiable burdens on society or potential psychosurgery patients. A recent Tennessee case could provide the rationale. The case involved the prohibition of the handling of snakes in religious ceremonies conducted by The Holiness Church of God in Jesus' Name. The court noted that while the First Amendment regarding freedom of religion was broad, it did not include the right to violate a statute or the right to commit or maintain a nuisance. In concluding that the handling of poisonous snakes by church members constituted an unlawful nuisance, the court said:

Tennessee has the right to guard against the unnecessary creation of widows and orphans. Our state and nation have *an interest in having a strong, healthy, robust, taxpaying citizenry* capable of bearing arms and adding to the resources and reserves of manpower. We, therefore, have a substantial and compelling state interest in the face of a clear and present danger so grave as to endanger paramount public interests . . . Yes, *the state has a right to protect a person from himself and to demand that he protect his own life* [emphasis added].[1]

---

[1] *Tennessee v. Pack,* 527 S.W.2d 99 (Tenn. 1975).

CHAPTER 26

My Case Against Psychosurgery

Gabe Kaimowitz

Let me tell you something about myself. It may help to know something about my prejudices and perceptions to understand why I took steps seven years ago to halt the practice of psychosurgery.

I was a journalist for nearly a decade, because I wanted to follow in the footsteps of one of my childhood heroes, the muckraker Lincoln Steffens. As a reporter and editor for various publications, I found myself at odds with the so-called objective school of reporting and writing prevalent in the fifties. Increasingly, I objected to a world view presented in the United States press that seemed to work against the working-class interests of my family and friends. So in the early sixties, after the assassination of President Kennedy, I decided to become an advocate for beliefs I could support, as opposed to those I was required to present by my employers. To do so, I went to law school, and I was graduated from New York University School of Law in 1967.

Since I am now trained in law, I will present a case to justify those actions of mine that brought the use of brain surgery for the control of human behavior to the attention of the public. I offer the evidence primarily to indicate how it affected the state of my mind when I decided to take legal action to bar the use of institutionalized persons as human subjects for medical research, and particularly for psychosurgery. I do not offer the content for its supposed truth.

Social and Ethical Concerns

I am deeply concerned about how much those of us outside the professional pale do not know about what is going on in scientific research because of what I perceive as barriers deliberately established between scientific investigators and the rest of us, who they do not think will understand anyway. What information has surfaced in the popular and political press about scientific exploration has compelled me to question the *process* by which any so-called scientific breakthrough has been accomplished. For example, I wonder how many mentally retarded people died or suffered unnecessary discomfort to develop a vaccine against serum hepatitis. I do know that such persons were used in the early stages of the development of such a vaccine at Michigan and New York state mental health facilities. How many persons will be used in experiments without their knowledge or consent so that we all can benefit from a control of cancerous cells? The stories of scientific breakthroughs rarely credit the humans who were subjected to unnamed horrors to produce some marvelous benefit for the populace. We all know about the Salk and Sabin vaccines, named for their primary medical investigators. But are we as familiar with the names of those subjected to various forms of such vaccines in the experimental stage to develop those protections against a dread condition? Obviously not. Simply put, how much is being done to advance science, and how much to advance a scientist, a theory, or the concerns of a pharmaceutical company? Certainly, little has been done to advance the present interests of human subjects used to determine *future* benefit of a particular form of medical procedure or treatment, given what we have learned from the scandals surrounding the evaluation of a syphilis treatment, or the practice of sterilization, or the less sophisticated form of psychosurgery known as lobotomy.

It is not only the process of involving human subjects in medical or other scientific research without their knowledge or assurance of adequate benefit and recognition that troubles me. The goals as well appear questionable. After six years of study and reading, I am convinced that professionals as a group, and many members of the scientific community, aspire to the creation of a world populated by humans they would regard as more perfect than those extant today. Whether by application of amniocentesis, or manipulation of genetic materials, or the application of psychosurgery, many want to bring about major changes in the human condition. I see no marked distinction between such dreams and the earlier aspirations, now publicly abhorrent, for the creation of a superman, or a master race.

As for "lower" forms of human life, I have heard professionals advocate the use of mentally defective persons for almost any form of research, on the grounds that such handicapped people thereby would make a material contribution to society and thus fulfill their human potential. I have listened to arguments that prisoners likewise should be used, to permit them to pay their "debt" to society or make expiation for their antisocial acts. Further, I have read that it would be difficult to eliminate physical and mental defects without the use of subjects from the lower depths of humankind, including the poor. To me, such suggestions bespeak a disregard for the common people, at best, and threaten their eventual elimination, at worst.

Of course, few of us participating in such discussions are likely to be categorized as somehow less than human, or "sacrificed" as human subjects. We are exempted by our own ability to voluntarily participate, or to withhold consent from such participation—unlike those who are under the control of the state, or who are dependent economically on public aid or charity. Let me be clear. Scientific investigators rarely exercise direct control over the lives of others. Therefore, they often consider themselves removed from the process of selecting human subjects for their research. Here, as in Nazi Germany, researchers rely on the state to supply them with subjects after these investigators dutifully inform some authority why the use of humans is needed. What investigators fail to realize is that in legal terms they are in most instances either acting directly or indirectly in a partnership or agency relationship with the state on which they rely for funding and/or for the supply of human subjects. Meanwhile, state representatives often seem to accept without question what the scientific investigators believe to be best, since the lawmakers seldom think they have the necessary specialized knowledge to judge for themselves.

It is the blindness in the scientific community to the relationship between its work and societal values as a whole that I would cure before permitting scientifically formulated and controlled research into the human condition. I would like nothing better than to see a moratorium on *all* such research until ethical guidelines are properly in place. Science can wait until we decide why something should or should not be done. For example, *why* do we want perfect humans?

Most attempts to develop a more perfect species have produced economic and social "side effects" resulting in suffering and even death, but the scientific community absolves itself of responsibility. Too broad a charge? Then let me be specific. If I were an unlicensed person who decided to help a child unable to function in society by cutting into him with a knife, and he died, surely I would be either locked up as a criminal or treated as a madman. However, if a licensed physician causes the death of that child by experimentally removing a part of the minor's brain, any culpability would have to be determined civilly. As long as the surgeon operates within his sphere of knowledge, no matter how little there may be, society will not hold him responsible, no matter how much damage, even death, he may inflict on another human being. After all, it is not murder; it simply is scientific progress at an experimental stage.

And if I wander the halls of a hospital and see individuals suffering from lack of motor control—not from the psychosis for which they are being treated, but from the alleviating medication—who can I hold responsible? If I had not intervened to stop a prisoner from being used as the subject of a surgical experiment and he had suffered paralysis, blindness, or even death, as the form requesting his consent said he might, who would have been accountable? Who would even have known about it? And today? Sadly, I have no reason to believe matters are different. Investigators have not stopped operating. They still decide what to report and how to present the information. Certainly, I have found no more willingness to disclose, for example, when children and mentally defective persons in Michigan facilities are being used as subjects for research today than I did six years ago. The only reason I have been able to detect scientific abuses at all is that occasionally a periscope appears in troubled waters where none is supposed to be. And I, for one, continue to look for them. I have become expert in recognizing them as signs of perhaps alien submarines. The tracking process of scientific abuses continues to be a hit-or-miss proposition.

Other contributors presumably will strive to be more objective and let the data they have accumulated and arranged speak for them. Many may believe their prejudices, races, ages, ethnic backgrounds, sexes or sexual preferences, family ties, comparative wealth, aspirations, and personalities simply would confuse the issues at hand. Rather, the contributors will display their educational and professional credentials and their previous publications. These are passports to credibility, at least among this assumed readership. For without these credentials, why would you listen to any of us, any more than you would want to read about the personal accounts of patients recuperating from operations in a hospital ward after surgery—unless, of course, you needed that information for research?

Given my admitted ignorance about psychosurgery seven years ago, when I took legal action to stop its use, how did I get a right to participate in this elite discussion? I intruded myself on behalf of a prisoner to prevent his subjection to brain surgery. I acted against his wishes! At the various seminars in law, medicine, and ethics I have attended since the legal action was initiated, the most vexing question put to me has been: "What gave you the right. . . ?" It is significant that I have yet to get an answer to my question: "What gave the investigators, the researchers, the right?" One could ask, for that matter, what gave the *Washington Post* the right to inquire what, or who, had the authority to hire hands to enter Democratic Party headquarters at the Watergate housing complex? Who in our society is or should be appointed to identify the nakedness of the emperor when he thinks he is wearing new clothes?

I acted on the basis of the belief that a wrong might be done without subjection to public scrutiny. I was not to make the decision, but I was qualified to present to our courts the issue as to whether incarcerated people can be given a choice between, as I saw it, the devil and the deep blue sea. At the time, I intended only to ask whether inmates being held indefinitely by the state could be "asked" to submit to either a surgical or a chemical process designed to inhibit their sexuality. If they refused, did they face unspoken penalties in the form of continued incarceration and disfavor from authorities who controlled their lives?

I already have said I do not regard myself as *professionally* qualified to ask such questions. Although I am an attorney, I acted not in that capacity but as an adult. Any adult in Michigan can object to the illegal detention, or incarceration for an unlawful purpose, of a human being. An individual in Michigan cannot submit himself to prison without question, or ask the state to commit mayhem on his person. In other words, the state where I reside recognizes John Stuart Mill's concept that an exception is made to the rule of liberty when people use that liberty to choose slavery. Such an exception is necessary to protect those who may be overborne by the state, rather than to protect the individual himself or herself.

But what has liberty to do with a physician offering to treat a person to relieve or cure an unwanted, definable ailment? The first judge I appealed to could see no issue when I asked him to apply state law to prevent this medically proposed intrusion on the person of a prisoner in the hands of the state. The inmate simply was consenting to help offered to him by a medical doctor. Apparently, the judge did not consider that a state-held inmate can hardly decide when to go to the bathroom, much less go for a walk or exercise rights of protest while under state control. How then can a prisoner voluntarily, knowingly, and competently consent to participate as a subject in state-financed and -directed research to permanently alter his behavior?

Few physicians or medical researchers with whom I subsequently have discussed the problems seem to understand the need for public scrutiny of any consensual arrangement between an individual, especially an inmate or a child, and an attending person, *as long as that person is licensed or authorized by the state to offer to inhibit or prevent an unwanted condition.* They do see the issue when people want to place their bodies in the hands of faith healers, or in the hands of midwives, or in the hands of the few licensed physicians who are willing to prescribe Laetrile for cancer; they do see the issue when people termed patients decide to refuse amputations or blood transfusions that the medicoscientific community believes to be in their interest. Scientists and doctors do seek to use the law and the court to prevent quackery or impose treatment, but they fail to understand that the essence for the judiciary very often is nothing more or less than state condonation by licensing or funding, and it has little to do with the condition to be treated *or the ethics of the practitioners.*

On the terms just set forth, the medicoscientific community gains more control of human behavior whenever it can label a condition as requiring its expertise rather than that of the economist, criminologist, sociologist, or even the politician (who, of course, is necessary at least to authorize the flow of funds). If that medicoscientific community determines that human aggressivity, or cigarette smoking, or alcoholism, or depression, or baldness, or homosexuality is a disease, it immediately begins to accumulate the expertise, through research and investigation, to control the conduct or condition it has deemed unwanted.

So the first critical question for me when I learned about the circumstances of the psychosurgery research project was whether investigators were attempting to study what I clearly could regard as a medical matter. My answer was no. And it still is.

I would hope to leave readers with serious doubts whether the issues of scientific advancement are within the sole, or even primary, purview of a given discipline or disciplines. The most useful way of approaching this question is to convene representatives of numerous disciplines and the community and determine how their education and experience might be applied to resolve a given issue. This was attempted at two symposia I attended in Pennsylvania in 1975—one on medical research and experimentation, at Duquesne University, and the other on "divergent attitudes which have been expressed toward treating or withholding treatment of severely defective newborn children," at Skytop. Particularly at the latter convening of physicians, investigators, lawyers, medical practitioners, social workers, sociologists, religious and secular ethicists, and several lay people, the question as well as the answers evoked by the quoted topic changed as divergent viewpoints were presented.

There are many questions that should be asked at such gatherings. What is a disease? What is treatment? Can withholding treatment be tantamount to murder? Can giving it? Can a family with an interest obviously conflicting with that of an individual member subject that person to suffering or death by granting or withholding treatment? What is a person? Can seriously defective individuals be used for medical research? How much does the economic status of the individual or his family determine the probability of his being kept alive or being used as a subject for future advances in medical knowledge? Do physicians who are responsible for creating life-sustaining, but often debilitating, conditions have more or less of a right to determine how their technological advances should be used? What positions should we take in regard to such unwanted conditions as an open spine at birth, which may heal itself or cause brain damage? Who should ultimately decide whether someone so "handicapped" would prefer to live or die? Who should have the biggest influence on the decision process? The family, informed of the economic and social costs if the defective individual is sustained? The physician, who might be required to maintain the defective individual? The social worker, who ultimately might be responsible for caring for these individuals and pleading with society to provide the needed resources? Or the lawyer, who might see any form of either withholding treatment or experimental intrusion as murder or an assault?

To me, the question of liberty lies at the core of such ethical issues. Liberty embodies the freedom to choose, and to the degree that society impinges on that freedom, it must justify its actions. Society cannot expand liberty, since to me "freedom" is an infinite concept. However, the state may make it possible for a person to choose by restoring physical or mental faculties. If a person is unable to render a choice at a given time, *society must act to sustain life and the possibility of choice*, or liberty, even if the consensus is that the person may never have the capacity to choose.

The Story Behind the Case

In the winter of 1972–1973, how did the issues outlined above bear on the question of psychosurgery being offered to a person in the hands of a state that wished to curb his supposedly unwanted condition? It should have been, but was not, obvious from the outset that a person in the hands of the state is in no position to choose, because the state limits the choice for him. The state could have acted to impose psychosurgery on the subject or to withhold it, as it could the infliction of capital punishment or the original incarceration. The fallacy of the procedure became clear when the state, through its officials and investigators, attempted to get his consent and that of his family for the surgical intrusion.

In effect, I am asserting that in actuality performing any surgical intrusion does not require the consent of an individual in the hands of the state. The choice to operate is the state's, not the inmate's, whose options are limited in most significant respects at the time of incarceration. The state may restrict access to physicians; it may decide that one inmate's condition is not as life-threatening as some other prisoner's and offer the limited services of the doctor to the latter. Simply, in the hands of the state, one does not choose even when to live or to die. For example, the state is troubled when a condemned Nazi like Hermann Goering or a condemned murderer like Gary Gilmore attempts to take his own life before a designated time of execution. The state will decide, not the person who has forfeited choice after the state assumes control over his entire life. This is not a situation I favor. It is the reality as I see it, here or in Nazi Germany, South Africa, or the Soviet Union.

I suggest to the reader, then, that a state offers consent options to people only when it does not want to be responsible for what happens to them. Consent that is in fact knowing, competent, and voluntary rarely is subject to question. The question of consent appears to be important only when an individual in a coma—even an adult like Karen Quinlan—or a person who is defective, or a Jehovah's Witness is not able to act or refuses to act in accordance with society's wishes. The offer of consent options to persons we know are incapable of consenting freely belies, rather than strengthens, our belief that people when capable to choose and not subject to punishment will act as we wish them to act.

Once having determined, as I did, that the prisoner's status rendered him incapable of providing informed consent, I would not tolerate the concept of substitute judgment for the good of the person or in his best interests. I have yet to see or hear of a situation where such substitution did not involve some potential conflict with the view of the human subject in question or where it did not give rise to a reasonable suspicion that the benefit of such choice would be for someone other than the person for whom judgment was being substituted. The reader by now should understand that I would not have intruded to have the offer of psychosurgery subverted if the state first had unconditionally released the prisoner or prisoners in question and then asked whether he or they wished to participate in the research project.

How, then, can society provide assistance, if that is what it intends to do, for individuals considered incapable of deciding for themselves by virtue of their mental or physical state, or imposed environment? I say *provide assistance* because I do not wish to include situations where the state chooses to confine someone believed to be dangerous to others, be it a person suffering from tuberculosis or schizophrenia, a leper, or an unruly child. If society, in open court, decides that John Doe should undergo psychosurgery to prevent him from being dangerous to others, I may not agree in some instances, but I would not intervene. The danger that appears greatest to me is when society, or the medicoscientific community, assists John Doe ostensibly for his benefit even though he made no cry for help except in response to inducement by the state. Society can impose its will on us within constitutional and statutory limits. But when it wants our "consent" that we cannot freely give, it is seeking a simple way to get around those rules—or an imposition people might find abhorrent if they thought about it.

I arrived at these premises largely as a result of my involvement with John Doe, who was the first person selected to participate in a research project designed to control human aggressivity, particularly related to male sexuality. The project was intended to involve twenty-four males confined indefinitely as criminal sexual psychopaths. A dozen would be subjected to psychosurgical exploration, the others to a drug-induced impotence. No control group was involved, and there was no promise to release any or all of the subjects to see whether the treatments affected behavior outside the prison walls. Ironically, an enlightened policy to release all but seventeen persons in Michigan classified as criminal sexual psychopaths was being carried out separately at the time of the project's creation, but the researchers were unaware that their sample population had been decimated until the project was under way. When the subjects were to be selected, John Doe was deemed the only suitable candidate. After the popular press publicized the study, thirteen of the sixteen other confined sexual psychopaths wrote to me to plead that none of them be offered the choice between surgery and medication; but in truth, none of them had been deemed suitable. It is possible that the target population would have been shifted to include persons said to be mentally ill or mentally retarded, but I cannot say so for a certainty.

As for John Doe, I have seen him only twice, once when he testified during the course of the trial that he no longer wanted surgical intervention, primarily because of what he had read in *Ebony* and other lay publications, and once after the trial during a panel discussion. On that panel, he expressed dismay that the surgery was intended to curb his sexuality, which he regarded as normal, as well as his aggressivity, which he did believe to be uncontrollable in some respects. However, I am satisfied that although John Doe might have been misled about the particulars, he did in fact agree to participate in research that might have placed him and his brain at risk. But as I have stated, I did not act to represent him. I moved to prevent the use of state-approved and -financed surgical intervention to control, manipulate, or direct human behavior. I was pleased that the three judges who heard the issues presented recognized this distinction from the outset and appointed counsel specifically to represent John Doe's interests.

My involvement with the issues I am discussing began in late 1972 when I attended a meeting of lawyers in Detroit who believed in the necessity for radical change in society, primarily to gain a redistribution of wealth. They invited people in the psychomedical fields who were said to be kindred spirits, to determine how members of each profession could assist the other. I went to the meeting primarily to gather information I might use in legal action I undertook in 1971 to prevent persons in state mental facilities from being subjected to unwanted institutionalization, medication, and electroshock treatment. I knew nothing about psychosurgery or lobotomy other than what I had read previously in Ken Kesey's novel *One Flew Over the Cuckoo's Nest*.

The night before the meeting, I coincidentally read the first part of Michael Crichton's novel *Terminal Man*, as it was being serialized in *Playboy* magazine. I was intrigued by what I then regarded as the pure fantasy of an engineer running amok because of his brain mal-functioning. I had no idea at the time that the author believed it to be based on a true case history of an individual who was subjected to psychosurgery to alleviate his outbursts of episodic violence, perhaps precipitated by a form of epilepsy. I was curious later when Crichton, who has a medical degree, recanted on the link he had made between aggressivity and epilepsy. Ironically, he recanted largely as a result of information obtained from Dr. Ernst Rodin, the principal defendant in the Michigan psychosurgery trial. Dr. Rodin generally saw no correlation between epilepsy and aggressivity, although he testified at one point that John Doe might be a sus-pected epileptic if an abnormality were needed to justify surgical intrusion into his brain. I never finished *Terminal Man*. I have yet to see Anthony Burgess' *Clockwork Orange* world of imposed behavior modification to curb human aggressivity. I no longer want to con-fuse "fact" with fiction in considering the applications of techniques used by society to control or modify human behavior.

At the 1972 meeting previously mentioned, my sensibilities were jarred when a resident psychiatrist indicated that someone was being held at the respected Lafayette Clinic research center in De-troit to determine the relationship between his brain activity and his criminal conduct. I knew Lafayette was a state-funded facility selec-tive about its patient intake, but little else. Though several others at the gathering were affiliated with Lafayette, none claimed to know about the brain research. The discussion easily shifted to other, seem-ingly more relevant topics about the relationship between law and psychiatry. After the meeting, I sought out the resident and started my own inquiry about the experiment. I learned a little more, in-cluding the fact that one person said to be an epileptic already had been subjected to surgical intrusion into his brain to control or change his behavior. Echoes of *Terminal Man* began to sound in my head.

Further questioning proved more disquieting. The resident had studied in Germany. He was of the opinion that the worldwide medical community was aware at the time of the experiments per-formed on politically deviant, mentally disabled, and terminally ill persons in Germany before World War II. Many of those experiments were similar to those tried later in the concentration camps when people were headed toward certain death. The experiments often caused pain and suffering, even death. Many of them, however, were expected to contribute to knowledge about eugenics and emergency treatment, such as operating without anesthesia on a battlefield. The research could be said to lead to the creation and preservation of a master race.

A master race created for political purposes? Horrifying, no doubt. But what if mankind could detect and eliminate, by sterilization or in-the-womb examination and abortion, the birth of people regarded as mentally or physically defective? What if retardation could be prevented? What if diseases could be eliminated after being induced and studied in some human subjects? What if murder, rape, assault, and other antisocial acts were the result of faulty genetic makeup or aberrant conditions of the brain and could be prevented by eliminating the carriers of the unwanted conditions? What if the Germans simply were mistaken about the Jews carrying unwanted characteristics and beliefs, but were right in the premise that certain groups did in fact contain seeds that grew to destroy the economic and social fabric of society? Imagine a society without crime or corruption! Where all the people truly were created equal without unwanted physical and mental defects because the state could eliminate deviancy! What if there were investigators in the worldwide medicoscientific community who believed in the ideology of creating a superior human species, but simply presumed the Nazis were going about it in the wrong way?

In that brief conversation with the resident, in which many of these concepts floated in my mind, I concluded that there were certain issues I did *not* want raised, certain values I would *never* uphold, certain discoveries I hoped *never* would be made. Although I am not religious, I began to wonder whether I would have fought the use of cadavers for research by physicians in the nineteenth century, on moral grounds, especially if I learned that the bodies had been unlawfully dug up from graves or, worse, if I learned that someone had been murdered to supply a body.

After my conversation with the resident, I hurried to my office and called Jo Thomas, a *Detroit Free Press* reporter. We had come to know one another earlier in the year at a conference in which noted antipsychiatrist Thomas Szasz preached against the myth of mental illness and inveighed against institutionalization of people considered deviant. Jo and I then found we shared with Dr. Szasz a similar distaste for the helping professions when they seemed likely to cause more harm than good.

Largely as a result of Jo's efforts, we learned that the Lafayette inmate was to be subjected to surgical intrusion into his brain to determine whether a murder he committed almost a generation earlier was the product of some kind of physical or mental defect controllable by brain surgery. John Doe had been taken from Ionia State Hospital for the Criminally Insane; he had been under study for some months, and the operation was imminent. Could we expose and prevent it by use of the press and the law?

As we gathered information, we learned that a select group of legislators, prominent physicians at Wayne State School of Medicine, several law professors and an entire class of law students at Wayne State, another *Detroit Free Press* reporter, and a psychiatrist known to question the use of lobotomy had all been let in on the "secret" during the preceding weeks. Each had been sworn to secrecy until the project was completed and the results were published. No one had spoken out. Later, similarly respected individuals and organizations, including the *New York Times*, proclaimed the virtues psychosurgery might accomplish and continued to question the need for public exposure of a research project accepted within the established medicoscientific community, until all of the results were available.

The silence surrounding the case was broken forever one morning by headlines splashed across the front page of a Sunday edition of the *Detroit Free Press*. The article reported that I was considering legal action to halt the project. In fact, I did not know at the time how I, or anyone, could raise the matter as a legal concern. With input from several colleagues, I developed theories based on laws permitting real property taxpayers to question the expenditure of public funds for projects violating public policy, and allowing individuals to object to someone being held in a public facility for an illegal purpose. But I still did not have a client, and I still did not have the facts. Then I got a break.

Dr. Ernst Rodin, the neurologist who conceived the project, Lafayette Clinic Director Jacques Gottlieb, and their colleague Elliot Luby, who organized most of the review efforts approving the project, decided to make available to Jo, Dolores Katz, also of the *Detroit Free Press*, and me the details, including protocols and correspondence, and signed consent forms, for the research project. Presumably, they hoped we would be persuaded about the efficacy of the work once the sensational aspects could be viewed in the clearer light of day, after nearly two years of "darkness." Dr. Rodin, especially, was convinced the project would be accepted, if not by us, then by a court of law.

Fortunately, from my point of view, he was wrong. Using the documents provided to me and the press, and information gathered primarily by Jo Thomas, I filed a legal action on behalf of myself and individual members of the Medical Committee for Human Rights, who I knew to be real property holders, to prevent the use of John Doe and twenty-three unnamed others as human subjects in a nearly $300,000 state-funded experiment to determine whether brain surgery or an impotence-inducing drug would be more effective in controlling human sexual aggressivity in males known to have committed antisocial acts. The rest is history.

Postscript: Pride and Prejudice

Since I regard this account as purely subjective, I have refrained from footnoting any statements. I do not regard this as a scholarly work, but as one simply setting forth the value system of an individual, who saw fit to intrude his views on the medicoscientific and legal communities and the public in general. I have made this contribution to this collection, not because I believe this volume to be representative of a spectrum of views on the issues raised by the editors and publisher surrounding the so-called psychosurgery controversy, but because most of the previous accounts of the Michigan psychosurgery case have been in error in assuming that the legal action was instituted by nationally recognized elements of the law, the community, and the press, including the Center on Social Policy and Law, the Medical Committee for Human Rights, and the *New York Times*, as well as the American Civil Liberties Union and related affiliates.

The very effort to place the case in the classic mold of a problem soluble by a profession, or professions acting within their respective fields, is indicative of the kind of thinking that denigrates deviancy from the norm—the kind of thinking that I believe produces the need for a psychosurgery case to bring into question the widespread belief that the medicoscientific community generally knows what it is doing.

CHAPTER 27

Organic Rehabilitation and Criminal Punishment

Richard Delgado

Organic therapies, such as psychosurgery, electrical stimulation of the brain, and chemical and pharmacological treatment, increasingly are being urged as treatments for aberrant or antisocial behavior, particularly impulsive violence (Delgado, 1969; Mark and Ervin, 1970; Schwitzgebel, 1969; Shapiro, 1974; Spece, 1972). When applied to captive populations, such as prison inmates or mental patients, such treatments raise serious moral and legal problems (Shapiro, 1974; Mason, 1974; Staff of Subcommittee, 1974). Until recently, the debate concerning such treatments centered around the rights to and against treatment.[1] This article suggests that the recent development of potent technologies for behavior control poses yet a third issue, which we may call the *right after treatment*. It assumes the following:

1. That technologies such as those mentioned above may in some cases alleviate the organic basis or substrate of criminal behavior, such as impulsive violence.

---

[1] *Knecht* v. *Gilman*, 488 F.2d 1136 (8th Cir. 1973) (instituting procedures under which inmates may consent to drug treatment); Cal. Penal Code SS 2670–2680 (West. Supp. 1976); Cal. Welf. and Inst. Code SS 5325–5326 (West Supp. 1976) (setting forth condi-

2. That such alleviation may subsequently be verified with the requisite degree of certainty.

3. That certain modes of treatment will operate more or less narrowly, excising particular criminogenic traits or propensities, while others will effect more broad-based changes in thinking, feeling, and behavior.

4. That convicted felons will gain access to such treatment, as a matter of constitutional right, or otherwise.

These assumptions are discussed in more detail in Delgado, 1977a.

The question then arises: What shall be done with such technologically "rehabilitated" individuals? Their disposition to commit violent crimes may have been reduced to normal, indeed below normal levels; yet they may still have lengthy prison sentences to serve. Such a case was described in an article that appeared in a West Coast newspaper (Shapiro, 1974, p. 337, n. 338). It contained a brief, unelaborated account of an inmate of a British prison who petitioned for release after undergoing successful brain surgery. Prison physicians had operated to correct a condition in which bone fragments exerted pressure on portions of the inmate's brain, resulting in episodes of uncontrolled violence. On recovering from the operation, the prisoner demanded release on the ground that the operation had not only relieved his violent propensities but had given him a new personality and outlook on life. Arguing, in effect, that he was a new man imprisoned in an old body, he requested release on the ground that, in his new identity, he had committed no crime.

More recent cases in American institutions suggest that similar claims may well arise here. Stereotaxic psychosurgery has been carried out on California prisoners at Vacaville (Aarons, 1972). A Mary-

---

tions under which prisoners and other institutionalized individuals may consent to organic therapy); Shapiro, 1974, 311–315, 324–336. The substantive right of access to treatment has been based on a number of legal theories, including (1) autonomy and freedom of mentation—see, for example, Shapiro, 1974, 255–273; the eighth amendment; *Martinez* v. *Mancusi,* 443 F.2d 921 (2d Cir. 1970); but see *Sawyer* v. *Sigler,* 445 F.2d 818 (8th Cir. 1971); and (2) due process or equal protection—see Comment, 1971, 233–243; compare *Rouse* v. *Cameron,* 373 F.2d 451 (D.C. Cir. 1966) (by implication); see generally *Pell* v. *Procunier,* 417 U.S. 817, 823 (1974); as well as on statutes, especially those setting out objectives of particular penal programs—see Comment, 1971a, 236–237; National Commission for the Protection of Human Subjects of Biomedical and Behavioral Research, Research Involving Prisoners: Report and Recommendations 9 (Draft, June 23, 1976) (viewing it as settled that prison inmates may consent to or refuse medical treatment). While the right of access to treatment has received increasing recognition, there has been a simultaneous increase in concern over freedom of choice and the problem of environmental and institutional coercion —for example, Gobert, 1975, 195; Shapiro, 1974, 316–320; Wexler, 1975.

land prisoner recently successfully sought the aid of a federal district court in obtaining access to chemical treatment for crimes of sexual violence (Colen, 1975; Delgado, 1977a, p. 230). Outside the prison walls, the demand for organic treatment for aberrant or impulsive behavior is increasing rapidly. Mark and Ervin have treated dozens of patients and report turning away hundreds more (Mark and Ervin, 1970). Other researchers treat a steady stream of patients concerned about gaining control over their own violent impulses (Mark and Ervin, 1970, pp. 85–86; Fields and Sweet, 1975). The current societal preoccupation with violent crime, and the solicitude that courts and legislatures have displayed toward the right of access of the institutionalized to medical treatment, suggest that prisoners will succeed in gaining access to organic therapies designed to eradicate the chemical, electrical, or hormonal basis for the violent acts that led to their incarceration.

The task, then, will be to assess the appropriate legal and societal response to such "new men." An earlier article by this author considered the applicability of current legal doctrine to release claims based on organic rehabilitation (Delgado, 1977a, pp. 238–250). This review concluded that current case law relating to limitations placed on particular rights of prisoners, such as the right to worship, to receive mail, and to petition the judiciary and the legislature for relief, holds that such limitations are justified only if it can be shown that they promote one of the classic rationales of criminal punishment, or else are necessary to an important institutional objective, such as order, discipline, or safety. In certain, somewhat rarer cases, courts have insisted on review of incarceration itself. As a consequence, it seems highly likely that courts will declare the continued confinement of a demonstrably "cured" inmate unconstitutional, unless one of the fundamental objectives of punishment can be shown to be served.

This chapter surveys the classic objectives of criminal punishment —deterrence, rehabilitation, retribution, and societal protection—in an effort to forecast the likely result of petitions for release brought by organically rehabilitated prisoners. Concluding that courts may well find such continued confinement unconstitutional, the discussion then suggests some attributes of ideal release machinery by which such claims might be heard. Throughout, two polar cases are distinguished: (1) the individual whose criminogenic substrate has been narrowly excised (Delgado, 1977a, pp. 251–254, 259–260) and (2) the individual whose treatment has resulted in broad personality changes along with removal of the offending behavioral trait or propensity (Delgado, 1977a, pp. 227–232, 233–236).

Deterrence and the "New Man"

A fundamental objective of the criminal justice system is deterrence. The spectacle of punishment meted out to wrongdoers is assumed to instill fear in potential wrongdoers, thereby deterring them from engaging in similar conduct (Andenaes, 1966).[2] This fear is intended to operate on two categories of individual: (1) the wrongdoer himself and (2) members of society at large. Deterrence of repeat acts of wrongdoing by the same offender is termed *specific deterrence;* that of members of society at large, *general deterrence.*[3]

Does the deterrent rationale support continued confinement of organically rehabilitated offenders? Specific deterrence is manifestly inapplicable: since the offender no longer has a propensity to repeat the offense, further punishment is no longer necessary to assure conformity with the law. (See the discussion of rehabilitation later in this chapter.) With regard to general deterrence, however, the issue is more complex. The early release of offenders who have committed violent crimes could be seen as condoning their behavior. The public's will to resist the temptation to commit such crimes could thereby be weakened.

Several considerations suggest that this need not result, however. First, the therapy itself could be seen as a form of deterrence (compare Gobert, 1975, and Shapiro, 1974, p. 292, n. 188). Few free individuals would care to undergo organic treatment, particularly by means of modalities such as psychosurgery, which can produce wide-ranging changes of personality and character (compare Shapiro, 1974, p. 337, n. 338, with Valenstein, 1973, pp. 294–336; Delgado, 1969, p. 214; Brody, 1973, pp. 151–152). Such treatments might be seen as a form of mini-death, in which the pre-treatment (offender) personality ceased to exist and a new identity arose in his place (Comment, 1976). This fear might prove as effective as incarceration in deterring individuals from committing violent crimes.

Further, continued punishment of organically rehabilitated offenders may violate one of the essential limiting principles of deterrence. Critics of this rationale have pointed out that deterrence might, in principle, justify the public flogging of an innocent person,

---

[2] *Sauer* v. *United States,* 241 F.2d 640, 648 (9th Cir. 1957).

[3] Specific deterrence consists of after-the-fact inhibition of the person punished. Specific deterrence rests on the assumption that the individual will avoid future conduct that is likely to subject him to imprisonment again (see Orland, 1973, p. 186). The first modern discussion of general deterrence is found in Bentham, 1962. The concept has received continual criticism (for example, Sellin, 1964, p. 274). The doctrine has been revitalized, however, by Andenaes.

if doing so served to discourage others from engaging in the criminal acts imputed to him. To avoid this possibility, modern proponents of deterrence have insisted that the object of punishment be personally deserving of punishment—that is, chosen from among the guilty (Packer, 1968, pp. 62–70; Delgado, 1977a, p. 252, n. 241). Where personality modification has been extreme, this condition may be unsatisfied, since the post-treatment individual's identity may differ significantly from that of the individual who committed the crime (Shapiro, 1974, p. 337, n. 338; Valenstein, 1973, pp. 294–336; Delgado, 1969, p. 214; Brody, 1973, pp. 151–152). Our legal system takes cognizance of many changes that occur naturally—fetuses reaching the stage of viability, juveniles attaining adulthood, aged individuals lapsing into senility[4]—which involve less drastic alterations than those that may result from organic treatments. If these naturally occurring changes can alter an individual's legal status, surely the potentially greater changes produced by organic treatment might also call for new legal responses. In particular, where identity change has been great, the rehabilitated offender may appear an inappropriate object of punishment under the deterrent model, since such punishment contravenes the principle that innocent persons should not be punished merely to discourage others.

When the treatment operates narrowly, however, affecting only a single trait or behavior, the deterrent rationale might appear to remain intact. The subject retains essentially the same personality structure he had before treatment. He has the same values, memories, and ways of speaking and acting. The sole difference is that a single criminogenic trait, or physical substrate, has been eliminated. It might be argued, with some plausibility, that such an individual may be punished in order to deter others from committing similar crimes.

While perhaps conceptually valid, such punishment still presents a number of difficulties. One concerns the matter of sentence length. As numerous critics of deterrence have written, this principle may tell us who should be punished, but it gives little assistance in calculating the proper length of such punishment.[5] To remedy this insufficiency, most proponents of deterrence resort to the prin-

---

[4] See, for example, *Roe* v. *Wade*, 410 U.S. 113, 164–166 (1973) (fetuses attaining viability); *Workman* v. *Commonwealth*, 429 S.W.2d 374, 377–378 (Ky. 1968) (juveniles attaining age of majority); see also *In re Gault*, 387 U.S. 1 (1967); *State* v. *Hadley*, 65 Utah 109, 234 P.940 (1925) (aged person declining into senile dementia).
[5] The empirical relationship between sentence length and deterrence is complex; long sentences do not always deter better than short ones (see Andenaes, 1966, pp. 964–970).

ciple of utility: Punishment should be imposed in such fashion as to produce the needed amount of deterrence, and no more. Since punishment is in itself an evil, it should continue no longer than necessary to discourage repeat offenses.[6] In the case of narrowly modified individuals, however, this might amount to no punishment at all. If the public knows that the offender has undergone treatment and is no longer a danger to himself or society, punishment may lose its exemplary effect. It may, indeed, have counter-utilitarian value, since it could discourage inmates in need of treatment from seeking it. Why undergo organic treatment if doing so can have no possible effect on one's sentence? (See Gobert, 1975, pp. 157–158.)

Considerations of the types of offense for which organic therapies are likely to be used yield further grounds for doubting the efficacy, in deterrence terms, of punishing rehabilitated offenders. Andenaes, a classic exponent of deterrence theory, has observed that the deterrent effect of punishment is a function of the type of crime (Andenaes, 1966, pp. 957–958). In punishing acts that are *mala in se* (wrong in themselves), the law supports an existing moral revulsion; even if the legal sanction were withdrawn, we would still continue to condemn such acts. With regard to acts that are *mala prohibita* (wrong only because prohibited by law), however, punishment is imposed only because the law proscribes them. Thus, if it somehow became possible to "cure" a propensity to engage in tax evasion by means of a simple operation, society might decide not to release these organically rehabilitated tax offenders to avoid weakening an already tenuous norm. In contrast, society might well decide to release a fully rehabilitated violent offender whose criminal acts resulted from a limbic system disorder that has now been remedied. The release of such an offender represents less of a risk to the vitality of the norm against crimes of violence since there already exists a strong community attitude of disapproval of such conduct. In general, the more rationally motivated and normal-seeming the conduct, the greater the need for the criminal sanction. Since acts of senseless violence perpetrated by individuals suffering organic pathology are not acts normal persons are tempted to imitate, shortening the sentences of small numbers of such individuals is not likely to encourage lawless behavior of this type.

It thus appears that specific deterrence offers no support for the continued confinement of organically rehabilitated offenders. Gen-

---

[6]See, for example, *Battle* v. *Norton,* 365 F. Supp. 925, 231 (D. Conn. 1973) (a parole board can refuse to grant parole in cases where early release would depreciate the seriousness of the offense in the eyes of the public—that is, where general deterrence might be harmed); Benn and Peters, 1959, 186–194.

eral deterrence remains valid only if the therapy itself is not seen as an adequate punishment, and even then only in cases where personality change is not so great as to blur the identity between the pre- and the post-treatment individual. In both cases, practical sentencing considerations obviate much of the need for continued punishment.

Rehabilitation

A number of the same considerations that militate against the deterrent rationale also operate to attenuate the rehabilitative principle. According to this principle, human behavior is the product of antecedent causes, many of which can be scientifically ascertained. In some cases, measures can be taken to treat these causes so that undesirable behavior is eliminated. This enterprise—sometimes termed the *therapeutic state*—is the only defensible reason, such proponents argue, for incarcerating human beings in a civilized society (Allen, 1959; Hart, 1968, pp. 158–210; Packer, 1968, pp. 9–71).

Rehabilitationists tend to see criminality as a type of sickness, over which the criminal has no more control than a person suffering from influenza or typhoid fever. Inflicting punishment on such persons is itself a crime, comparable to flogging persons for having contracted rheumatic fever or suffered a broken leg (Menninger, 1968, p. 254). Criminality has been viewed in essentially moralistic terms only because, until recently, medical science has been powerless to treat it. But now that physicians have learned to alter the psychological or physical bases of certain forms of criminality, refusal to accept the rehabilitative model is as irrational as the resistance, two centuries ago, to seeing insanity as a form of illness (Menninger, 1968, p. 258). Before the rehabilitative ideal can be accepted, its advocates assert, correctional institutions will need to adopt a "therapeutic attitude" and cease regarding criminals as objects of hatred and contempt (Menninger, 1968, p. 262). Although stern punishment may have some therapeutic effect on hardened offenders who need to have the poverty of their ways demonstrated to them as a precondition of treatment (Delgado, 1977a, p. 256), suffering should not be imposed for its own sake.

Although this view has not escaped criticism (Allen, 1959; Dershowitz, 1974; Stender, 1974), the rehabilitative position is consistent with a long developmental trend in American penological thinking and appears unlikely to recede in importance in the foreseeable future (Dershowitz, 1974, pp. 304–315; American Correctional Association, 1966, pp. 10–20; Comment, 1971a). Indeed, prison reformers have begun to press for recognition of rehabilitation as a constitutional right of prisoners, comparable to the "right to treatment" that some courts and statutes have recognized for involuntarily committed mental patients (Comment, 1971a; Comment, 1971b, p. 545).

Whether or not rehabilitation should be accepted as the preeminent principle its advocates urge, the question remains whether the rehabilitative principle can justify incarceration for organically induced "new men." Since the object of rehabilitation is to produce an individual whose propensity to commit crimes of certain types has been reduced to acceptable levels, it would appear that the rehabilitative principle cannot justify the continued confinement of one whose treatment has excised the organic substrate responsible for his past crimes. As was observed in connection with deterrence, such incarceration can frustrate the rehabilitative ideal by exposing the prisoner to corrupting influences inherent in prison life (Spece, 1972, pp. 657–658; Shapiro, 1972, pp. 59–63). Moreover, the prisoner might feel justifiable bitterness at being punished even though he is no longer a threat to society.

Some commentators have disputed the propriety of applying the description "rehabilitated" to persons whose reformation has been effectuated by organic means. Rehabilitation, they argue, requires *self*-control and *self*-restraint.[7] The organically rehabilitated offender can demonstrate neither; he has simply been rendered incapable of breaking the law (Shapiro, 1972, p. 60). Such reconstitution is, at best, morally neutral. The status of such persons is thus radically different from that of prisoners who have repented their deeds and voluntarily embarked on programs designed to make them better persons.

There are two responses to this objection. First, when organic treatment is undertaken—as it ordinarily will be—at the prisoner's initiative, the changes that result become morally significant and may be taken as evidence of the prisoner's moral reformation. Second, the argument, to the extent that it is persuasive, rests on equivocation between means and ends, or processes and goals—a confusion invited by the twin meanings of "rehabilitation," which can refer both to cures and to treatments. When courts assess prison action that encroaches on fundamental liberties of inmates, they normally are concerned with the effect on ends, not means. Expressed differently, such courts look to the regulation's tendency

---

[7] See *Holt* v. *Sarver*, 309 F. Supp. 362 (E.D. Ark 1970).

to promote certain objectives of the criminal justice system, rather than its characterization as an acceptable means or type of intervention. When it is seen that the word "rehabilitation" has both a means and an ends sense, the confusion vanishes. Penal systems can no more rationally refuse to release an inmate who is reformed and otherwise entitled to release simply because he has undergone rehabilitation of one type rather than another than they can deny release to a convict who has served his full sentence on the grounds that he spent the entire time in a state of reverie or self-induced trance. Where rehabilitation is used to justify incarceration, the state has no business ruling certain avenues to rehabilitation out of bounds; if it does, the justification must come from a source outside the rehabilitative principle itself.[8]

Retribution

The retributive rationale has been formulated in a variety of ways. At their core is the insistence that punishment is justified, not because of some future gain expected to result from inflicting it, but because of the historical fact that the actor has committed some wrong (Mabbott, 1939; Ewing, 1929, p. 13). Perhaps the earliest known formulation is the *lex talionis*—the Old Testament "eye for an eye, tooth for a tooth."[9] Retribution looks backward, unlike utilitarian justifications, such as deterrence. Because the offender has taken what is not his to take, something must be taken from him in return.

Classical formulations of the retributive principle ring sternly to modern ears. Kant, for example, in his *Philosophy of Law*, declares that "punishment . . . must in all cases be imposed only because the individual on whom it is inflicted *has committed a Crime*" (Kant, 1974 ed., p. 195, emphasis in original). More recent proponents have sought to temper the retributive demand with an admixture of moral or humanitarian concerns. Fyodor Dostoyevsky wrote that criminal punishment was due as much as a matter of moral

---

[8] A refusal to recognize as rehabilitated those individuals whose cure has been effected by organic means, like denial of release to the prisoner who spends his days in a state of trance, may well reflect a concern deriving from retributivism. Because such a prisoner's "rehabilitation" has been made easy, he has not yet fully paid his debt to society. When addressed strictly in rehabilitative terms, however, this objection offers no justifiable basis for refusing to recognize as reformed individuals who have undergone organic therapy that has demonstrably reduced their potential for violence to normal levels.

[9] *Exodus* 21:23–25; see 4 W. Blackstone, *Commentaries* *12.

insight as of impersonal justice, since the offender becomes morally rehabilitated through deprivation and suffering (see Gerber and McAnany, 1972, p. 40; Pope Pius XII, 1960, pp. 97–100 and 108–109). Others, however, resist any attempt to combine retribution with other concerns, arguing that this dilutes the moral basis of punishment. Sir Walter Moberly, for example, writes that retributivists reject the notion that punishment should be inflicted for utilitarian reasons such as deterrence or reformation; such punishment degrades the victim since it treats him as a means rather than an end in himself (Moberly, 1968, pp. 109–110 and 117).

Courts have given retribution a mixed reception. Some have rejected it as an expression of primitive bloodlust.[10] Others, including Justice Stewart's concurring opinion in the death penalty case of *Furman* v. *Georgia*,[11] find the retributive instinct an essential expression of moral feeling.

Because retribution is, in principle, retrospective, it might appear an unassailable justification for continuing to punish organically rehabilitated offenders. If the prime reason for inflicting punishment is a past event—the prisoner's crime—it is difficult to see how a subsequent event—his alleged rehabilitation—can affect the moral rightness of his sentence. Such sentences, if properly imposed in the first instance, cannot become any more or less so in light of later occurring events.

Nevertheless, even granting the retributivist premise, such punishment can be criticized. First, a number of retributive theorists believe that moral condemnation—our instinctive hatred of those who violate our law—is essential to retributive punishment (Durkheim, 1933, pp. 108–109; Hart, 1958, pp. 404–405). Punishment of such offenders expresses and gives tangible form to our sense of outrage, thereby solidifying societal consensus and strengthening the general will to obey the law (Durkheim, 1933, pp. 108–109).[12]

To the extent that moral outrage is central to retributivism, this basis for punishment may be attenuated in the case of organically rehabilitated offenders. The fact of an organic cure constitutes a vivid reminder that the offender's act stems from organic causes, perhaps beyond his willed control. In such cases, anger might seem an inappropriate response; the actor is more to be pitied than

---

[10] See *Commonwealth* v. *Ritter*, 13 Pa. D. and C. 285, 290–291 (1930); compare *Williams* v. *New York*, 337 U.S. 241, 248 (1949) (retribution no longer the dominant objective of the criminal law).

[11] *Furman* v. *Georgia*, 408 U.S. 238, 308 (1972) (Stewart, J., concurring).

[12] *Ibid.*

blamed.[13] Moral outrage might also appear inappropriate because of drastic changes between the pre-treatment and the post-treatment personalities. If moral outrage requires a present target, as opposed to a past one, the reason for outrage could be seen to disappear when the target is transformed. Retribution requires an identity between the person punished and the individual who committed the offense (Moberly, 1968, p. 116). "[A] criminal cannot substitute another to undergo his punishment" (Hall, 1947, p. 318; Flew, 1954, pp. 293–294); unlike money debts, these are moral obligations that can only be paid by the criminal himself. If organic treatment can, on occasion, produce extensive personality changes calling into question the continuity of the pre-treatment identity, the grounds for retributive punishment may disappear. If we punish because there is a debt to be paid, when the person owing the debt is no longer present the debt may simply become uncollectible.

A final difficulty in applying the retributive rationale to "new men," similar to that discussed earlier in connection with deterrence, consists in determining the appropriate degree of punishment. Most retributivist writers have rejected the notion that offenders must be made to suffer in proportion to the suffering they have caused. Instead, they urge only that punishment not be "excessive" (compare Walker, 1972, p. 85, and Mabbott, 1939, pp. 152–154). But what was a retributively just sentence at the time of imposition might appear excessive in light of later events—in particular, the individual's organic rehabilitation. A retributivist may, of course, avoid this objection by insisting that excessiveness is to be measured, once and for all, at the time of the trial and that a sentence that is retributively just when imposed remains so forever. In such a case, the only recourse would lie in persuading him that the person being punished is not the one whose past contains the punishable offense, or, less paradoxically, that the two individuals are insufficiently alike to warrant continued punishment for retribution's sake.

In sum, the retributive rationale seems greatly, perhaps fatally, eroded in cases of organic rehabilitation. At most, it would appear to

---

[13] Sleepwalkers, for example, are no longer punished. See Fox, 1963, pp. 652–656; *Fain* v. *Commonwealth*, 78 Ky. 183 (1879); *Bradley* v. *State*, 277 S.W. 147 (Tex. Crim. 1925); Model Penal Code S2.01 (Proposed Official Draft 1962). Nor are epileptics condemned for actions carried out during seizures. See, for example, *People* v. *Decina*, 2 N.Y.2d 133, 146, 138 N.E.2d 799, 807, 157 N.Y.S.2d 558, 570 (1956) (Desmond, J., concurring in part, dissenting in part). The language we use to describe such individuals betrays our feeling that their acts are blameless. Similarly, moral outrage could seem inappropriate when the offense is the result of a treatable chemical imbalance, neurological anomaly, or other physical disorder, particularly when the violent impulse is irresistible.

justify brief sentences imposed in response to the community's felt need for vengeance. The need for even such brief sentences may well disappear when the organic bases of certain types of criminal behavior become known and the acts themselves appear proportionately less free.

Societal Protection

A final rationale is societal protection, the notion that society is justified in incarcerating offenders to guard against the possibility of their inflicting additional harm (see Packer, 1968, p. 49). This rationale is predictive in nature. One crime is likely to be followed by others of the same type; an individual who has demonstrated himself to be dangerous in the past is likely to be dangerous in the future.

Societal protection appears to play an important role in sentencing determinations, especially in cases involving violent crime. Individuals who have behaved violently, and who are therefore considered to be social risks, are apt to be "sent away" for long prison terms (Gerber and McAnany, 1972, pp. 129–130; National Council on Crime and Delinquency, 1969, pp. 1–5). In contrast, persons who have no history of violent crime or whose acts appear to have been the product of unique circumstances unlikely to be repeated are apt to receive lenient treatment. The interest in societal protection has been cited with approval by a number of courts[14] and has been recognized by several model statutes.[15] Typically, these statutes recite the importance of a determination of dangerousness and emphasize the need for psychiatric and neurological work-ups and other evidence prior to imposing sentence.

Societal protection would seem to be, at best, minimally furthered by incarceration of persons who have undergone successful organic rehabilitation. Since such individuals have been treated and certified as having a probability of recidivism below a certain safety level (Delgado, 1977a, pp. 231–232), the interest in societal protection can scarcely be furthered by additional punishment. It might be argued that the "new man," having already violated the law, should be held to a higher standard than mere safety. But in terms of societal pro-

---

[14] For example, *United States* v. *Brown*, 381 U.S. 437, 458 (1965); *Berrigan* v. *Norton*, 322 F. Supp. 46, 51 (D. Conn. 1971).

[15] Model Penal Code S 7.01 (Proposed Official Draft 1962); ABA Project on Minimum Standards for Criminal Justice, Sentencing Alternatives and Procedures SS 2.1-2.2 and Commentary (Approved Draft 1968); National Council on Crime and Delinquency, Model Sentencing Act SS 5-6 (1963).

tection, this demand would be misconceived. If it is an expression of the feeling that evildoers should redeem themselves through a painful and difficult process, it responds more appropriately to the retributive impulse. Insofar as it expresses a concern that moral values will decline if criminals go free too easily, it is more properly addressed to general deterrence. To the extent that it seeks to build in a safety margin, it misconceives the nature of the certification process, which is by its very nature probabilistic.

In societal protection terms, the appropriate sentence for the organically rehabilitated offender is no sentence at all: societal protection has already been achieved. Concededly, most sentencing decisions reflect a mixture of motives. In cases involving violent crime, the sentence often has (whether recognized or not) two components: (1) time to be served because of what the defendant has done and (2) time to be served as protection against what he might do in the future (Silving, 1961, p. 77). When the prisoner has been freed of his violent propensities as a result of physical treatment, the second component should drop out. The sentence would then depend on other factors, principally retribution. The extent to which retribution remains viable would, in turn, depend on the factors discussed earlier, principally the degree of identity change. In itself, however, societal protection offers scant support for continued confinement of "new men."

Remedies

If, as the above review of sentencing rationales suggests, punishment of organically rehabilitated offenders does not serve to advance the traditional rationales of criminal punishment, courts may be expected to prove receptive to release claims pressed by inmates who have undergone such reconstruction. Indeed, as has been argued elsewhere, release may well be held a constitutional or statutory necessity (Delgado, 1977a, pp. 239–250). Presently existing remedies, which include appellate review of sentence, motions to reduce sentence, state and federal habeas corpus, pardon and commutation of sentence, are not ideally suited to hearing challenges based on organic reformation, and new procedural channels will need to be developed (Delgado, 1977a, pp. 253–264). Existing remedies may have restrictive limitations on time of filing. Some are highly discretionary, or impose an unreasonably heavy burden of proof on the petitioner. Others have jurisdictional or evidentiary restrictions that limit their usefulness. Although most of the traditional remedies are probably capable of being modified to suit the unique circumstances of the organically rehabilitated offender, a new remedy would avoid the necessity of tortured interpretation or judge-made extension of legislative enactments. Such a remedy would seem to require provision for at least the following elements:

Prima Facie Case

The "new man" who seeks release must establish that he has undergone the necessary degree of change. This requirement can be satisfied by offering medical evidence that his dangerous tendencies have been alleviated and are unlikely to return. If the offender is not presently dangerous but requires additional treatment or observation to ensure that his symptoms will not recur, he will need to convince the court that if released he will continue to cooperate with treatment.

He will then need to persuade the court that the change he has undergone invalidates the grounds of his sentence.[16] If the prisoner is only seeking to demonstrate that his violent propensity has been narrowly treated, the arguments will center around general deterrence and retribution. If the sentencing record is unclear concerning the relative weights of the interests that entered into the sentencing decision, the inmate may argue that these rationales—especially retribution—have been disapproved by court or legislative action in his jurisdiction.[17] If his jurisdiction provides minimum sentences and he has already served the minimum term, he may argue that such sentence represents the extent of the state's interest in retrib-

[16] Where relapse is possible, such as following psychosurgery, a court might reasonably require the prisoner to submit to an extended period of observation and testing before ordering release (Delgado, 1977a, pp. 236–238).

[17] Deterrence has been criticized as a basis for punishment on the ground that the fear of sanction rarely deters potential offenders, while retribution has been characterized as an anachronistic expression of the instinct for tribal vengeance and as inconsistent with the goal of rehabilitation. See, for example, *Williams* v. *New York*, 337 U.S. 241 (1949); Gerber and McAnany, 1972, pp. 39–40 and 93–95. State constitutions, statutes, or enabling legislation relating to particular criminal institutions may refer to rehabilitation as the principal aim of confinement, thereby implicitly excluding deterrence and retribution. See, for example, Ind. Const. art. 1, S 18 ("The penal code shall be founded on the principles of reformation and prevention."); Cal. Penal Code SS 2002, 2032 (West 1970) (rehabilitation is the primary purpose of penal institutions); see also Colo. Rev. Stat. S 39-10-1 (1965) (setting out purpose of a particular penal program). Courts have cited these and similar statutes in striking down institutional programs that were not conducive to the advancement of statutorily defined objectives. See, for example, *Millard* v. *Cameron*, 373 F.2d 468, 472–473 (D.C. Cir. 1966); *United States* v. *Alsbrook*, 336 F. Supp. 973, 979–981 (D.D.C. 1971). See also Rubin, 1973, p. 740; Comment, 1971b.

ution.[18] On the other hand, if the inmate proves that his modification has amounted to an identity change, this second step will be unnecessary, since this degree of change renders the retributive rationale inapplicable.

The Appropriate Forum

Decisions concerning the release of organically rehabilitated inmates ideally should be made by the court that imposed the original sentence. The sentencing court is in the best position to know the manner in which the various sentencing rationales entered into the decision to punish, and to evaluate the extent to which these have been satisfied by the inmate's treatment. If it becomes necessary to recall witnesses, these will be more conveniently available in the original court than elsewhere. To protect against possible prejudice because the site of review and that of the original sentencing are the same, change of venue can be provided for.

Period of Limitations

A number of currently available release procedures require that the inmate file for relief within a certain specified time of beginning the sentence; others require that he first serve a minimum term.[19] These limitations, which may make sense in other contexts, are less easily justified in the case of organic rehabilitation. Organic rehabilitation may be administered at any point in the prisoner's sentence; when it is successful, the justification for further punishment may cease. Accordingly, it seems best to make release available whenever the inmate can show that physical correction of an organic anomaly has dissipated the original grounds of commitment.

Burden of Proof

Many release procedures are highly discretionary; parole board determinations, for example, are rarely overturned on substantive

---

[18] See ABA Project on Minimum Standards for Criminal Justice, Standards Relating to Sentencing Alternatives and Procedures SS 2.2, 2.5 (Approved Draft 1968) (suggesting that a minimum sentence might be necessary in certain cases in response to the "gravity" of the offense).

[19] See, for example, Fed. R. Crim. P. 33 (two-year limitation on motion for new trial on newly discovered evidence); Fla. Stat. Ann. (R. Crim. Proc.) 3.800(b) (1975) (time limitations on motion to reduce sentence); Wyo. Stat. S 7-408.1 (Supp. 1975) (five-year limitation on statutory postconviction remedy). See also 4 Attorney General's Survey of Release Procedures 4 (1939) (fixed minimum sentences).

grounds.[20] These decisions are considered to fall in an area of intuitive judgment, in which the parole board's expertise is given great weight. Where rehabilitation is no longer a matter of intuition and insight, but is susceptible of objective demonstration, the need for judicial deference is less compelling. Accordingly, courts should not be reluctant to entertain evidently meritorious claims even if doing so runs counter to an earlier negative determination by penal authorities, provided this determination antedated the organic treatment on which the release claim is based.

Framing the Relief

Most currently available postconviction procedures are limited in the forms of relief available under them. Depending on the remedy the inmate pursues, relief can range from outright or conditional release to a simple reduction of sentence (Singer and Statsky, 1974, pp. 1059–1093 and 1217). The civil disabilities that accompany successful application also vary (Singer and Statsky, 1974, pp. 1095–1134). Because the proposed remedy contemplates the postconviction review function as an extension of the sentencing process, it seems advisable to permit the court to select any of the sentencing options that were open to the court at the time of the original sentence. For organically reformed prisoners, these could include outright discharge, release on the condition that the individual submit to periodic treatment or observation, or release at an early specified date.[21] They could include an order that the prisoner undergo further observation or testing while still in prison, or that a "postsentencing investigation" be carried out to ascertain more certainly the fitness of the inmate to reenter society and the ability of his community and family to accept him and assist him in his adjustment.

Conclusion

Progress in several biomedical modalities suggests that propensities for certain types of behavior now punishable under the criminal law

---

[20] See, for example, *Hines* v. *State Bd. of Parole*, 293 N.Y. 254, 257–258, 56 N.E.2d 572, 573–574 (1944).

[21] See the National Advisory Comm'n on Criminal Justice Standards and Goals, Corrections (1973), Standard 5.2 (1973) (nondangerous offenders should be given the sentence alternatives that are the least drastic limitations on their freedom, consistent with the public safety). Where the prisoner's rehabilitation is very uncertain and release seems unwise, the inmate can be retained in the institution for an additional period of study and observation. During this time, a lighter disciplinary regime might well be appropriate, as well as useful in gauging the extent of the individual's return to normalcy.

are capable of being modified or eliminated. Such therapies as electronic brain stimulation, pharmacological treatment, and psychosurgery raise the possibility that a number of assumptions integral to our concept of criminal responsibility will give way, including the assumptions that (1) the moral justification for punishment remains constant during a prisoner's confinement, and (2) an offender's identity remains unchanged during the same period. Any significant erosion of these assumptions necessarily weakens the connection between punishment and the traditional goals and objectives that punishment is designed to serve.

Close scrutiny by courts of the efficacy and procedural regularity of prison programs and regimes, together with increased willingness to scrutinize prison sentences themselves under such theories as cruel and unusual punishment, therapeutic incarceration, and a more stringent construction of legislative intent, suggests that the courts may come to recognize a constitutional right to release. Presently existing channels are not ideally suited to consider such claims for release. The minimum requirements of any new remedy are outlined in this chapter.

Recognition of a release right for organically rehabilitated offenders is consistent with the view that punishment should serve rehabilitative ends. At the same time, it recognizes that punishment reflects interests other than rehabilitation and demands a consideration in each case of the extent to which other interests militate for or against release. The need to determine more precisely the social interests at stake in connection with such rationales as general deterrence and retribution will call for greater attention by courts and commentators to these interests than they have recently received. This inquiry should begin soon. Although the number of cases that have raised issues of organic rehabilitation has so far been small, the inexorable advance and dissemination of biotechnological treatments mean that this inquiry cannot be safely delayed much longer. Unless such questions are to be resolved haphazardly, as they arise, it is better that they be considered now while the law relating to organic rehabilitation is still being formulated.

CHAPTER 28

The Captive Patient: A Forgotten Man

M. Hunter Brown

The most unfortunate segment of humanity in our society are those who have major neuropsychiatric illness and are held in a state or federal institution. A considerable number of captive patients in prisons or mental hospitals suffer from schizophrenia, episodic impulse dyscontrol, temporal lobe epilepsy, organic brain syndrome, or manic-depressive disease. Their plight results from several factors: There is public indifference and hostility that stem from a natural revulsion against antisocial behavior; then follows a logical interest to restrain the increased use of tax monies to further such purpose; inadequate professional and paraprofessional staffing is a common feature, intensified by political control that ties the hands of dedicated scientists; indicated treatments are denied under the guise of "protection of patients' rights" and the impossibility of freely informed consent; and those who make our laws are well aware that prisoner-patients have no clout as a voting bloc.

The antipsychiatry movement is composed largely of corrections officials, courts and legislatures, ethicists and politicians—groups who never have to deal realistically with a composite amount of

537

human misery that is difficult to portray in words; if one never grapples with daily problems of suicide, homicide, depression, paranoia, or self-mutilation, abstractions are not hard to come by and tortured ambiguity easily reinforces preexisting bias or rationalization. The subject of psychiatric surgery for involuntary patients seems particularly tempting to those who like to be judgmental with little foundation in fact and none at all in science. In contrast, the propsychiatry movement is peopled almost entirely by scientists who have weathered more than a quarter century of social and political abuse in their efforts to help the mentally ill.

The great challenge to neuropsychiatry in this century is the development of a safe and effective treatment for established schizophrenia, and increasingly society is faced with a major escalation of violence. Often these two conditions overlap. At this point in time there is a consensus that present policies of the states and of the federal government in this field have been a disaster, that a fresh approach is needed and not more of the same. At least we have general agreement that institutional rehabilitation of the captive patient is a statistical myth when rates of recidivism approximate two cases out of three for crimes of aggression. Widespread political strictures exist on such established techniques as chemotherapy, electrotherapy, surgical therapy, and behavior modification. These ensure the captive patient's right either to a living death behind walls and bars on the one hand or to release without treatment to prey again on society under policies of determinate sentencing on the other. Realistically most "civilized nations" operate under a double standard, a two-tier system of free choice, due process, and the constitutional right of treatment for humans in the private sector in contrast to custodial indifference meted out in the public sector as if to subhumans. Neuroscience has an ethical mandate to propose more positive solutions. Countless lives depend on how well we meet this challenge.

Historical Background

During the past thirty years neurosurgery has witnessed steady progress in the development of more localized and refined targets for psychiatric treatment. The thrust has been to adjust such targets to the nature of the illness and to individual psychodynamics presented by the patient. Advances in stereotaxic technology using more precise single- and double-probe guides, as well as the development of the radiofrequency generator, have refined the art in terms of safety and predictability. Today the mortality worldwide is a miniscule two-tenths of 1 percent and significant benefit or recovery, in the writer's experience, occurs in nine cases out of ten while 10 percent of patients are no better or no worse. The risk-benefit ratio in target neurosurgery for psychiatric purposes is unsurpassed by any other procedure in neurological surgery, more impressive when one considers that these patients comprise the worst group of psychiatric failures. This chapter does not cover technical details that are well documented by the writer and many other colleagues elsewhere (Ballantine et al., 1967; Brown, 1972b; Narabayashi, 1969).

In recent years there has been a rapid acceleration of new developments in neurochemical transmitter substances, antipsychotic medications, implanted electrodes and pacemakers, as well as in target treatment. We have arrived at a biological consensus anticipated by such pioneers as Kraepelin and Freud. In 1892 Kraepelin postulated that future scientists would see that the particular effect of an already well-known drug on a particular mental process would lead to the possibility of better recognizing the true nature of that process. In 1977 Carlsson stated as follows: Every antipsychotic drug known at present possesses antidopaminergic properties and the converse is also true, an important statement that relates to the etiology of schizophrenia. Today a sound extension of this thesis is possible: From the particular effect of neurosurgical targets on a particular mental process, we are better able to recognize its true nature and gain insight into the cerebral localization of personality. Sigmund Freud fathered the concept of the unconscious drive, yet never wavered in the belief that it would be understood in purely biological terms at some time in the future. The work of Heath (1971), Mark, Sweet, and Ervin (1972), Walker (1973), and Sem-Jacobsen and Styri (1972) on depth-electrode recordings and cerebellar pacemakers has served to bridge the gap between the psychic brain and the somatic brain, if indeed such neat segregation were ever possible. Penfield's lifelong studies pinpointed localization of recent memory and recall in the mesial portion of the temporal lobe, which has obvious environmental implications (Penfield and Mathieson, 1974). Friedhoff (1973) maintained that the dichotomy between organic and functional psychosis is now largely meaningless, and our own experience supports his point of view. Today it is difficult if not impossible to quarrel with the conclusion that all human thought, feeling, mood, and behavior often have a genetic predisposition with final summation by neurochemical control at the synaptic junction, neuroelectrical control at the neurone, and electrochemical engrams that result from important environmental input. Opposing arguments would presuppose that brain control is monitored by a vacuum.

Behavioral change with temporal lobe epilepsy has been recognized for many years. Usually it is interictal with some suggestion of hemispheric asymmetry, and a so-called mirror focus is not uncommon. During recent years there has been an outpouring of data to further verify these well-known clinical observations (Baer and Fedio, 1977; Geschwind, 1977a). The behavioral changes vary all the way from minor emotional states to major schizophreniform-like psychoses. Geschwind (1977a) states that personality change in temporal lobe epilepsy may well be the most important single set of clues we possess to decipher neurological systems that underlie the emotional forces guiding behavior. Additionally, the impulse-dyscontrol syndrome often shows temporal slow wave or seizure activity in the electroencephalographic tracings, a dyslepsia without overt epilepsy. In this vein, Walker's (1973) observations following personal experience with some 3,000 depth-electrode studies are pertinent: For every overt seizure there are literally hundreds of subclinical covert discharges. All studies substantiate his original thesis that chronic irritation of the temporal lobes has a devastating effect on limbic balance. The evidence for a physical basis of behavior as drawn from these investigations hardly requires further comment.

Guidelines for Consent

Problems of informed consent in the captive patient have certain similarities as well as differences from those in the private sector. The most common concerns relate to possible coercion by their captors in two directions: (1) punitive reprisals in the event of patient refusal after medical advisers have recommended a course of action, or (2) the hope of possible recovery, even ultimate freedom, used as bait to influence a patient's decision. Opponents of surgery for major neuropsychiatric illness have harped on both themes ad nauseam. In the writer's assessment these arguments are straw men. The first potential abuse is easily answered by appointment of an ombudsman or advocate's committee in each state to interview candidates with respect to their true wishes and eliminate any chance of coercion by corrections officials or state mental hospital administrators; such persons should be of unquestioned integrity and immune to political influence. Clergymen appointed by a joint committee of the state bar and state medical associations would seem ideally suited for this service. Naturally, such functions would be separate from any scientific decision-making.

The second straw man rests on the desire for improvement or recovery, even the possibility of ultimate freedom. Objectors on these grounds are more to be pitied than scorned. The only moral and ethical imperative is that study and treatment should have an excellent possibility of benefit, which in the writer's experience has been firmly established (Cox and Brown, 1977). In this vein, the public posture of Chief Justice Warren Burger supports the concept that if society puts a man behind walls and bars, it has a collective moral responsibility to change his behavior favorably if possible. Ethical scientists have subscribed to this point of view without qualification. Man's desire for freedom is as normal and natural as the air he breathes, and to suggest otherwise literally stands truth on its head.

Similarities between captive patients and those in the private sector should be noted. Clearly each case should be studied and treated as an individual problem, and treatment in the mass avoided at all costs. Restrictions of psychosis or mental retardation limit the possibility of informed consent in some patients of both groups. In such instances medical advice must be weighed by the private or public guardian on the one hand or by parents in the case of minors on the other. Rarely, if ever, should a situation arise in which a court order is required from our overcrowded judicial system.

In the past demagogues have used political and racist innuendos as a tactic to prey on public anxiety. In the absence of any shred of evidence to support this claim, their strategy has died a natural death. The change was a studied insult to every ethical neuroscientist, paranoid prattling at its worst, and a disservice to all races. However, a statistical backlash developed as testimony of black neurosurgeons before the National Commission for the Protection of Human Subjects of Biomedical and Behavioral Research in 1976 indicated there *was* discrimination—that poor, marginal, and minority families were denied indicated treatment by adverse public policy. Four years ago Dr. H. Thomas Ballantine, Jr., and the writer pooled some 600 psychosurgery patients; ethnic distribution disclosed only six Hispanic and two Oriental-American cases with a single black patient—a finding that speaks for itself. Both Medicaid and Medicare often deny such benefits and, once again, we see a blatant double standard that mocks human rights in the private sector as well as in the public. Free choice joined to economic coercion is a charade.

Various current proposals suggest review boards in institutions or a national commission to monitor case selection; some favor lay control heavily manned with lawyers, ethicists, consumer advocates, clergymen, and the like. Clearly, lay persons should not get into a scientific act in which they have no competence, as informed decisions are not possible from uninformed persons. Disclosure of private material without the patient's consent is both unethical and illegal, most particularly in sensitive neuropsychiatric illness. The proper role of a review board is to monitor quality by outcome assessments in each institution, similar to peer review in all other departments. Authority in decision-making cannot be divorced from responsibility for treatment by mandatory *prospective* judgments of an uninformed committee. The Supreme Court clearly stated this principle in *Doe* v. *Bolton*, 410 U.S. 179 (1973): "If a physician is licensed by the State, he is recognized by the State as capable of exercising acceptable judgment. If he fails, professional censure and deprivation of his license are available remedies. *Required acquiescense by copractitioners* has no rational connection with a patient's needs and unduly infringes on the physician's right to practice."

Restrictive legislation in several states has caused a nightmare of bureaucratic obstacles, and the experience of others was well stated by the late Paul H. Blachly, Professor of Psychiatry at the University of Oregon: "In recommending a national psychosurgery review board the National Commission will for practical purposes eliminate the procedure after extensive studies gave highly favorable results." They mention, with seeming approval, legislation that set up such a board but failed to mention that since that time not one case has been so treated in Oregon (six years). Indeed some board members indicate that it would be impossible to ever get a case approved, such are the administrative impediments. A previous similar statute in California, A.B. 4481, was found unconstitutional, and currently its successor, A.B. 1032, is under legal attack after two years of nontreatment for patients suffering with life-threatening illnesses in addition to millions of dollars in wasted hospital costs.

It is proper that guidelines be determined by the relevant medical community. In March 1977 the position of the American Association of Neurological Surgeons was summarized by its president: Limbic target surgery is not performed for research and investigative purposes, it is not experimental, and it can be considered treatment for chronic schizophrenia. Lesions have been placed bilaterally in all of these anatomic areas for the treatment of psychiatric illness for more than a quarter of a century. In the framework of AANS policy, repressive legislation that turns out the light of science is an improper and illegal exercise of state police power.

Discussion

For some years I have urged my colleagues worldwide to support positive programs for the precise study and treatment of captive patients as only one feature of overall prison reform. It is proper to ask how best to manage the informed and competent prisoner who does *not* desire treatment as advised by his physicians. I suggest consideration of the penal island in lieu of the penal institution as a far more humane and practical alternative.

More than 190 years ago shiploads of prisoners left Great Britain for a distant land; they forged their own culture, and their descendants created the great continent we know as Australia. Lessons of history should not go unheeded. I have in mind large, habitable islands in which prisoners could live, work, farm, and fish, and be with their wives and children—an operation monitored by overwater and underwater techniques with no guards required. Excellent sites are available for the United States in the Caribbean and for Canada off the coast of British Columbia. This approach warrants serious attention when balanced against prison breaks, murder of guards and inmates, and the enormous tax costs of our present system. The island of San Lucas is used successfully by Costa Rica for this purpose.

If surgery is carried out, it seems preferable in the present climate to have this treatment in a nearby facility, not within the confines of the prison hospital. Often this requires an attendant, at least preoperatively. Cases that involve major violence should be returned for at least a year of postoperative observation, psychiatric supervision, and vocational rehabilitation as indicated. At the end of this time, appraisal by psychological, electrical, and psychiatric testing affords a basis for a future disposition as a supplement to the patient's behavior during this period.

Bluglass (1977) reported that the proportion of individuals serving a prison sentence in Great Britain who could be identified as having mental illness is recognized to be high, about one-third of the prison population. He also called attention to the long-standing principle (Penrose's law) that the size of the prison population and the size of the mental hospital population in Western countries is inversely proportional; that is, if one drops for whatever reason, the other rises and vice versa. In this context, the need for appropriate and effective therapy is quite clear. The writer is aware that for reasons of excessive constraint or timidity, certain of his colleagues do not favor stereotaxic treatment in captive cases. However, we all agree that men do sicken, suffer, and die in a prison setting as well as in a private setting, and constructive proposals are needed.

Most of these patients are young, and successful treatment can bring a happy combination of long-lasting individual, economic, and social benefits. A single case illustrates the gain that has been obtained by the writer in a number of such patients treated when under the jurisdiction of the court:

M.K., male, 29 years.
Diagnosis: (1) Schizophrenic psychosis. (2) Borderline mental retardation with impulse dyscontrol.

Early history indicated slow development following a difficult birth with likely trauma. There was inadequate progress in grammar school and education ceased at the twelfth grade. Aggressive behavior began coincident with puberty despite psychotherapy and chemotherapy. There were multiple hospitalizations in Ohio and Arizona. Often this illness became of psychotic proportions with restlessness, agitation, suspicion, hostility, and unpredictable behavior. Declared incompetent in 1969, he was released with his father as permanent guardian. Matters worsened and the neighborhood became terrorized by overt dangerousness until his arrest early in 1976 for attempted murder.

Psychometric examination indicated a schizophrenic reaction with paranoid elements and a full-scale IQ of 75. Following thorough psychiatric documentation, the patient received a bilateral six-target cingulo-innomino-amygdalotomy. Court examinations this year indicated remarkable improvement in behavior; the charges against him were dismissed in 1977 with the understanding that at the end of another year progress would be reviewed and determination made as to whether the case should remain dismissed or be refiled. In 1978 the case was dismissed and now he is doing well in a training center working in a program of supervised rehabilitation.

Shuman (1974) gave a brilliant exposé of the reasoning that afflicts opponents of surgery for psychiatric purposes in the prisoner-patient. To paraphrase his argument: Legislators or courts may appear to say that because, as a matter of law, a prisoner cannot consent to psychosurgery, he lacks the requisite capacity. But, of course, the patient lacks the capacity only after their decision. Presuming the answer to the question by posing the question is not a model for rational judicial decision-making, and one has to wince at such substitute for argument.

Society remains trapped in a situation wherein the captive who faces a life sentence for a crime resulting from such illness as paranoid schizophrenia or temporal lobe epilepsy is free to tell himself each day as he stares out from behind the bars: "See, the ever-vigilant government in this great land of ours has guaranteed that I may spend the rest of my natural life in confinement, safe in the comforting knowledge that no one took advantage of my legally manufactured incompetence to consent." The hypocrisy of this reasoning needs little elaboration.

Experience of more than a quarter century indicates that apprehension concerning modern psychiatric surgery is unwarranted, often fabricated, and unsubstantiated by any scientific evidence. Denial of such benefits to humanity should pose moral and ethical problems for the public conscience.

Epilogue

There will be many readers of this book who strongly disagree, as does the editor, with some of the views expressed in one or more of the chapters. As editor, not only do I have no regrets, but I am actually pleased about the possibility that such disagreements may catalyze more discussion of the issues.

It is not surprising that so many opposing views have been expressed. Most of the contributors have been active protagonists in "the psychosurgery debate." Among them, there are physicians (including neurosurgeons), behavioral and brain scientists, and lawyers. In short, those who treat patients, those who study them, those who defend their rights, and those who are struggling to understand how their brains function. However, the degree of dissension cannot be attributed solely to the various perspectives of separate disciplines. This book illustrates that differences of opinion can be very large within the same discipline, for example, among lawyers, and they can also be very considerable even among the neurosurgeons who perform psychosurgery. I have concluded that only part of the conflict can be attributed to arguments about the data.

Perhaps more significant are the divergent views of human nature and of the proper relationship between the individual and society. Such contrasting views often generate strong passions.

Ours is a pluralistic society, so that opinions and the manner of expressing opinions differ widely. Anyone who would grapple with similar debates in the future must be prepared to cope with such diversity.

June 1980   Elliot S. Valenstein

Bibliography

Aarons, L. 1972. Brain surgery is tested on three California convicts. *Washington Post*, February 25, p. 1.

Adams, J. E. 1973. Lobectomy ends violent episodes in two patients. *J. Am. Med. Assoc.*, 266, 19–20.

Akiskal, H. S., and McKinney, W. T. 1975. Overview of recent research in depression: Integration of ten conceptual models into a comprehensive clinical frame. *Arch. Gen. Psychiatry*, 32, 285–305.

Allen, F. A. 1959. Criminal justice, legal values, and the rehabilitative ideal. *J. Criminal Law*, 50, 226–232.

Alpers, B. J. 1937. Relation of the hypothalamus to disorders of personality: Report of a case. *Arch. Neurol. Psychiatry*, 38, 291–303.

American College of Neuropsychopharmacology, Food and Drug Administration Task Force. 1973. Special report: Neurological syndromes associated with anti-psychotic drug use. *Arch. Gen. Psychiatry*, 28, 463–467.

American Correctional Association. 1966. *Correctional standards*. New York: American Correction Association.

American Medical Association. 1977. *AMA Drug Evaluations*. Littleton, Mass.: PSG Publishing Co.

American Psychiatric Association, Task Force on Electroconvulsive Therapy. 1978. *Electroconvulsive therapy* (Task Force Report 14). Washington, D.C. American Psychiatric Association, 1978.

Andenaes, J. 1952. General prevention—Illusion or reality? *J. Criminal Law, Criminology, and Police Science, 43,* 176–198.

———. 1966. The general preventive effects of punishment. *Univ. Penn. Law Rev., 114,* 949–983.

Andersen, R. 1972. Differences in the course of learning as measured by various memory tasks after amygdalectomy in man. In E. Hitchcock, L. Laitinen, and K. Vaernet (Eds.), *Psychosurgery.* Springfield, Ill.: Charles C Thomas. Pp. 177–183.

Andy, O. J. 1966. Neurosurgical treatment of abnormal behavior. *Am. J. Med. Sci., 252,* 232–238.

———. 1970. Thalamotomy in hyperactive and aggressive behavior. *Confinia Neurologica, 32,* 322–325.

———. 1971. Testimony given in hearings on S.974, S.878, and S.J. Res. 71 before Subcommittee on Health, Senate Committee on Labor and Public Welfare, 93rd Congress, pt. 2, pp. 348–357.

Annas, G. J. 1976. *In re* Quinlan: Legal comfort for doctors. *Hastings Center Rpt., 6,* 29–31.

———. 1977. Law and the life sciences: Psychosurgery: Procedural safeguards. *Hastings Center Rpt., 7,* 11–13.

Annas, G. J., and Glantz, L. 1974. Psychosurgery: The law's response. *Boston Univ. Law Rev., 54,* 249–267.

Annas, G. J.; Glantz, L. H.; and Katz, B. F. 1977. *Informed consent to human experimentation: The subject's dilemma.* Cambridge, Mass.: Ballinger.

Arieti, S. 1967. *The intrapsychic self: Feeling, cognition, and creativity in health and mental illness.* New York: Basic Books.

———. 1974. *Interpretation of schizophrenia.* New York: Basic Books.

Bailey, H. R.; Dowling, J. L.; and Davies, E. 1973. Studies in depression: III. The control of affective illness by cingulotractotomy: A review of 150 cases. *Med. J. Australia, 2,* 366–371.

Bailey, H. R.; Dowling, J. L.; Swanton, C. H.; and Davies, E. 1971. Studies in depression: I. Cingulotractotomy in the treatment of severe affective illness. *Med. J. Australia, 1,* 8–12.

Balasubramaniam, V. 1972. Surgery for behavioural disorders. *Institute of Neurology, Madras, Proceedings, 2,* 1–6.

Balasubramaniam, V., and Kanaka, T. S. 1975. Amygdalotomy and hypothalatomy—A comparative study. *Confinia Neurologica, 37,* 195–201.

———. 1976. Hypothalamotomy in the management of aggressive behavior. In T. P. Morley (Ed.), *Current controversies in neurosurgery.* Philadelphia: W. B. Saunders. Pp. 768–777.

Balasubramaniam, V.; Kanaka, T. S.; and Ramanujam, P. B. 1973. Stereotaxic cingulotomy for drug addiction. *Neurology India, 21,* 63–66.

Balasubramaniam, V.; Kanaka, T. S.; Ramanujam, P. V.; and Ramamurthi, D. 1969. Sedative neurosurgery. *J. Ind. Med. Assoc., 53,* 377–381.

Balasubramaniam, V.; Kanaka, T. S.; Ramanujam, P. V.; and Ramamurthi, D. 1970. Surgical treatment of hyperkinetic and behavior disorders. *International Surgery, 54,* 18–34.

Balasubramaniam, V.; Kanaka, T. S.; Ramanujam, P. B.; and Ramamurthi, B. 1971. Stereotaxic hypothalamotomy. *Ind. J. Surgery, 33,* 227–230.

Balasubramaniam, V.; Kanaka, T. S.; Ramanujam, P. B.; and Ramamurthi,

B. 1973. Stereotaxic hypothalamotomy. *Confinia Neurologica, 35,* 138–143.

Balasubramaniam, V.; Ramanujam, P. B.; Kanaka, T. S.; and Ramamurthi, B. 1972. Stereotaxic surgery for behavior disorders. In E. Hitchcock, L. Laitinen, and K. Vaernet (Eds.), *Psychosurgery.* Springfield, Ill.: Charles C Thomas. Pp. 156–163.

Ballantine, H. T., Jr.; Cassidy, W. L.; Brodeur, J.; and Giriunas, I. 1972. Frontal cingulotomy for mood disturbance. In E. Hitchcock, L. Laitinen, and K. Vaernet (Eds.), *Psychosurgery.* Springfield, Ill.: Charles C Thomas. Pp. 221–229.

Ballantine, H. T., Jr.; Cassidy, W. L.; Flanagan, N. W.; and Marino, R., Jr. 1967. Stereotaxic anterior cingulotomy for neuropsychiatric illness and intractable pain. *J. Neurosurgery, 26,* 488–495.

Ballantine, H. T., Jr.; Levy, B. S.; Dagi, T.; and Giriunas, I. B. 1977. Cingulotomy for psychiatric illness: Report of 13 years experience. In W. H. Sweet, S. Obrador and J. G. Martin-Rodriguez (Eds.), *Neurosurgical treatment in psychiatry, pain, and epilepsy.* Baltimore: University Park Press. Pp. 333–353.

Bandura, A. 1969. *Principles of behavior modification.* New York: Holt, Rinehart and Winston.

Bandura, A.; Blanchard, E. G.; and Ritter, B. 1969. Relative efficacy of desensitization and modeling approaches for inducing behavioral, affective, and attitudinal changes. *J. Personality and Soc. Psychology, 13,* 173–199.

Barlow, D. H.; Agras, W. S.; Leitenberg, H.; and Wincze, J. P. 1970. An experimental analysis of the effectiveness of "shaping" in reducing maladaptive avoidance behavior. *Behavior Research and Therapy, 8,* 165–173.

Barnhart, B. A.; Pinkerton, M. L.; and Roth, R. T. 1977. Informed consent to organic behavior control. *Santa Clara Law Rev., 17,* 39–83.

Barrett, C. L. 1969. Systematic desensitization versus implosive therapy. *J. Abnormal Psychology, 74,* 587–592.

Bateson, G.; Jackson, D. D.; Haley, J.; and Weakland, J. H. 1956. Toward a theory of schizophrenia. *Behavioral Science, 1,* 251–264.

Bear, D. M. 1977. The significance of behavioral change in temporal lobe epilepsy. *McLean Hosp. J.,* Special Issue, June, pp. 9–21.

Bear, D. M., and Fedio, P. 1977. Quantitative analysis of interictal behavior in temporal lobe epilepsy. *Arch. Neurology, 34,* 454–464.

Bechtereva, N. P.; Bondartchuk, A. N.; Smirnov, V. M.; Meliutcheva, L. A.; and Shandurina, A. N. 1975. Method of electrostimulation of the deep brain structures in treatment of some chronic diseases. *Confinia Neurologica, 37,* 136–140.

Bechtereva, N. P., and Bundzen, P. V. 1973. Neurophysiological organization of mental activity in man. In S. Bogoch (Ed.), *Biological diagnosis of brain disorders.* New York: Spectrum. Pp. 3–23.

Bechtereva, N. P.; Kambarova, D. K.; Smirnov, V. M.; and Shandurina, A. N. 1977. Using the brain's latent abilities for therapy: Chronic intracerebral electrical stimulation. In W. H. Sweet, S. Obrador, and J. G. Martin-Rodriguez (Eds.), *Neurosurgical treatment in psychiatry, pain, and epilepsy.* Baltimore: University Park Press. Pp. 581–613.

Beech, H. R. 1974. *Obsessional states.* London: Methuen.

Beecher, H. K. 1961. Surgery as placebo. A quantitative study of bias. *J. Am. Med. Assoc., 176,* 1102–1107.

Beecher, H. K. 1962. The placebo effect and sound planning in surgery. *Surg., Gynecol. Obstet.*, *114*, 507–509.

Benn, S., and Peters, R. 1959. *Social principles and the democratic state.* London: Allen & Unwin.

Bentham, J. 1962. Principles of penal law. In J. Bowring (Ed.), *Works.* New York: Russell & Russell. Pp. 367–580.

Benton, A. L. 1974. *Revised visual retention test.* New York: Psychological Corp.

Berger, P. A.; Elliot, G. R.; and Barchas, J. D. 1978. Neuroregulators and schizophrenia. In M. A. Lipton, A. DiMascio, and K. F. Killam (Eds.), *Psychopharmacology: A generation of progress.* New York: Raven Press. Pp. 1071–1082.

Bergman, P., and Escalona, S. K. 1949. Unusual sensitivities in very young children. *The psychoanalytic study of the child, Vol. III/IV.* New York: International University Press. Pp. 333–352.

Bernard, C. 1961. *An introduction to the study of experimental medicine.* New York: Collier Books. Original publication 1865.

Bernstein, I.; Callahan, W.; and Jaranson, J. 1975. Lobotomy in private practice. *Arch. Gen. Psychiatry, 32,* 1041–1047.

Bingley, T.; Leksell, L.; Meyerson, B. A.; and Rylander, G. 1977. Long-term results of stereotactic anterior capsulotomy in chronic obsessive-compulsive neurosis. In W. H. Sweet, S. Obrador, and J. G. Martin-Rodriguez (Eds.), *Neurosurgical treatment in psychiatry, pain, and epilepsy.* Baltimore: University Park Press. Pp. 287–299.

Bird, D. 1968. More stress urged on cause of civil disorders. *New York Times*, August 14, p. 19.

Birley, J. 1964. Modified frontal leucotomy: A review of 106 cases. *Brit. J. Psychiatry, 110,* 211–221.

Blaney, P. H. 1975. Implications of the medical model and its alternatives. *Am. J. Psychiatry, 132,* 911–914.

Bluglass, R. 1977. Current developments in forensic psychiatry in the United Kingdom, *Psychiatry J. Univ. Ottawa, 2,* 53–62.

Blumer, D. P.; Williams, H. W.; and Mark, V. H. 1974. The study and treatment, on a neurological ward, of abnormally aggressive patients with focal brain disease. *Confinia Neurologica, 36,* 125–176.

Boersma, K.; Den Hengst, S.; Dekker, J.; and Emmelkamp, P. 1976. Exposure and response prevention in the natural environment: A comparison with obsessive-compulsive patients. *Behaviour Research and Therapy, 14,* 19–24.

Bohm, D., and Hiley, B. 1975. On the intuitive understanding of nonlocality as implied by quantum theory. *Found. of Physics, 5,* 102.

Bond, E. D., and Braceland, F. J. 1937. Prognosis in mental disease. *Am. J. Psychiatry, 94,* 263–274.

Boulougouris, J.; Rabavilas, A.; and Stefanis, C. 1977. Psychophysiological responses in obsessive-compulsive patients. *Behaviour Research and Therapy, 15,* 221–230.

Braginsky, B. M., and Braginsky, D. D. 1974. *Mainstream psychology: A critique.* New York: Holt, Rinehart & Winston.

Brakel, S. J., and Rock, R. S. (Eds.). 1971. *The mentally disabled and the law.* Chicago: University of Chicago Press.

Braunwald, E. 1977. Coronary artery surgery at the crossroads. *New Engl. J. Med., 297,* 661–663.

Breggin, P. L. 1974. Is psychosurgery an acceptable treatment for "hyperactive" children? *M/H (Mental Health)*, *58*, 19–21.

Breggin, P. R. 1964. Coercion of voluntary patients in an open hospital. *Arch. Gen. Psychiatry*, *10*, 173–181.

———. 1971a. *The crazy from the sane.* New York: Lyle Stuart.

———. 1971b. Psychotherapy as applied ethics. *Psychiatry*, *34*, 59–75.

———. 1971c. Testimony given in Hearings on S.974 before Subcommittee on Health, Senate Committee on Labor and Public Welfare, 93rd Congress, 1st Session, pt. 2, pp. 357–363.

———. 1972a. The return of lobotomy and psychosurgery. *Congressional Record*, February 24, E1602–E1612.

———. 1972b. Lobotomy is still bad medicine. *Medical Opinion*, *8*, 32–36.

———. 1972c. The politics of therapy. *M/H (Mental Health)*, *56*, 9–13.

———. 1972d. Lobotomy: An alert. *Am. J. Psychiatry*, *129*, 98–99.

———. 1972e. The revival of lobotomy (an interview). *Liberation*, October, p. 15.

———. 1972f. Letter to the editor on psychosurgery. *Science News*, April 15, p. 242.

———. 1973a. Psychosurgery. *J. Am. Med. Assoc.*, *226*, 1121.

———. 1973b. Federal funding for lobotomies. *Human Events*, May 5, p. 12.

———. 1973c. An independent follow-up of a person operated upon for violence and epilepsy. *Rough Times*, November–December, p. 8.

———. 1973d. Testimony given in *Kaimowitz* v. *Department of Mental Health.* Civil No. 73-19, 434-AW (Cir. Ct. Wayne Co., Michigan), July 10.

———. 1973e. The second wave of psychosurgery. *M/H (Mental Health)*, *57*, 10–13.

———. 1974. Therapy as applied utopian politics. *Mental Health and Society*, *1*, 129–146.

———. 1975a. Psychosurgery for political purposes. *Duquesne Law Rev.*, *13*, 841–862.

———. 1975b. Psychosurgery for the control of violence: A critical review. In W. Fields and W. Sweet (Eds.), *Neural bases of violence and aggression.* St. Louis: Warren H. Green. Pp. 350–391.

———. 1975c. Psychiatry and psychotherapy as political processes. *Am. J. Psychotherapy*, *29*, 369–382.

———. 1975d. Needed: Voluntaristic psychiatry. *Reason*, September, p. 7.

———. 1977a. Why we consent to oppression. *Reason*, September, p. 28.

———. 1977b. If psychosurgery is wrong in principle? *Psychiatric Opinion*, *14*, 23–27.

———. 1979. *Electroshock: Its brain-disabling effects.* New York: Springer.

———. In press. *The psychology of freedom.* New York: Prometheus Books.

Breggin, P. R., and Greenberg, D. 1972. Return of the lobotomy. *Washington Post*, March 12, p. C.1.

Bridges, P. K., and Bartlett, J. R. 1977. Psychosurgery: Yesterday and today. *Brit. J. Psychiatry*, *131*, 249–260.

Bridges, P. K.; Goktepe, E.; and Maratos, J. 1973. A comparative review of patients with obsessional neurosis and with depression treated by psychosurgery. *Brit. J. Psychiatry*, *123*, 663–674.

Brody, E. B. 1973. On the legal control of psychosurgery: An editorial. *J. Nervous and Mental Disease*, *157*, 151–153.

Brown, B. S.; Wienckowski, L. A.; and Bivens, L. W. 1973. *Psychosurgery:*

Perspective on a current issue. Department of Health, Education and Welfare, Pub. No. HSM 73-9119, U.S. Government Printing Office.

Brown, J. 1958. Some tests of the decay theory of immediate memory. *Quarterly J. Exp. Psychology, 10,* 12–21.

Brown, M. H. 1972a. The changing role of cingulate surgery. Unpublished speech delivered at Symposium on the Cingulate Gyrus, Hahneman Medical College and Hospital, Philadelphia, June 16.

————. 1972b. Double lesions of the limbic system in schizophrenia and psychopathy. In E. Hitchcock, L. Laitinen, and K. Vaernet (Eds.), *Psychosurgery.* Springfield, Ill.: Charles C Thomas. Pp. 195–203.

————. 1973. Further experience with multiple limbic targets for schizophrenia and aggression. In L. Laitinen and K. Livingston (Eds.), *Surgical approaches in psychiatry.* Baltimore: University Park Press. Pp. 189–195.

————. 1975. Multi-target neurosurgery in the treatment of schizophrenia and violence. *Psychiatric J. Univ. Ottawa, 2,* 29–36.

————. 1977. Neurosurgical intervention or a lifetime in prison or hospital? *Roche Report: Frontiers of Psychiatry.* Nutley, N.J.: Division of Hoffman–LaRoche. Pp. 5–11.

Brownfeld, A. C. 1973. Psychosurgery: Mental progress or medical nightmare? *Private Practice,* June, p. 45.

Burckhardt, G. 1891. Über Rindenexcisionen, als Beitrag zur operativen Therapie der Psychosen. *Allegemaine Zeitschrift für Psychiatrie, 47,* 463–548.

Capstick, N. 1975. Clomipramine in the treatment of obsessional states. *Psychosomatics, 16,* 21–25.

Carlsson, A. 1978. Does dopamine play a role in schizophrenia? *J. Society of Biological Psychiatry, 13,* 3–21.

Cartwright, S. A. 1851. Report on the diseases and physical peculiarities of the Negro race. *New Orleans Medical and Surgical J.,* May.

Casper, B. M. 1976. Technology and policy and democracy. *Science, 194,* 29–35.

Cassidy, W. L.; Ballantine, H. T., Jr.; and Flanagan, N. B. 1965–66. Frontal cingulotomy for affective disorders. *Recent Advances in Biol. Psychiatry, 8,* 269–275.

Cassidy, W. L.; Flanagan, N. B.; Spellman, M.; and Cohen, M. E. 1957. Clinical observations in manic-depressive disease. *J. Am. Med. Assoc., 164,* 1535–1546.

Catts, S., and McConaghy, N. 1975. Ritual prevention in the treatment of obsessive-compulsive neurosis. *Austral. and New Zealand J. Psychiatry, 9,* 37–41.

Cawley, R. H. 1974. Psychotherapy and obsessional disorders. In H. R. Beech (Ed.), *Obsessional states.* London: Methuen. Pp. 259–290.

Cheng, S.; Tait, H.; and Freeman, W. 1956. Transorbital lobotomy vs. electroconvulsive shock therapy in the treatment of mentally ill tuberculosis patients. *Am. J. Psychiatry, 113,* 32–56.

Chesser, E. S. 1976. Behaviour therapy: Recent trends and current practice. *Brit. J. Psychiatry, 129,* 289–276.

Cheyfitz, K. 1976. 13 given mind-altering operations. *Detroit Free Press,* April 11, p. 1.

Chorover, S. L. 1966. The psychophysiology of memory. *Technology Rev.*, 69, 17–23.

———. 1973. Big brother and psychotechnology. *Psychology Today*, 7, 43–54.

———. 1974 Psychosurgery: A neuropsychological perspective. *Boston Univ. Law Rev.*, 54, 231–248.

———. 1976a. An experimental critique of "consolidation" studies and an alternative model systems approach to the psychobiology of memory. In M. R. Rosenzweig and E. L. Bennett (Eds.), *Neural mechanisms of learning and memory.* Cambridge, Mass.: M.I.T. Press. Pp. 561–582.

———. 1976b. The pacification of the brain: From phrenology to psychosurgery. In T. P. Morley (Ed.), *Current controversies in neurosurgery.* Philadelphia: W. B. Saunders. Pp. 730–767.

———. 1979. *From genesis to genocide: The meaning of human nature and the power of behavior control.* Cambridge, Mass.: M.I.T. Press.

Clark, K. B. 1971. The pathos of power: A psychological perspective. *Am. Psychol.*, 26, 1047–1057.

Cochrane, A. L. 1972. *Effectiveness and efficiency: Random reflections on health services.* Abington, Berks, England: Burgess and Son.

Cole, J. O., and Davis, J. M. 1975. Antidepressant drugs. In A. M. Freedman, H. I. Kaplan, and B. J. Sadock (Eds), *Comprehensive textbook of psychiatry.* Baltimore: Williams & Wilkins. Pp. 1941–1956.

Colen, B. D. 1975. Drug for sex offenders called success. *Washington Post*, November 30, Section B, p. 3, Column 1.

Comment. 1971a. A jam in the revolving door: A prisoner's right to rehabilitation. *Georgetown Law J.*, 60, 225–247.

Comment. 1971b. A statutory right to treatment for prisoners: Society's right of self-defense. *Neb. Law Rev.*, 50, 543-566.

Comment. 1976. The limits of state intervention: Personal identity and ultrarisky actions. *Yale Law J.*, 85, 826–846.

Cooper, I. S. 1973. *The victim is always the same.* New York: Harper & Row.

Corkill, G.; Ratcliff, E.; and Simpson, R. C. 1973. Leucotomy in the 1970s. *Med. J. Australia*, 1, 442–443.

Corkin, S. 1965. Tactually-guided maze learning in man: Effects of unilateral cortical excisions and bilateral hippocampal lesions. *Neuropsychologia*, 3, 339–351.

———. 1979. Hidden-figures-test performance: Lasting effects of unilateral penetrating head injury and transient effects of bilateral cingulotomy. *Neuropsychologia*, 17, 585–605.

Corkin, S.; Twitchell, T. E.; and Sullivan, E. V. 1977. A study of cingulotomy in man. Second Interim Report (unpublished). Prepared for the National Commission for the Protection of Human Subjects of Biomedical and Behavioral Research.

———. 1979. Safety and efficacy of cingulotomy for pain and psychiatric disorder. In E. R. Hitchcock, H. T. Ballantine, Jr., and B. A. Meyerson (Eds.), *Modern concepts in psychiatric surgery.* Amsterdam: Elsevier/ North Holland Biomedical Press. Pp. 253–271.

Costello, C. G. 1976. Electroconvulsive therapy: Is further investigation necessary? *Can. Psychiatric Assoc. J.*, 21, 61–66.

Cousins, N. 1979. *Anatomy of an illness.* New York: Norton.

Cox, A. W., and Brown, M. H. 1977. Results of multi-target limbic surgery in the treatment of schizophrenia and aggressive states. In W. H. Sweet, S. Obrador, and J. G. Martin-Rodriguez (Eds.), *Neurosurgical treatment in psychiatry, pain, and epilepsy.* Baltimore: University Park Press. Pp. 469–479.

Crane, G. 1973. Clinical psychopharmacology in its 20th year. *Science, 181,* 124–128.

Crowe, M. J.; Marks, I. M.; Agras, W. S.; and Leitenberg, H. 1972. Time-limited desensitization, implosion, and shaping for phobic patients: A cross-over study. *Behaviour Research and Therapy, 10,* 319–328.

Culliton, B. J. 1976. Psychosurgery: National commission issues surprisingly favorable report. *Science, 194,* 299–301.

Cushing, H. 1929. *The pituitary body and hypothalamus.* Springfield, Ill.: Charles C Thomas.

D'Arazien, S. 1972. The new lobotomists. *Boston After Dark,* March 7–13, p. 1.

Davis, J. M., and Cole, J. O. 1975. Antipsychotic drugs. In A. M. Freedman, H. I. Kaplan, and B. J. Saddock (Eds.), *Comprehensive textbook of psychiatry.* Baltimore: Williams & Wilkins. Pp. 1921–1941.

Dawidoff, D. J. 1973. *The malpractice of psychiatrists.* Springfield, Ill.: Charles C Thomas.

Dax, E. C. 1977. The history of prefrontal leucotomy. In J. S. Smith and L. G. Kiloh (Eds.), *Psychosurgery and society.* New York: Pergamon Press. Pp. 19–24.

DeBakey, M. E., and Lawrie, G. M. 1978. Aortocoronary-artery bypass: Assessment after 13 years. *J. Am. Med. Assoc., 239,* 837–839.

Delgado, J. 1969. *Physical control of the mind: Toward a psychocivilized society.* New York: Harper & Row.

———. 1973. Physical manipulation of the brain. *Hastings Center Rpt., 3,* Special Supplement.

Delgado, R. 1977a. Organically induced behavioral change in correctional institutions: Release decisions and the "new man" phenomenon. *S. Calif. Law Rev., 50,* 215–270.

———. 1977b. Religious totalism: Gentle and ungentle persuasion under the first amendment. *S. Calif. Law Rev., 51,* 1–98.

Department of Health, Education and Welfare. 1977. Use of psychosurgery in practice and research: Report and recommendations for public comment. *Federal Register, 42,* 26318–26332.

Derogatis, L. R.; Lipman, R. S.; Rickles, K.; Uhlenhuth, E. H.; and Covi, L. 1974. Hopkins symptom checklist (HSCL). In P. Tichot (Ed.), *Psychological measurements in psychopharmacology.* Paris: Carger. Pp. 79–110.

Dershowitz, S. 1974. Indeterminate confinement: Letting the therapy fit the harm. *Univ. Penn. Law Rev., 123,* 296–339.

Dickens, B. 1975. What is a medical experiment? *Can. Med. Assoc. J., 4,* 635–639.

Dickson, D. 1979. Psychosurgery supporters sued for malpractice. *Nature, 277,* 164–165.

Dieckmann, G., and Hassler, R. 1975. Unilateral hypothalamotomy in sexual delinquents. *Confinia Neurologica, 37,* 177–186.

———. 1977. Treatment of sexual violence by stereotactic hypothalamotomy. In W. H. Sweet, S. Obrador, and J. G. Martin-Rodriguez (Eds.),

Neurosurgical treatment in psychiatry, pain, and epilepsy. Baltimore: University Park Press. Pp. 451–462.

Dietz, J. 1972. Senate urged to kill brain study. *Boston Sunday Globe,* September 24, p. 38.

———. 1973a. Boston's psychosurgery: Success and controversy. *Boston Sunday Globe,* January 21, p. A-1.

———. 1973b. Opponent sees "grave danger" in new psychosurgery effort by Hub team. *Boston Globe,* May 24, p. 43.

DiMascio, A., and Shader, R. 1968. Behavioral toxicity. In D. Efron (Ed.), *Psychopharmacology: A review of progress, 1957–1967.* Rockville, Md.: U.S. Public Health Service Pub. No. 1836, pp. 551–560.

DiPalma, J. 1971. *Drill's pharmacology in medicine.* New York: McGraw-Hill.

Donnelly, J. 1978. The incidence of psychosurgery in the United States, 1971–1973. *Am. J. Psychiatry, 135,* 1476–1480.

Dorus, E.; Pandey, G. N.; Shaughnessy, R.; Val, M. G.; Erickson, S.; and Davis, J. M. 1979. Lithium transport across red cell membrane: A cell membrane abnormality in manic-depressive illness. *Science, 205,* 932–934.

Dow, R. S.; Grimm, R. J.; and Rushmer, D. S. 1975. Psychosurgery and brain stimulation: The legislative experience in Oregon in 1973. In I. S. Cooper, M. Riklan, and R. S. Snider (Eds.), *The cerebellum, epilepsy, and behavior.* New York: Plenum. Pp. 367–389.

Draper, P. A. 1947. Prefrontal lobotomy: A new type of brain surgery. *Your Mind: Psychology Digest,* June, 3–7.

Drewe, E. A. 1974. The effect of type and area of brain lesion on Wisconsin card sorting test performance. *Cortex, 10,* 159–170.

Durell, J. 1973. Introduction. In J. Mendels (Ed.), *Biol. psychiatry.* New York: Wiley. Pp. 1–13.

Durkheim, E. 1933. *The division of labor in society.* New York: Free Press.

Dworkin, G. 1976. Autonomy and behavior control. *Hastings Center Rpt., 6,* 23–28.

Edgar, H. 1975. Regulating psychosurgery: Issues of public policy and law. In W. Gaylin, J. S. Meister, and R. C. Neville (Eds.), *Operating on the mind: The psychosurgery debate.* New York: Basic Books. Pp. 117–168.

Editorial. 1972. Psychosurgery. *Lancet*/Part ii, 69–70.

Emmelkamp, P. M. G., and Kraanen, J. 1977. Therapist-controlled exposure versus self-controlled exposure. *Behaviour Research and Therapy, 15,* 491–496.

Emmelkamp, P. M. G., and Kwee, K. G. 1977. Obsessional ruminations: A comparison between thought-stopping and prolonged exposure in imagination. *Behaviour Research and Therapy, 15,* 441–444.

Emmelkamp, P. M. G., and Wessels, H. 1975. Flooding in imagination vs. flooding *in vivo:* A comparison with agoraphobics. *Behaviour Research and Therapy, 13,* 7–15.

Engelhardt, H. T., Jr. 1975. The concepts of health and disease. In H. T. Engelhardt, Jr. and S. F. Spicker (Eds.), *Evaluation and explanation in the biomedical sciences.* Boston: D. Reidel. Pp. 125–141.

Ennis, B. 1972. *Prisoners of psychiatry: Mental patients, psychiatrists, and the law.* New York: Harcourt Brace Jovanovich.

Ennis, B. J., and Litwack, T. R. 1974. Psychiatry and the presumption of expertise: Flipping coins in the courtroom. *Calif. Law Rev.*, *62*, 693–752.

Ervin, F. R. 1976. Evaluation of organic factors in patients with impulse disorders and episodic violence. In W. L. Smith and A. Kling (Eds.), *Issues in brain/behavior control.* New York: Spectrum. Pp. 23–32.

Ervin, F. R.; Brown, C. E.; and Mark, V. H. 1966. Striatal influence on facial pain. *Confinia Neurologica*, *27*, 75–86.

Ervin, F. R.; Mark, V. H.; and Sweet, W. H. 1969. Focal cerebral disease, temporal lobe epilepsy, and violent behavior. *Trans. Am. Neurol. Assoc.*, *94*, 253–256.

Escobar, J. I., and Shandel, V. 1977. Nuclear symptoms of schizophrenia after cingulotomy: A case report. *J. Am. Psychiatric Assoc.*, *134*, 1304–1306.

Escobedo, F.; Fernandez-Guardiola, A.; Contreras, C.; and Solis, H. 1977. Electrical stimulation of the cerebellum in humans related to behavioral disorders. In W. H. Sweet, S. Obrador, and J. G. Martin-Rodriguez (Eds.), *Neurosurgical treatment in psychiatry, pain, and epilepsy.* Baltimore: University Park Press. Pp. 527–537.

Escobedo, F.; Fernandez-Guardiola, A.; and Solis, G. 1973. Chronic stimulation of the cingulum in humans with behavior disorders. In L. Laitinen and K. Livingston (Eds.), *Surgical approaches in psychiatry.* Baltimore: University Park Press. Pp. 65–68.

Ewing, A. 1929. *The morality of punishment.* Montclair, N.J.: Patterson Smith.

Eysenck, H. J. 1965. The effects of psychotherapy. *Int. J. Psychiatry*, *1*, 99–142.

Eysenck, H. J., and Eysenck, S. G. G. 1968. *Eysenck Personality Inventory.* San Diego, Calif.: Educational and Industrial Testing Service.

Falconer, M. A. 1973. Reversibility by temporal lobe resection of the behavioral abnormalities of temporal lobe epilepsy. *New Eng. J. Med.*, *289*, 451–455.

Falconer, M. A., and Serafetinides, E. A. 1963. A follow-up study of surgery in temporal lobe epilepsy. *J. Neurology, Neurosurgery, and Psychiatry*, *26*, 154–165.

Falconer, M. A.; Hill, D.; Meyer, A.; and Wilson, J. A. 1958. Clinical, radiological and EEG correlations with pathological changes in temporal lobe epilepsy and their significance in surgical treatment. In M. Baldwin and P. Baily (Eds.), *Temporal lobe epilepsy.* Springfield, Ill.: Charles C Thomas.

Farina, A.; Gliha, D.; Boudreau, L. A.; Allen, J. G.; and Sherman, M. 1971. Mental illness and the impact of believing others know about it. *J. Abnormal Psychology*, *77*, 1–5.

Fields, W., and Sweet, W. (Eds.), 1975. Neural bases of violence and aggression. St. Louis: Warren H. Green.

Fink, M. 1978. Efficacy and safety of induced seizures (EST) in man. *Comprehensive Psychiatry*, *19*, 1–18.

Flew, A. 1954. The justification of punishment. *Philosophy*, *29*, 291–307.

Flor-Henry, P. 1969. Psychosis and temporal lobe epilepsy: A controlled investigation. *Epilepsia* (Amsterdam), *10*, 363–395.

―――. 1975. Psychiatric surgery—1935–1973. *Can. Psychiatric Assoc. J.*, *20*, 157–167.

Foa, E. B., and Goldstein, A. 1978. Prolonged exposure and strict response prevention in the treatment of obsessive-compulsive neurosis. *Behavior Therapy, 8,* 821–829.

Foltz, E. L., and White, L. E. 1962. Pain "relief" by frontal cingulotomy. *J. Neurosurgery, 19,* 89–100.

Fox, S. 1963. Physical disorder, consciousness, and criminal liability. *Columbia Law Rev., 63,* 645–668.

Frank, G. 1975. *Psychiatric diagnosis: A review of research.* Oxford: Pergamon Press.

Frankena, W. K. 1973. *Ethics.* Englewood Cliffs, N.J.: Prentice-Hall.

Freedman, A. M.; Kaplan, H. I.; and Sadock, B. J. (Eds.). 1975. *Comprehensive textbook of psychiatry.* Baltimore: Williams & Wilkins.

Freeman, W. 1959. Psychosurgery. In S. Arieti (Ed.), *American handbook of psychiatry, II.* New York: Basic Books. Pp. 1521–1540.

————. 1968. *The psychiatrist: Personalities and patterns.* New York: Grune & Stratton.

————. 1971. Frontal lobotomy in early schizophrenia: Long follow-up in 415 cases. *Brit. J. Psychiatry, 119,* 621–624.

Freeman, W., and Watts, J. W. 1942. 2nd ed. 1950. *Psychosurgery.* Springfield, Ill.: Charles C Thomas.

————. 1944. Physiological psychology. In J. M. Luck and V. E. Hall (Eds.), *Annual review of psychology,* Vol. VI. Stanford, Calif.: American Physiological Society and Annual Reviews. Pp. 517–542.

Freidberg, J. 1977. Shock treatment, brain damage, and memory loss: A neurological perspective. *Am. J. Psychiatry, 134,* 1010–1014.

Freud, S. 1964. *The question of lay analysis, with Freud's 1927 postscript.* Translated and edited by J. Strachez. Garden City, N.Y.: Doubleday Anchor Books.

Fried, C. 1973. Introduction: The need for a philosophical anthropology. *Indiana Law J., 48,* 527–532.

Friedhoff, R. J. 1973. Biogenic amines and schizophrenia. In J. Mendels (Ed.), *Biological psychiatry.* New York: Wiley. Pp. 113–129.

Fulton, J. F. 1948. Surgical approach to mental disorder. *McGill Med. J., 17,* 133–145.

————. 1951. *Frontal lobotomy and affective behavior: A neurophysiological analysis.* New York: Norton.

Gardner, E. A. 1974. Implications of psychoactive drug therapy. *New Eng. J. Med., 290,* 800–801.

Gastaut, H.; Morin, G.; and Lesèvre, M. 1955. Étude du comportement d'épileptiques psychomoteurs dans l'intervalle de leurs crises, les troubles de l'activité globale et de la sociabilité. *Ann. Med. et Psychol., 113,* 1–27.

Gaylin, W. M. 1975. The problem in psychosurgery. In W. M. Gaylin, J. S. Meister, and R. C. Neville (Eds.), *Operating on the mind: The psychosurgery debate.* New York: Basic Books. Pp. 3–23.

Gazzaniga, M. S.; Bogen, J. E.; and Sperry, R. W. 1963. Laterality effects in somesthesis following cerebral commissurotomy in man. *Neuropsychologia, 1,* 209–215.

Gerber, R., and McAnany, P. (Eds.). 1972. *Contemporary punishment.* North Bend, Ind.: University of Notre Dame Press.

Geschwind, N. 1977a. Behavioral change in temporal lobe epilepsy. *Arch. Neurology, 34,* 453.

————. 1977b. Introduction: Psychiatric complications in the epilepsies:

Current research and treatment. *McLean Hosp. J.*, Special Issue, June, pp. 6–8.

Gildenberg, P. L. 1975. Survey of stereotaxic and functional neurosurgery in the United States and Canada. *Appl. Neurophysiology, 38,* 31–37.

Gobert, J. 1975. Psychosurgery, conditioning, and the prisoner's right to refuse "rehabilitation." *Virginia Law Rev., 61,* 155–196.

Goktepe, E.; Young, L.; and Bridges, P. 1975. A further review of the results of stereotactic subcaudate tractotomy. *Brit. J. Psychiatry, 126,* 270–280.

Goldberg, S. C.; Frosch, W. A.; Drossman, A. K.; Schooler, N. R.; and Johnson, G. F. S. 1972. Prediction of response to phenothiazines in schizophrenia: A cross-validation study. *Arch. Gen. Psychiatry, 26,* 367–373.

Goldman, P. S.; Crawford, H. T.; Stokes, L. P.; Galkin, T. W.; and Rosvold, H. E. 1974. Sex-dependent behavioral effects of cerebral cortical lesions in the developing rhesus monkey. *Science, 186,* 540–542.

Goldstein, J. 1978. On the right of the "institutionalized mentally infirm" to consent to or refuse to participate as subjects in biomedical and behavioral research. Report to the National Commission for the Protection of Human Subjects of Biomedical and Behavioral Research. *Appendix: Research involving those institutionalized as mentally infirm.* Department of Health, Education and Welfare, Pub. No. (OS) 78-0007, U.S. Government Printing Office, pp. 2-1 to 2-39.

Goldstein, K. 1950. Prefrontal lobotomy: Analysis and warning. *Scientific American, 182,* 44–47.

Goldstein, M. N.; Joynt, R. J.; and Hartley, R. B. 1975. The long-term effects of callosal sectioning. Report of a second case. *Arch. Neurology, 32,* 52–53.

Goodman, L., and Gillman, A. 1956. *The pharmacological basis of therapeutics.* New York: Macmillan.

Grant, D. A., and Berg, E. A. 1948. A behavioral analysis of degree of reinforcement and ease of shifting to new responses in a Weigl-type card-sorting problem. *J. Exp. Psychology, 38,* 404–411.

Greenblatt, M.; Arnot, R.; and Solomon, H. 1950. *Studies in lobotomy.* New York: Grune & Stratton.

Grenell, R. G., and Gabay, S. (Eds.). 1976. *Biological foundations of psychiatry.* New York: Raven Press.

Grimm, R. J. 1976. Brain control in a democratic society. In W. L. Smith and A Kling (Eds.), *Issues in brain/behavior control.* New York: Halsted. Pp. 109–149.

Griponissiotis, B., and Tavridis, G. 1972. Open technique of selective leucotomy as an improved step in psychosurgery. In I. Fusek and Z. Kunc (Eds.), *Present limits of neurosurgery.* Prague: Avicenum. Pp. 491–493.

Gross, M. D., and Wilson, C. W. 1974. *Minimal brain dysfunction.* New York: Brunner-Mazel.

Grosser, G. H.; Pearsall, D. T.; Fisher, C. L.; and Geremonte, L. 1974. The regulation of electro-convulsive treatment in Massachusetts: A follow-up. Department Report of the Department of Mental Health of the State of Massachusetts.

Group for the Advancement of Psychiatry, Committee on Research. 1975. *Pharmacotherapy and psychotherapy: Paradoxes, problems and progress.* New York: Mental Health Materials Center.

Gurland, B. J.; Fleiss, J. L.; Cooper, J. E.; Sharpe, L.; Kendell, R. E.; and

Roberts, P. 1970. Cross-national study of diagnosis of mental disorders. *Comprehensive Psychiatry, 11,* 18–25.

Guttman, E.; Mayer-Gross, W.; and Slater, E. T. O. 1939. Short-distance prognosis of schizophrenia. *J. Neurol. Psychiatry, 2,* 25–34.

Guze, S. B., and Robins, E. 1970. Suicide and primary affective disorders. *Brit. J. Psychiatry, 117,* 437–438.

Hackmann, A., and McClean C. 1975. A comparison of flooding and thought-stopping treatment. *Behavior Research and Therapy, 13,* 263–269.

Hall, J. 1947. *General principles of criminal law.* Indianapolis: Bobbs-Merrill.

Hampton, J. 1972. Eerie brain surgery. *National Observer,* March 25, p. 1.

Hanaway, J.; Scott, W. R.; and Strother, C. M. 1977. *Atlas of the human brain and the orbit for computed tomography.* St. Louis: Warren H. Green.

Hart, H. L. A. 1958. The aims of criminal law. *Law and Contemp. Problems, 23,* 401–441.

———. 1968. *Punishment and responsibility.* New York: Oxford University Press.

Hartelius, H. 1952. Cerebral changes following electrically induced convulsions. *Acta Psychiatr. Scand., 77,* 1–128.

Hathaway, S. R., and McKinley, J. C. 1967. *Minnesota Multiphasic Personality Inventory.* New York: Psychological Corp.

Heath, R. G. 1971. Depth recording and stimulation studies in patients. In A. Winter (Ed.), *The surgical control of behavior: A symposium.* Springfield, Ill.: Charles C Thomas. Pp. 21–37.

Heimburger, R. F.; Small, I. F.; Small, J. G.; Milstein, V.; and Moore, C. 1978. Stereotactic amygdalotomy for convulsive and behavioral disorders. *Appl. Neurophysiology, 41,* 43–51.

Heisenberg, W. 1958. *Physics and philosophy.* New York: Harper Torchbooks.

Helzer, J. E.; Clayton, P. J.; Pambakian, R.; Reich, T.; Woodruff, R. A., Jr.; and Reveley, M.A. 1977b. Reliability of psychiatric diagnoses: II. The test/retest reliability of diagnostic classification. *Arch. Gen. Psychiatry, 34,* 136–141.

Helzer, J. E.; Robins, L. N.; Taibleson, M.; Woodruff, J. A., Jr.; Reich, T.; and Wish, E. D. 1977a. Reliability of psychiatric diagnoses: I. A methodological review. *Arch. Gen. Psychiatry, 34,* 129–135.

Henkin, L. 1974. Privacy and autonomy. *Columbia Law Rev., 74,* 1410–1433.

Hersen, M., and Bellack, A. S. (Eds.), 1978. *Behavior therapy in the psychiatric setting.* Baltimore: Williams & Wilkins.

Hersen, M.; Eisler, R. M.; Alford, G. S.; and Agras, W. S. 1973. Effects of token economy on neurotic depression: An experimental analysis. *Behavior Therapy, 4,* 392–397.

Hetherington, R. F.; Haden, P.; and Craig, W. J. 1972. Neurosurgery in affective disorder. In E. Hitchcock, L. Laitinen, and K. Vaernet (Eds.), *Psychosurgery.* Springfield, Ill.: Charles C Thomas. Pp. 332–345.

Heyse, H. 1975. Response prevention and modelling in the treatment of obsessive-compulsive neurosis. In J. Brengelmann (Ed.), *Progress in be-*

haviour therapy. Berlin: Springer-Verlag. Pp. 53–58.

Hiatt, H. 1977. Lessons of the coronary bypass debate. *New Eng. J. Med.,* 297, 1462–1464.

Hill, D. 1944. Cerebral dysrhythmia: Its significance in aggressive behavior. *Proc. Royal Soc. Med., 37,* 317–330.

Hirose, S. 1972. The case selection of mental disorder for orbitoventrome-dial undercutting. In E. Hitchcock, L. Laitinen, and K. Vaernet (Eds.), *Psychosurgery.* Springfield, Ill.: Charles C Thomas. Pp. 291–303.

————. 1973. Long-term evaluation of orbito-ventromedial undercuttings in "atypical" schizophrenic patients. In L. Laitinen and K. Livingston (Eds.), *Surgical approaches in psychiatry.* Baltimore: University Park Press. Pp. 196–205.

————. 1977. Psychiatric evaluation of psychosurgery. In W. H. Sweet, S. Obrador, and J. G. Obrador (Eds.), *Neurosurgical treatment in psychiatry, pain, and epilepsy.* Baltimore: University Park Press. Pp. 203–209.

————. 1979. Past and present trends of psychiatric surgery in Japan. In E. R. Hitchcock, H. T. Ballantine, Jr., and B. A. Meyerson (Eds.), *Modern concepts in psychiatric surgery.* New York: Elsevier/North-Holland Biomedical Press. Pp. 349–357.

Hirsch, S. R. 1979. Do parents cause schizophrenia? *Trends in neuroscience, 2* (No. 2), 49–52.

Hitchcock, E., and Cairns, V. 1973. Amygdalotomy. *Postgrad. Med. J., 49,* 894–904.

Hoch, P. 1959. Drug therapy. In S. Arieti (Ed.), *The American handbook of psychiatry, II.* New York: Basic Books. Pp. 1541–1551.

Hodgson, R.; Rachman, S.; and Marks, I. M. 1972. The treatment of chronic obsessive-compulsive neurosis: Follow-up and further findings. *Behaviour Research and Therapy, 10,* 181–189.

Holder, A. R. 1978. *Medical malpractice law.* New York: Wiley.

Hollingshead, A. B. 1977. *Four factor index of social status.* New Haven: Author.

Hunt, R. C.; Feldman, H.; and Fiero, R. P. 1938. "Spontaneous" remissions in dementia praecox. *Psychiatric Quarterly, 12,* 414–425.

Hunter, R., and Macalpine, I. 1963. *Three hundred years of psychiatry: 1535–1860.* London: Oxford University Press.

Hutton, E. L.; Fleming, G. W. T. H.; and Fox, F. E. 1941. Early results of prefrontal leucotomy. *Lancet, 2,* 3–7.

Ingelfinger, F. J. 1972. Informed (but uneducated) consent. *New Eng. J. Med., 287,* 465–466.

Ingraham, B. L., and Smith G. W. 1972. The use of electronics in the observation and control of human behavior and its possible use in rehabilitation and parole. *Issues in Criminology, 7,* 35–53.

Ingram, J. M. 1961. Obsessional illness in mental hospital patients. *J. Mental Sci., 107,* 382–402.

Jacobsen, C. F. 1936. Studies of cerebral function in primates: I. The functions of the frontal association areas in monkeys. *Comp. Psychology Monographs, 13,* 3–60.

Janis, I. L. 1948. Memory loss following electric convulsive treatments. *J. Personality, 17,* 29–32.

————. 1950. Psychological effects of electric convulsive treatments. *J. Nervous and Mental Disease, 111*, 359–397, 469–489.

Janis, I. L., and Astrachan, M. 1951. The effect of electro-convulsive treatments on memory efficiency. *J. Abnormal Psychology, 46*, 501–511.

Jarvick, M. 1970. Drugs used in the treatment of psychiatric disorders. In L. Goodman and H. Gilman (Eds.), *The pharmacological basis of therapeutics.* New York: Macmillan. Pp. 159–214.

Jonas, H. 1970. Philosophical reflections on experimenting with human subjects. In P. A. Freund (Ed.), *Experimentation with human subjects.* New York: George Braziller. Pp. 1–31.

Jurko, M. F., and Andy, O. J. 1973. Psychological changes correlated with thalamotomy site. *J. Neurology, Neurosurgery, and Psychiatry, 36*, 846–852.

Kadish, S. H., and Paulsen, M. G. 1975. *Criminal law and its processes: Cases and materials.* Boston: Little, Brown.

Kalinowsky, L. B. 1975. The convulsive therapies. In A. M. Freeman, H. I. Kaplan, and B. J. Sadock (Eds.), *Comprehensive textbook of psychiatry.* Baltimore: Williams & Wilkins. Pp. 1969–1978.

Kant, I. 1974. *Philosophy of law.* W. Hastie (Trans.) Fairfield, N.J.: Augustus M. Kelley.

Kaplan, E. L.; Anthony, B. F.; Bisno, A.; Durack, D.; Houser, H.; Millard, D.; Sanford, J.; Shulman, S. T.; Stillerman, M.; Taranta, A.; and Wenger, N. 1977. Prevention of bacterial endocarditis. *Circulation, 56*, 139A–143A.

Katz, J. 1969. The right to treatment—An enchanting legal fiction? *Univ. of Chicago Law Rev., 36*, 755–783.

Katz, M. M.; Cole, J. O.; and Lowery, H. A. 1964. Nonspecificity of diagnosis of paranoid schizophrenia. *Arch. Gen. Psychiatry, 11*, 197–202.

Kazdin, A. E. 1977. *The token economy: A review and evaluation.* New York: Plenum.

Kazdin, A. E., and Wilson, G. T. 1978. *Evaluation of behavior therapy: Issues, evidence, and research strategies.* Cambridge, Mass.: Ballinger.

Kelley, P. M. 1978. Prisoner access to psychosurgery: A constitutional perspective. *Pacific Law J., 9*, 249–280.

Kelly, D. 1973. Psychosurgery and the limbic system. *Postgrad. Med. J., 49*, 825–833.

————. 1975. What's new in psychosurgery? In S. Arieti (Ed.), *New dimensions in psychiatry: A world view.* New York: Wiley. Pp. 114–141.

————. 1976. Psychosurgery in the '70s. *Brit. J. Hosp. Med., 16*, 165–174.

Kelly, D., and Mitchell-Heggs, N. 1973. Stereotactic limbic leucotomy—A follow-up study of thirty patients. *Postgrad. Med. J., 49*, 865–882.

Kelly, D.; Richardson, A.; Mitchell-Heggs, N.; Greemy, J.; Chen, D.; and Hafner, R. 1973. Stereotactic limbic leucotomy. *Brit. J. Psychiatry, 123*, 141–148.

Kendell, R. E. 1975. *The role of diagnosis in psychiatry.* Oxford: Blackwell Scientific Publications.

Kety, S. S.; Rosenthal, D.; Wender, P. H.; and Schulsinger, F. 1968. The types and prevalence of mental illness in the biological and adopted families of schizophrenics. In D. Rosenthal and S. S. Kety (Eds.), *The transmission of schizophrenia.* New York: Pergamon. Pp. 345–362.

Khachaturyan, A. A. *Neuropatologiya i Psichiatriya, 20*, 18–22. Microfilmed English translation, Library of Congress, TT60-13724.

Kimura, D. 1963. Right temporal lobe damage. *Arch. Neurology, 8,* 264 –271.

King, J. H., Jr. 1977. *The law of medical malpractice in a nutshell.* St. Paul: West Publishing Co.

Kittrie, N. N. 1971. *The right to be different: Deviance and enforced therapy.* Baltimore: Johns Hopkins Press.

Klein, D. F., and Davis, J. M. 1969. *Diagnosis and drug treatment of psychiatric disorders.* Baltimore: Williams & Wilkins.

Klerman, G. L. 1970. Clinical efficacy and actions of antipsychotics. In A. DiMascio and R. Shader (Eds.), *Clinical handbook of psychopharmacology.* New York: Science House. Pp. 40–56.

——— . 1975. Overview of depression. In A. M. Freedman, H. I. Kaplan, and B. J. Sadock (Eds.), *Comprehensive textbook of psychiatry.* Baltimore: Williams & Wilkins. Pp. 1003–1012.

Knight, G. 1964. The orbital cortex as an objective in surgical treatment of mental illness. *Brit. J. Surgery, 51,* 114–124.

——— . 1965. Stereotactic tractotomy in the surgical treatment of mental illness. *J. Neurology, Neurosurgery, and Psychiatry, 28,* 257–266.

——— . 1973. Further observations from an experience of 660 cases of stereotactic tractotomy. *Postgrad. Med. J., 49,* 845–854.

Knowles, S. 1975. Beyond the "Cuckoo's Nest": A proposal for federal regulation of psychosurgery. *Harvard J. of Legislation, 12,* 610–667.

Kolb, L. 1973. *Modern clinical psychiatry. 8th ed.* Philadelphia: W. B. Saunders.

Kornetov, A. N. 1972. Some data on long-term catamnesis of pernicious schizophrenic patients subjected to prefrontal leucotomy. In I. Fusek and Z. Kunc (Eds.), *Present limits of neurosurgery.* Prague: Avicenum. Pp. 475–476.

Koskoff, Y. D., and Goldhurst, R. 1968. *The "dark side of the house."* New York: Dial Press.

Kramer, M. 1954. The 1951 survey of the use of psychosurgery. In W. Overholser (Ed.), *Proceedings of the Third Research Conference on Psychosurgery, 1951.* Bethesda, Md.: National Institutes of Health, U.S. Public Health Service Pub. No. 221. Pp. 159–168.

——— . 1969. Cross-national study of diagnosis of the mental disorders: Origin of the problem. *Am. J. Psychiatry, 125,* 1–11.

Kuhn, T. S. 1970. *The structure of scientific revolutions.* Chicago: University of Chicago Press.

LaFave, W. R., and Scott, A. W., Jr. 1972. *Handbook on criminal law.* St. Paul: West Publishing Co.

Laing, R. D. 1967. *The politics of experience.* New York: Ballantine.

——— . 1971. *The politics of the family and other essays.* New York: Pantheon Books.

Laitinen, L. V. 1977 Ethical aspects of psychiatric surgery. In W. H. Sweet, S. Obrador, and J. G. Martin-Rodriguez (Eds.), *Neurosurgical treatment in psychiatry, pain, and epilepsy.* Baltimore: University Park Press. Pp. 483–488.

Landis, C.; Zubin, J.; and Mettler, F. 1950. The functions of the human frontal lobe. *J. Psychology, 30,* 123–138.

Lansdell, H. 1968. The use of factor scores from the Wechsler-Bellevue Scale of Intelligence in assessing patients with temporal lobe removals. *Cortex, 4,* 257–268.

Le Beau, J., and Pecker, J. 1950. Étude de certaines formes d'agitation psychomotrice au cours de l'épilepsie et de l'arriération mentale, traitées par la topectomie péri-calleuse antérieure bilatérale. *Semaine des Hôpitaux de Paris, 26,* 1536–1551.

Lehmann, H. E. 1955. Therapeutic results with chlorpromazine (largactile) in psychiatric conditions, *Can. Med. Assoc. J., 72,* 91–99.

———. 1975. Schizophrenia: Clinical features. In A. M. Freedman, H. I. Kaplan, and B. J. Sadock (Eds.), *Comprehensive textbook of psychiatry.* Baltimore: Williams & Wilkins. Pp. 890–923.

Lehmann, H., and Hanrahan, G. 1954. Chlorpromazine, a new inhibiting agent for psychomotor excitement and manic states. *Arch. Neurology and Psychiatry, 71,* 227–237.

Lehmann, H. E., and Ostrow, D. E. 1973. Quizzing the expert: Clinical criteria for psychosurgery. *Hosp. Physician, 9,* 24–31.

Leinwand, S. N. 1976. Aversion therapy: Punishment as treatment and treatment as cruel and unusual punishment. *S. Calif. Law Rev., 49,* 880–983.

Leitenberg, H. 1976. Behavioral approaches to treatment of neuroses. In H. Leitenberg (Ed.), *Handbook of behavior modification and behavior therapy.* Englewood Cliffs, N.J.: Prentice-Hall. Pp. 124–167.

Lesser, R. P., and Fahn, S. 1978. Dystonia: A disorder often diagnosed as a conversion reaction. *Am. J. Psychiatry, 135,* 349–352.

Levine, J. D.; Gordon, N. C.; and Fields, H. L. 1978. Evidence that the analgesic effect of placebo is mediated by endorphins (Abstract). Paper presented at the Second World Congress on Pain, Montreal, August.

Levine, R. J. 1975. Boundaries between research involving human subjects and accepted routine professional practices. In R. L. Bogomolny (Ed.), *Human experimentation.* Dallas: Southern Methodist University Press. Pp. 3–20.

Lewin, W. 1961. Observations on selective leucotomy. *J. Neurology, Neurosurgery, and Psychiatry, 24,* 37–44.

Lewinsohn, P. M. 1975. The behavioral study and treatment of depression. In M. Hersen, R. M. Eisler, and P. M. Miller (Eds.), *Progress in behavior modification, Vol. I.* New York: Academic Press. Pp. 19–64.

Lewontin, R. C. 1977. Biological determinism as a social weapon. In Ann Arbor Science for the People Editorial Collective (Eds.), *Biology as a social weapon.* Minneapolis: Burgess. Pp. 6–18.

Lidz, T. 1968. The family, language, and the transmission of schizophrenia. In D. Rosenthal and S. Kety (Eds.), *The transmission of schizophrenia.* New York: Pergamon. Pp. 175–184.

Lidz, T.; Flick, S.; and Cornelison, A. R. 1965. *Schizophrenia and the family.* New York: International University Press.

Lilly, J. C. 1978. *The scientist: A novel autobiography.* Philadelphia: Lippincott.

Limburg, C. C. 1951. A survey of the use of psychosurgery with mental patients. In N. Bigelow (Ed.), *Proceedings of the First Research Conference on Psychosurgery, 1949.* Bethesda, Md.: National Institutes of Health, U.S. Public Health Service Pub. No. 16. Pp. 165–173.

Lisowski, F. P. 1967. Prehistoric and early historic trepanation. In D. Broth-well and A. T. Sandison (Ed.), *Diseases in antiquity*. Springfield, Ill.: Charles C Thomas. Pp. 651–672.

Livingston, K. E. 1953. Cingulate cortex isolation for the treatment of psychoses and psychoneuroses. *Research Publications, Assoc. for Research in Nervous and Mental Disease, 31*, 374–378.

————. 1973. Neurological aspects of primary affective disorders. In J. R. Youmans (Ed.), *Neurological Surgery, Vol. 3*. Philadelphia: W. B. Saunders. Pp. 1881–1900.

————. 1975. Surgical contributions to psychiatric treatment. In S. Arieti (Ed.), *American handbook of psychiatry, Vol. 5*. New York: Basic Books. Pp. 548–563.

Lo, W. 1967. A follow-up study of obsessional neurotics in Hong Kong Chinese. *Brit. J. Psychiatry, 113*, 823–832.

Loevenhart, A. S.; Lorenz, W. F.; and Waters, R. M. 1929. Cerebral stimulation. *J. Am. Med. Assoc., 92*, 880–883.

London, P. 1969. *Behavior control*. New York: Harper & Row.

López-Ibor, J. J., and López-Ibor Aliño, J. J. 1977. Selection criteria for patients who should undergo psychiatric surgery. In W. H. Sweet, S. Obrador, and J. G. Martin-Rodriguez (Eds.), *Neurosurgical treatment in psychiatry, pain, and epilepsy*. Baltimore: University Park Press. Pp. 151–162.

Louisell, D. W., and Williams H. 1970–1977. *Medical malpractice*. New York: Matthew Bender.

Lowenbach, H., and Stainbrook, L. T. 1942. Observations on mental patients after electroshock. *Am. J. Psychiatry, 98*, 828–831.

Luria, R. E., and Berry, R. 1979. Reliability and descriptive validity of PSE syndromes. *Arch. General Psychiatry, 36*, 1187–1195.

Mabbott, J. 1939. Punishment. *Mind, 48*, 152–167.

McCance, R. A. 1951. The practice of experimental medicine. *Proc. Royal Soc. Med., 44*, 189–194.

McLaurin, R. L., and Heimer, F. 1965. The syndrome of temporal lobe contusion. *J. Neurosurgery, 23*, 296–304.

MacLean, P. D. 1958. Contrasting functions of limbic and neocortical systems of the brain and their relevance to psychophysiological aspects of medicine. *Am. J. Med., 25*, 611–626.

McNair, D. M.; Lorr, M.; Droppleman, L. F. 1971. *Profile of mood states*. San Diego, Calif.: Educational and Industrial Test Service.

McNeil, E. B. 1970. *The psychoses*. Englewood Cliffs, N.J.: Prentice-Hall.

Malamud, N. 1967. Psychiatric disorder with intracranial tumors of the limbic system. *Arch. Neurology, 17*, 113–123.

Marholin, D., II; Siegel, L. J.; and Phillips, D. 1976. Treatment and transfer: A search for empirical procedures. In M. Hersen, R. M. Eisler, and P. M. Miller (Eds.), *Progress in behavior modification, Vol. 3*. New York: Academic Press. Pp. 293–342.

Mark, V. H. 1973. Brain surgery in aggressive epileptics. *Hastings Center Rpt., 3*, 1–5.

————. 1974. A psychosurgeon's case for psychosurgery. *Psychology Today, 8*, 28–86.

————. In press. The sociobiological theory of abnormal aggression. In I. L.

Kutash, S. B. Kutash, and L. B. Schlesinger (Eds.), *Violence: Perspectives on murder and aggression.* San Francisco: Jossey-Bass.

Mark, V., and Ervin, F. 1968. Is there a need to evaluate the individuals producing human violence? *Psychiatric Opinion,* August, p. 32–34.

———. 1970. *Violence and the brain.* New York: Harper & Row.

Mark, V. H.; Folkman, J.; Ervin, F. R.; and Sweet, W. H. 1969. Focal brain suppression by means of a silicone rubber chemode: Technical note. *J. Neurosurgery, 30,* 195–199.

Mark, V. H., and Neville, R. 1973. Brain surgery in aggressive epileptics. Social and ethical implications. *J. Am. Med. Assoc., 226,* 765–772.

Mark, V. H., and Ordia, I. J. 1976. The controversies over the use of neurosurgery in aggressive states and an assessment of the critics of this kind of surgery. In T. P. Morley (Ed.), *Current controversies in neurosurgery.* Philadelphia: W. B. Saunders. Pp. 722–729.

Mark, V. H., and Sweet, W. H. 1974. The role of limbic brain dysfunction in aggression. In S. H. Frazier (Ed.), *Aggression.* Baltimore: Williams & Wilkins. Pp. 186–200.

Mark, V.; Sweet, W. H.; and Ervin. F. R. 1967. The role of brain disease in riots and urban violence. *J. Am. Med. Assoc., 201,* 895.

Mark, V. H.; Sweet, W. H.; and Ervin, F. R. 1972. The effect of amygdalectomy on violent behavior in patients with temporal lobe epilepsy. In E. Hitchcock, L. Laitinen, and K. Vaernet (Eds.), *Psychosurgery.* Springfield, Ill.: Charles C Thomas. Pp. 139–155.

Marks, I. M. 1975. Behavioral treatments of phobic and obsessive-compulsive disorders: A critical appraisal. In M. Hersen, R. M. Eisler, and P. M. Miller (Eds.), *Progress in behavior modification, Vol. 1.* New York: Academic Press. Pp. 65–158.

Marks, I. M.; Hallam, R.; Connolly, J.; and Philpott, R. 1976. *Nursing in behavioural psychotherapy.* London: Royal College of Nursing.

Marks, I. M.; Hodgson, R.; and Rachman, S. 1975. Treatment of chronic obsessive-compulsive neurosis by in-vivo exposure, *Brit. J. Psychiatry, 127,* 349–364.

Marshall, J. F. 1974. Stereotaxy for obesity. *Lancet, 2,* 106.

Marslen-Wilson, W. D., and Teuber, H.-L. 1975. Memory for remote events in anterograde amnesia: Recognition of public figures from news photographs. *Neuropsychologia, 13,* 353–364.

Mason, B. J. 1973. New threat to blacks: Brain surgery to control behavior. *Ebony,* February, pp. 63–72.

Mason, J. R. 1974. *Kaimowitz* v. *Department of Mental Health:* A right to be free from experimental psychosurgery? *Boston Univ. Law Rev., 54,* 301–339.

Maudsley, H. 1874. *Responsibility in mental disease.* New York: Appleton.

Mauriac, C. 1959. *The new literature.* New York: George Braziller.

May, P. R. A., and Van Putten, T. 1974. Treatment of schizophrenia: II. A proposed rating scale of design and outcome for use in literature surveys. *Comprehensive Psychiatry, 15,* 267–275.

Mayer, E. E. 1947–48. Prefrontal lobotomy and the courts. *J. Criminal Law and Criminology, 38,* 576–583.

Medvedev, Z., and Medvedev, R. A. A. 1979. *Question of madness.* New York: Norton.

Meisel, A.; Roth, L. H.; and Lidz, C. W. 1977. Toward a model of the legal doctrine of informed consent. *Am. J. Psychiatry, 134,* 285–289.

Melzack, R. 1975. The McGill pain questionnaire: Major properties and scoring methods. *Pain, 1,* 277–299.

Mendels, J. (Ed.). 1973. *Biological psychiatry.* New York: Wiley.

Mendlewicz, J. 1977. Applications of genetic techniques to psychiatric research. In A. Frazer and A. Winokur (Eds.), *Biological bases of psychiatric disorders.* New York: Spectrum. Pp. 79–88.

Menninger, K. 1968. *The crime of punishment.* New York: Viking Press.

Methvin, E. H. 1979. Should we halt the brain-probers? *Reader's Digest, 114,* 123–126.

Mettler, F. A. (Ed.). 1952. *Psychosurgical Problems* (The Columbia Greystone Associates, Second Group). New York: Blakiston.

Meyer, V. 1966. Modification of expectations in cases with obsessional rituals. *Behaviour Research and Therapy, 4,* 273–280.

Meyer, V.; Levy, R.; and Schnurer, A. 1974. The behavioural treatment of obsessive-compulsive disorder. In H. R. Beech (Ed.), *Obsessional States.* London: Methuen. Pp. 233–258.

Milgram, S. 1974. *Obedience to authority.* New York: Harper & Row.

Mills, H.; Agras, S.; Barlow, D.; and Mills, J. 1973. Compulsive rituals treated by response prevention. *Arch. Gen. Psychiatry, 28,* 524–529.

Milner, B. 1958. Psychological defects produced by temporal lobe excision. In *The brain and human behavior.* Proceedings of the Association for Research in Nervous and Mental Disease, Vol. 36. New York: Hafner. Pp. 244–257.

———. 1963. Effects of different brain lesions on card sorting. *Arch. Neurology, 9,* 90–100.

———. 1965. Visually-guided maze learning in man: Effects of bilateral hippocampal, bilateral frontal, and unilateral cortical cerebral lesions. *Neuropsychologia, 3,* 317–338.

Milner, B., and Teuber, H.-L. 1968. Alteration of perception and memory in man: Reflection on methods. In L. Weiskrantz (Ed.), *Analysis of behavioral change.* New York: Harper & Row. Pp. 268–375.

Mirsky, A. 1970. Neuroelectrophysiologic studies of centrally acting drugs: An overview. In A. DiMascio and R. Shader (Eds.), *Clinical handbook of psychopharmacology.* New York: Science House. Pp. 121–136.

Mirsky, A. F., and Orzack, M. H. 1976. Final report on psychosurgery pilot study. August 6 (typescript copy). Report to The National Commission for the Protection of Human Subjects of Biomedical and Behavioral Research. Bethesda, Md.: National Institutes of Health.

———. 1977. Final report on psychosurgery pilot study. Report to The National Commission for the Protection of Human Subjects of Biomedical and Behavioral Research. *Appendix: Psychosurgery.* Department of Health, Education and Welfare, Publ. No. (OS) 77-0002, U.S. Government Printing Office. Sec. II, pp. 1–167.

Mishkin, M. 1957. Effects of small frontal lesions on delayed alteration in monkeys. *J. Neurophysiology, 20,* 615–622.

Mitchell-Heggs, N.; Kelly, D.; and Richardson, A. 1976. Stereotactic limbic leucotomy. *Brit. J. Psychiatry, 128,* 226–240.

———. 1977. Stereotactic limbic leucotomy: Clinical, psychological, and physiological assessment at 16 months. In W. H. Sweet, S. Obrador, and J. G. Martin-Rodriguez (Eds.), *Neurosurgical treatment in psychiatry, pain, and epilepsy.* Baltimore: University Park Press. Pp. 367–379.

Moberly, W. 1968. *The ethics of punishment.* Hamden, Conn.: Shoe String Press.

Moniz, E. 1936. *Tentatives operatories dans le traitement de certaines psychoses.* Paris: Masson.

————. 1956. How I succeeded in performing the prefrontal leukotomy. In A. Sackler, M. Sackler, R. Sackler, and F. Marti-Ibanez (Eds.), *The great psychodynamic therapies in psychiatry.* New York: Paul Hoeber Med. Div., Harper & Row. Pp. 131–137.

Moore, F. D. 1975. Perspectives of biomedical research: A cultural and historical view. In F. C. Robbins (Ed.), *Experiments and research with humans: Values in conflict.* Washington, D.C.: National Academy of Sciences. Pp. 15–30.

Moore, M. S. 1975. Some myths about "mental illness." *Arch. Gen. Psychiatry, 32,* 1483–1497.

Morris, N. E. 1975. A group self-instruction method for the treatment of depressed outpatients. Unpublished doctoral dissertation, University of Toronto.

Morse, S. J. 1978. Crazy behavior, morals, and science: An analysis of mental health law. *S. Calif. Law Rev., 51,* 527–654.

Morse, S. J., and Watson, R. I., Jr. (Eds.). 1977. *Psychotherapies.* New York: Holt, Rinehart and Winston.

Moser, M.; Guyther, J. R.; Finnerty, F., Jr.; Richardson, D. W.; Langford, H.; Perry, H. M., Jr.; Wood, D. E.; Krishan, I.; Branche, G. C., Jr.; and Smith, W. M. 1977. Report of the Joint National Committee on Detection, Evaluation, and Treatment of High Blood Pressure. Department of Health, Education and Welfare, Pub. No. (NIH) 77-1088, U.S. Government Printing Office.

Mullan, J. 1971. Violent behavior. A case report presented at the Central Neurosurgical Society, Chicago, March.

Müller, D.; Roeder, F.; and Orthner, H. 1973. Further results of stereotaxis in human hypothalamus in sexual deviations: First use of this operation in addiction to drugs. *Neurochirurgia (Stuttgart), 16,* 113–126.

Murphy, J. M. 1976. Psychiatric labeling in cross-cultural perspective, *Science, 191,* 1019–1028.

Murphy, M. L.; Hultgren, H. N.; Detre, K.; Thomsen, J.; and Takaro, T. 1977. Treatment of chronic stable angina. *New Eng. J. Med., 297,* 621–627.

Myers, M. J. 1967. Informed consent in medical malpractice. *Calif. Law. Rev., 55,* 1396–1418.

Nádvorník, P., Pogády, J.; and Šramka, M. 1973. The results of stereotactic treatment of the aggressive syndrome. In L. Laitinen and K. Livingston (Eds.), *Surgical approaches in psychiatry.* Baltimore: University Park Press. Pp. 125–128.

Nádvorník, P.; Šramka, M.; and Patoprstá, G. 1977. Transventricular anterior hypothalamotomy in stereotactic treatment of hedonia. In W. H. Sweet, S. Obrador, and J. G. Martin-Rodriguez (Eds.), *Neurosurgical treatment in psychiatry, pain, and epilepsy.* Baltimore: University Park Press. Pp. 445–449.

Nádvorník, P.; Šramka, M.; Pogády, J.; and Patoprstá, G. 1974. Stereotactic treatment of some psychoses—Survey of results. *Acta Nervosa Superior (Praha), 16,* 124.

Narabayashi, H. 1969. Stereotaxic amygdalectomy (its long-term results). *Excerpta Medica International Congress Series, 8,* 193–198.

———. 1972. Stereotaxic amygdalectomy. In B. E. Eleftheriou (Ed.), *The neurobiology of the amygdala.* New York: Plenum. Pp. 459–483.

———. 1973. Stereotaxic operations for behavior disorders. *Progress in Neurol. Surgery, 5,* 113–158.

Narabayashi, H., and Shima, F. 1973. Which is the better amygdala target, the medial or lateral nuclei? In L. Laitinen and K. Livingston (Eds.), *Surgical approaches in psychiatry.* Baltimore: University Park Press. Pp. 129–134.

National Commission for the Protection of Human Subjects of Biomedical and Behavioral Research. 1976. *Research involving prisoners: Report and recommendations.* Department of Health, Education and Welfare, Pub. No. (OS) 76-131, U.S. Government Printing Office.

———. 1977. *Report and recommendations: Psychosurgery.* Department of Health, Education and Welfare, Pub. No. (OS) 77-0002, U.S. Government Printing Office.

National Council on Crime and Delinquency, Council of Judges. 1969. *Guides to sentencing the dangerous offender.* New York: National Council on Crime and Delinquency.

Nauta, W. J. H. 1958. Hippocampal projections and related neural pathways to the midbrain in the cat. *Brain, 81,* 319–340.

Nauta, W. J. H., and Domesick, V. B. 1979. Neural associations of the limbic system. In A. Beckman (Ed.), *Neural basis of behavior: Proceedings of the DuPont symposium on neural substrates of behavior.* New York: Spectrum.

Neville, R. C. 1974. Pots and black kettles: A philosopher's perspective on psychosurgery. *Boston Univ. Law Rev., 54,* 340–353.

———. 1975. Zalmoxis or the morals of ESB and psychosurgery. In W. Gaylin, J. Meister, and R. Neville (Eds.), *Operating on the mind.* New York: Basic Books. Pp. 87–116.

Newcombe, F. 1969. *Missile wounds of the brain: A study of psychological deficits.* London: Oxford University Press.

Newman, P. 1965. *The theory of exchange.* Englewood Cliffs, N.J.: Prentice-Hall.

Nicola, G. C., and Nizzoli, V. 1972. Psychosurgery: Experience with 95 consecutive cases (preliminary report). In I. Fusek and Z. Kunc (Eds.), *Present limits of neurosurgery.* Prague: Avicenum. Pp. 471–473.

Norris, N. E. 1975. A group self-instruction method for the treatment of depressed outpatients. Unpublished doctoral dissertation, University of Toronto.

Note. 1974. Developments in the law—Civil commitment of the mentally ill. *Harvard Law Rev., 87,* 1190–1406.

Noyes, A., and Kolb, L. 1958. *Modern clinical psychiatry.* Philadelphia: W. B. Saunders.

Nozick, R. 1974. *Anarchy, state, and utopia.* New York: Basic Books.

Obrador, S. 1977. Opening remarks in W. H. Sweet, S. Obrador and J. G. Martin-Rodriguez (Eds.), *Neurosurgical treatment in psychiatry, pain, and epilepsy.* Baltimore: University Park Press. P. xxv.

O'Donnell P. 1974. Ethical concepts of consent. In F. Ayd (Ed.), *Medical, moral and legal issues in mental health care.* Baltimore: Williams & Wilkins. Pp. 1–6.

Offer, D., and Sabshin, M. 1974. *Normality: Theoretical and clinical concepts of mental health.* New York: Basic Books.

Older, J. 1974. Psychosurgery: Ethical issues and a proposal for control. *Am. J. Orthopsychiatry, 44,* 661–674.

Olsenes, K.; Luczywek, E.; and Mempel, E. 1976. Wplyw amygdalotomii na pamiec I uczenie sie u chorych operowanych z powodu padaczki. *Neur. Neurochir. Pol.,* t X (XXVI), no. 6.

O'Neill, D. 1977. Psychosurgery denied murderer. *Sacramento Bee,* September 1, p. AA5.

Oppenheimer, J. R. 1956. Analogy in science. *Am. Psychologist, 11,* 127–135.

Orland, L. 1973. *Justice, punishment, treatment.* Riverside, N.J.: Free Press.

Orthner, H.; Müller, D.; and Roeder, F. 1972. Stereotaxic psychosurgery: Techniques and results since 1955. In E. Hitchcock, L. Laitinen, and K. Vaernet (Eds.), *Psychosurgery.* Springfield, Ill.: Charles C Thomas. Pp. 377–390.

Osterrieth, P., and Rey, A. 1944. Le test de copie d'une figure complexe. *Archives de Psychologie, 30,* 205–356.

Ounstead, C.; Lindsay, J.; and Norman, R. 1966. *Biological factors in temporal lobe epilepsy.* London: Heinemann.

Overall, J.; Pull, C.; Carranza, J.; and Cassano, G. 1977. Phenomenological classification of syndrome interpretation by psychiatrists in Italy, France, Mexico, and the United States. *J. Psychiatric Research, 13,* 225–236.

Packer, H. 1968. *The limits of the criminal sanction.* Stanford, Calif.: Stanford University Press.

Pandya, D. N.; Dye, P.; and Butters, N. 1971. Efferent cortico-cortical projections of the prefrontal cortex in the rhesus monkey. *Brain Research, 31,* 35–46.

Pandya, D. N., and Kuypers, H. G. J. M. 1969. Cortico-cortical connections in the rhesus monkey. *Brain Research, 13,* 13–36.

Pandya, D. N., and Vignolo, L. A. 1971. Intra- and inter-hemispheric projections of the precentral, premotor and arcuate areas in the rhesus monkey. *Brain Research, 26,* 217–233.

Paniagua, J. L.; Jimeno, A. L.; and Diaz-Aramendi, A. 1977. Stereotactic cingulotomy in aggression. In W. H. Sweet, S. Obrador, and J. G. Martin-Rodriguez (Eds.), *Neurosurgical treatment in psychiatry, pain, and epilepsy.* Baltimore: University Park Press. Pp. 399–400.

Papandreou, A. G. 1958. *Economics as a science.* Chicago: Lippincott.

——— . 1962. *Fundamentals of model construction in macro-economics.* Athens, Greece: C. Serbinis Press.

Papez, J. W. 1937. A proposed mechanism of emotion. *Arch. Neurology and Psychiatry, 38,* 725–743.

Parachini, A. 1973. Mind study: "Front" or frontier? *Los Angeles Herald Examiner,* April 15, p. 1.

Patterson, G. R. 1974. Interventions for boys with conduct problems: Multiple settings, treatments, and criteria. *J. Consulting and Clinical Psychology, 42,* 471–481.

Paul, G. L. 1967. Insight vs. desensitization in psychotherapy two years after termination. *J. Consulting Psychology, 31*, 333–348.

———. 1969. Outcome of systematic desensitization II: Controlled investigations of individual treatment; technique variations, and current status. In C. M. Franks (Ed.), *Behavior therapy: Appraisal and status.* New York: McGraw-Hill. Pp. 105–159.

Paul, G. L., and Shannon, D. T. 1966. Treatment of anxiety through systematic desensitization in therapy groups. *J. Abnormal Psychology, 71*, 124–135.

Pelletier, K. R. 1979. Holistic medicine: From pathology to optimum health. New York: Delacorte.

Penfield, W. 1978. *The mystery of the mind.* Princeton, N.J.: Princeton University Press.

Penfield, W., and Mathieson, G. 1974. Memory. *Arch. Neurology, 31*, 145–154.

Peraita, P., and Lopez de Lerma, J. 1977. Frontal psychosurgery—A review of 424 cases. In W. H. Sweet, S. Obrador, and J. G. Martin-Rodriguez (Eds.), *Neurosurgical treatment in psychiatry, pain, and epilepsy.* Baltimore: University Park Press. Pp. 211–215.

Peszke, M. A. 1975. Is dangerousness an issue for physicians in emergency commitment? *Am. J. Psychiatry, 132*, 825–828.

Peterson, L. R., and Peterson, M. J. 1959. Short-term retention of individual verbal items. *J. Exp. Psychology, 58*, 193–198.

Peterson, S. A., and Somit A. 1978. Methodological problems associated with a biologically-oriented social science. *J. Social. Biol. Struct., 1*, 11–25.

Physicians' Desk Reference. 1978. 32nd ed. Oradell, N.J.: Medical Economics Co.

Pilcher, C. 1937. Recent advances in neurosurgery. *Surgery, 1*, 131–143.

Plutchik, R.; Climent, C.; and Ervin, F. 1976. Research strategies for the study of human violence. In W. L. Smith and A. Kling (Eds.), *Issues in brain/behavior control.* New York: Spectrum. Pp. 69–94.

Pohl, W. 1973. Dissociation of spatial discrimination deficits following frontal and parietal lesions in monkeys. *J. Comp. and Physiol. Psychology, 82*, 227–239.

Pollitt, J. 1957. Natural history of obsessional states. *Brit. Med. J., 1*, 195–198.

Pope Pius XII, 1960. Crime and punishment. *Catholic Law, 6*, 92–109.

Poppen, J. L. 1948. Technic of prefrontal lobotomy. *J. Neurosurgery, 5*, 514–520.

Popper, K. R., and Eccles, J. C. 1977. *The self and its brain: An argument for interaction.* New York: Springer-Verlag.

Porteus, S. D. 1965. *Porteus Maze Test: Fifty years' application.* Palo Alto, Calif.: Pacific Books.

Porteus, S. D., and Kepner, R. D. 1944. Mental changes after bilateral prefrontal lobotomy. *Genetic Psychology Monographs, 29*, 3–115.

Post, F.; Rees, W.; and Schurr, P. 1968. An evaluation of bimedial leucotomy. *Brit. J. Psychiatry, 114*, 1223–1246.

Post, F., and Schurr, P. H. 1977. Changes in the pattern of diagnosis of patients subjected to psychosurgical procedures, with comments on their use in the treatment of self-mutilation and anorexia nervosa. In W. H. Sweet, S. Obrador, and J. G. Martin-Rodriguez (Eds.), *Neurosurgical treat-*

ment in psychiatry, pain, and epilepsy. Baltimore: University Park Press. Pp. 261–266.

Potkin, S. G. 1978. Are paranoid schizophrenics biologically different from other schizophrenics? *New Eng. J. Med., 298*, 61–66.

Potter, H., and Butters, N. In press. An assessment of olfactory deficits in patients with damage to prefrontal cortex. *Neuropsychologia.*

Prichard, A. 1896. A few medical and surgical reminiscences. Bristol, England: Arrowsmith. Pp. 19–20.

Project. 1968. The computerization of government files: What impact on the individual? *UCLA Law Rev., 15*, 1371–1498.

Puusepp, L. 1937. Alcune considerazioni sugli interventi chirurgici nelle malattie mentali. *Giornale della Accademia di medicina di Torino, 100*, 3–16.

Quaade, F. 1974. Stereotaxy for obesity. *Lancet, 1*, 267.

Quaade, F.; Vaernet, K.; and Larsson, S. 1974. Stereotaxic stimulation and electrocoagulation of the lateral hypothalamus in obese humans. *Acta Neurochirurgia (Vienna), 30*, 111–117.

Rabavilas, A., and Boulougournis, J. 1974. Physiological accompaniments of ruminations flooding and thought-stopping in obsessive patients. *Behaviour Research and Therapy, 12*, 239–243.

Rachman, S. 1971. *The effects of psychotherapy.* Oxford: Pergamon Press.
——— . 1976. Observational learning and therapeutic modeling. In M. P. Feldman and A. Broadhurst (Eds.), *Theoretical and experimental bases of the behaviour therapies.* London: Wiley. Pp. 193–226.

Rachman, S., and Hodgson, R. 1980. *Obsessions and compulsions.* Englewood Cliffs, N.J.: Prentice-Hall.

Rachman, S.; Hodgson, R.; and Marks, I. M. 1971. Treatment of chronic obsessive-compulsive neurosis. *Behaviour Research and Therapy, 9*, 237–247.

Rachman, S.; Hodgson, R.; and Marzillier, J. 1970. The treatment of an obsessional-compulsive disorder by modelling. *Behaviour Research and Therapy, 8*, 385–392.

Rachman, S.; Marks, I.; and Hodgson, R. 1973. The treatment of chronic obsessive-compulsive neurosis by modelling and flooding in vivo. *Behaviour Research and Therapy, 11*, 463–471.

Ramamurthi, B., and Davidson, A. 1975. Central median lesions—Analysis of 89 cases. *Confinia Neurologica, 37*, 63–72.

Ramsay, R., and Sikkel, R. 1971. Behaviour therapy and obsessive neurosis. Paper presented at the European Conference on Behaviour Therapy, Munich.

Rapoport, J. L.; Buchsbaum, M. S.; Zahn, T. P.; Weingartner, H.; Ludlow, C.; and Mikkelsen, E. J. 1978. Dextroamphetamine: Cognitive and behavioral effects in normal prepubertal boys. *Science, 199*, 560–563.

Raskin, A. 1974. A guide for drug use in depressed disorders. *Am. J. Psychiatry, 131*, 181–185.

Rawls, J. 1971. *A theory of justice.* Cambridge, Mass.: Belknap Press of Harvard University Press.

Reeves, A. G., and Plum, F. 1969. Hyperphagia, rage, and dementia accompanying a ventromedial hypothalamic neoplasm. *Arch. Neurology, 20*, 616–624.

Retterstol, N. 1975. Scandinavia and Finland. In J. G. Howells (Ed.), *World history of psychiatry*. New York: Brunner/Mazel. Pp. 207–237.

Rey, A. 1942. L'examen psychologique dans les cas d'encéphalopathie traumatique. *Archives de Psychologie, 28,* 286–340.

Richardson, A. E.; Kelly, D.; and Mitchell-Heggs, N. 1976. Lesion site determination in stereotactic limbic leucotomy. In W. H. Sweet (Ed.), *Neurosurgical Treatment in Psychiatry*. Baltimore: University Park Press. Pp. 363–365.

Robin, A., and Macdonald, D. 1975. *Lessons of leucotomy*. London: Henry Kimpton.

Robinson, M. F.; Freeman, W.; and Watts, J. W. 1951. Personality changes after psychosurgery. In N. Bigelow (Ed.), *Proceedings of the First Research Conference on Psychosurgery, 1949*. Bethesda, Md.: National Institutes of Health, U.S. Public Health Service Pub. No. 16. Pp. 159–162.

Rodin, E. 1973. A neurological appraisal of some episodic behavioral disturbances with special emphasis on aggressive outbursts. Exhibit AC-4 in *Kaimowitz* v. *Department of Mental Health*, Civil No. 73-19434-AW (Cir. Ct., Wayne Co., Mich.). July 10.

Rodriguez-Burgos, F.; Arjona, V.; and Rubio, E. 1977. Stereotactic cryothalamotomy for pain. In W. H. Sweet, S. Obrador, and J. G. Martin-Rodriguez (Eds.), *Neurosurgical treatment in psychiatry, pain, and epilepsy*. Baltimore: University Park Press. Pp. 679–683.

Roeder, F. D. 1966. Stereotaxic lesion of the tuber cinereum in sexual deviation. *Confinia Neurologica, 27,* 162–163.

Roeder, F. D.; Orthner, H.; and Müller, D. 1972. The stereotaxic treatment of pedophilic homosexuality and other sexual deviations. In E. Hitchcock, L. Laitinen, and K. Vaernet (Eds.), *Psychosurgery*. Springfield, Ill.: Charles C Thomas. Pp. 87–111.

Roger, A., and Dongier, S. 1950. Correlations electrocliniques chez 50 épileptiques internes. *Revue Neurologique, 83,* 593–596.

Röper, G.; Rachman, S.; and Marks, I. M. 1975. Passive and participant modeling in exposure treatment of obsessive-compulsive neurotics. *Behaviour Research and Therapy, 13,* 271–279.

Rorvik, D. 1969. Someone to watch over you (for less than 2 cents a day). *Esquire*, December, p. 164.

Rosen, G. M.; Glasgow, R. E.; and Barrera, M., Jr. A controlled study to assess the clinical efficacy of totally self-administered systematic desensitization. *J. Consulting and Clinical Psychology, 44,* 208–217.

Rosenfeld, A. 1968. The psychobiology of violence. *Life*, June 21, pp. 68–71.

Rosenhan, D. L. 1973. Being sane in insane places. *Science, 179,* 250–258.

Rosenthal, T. L., and Bandura, A. 1978. Psychological modeling: Theory and practice. In S. L. Garfield and A. E. Bergin (Eds.), *Handbook of psychotherapy and behavior change*. 2nd ed. New York: Wiley.

Rosvold, H. E.; Mirsky, A. F.; Sarson, I.; Bransome, E. B., Jr.; and Beck, L. H. 1956. A continuous performance test of brain damage. *J. Consulting Psychology, 20,* 343–350.

Rosvold, H. E., and Mishkin, M. 1950. Evaluation of the effects of prefrontal lobotomy on intelligence. *Can. J. Psychology, 4,* 122–126.

Rothman, L. M.; Sher, J.; Quencer, R. M.; and Tenner, M. S. 1976. Intracranial ectopic pituitary adenoma: Case report. *J. Neurosurgery, 44,* 96–99.

Royal College of Psychiatrists. 1977. Memorandum on the use of electroconvulsive therapy. *Brit. J. Psychiatry, 131,* 261–272.

Rubin, S. 1973. *The law of criminal corrections.* St. Paul: West Publishing Co.

Rubio, E.; Arjona, V.; and Rodriguez-Burgos, F. 1977. Stereotactic cryohypothalamotomy in aggressive behavior. In W. H. Sweet, S. Obrador, and J. G. Martin-Rodriguez (Eds.), *Neurosurgical treatment in psychiatry, pain, and epilepsy.* Baltimore: University Park Press. Pp. 439–444.

Rush, A. J.; Beck, A. T.; Kovacs, M.; and Hollon, S. 1977. Comparative efficacy of cognitive therapy and pharmacotherapy in the treatment of depressed outpatients. *Cognitive Therapy and Research, 1,* 17–37.

Ryan, W. 1976. *Blaming the victim.* New York: Vintage.

Rylander, G. 1948. Personality analysis before and after frontal lobotomy. In *Association for Research in Nervous and Mental Disease, the Frontal Lobes, 27,* 691–705.

Sadow, L., and Suslick, A. 1961. Simulation of a previous psychotic state. *Arch. General Psychiatry, 4,* 452–458.

Sano, K. 1975. Posterior hypothalamic lesions in the treatment of violent behavior. In W. S. Fields and W. H. Sweet (Eds.), *Neural bases of violence and aggression.* St. Louis: Warren H. Green. Pp. 401–420.

Sano, K.; Sekino, H.; Hashimoto, I.; Amano, K.; and Sugiyama, H. 1975. Posteromedial hypothalamotomy in the treatment of intractable pain. *Confinia Neurologica, 37,* 285–290.

Sano, K.; Sekino, H.; and Mayanagi, Y. 1972. Results of stimulation and destruction of the posterior hypothalamus in cases with violent aggressive or restless behaviors. In E. Hitchcock, L. Laitinen, and K. Vaernet (Eds.), *Psychosurgery.* Springfield, Ill.: Charles C Thomas. Pp. 57–75.

Sargant, W., and Slater, E. 1963. *An introduction to physical methods of treatment in psychiatry.* 5th ed. London: Churchill Livingstone.

Sargant, W.; Slater, P.; and Kelly, D. 1972. *An introduction to physical methods of treatment in psychiatry.* 5th ed. London: Churchill Livingstone.

Scheff, T. J. 1963. Cultural stereotypes and mental illness. *Sociometry, 26,* 438–452.

Scheff, T. J. 1966. *Being mentally ill: A sociological theory.* Chicago: Aldine.

Scheflin, A. W., and Opton, E. M., Jr. 1978. *The mind manipulators.* New York: Paddington Press.

Schildkraut, J. J. 1978. Current status of the catecholamine hypothesis of affective disorders. In M. A. Lipton, A. DiMascio, and K. F. Killam (Eds.), *Psychopharmacology: A generation of progress.* New York: Raven Press. Pp. 1223–1234.

Schneider, H. 1977. Psychic changes in sexual delinquency after hypothalamotomy. In W. H. Sweet, S. Obrador, and J. G. Martin-Rodriguez (Eds.), *Neurosurgical treatment in psychiatry, pain, and epilepsy.* Baltimore: University Park Press. Pp. 463–468.

Schvarcz, J. R. 1977. Results of stimulation and destruction of the posterior hypothalamus: A long-term evaluation. In W. H. Sweet, S. Obrador, and J. G. Martin-Rodriguez (Eds.), *Neurosurgical treatment in psychiatry, pain, and epilepsy.* Baltimore: University Park Press. Pp. 429–438.

Schvarcz, J. R.; Driollet, R.; Rios, E.; and Betti, O. 1972. Stereotaxic hypothalamotomy for behavior disorders. *J. Neurol. Neurosug., Psychiatry, 35,* 356–359.

Schwitalla, A. M. 1929. The real meaning of research and why it should be encouraged. *Modern Hospital, 33,* 77–80.

Schwitzgebel, R. 1969. Issues in the uses of an electronic rehabilitation system with chronic recidivists. *Law and Society Rev., 3,* 597–610.

Scoville, W. B. 1971. The effect of surgical lesions of the brain on psyche and behavior in man. In A. Winter (Ed.), *The surgical control of behavior.* Springfield, Ill.: Charles C Thomas. Pp. 53–68.

———— . 1972. Psychosurgery and other lesions of the brain affecting human behavior. In E. Hitchcock, L. Laitinen, and K. Vaernet, *Psychosurgery.* Springfield, Ill.: Charles C Thomas. Pp. 5–21.

———— . 1973. Surgical locations for psychiatric surgery with special reference to orbital and cingulate operations. In L. Laitinen and K. Livingston (Eds.), *Surgical approaches in psychiatry.* Baltimore: University Park Press. Pp. 29–36.

Scoville, W. B., and Bettis, D. B. 1977. Results of orbital undercutting today: A personal series. In W. H. Sweet, S. Obrador, and J. G. Martin-Rodriguez (Eds.), *Neurosurgical treatment in psychiatry, pain, and epilepsy.* Baltimore: University Park Press. Pp. 189–202.

Sellin, J. 1964. Death and imprisonment as deterrents to murder. In H. Bedau (Ed.), *The death penalty in America.* Garden City, N.Y.: Anchor Books. Pp. 274–284.

Sem-Jacobsen, C. W., and Styri, O. B. 1972. Depth-electrographic stereotaxic psychosurgery. In E. Hitchcock, L. Laitinen, and K. Vaernet (Eds.), *Psychosurgery.* Springfield, Ill.: Charles C Thomas. Pp. 76–82.

Semmes, J.; Weinstein, S.; Ghent, L.; and Teuber, H.-L. 1963. Correlates of impaired orientation in personal and extrapersonal space. *Brain, 86,* 747–772.

Shapiro, M. H. 1972. The uses of behavior control technologies: A response. *Issues in Criminology, 7,* 55–93.

———— . 1974. Legislating the control of behavior control: Autonomy and the coercive use of organic therapies. *S. Calif. Law Rev., 47,* 237–356.

———— . 1975. Therapeutic justification for intervention into mentation and behavior. *Duquesne Law Rev., 13,* 673–781.

Shaw, B. F. 1977. A comparison of cognitive therapy and behavior therapy in the treatment of depression. *J. Consulting and Clinical Psychology, 45,* 543–551.

Shaw, G. B. 1963. Preface on doctors. In *Bernard Shaw: Complete plays with prefaces.* New York: Dodd, Mead.

Sherman, A. R. 1972. Real-life exposure as a primary therapeutic factor in the desensitization treatment of fear. *J. Abnormal Psychology, 79,* 19–28.

Shuman, S. I. 1974. The emotional, medical, and legal reasons for the special concern about psychosurgery. In F. J. Ayd, Jr. (Ed.), *Medical, moral and legal issues in mental health care.* Baltimore: Williams & Wilkins. Pp. 48–80.

———— . 1977. *Psychosurgery and the medical control of violence.* Detroit: Wayne State University Press.

Siegel, S. 1956. *Nonparametric statistics.* New York: McGraw-Hill.

Siegler, M., and Osmond, H. 1974. *Models of madness, models of medicine.* New York: Macmillan.

Siegler, M.; Osmond, H.; and Newell, S. 1974. Models of alcoholism (Appendix II). In M. Siegler and H. Osmond (Eds.), *Models of madness, models of medicine.* New York: Macmillan. Pp. 243–266.

Sifneos, P. E. 1972. The prevalence of "alexithymic" characteristics in psychosomatic patients. In H. Freyberger (Ed.), *Topics of psychosomatic research.* Basel: Karger. Pp. 255–262.

Silving, H. 1961. "Rule of Law" in criminal justice. In G. Mueller (Ed.), *Essays in criminal science.* Hackensack, N.J.: Rothman. Pp. 77–154.

Singer, R., and Statsky, W. 1974. *Rights of the imprisoned.* Indianapolis: Bobbs-Merrill.

Small, I. F.; Heimburger, R. F.; Small, J. G.; Milstein, V.; and Moore, D. F. 1977. Follow-up of stereotaxic amygdalotomy for seizure and behavior disorders. *Biol. Psychiatry, 12,* 401–411.

Smith, A. 1964. Changing effects of frontal lesions in man. *J. Neurol. Neurosurg., Psychiatry, 27,* 511–515.

Smith, A., and Kinder, E. F. 1959. Changes in psychological test performances of brain operated schizophrenics after 8 years. *Science, 129,* 149–150.

Smith, J. S. 1977. The treatment of anxiety, depression and obsessionality. In J. S. Smith and L. G. Kiloh (Eds.), *Psychosurgery and society.* New York: Pergamon Press. Pp. 25–35.

Smith, J. S., and Kiloh, L. G. 1977. *Psychosurgery and society.* New York: Pergamon Press.

Smith, J. S.; Kiloh, L. G.; Cochrane, N.; and Klijajic, I. 1976. A prospective evaluation of open prefrontal leucotomy. *Med. J. Australia, 1,* 731–735.

Snyder, S. H. 1974. *Madness and the brain.* New York: McGraw-Hill.

Snyder, S. H., and Matthysse, S. 1975. Opiate receptor mechanisms. *Neurosciences Res. Program Bull., 13,* 1–166.

Sociobiology Study Group. 1977. Sociobiology: A new biological determinism. In Ann Arbor Science for the People Editorial Collective (Eds.), *Biology as a social weapon.* Minneapolis: Burgess. Pp. 133–149.

Spece, R. G. 1972. Note. Conditioning and other technologies used to "treat?" "rehabilitate?" "demolish?" prisoners and mental patients. *Calif. Law Rev., 45,* 616–684.

Special Report. 1973. Neurological syndromes associated with antipsychotic drug use. *Arch. Gen. Psychiatry, 28,* 463–467.

Spiegel, E. A.; Wycis, H. T.; and Freed, H. 1949. Thalatomy: Neuropsychiatric aspects. *N.Y. State J. Med., 49,* 2273–2274.

Spitzer, R. L.; and Endicott, J. 1970. *Problem Appraisal Scale (PAS).* New York: State Department of Mental Hygiene.

Spitzer, R. L.; Endicott, J.; Fleiss, J. L.; and Cohen, J. 1970. The psychiatric status schedule. *Arch. Gen. Psychiatry, 23,* 41–55.

Spitzer, R. L.; Endicott, J.; and Robins, E. 1975. Clinical criteria for psychiatric diagnosis DSM III. *Am. J. Psychiatry, 132,* 1187–1192.

Spitzer, R. L., and Fleiss, G. L. 1974. A re-analysis of the reliability of psychiatric diagnosis. *Brit. J. Psychiatry, 125,* 341–347.

Šramka, M., and Nádvorník, P. 1975. Surgical complication of posterior hypothalamotomy. *Confinia Neurologica, 37,* 193–194.

Šramka, M.; Sedlak, P.; and Nádvorník, P. 1977. Observation of kindling phenomenon in treatment of pain by stimulation in thalamus. In W. H. Sweet, S. Obrador, and J. G. Martin-Rodriguez (Eds.), *Neurosurgical treatment in psychiatry, pain, and epilepsy.* Baltimore: University Park Press. Pp. 651–654.

Srole, L.; Langner, T. S.; Michael, S. T.; Opler, M. K.; and Rennie, T. A. C. 1962. *Mental health in the metropolis: The Midtown Manhattan Study.* New York: McGraw-Hill.

Staff of Subcommittee on Constitutional Rights of the Senate Committee on the Judiciary. 1974. Individual rights and the federal role in behavior modification. 93rd Congress, 2nd Session, Committee Print.

Stapp, H. P. 1971. S-matrix interpretation of quantum theory. *Physical Rev., D3,* 1303–1320.

Stender, F. 1974. The need to abolish "corrections." *Santa Clara Lawyer, 14,* 793–809.

Stern, R., and Marks, I. M. 1973. Brief and prolonged flooding. *Arch. Gen. Psychiatry, 28,* 270–276.

Sternberg, M. 1974. Physical treatments in obsessional disorders. In H. R. Beech (Ed.), *Obsessional states.* London: Methuen. Pp. 291–306.

Stevens, J. C., and Mack, J. D. 1959. Scales of apparent force. *J. Exp. Psychology, 5,* 405.

Stokes, T. F., and Bear, D. M. 1977. An implicit technology of generalization. *J. Appl. Behavior Analysis, 10,* 349–367.

Stone, A. 1975. Psychosurgery in Massachusetts: A task force report. *Mass. J. Mental Health, 5,* 26.

Ström-Olsen, R., and Carlisle, S. 1971. Bifrontal stereotactic tractotomy. *Brit. J. Psychiatry, 118,* 141–154.

Ström-Olsen, R., and Carlisle, S. 1972. Bifrontal stereotaxic tractotomy. In E. Hitchcock, L. Laitinen, and K. Vaernet (Eds.), *Psychosurgery.* Springfield, Ill.: Charles C Thomas. Pp. 278–288.

Stroufe, L. A., and Steward, M. A. 1973. Treating problem children with stimulant drugs. *New Eng. J. Med., 289,* 407–412.

Sweet, W. H. 1970. Foreword. In V. H. Mark and F. R. Ervin, *Violence and the brain.* New York: Harper & Row. P. vii.

——— . 1973. Treatment of medically intractable mental disease by limited frontal leucotomy—justifiable? *New Eng. J. Med., 289,* 1117–1125.

Sweet, W. H.; Ervin, F.; and Mark, V. H. 1969. The relationship of violent behavior to focal cerebral disease. In S. Garattini and E. B. Sigg (Eds.), *Aggressive behavior.* New York: Wiley. Pp. 336–352.

Sykes, M., and Tredgold, R. 1964. Restricted orbital undercutting. *Brit. J. Psychiatry, 110,* 609–640.

Szasz, T. S. 1960. The myth of mental illness. *Am. Psychologist, 15,* 113–118.

——— . 1961. Rev. ed. 1974. *The myth of mental illness: Foundations of a theory of personal conduct.* New York: Harper & Row.

——— . 1963. *Law, liberty and psychiatry.* New York: Macmillan.

——— . 1965. *Psychiatric justice.* New York: Collier Books.

——— . 1970. *The manufacture of madness: A comparative study of the inquisition and the mental health movement.* New York: Harper & Row.

——— . 1972. Introduction. In B. J. Ennis (Ed.), *Prisoners of psychiatry: Mental patients, psychiatrists and the law.* New York: Harcourt Brace Jovanovich. Pp. xi–xix.

——— . 1977. Aborting unwanted behavior: The controversy on psychosurgery. *The Humanist, 37* (No. 4), 7–11.

————. 1978. *The myth of psychotherapy*. Garden City, N.Y.: Anchor Press/Doubleday.

Tan, E.; Marks, I.; and Marset, P. 1971. Bimedial leucotomy in obsessive-compulsive neurosis: A controlled serial enquiry. *Brit. J. Psychiatry, 118,* 155–164.

Task Force of the Presidential Advisory Group on Anticipated Advances in Science and Technology. 1976. The science court experiment: An interim report. *Science, 193,* 653–656.

Taylor, L. B. 1969. Localization of cerebral lesions by psychological testing. *Clinical Neurosurgery, 16,* 269–287.

Taylor, M. A.; Gaztanaga, P.; and Abrams, R. 1974. Manic-depressive illness and acute schizophrenia: A clinical, family history, and treatment-response study. *Am. J. Psychiatry, 131,* 678–682.

Tecce, J.; Orzack, M. H.; and Mirsky, A. F. In press. Absence of CNV rebound in psychosurgery patients. In D. A. Otto (Ed.), *Multi-disciplinary perspectives in event related brain potential research*. Washington, D.C.: U.S. Government Printing Office.

Teuber, H.-L.; Battersby, W. A.; and Bender, M. B. 1951. Performance of complex visual tasks after cerebral lesions. *J. Nervous and Mental Disease, 114,* 413–429.

Teuber, H.-L.; Corkin, S. H.; and Twitchell, T. E. 1977a. Study of cingulotomy in man: A summary. In W. H. Sweet, S. Obrador, and J. G. Martin-Rodriquez (Eds.), *Neurosurgical treatment in psychiatry, pain, and epilepsy*. Baltimore: University Park Press. Pp. 355–362.

————. 1977b. A study of cingulotomy in man. Report to The National Commission for the Protection of Human Subjects of Biomedical and Behavioral Research. *Appendix: Psychosurgery*. Department of Health, Education and Welfare, Pub. No. (OS) 77-0002, U.S. Government Printing Office. Sec. III, pp. 1–115.

Teuber, H.-L., and Mishkin, M. 1954. Judgment of visual and postural vertical after brain injury. *J. Psychology, 38,* 161–175.

Thurstone, L. L. 1944. *A factorial study of perception*. Chicago: University of Chicago Press.

Titmus, R. M. 1971. *The gift relationship*. New York: Pantheon Books.

Tooth, G. C., and Newton, M. P. 1961. Leucotomy in England and Wales 1942–1954. *Great Britain Ministry of Health Reports on Public Health and Medical Subjects*, No. 104. London: Her Majesty's Stationery Office.

Torrey, E. F. 1974. *The death of psychiatry*. Radnor, Pa.: Chilton.

Tow, P. M. 1952. Therapeutic trauma of the brain. *Lancet, 2,* 253–255.

————. 1955. *Personality changes following frontal leucotomy*. London: Oxford University Press.

Tribe, L. H. 1978. *American constitutional law*. Mineola, N.Y.: Foundation Press.

Trotter, R. J. 1973a. Psychosurgery: The courts and Congress, *Science News*, May 12, pp. 310–311.

————. 1973b. Peter Breggin's private war. *Human Behavior*, November, pp. 50–57.

Turek, I. S., and Hanlon, T. E. 1977. The effectiveness and safety of electroconvulsive therapy (ECT). *J. Nervous and Mental Disease, 164,* 419–431.

Turnbull, F. 1969. Neurosurgery in the control of unmanageable affective reactions: A critical review. In *Clinical neurosurgery, Vol. 16.* Baltimore: Williams & Wilkins. Pp. 218–233.

Turner, E. 1973a. The concept of diencephalic instability. In L. Laitinen and K. Livingston (Eds.), *Surgical approaches in psychiatry.* Baltimore: University Park Press. Pp. 237–241.

——. 1973b. Custom psychosurgery. *Postgrad. Med. J.,* 49, 834–844.

Ulett, G. A. 1972. *A synopsis of contemporary psychiatry.* St. Louis: C. V. Mosby.

Ullmann, L. P., and Krasner, L. 1969. *A psychological approach to abnormal behavior.* Englewood Cliffs, N.J.: Prentice-Hall.

Umbarger, D.; Dalsimer, J.; Morrison, A.; and Breggin, P. 1962. *College students in a mental hospital.* New York: Grune & Stratton.

Usdin, E.; Hamburg, D. A.; and Barchas, J. D. (Eds.). 1977. *Neuroregulators and psychiatric disorders.* New York: Oxford University Press.

Vaernet, K. 1973. Behavior disorders—Neurosurgical therapy. Paper given before the American Association of Neurological Surgeons, Los Angeles, April.

Vaernet, K., and Madsen, A. 1970. Stereotaxic amygdalotomy and basofrontal tractotomy in psychotics with aggressive behavior. *J. Neurology, Neurosurgery, and Psychiatry,* 33, 858–863.

——. 1972. Lesions in the amygdala and the substantia innominata in aggressive psychotic patients. In E. Hitchcock, L. Laitinen, and K. Vaernet (Eds.), *Psychosurgery.* Springfield, Ill.: Charles C Thomas. Pp. 187–194.

Valenstein, E. S. 1973. *Brain control: A critical examination of brain stimulation and psychosurgery.* New York: Wiley.

——. 1975. Persistent problems in the physical control of the brain. Forty-fourth James Arthur Lecture on the Evolution of the Human Brain. New York: American Museum of Natural History.

——. 1976. Brain stimulation and the origin of violent behavior. In W. L. Smith and A. Kling (Eds.), *Issues in brain/behavior control.* New York: Spectrum. Pp. 33–48.

——. 1977. The practice of psychosurgery: A survey of the literature (1971–1976). Report to The National Commission for the Protection of Human Subjects of Biomedical and Behavioral Research. *Appendix: Psychosurgery.* Department of Health, Education and Welfare, Pub. No. (OS) 77-0002, U.S. Government Printing Office, Pp. I-1 to I-183.

——. 1978. Science-fiction fantasy and the brain. *Psychology Today,* 12 (No. 2), 28–39.

Valla, L. 1967. On free will. In A. B. Fallico and H. Shapiro (Eds.), *Rennaissance philosophy I.* New York: Random House. Pp. 41–65.

Van Rensburg, M. J.; Proctor, N. S. F.; Danziger, J.; and Orelowitz, M. S. 1975. Temporal lobe epilepsy due to an intracerebral schwannoma: Case report. *J. Neurology, Neurosugery, and Psychiatry,* 38, 703–709.

Vaughan, H. G. 1975. Psychosurgery and brain stimulation in historical perspective. In W. M. Gaylin, J. S. Meister, and R. C. Neville (Eds.), *Operating on the mind.* New York: Basic Books. Pp. 24–72.

Veatch, R. M. 1977. *Case studies in medical ethics.* Cambridge, Mass.: Harvard University Press.

Vonderahe, A. H. 1940. Forebrain and rage reaction. *Trans. Am. Neurol. Assoc., 66*, pp. 127–131.

von Hoffman, N. 1971. Brain maim. *Washington Post,* July 16, p. B1.

Vosburg, R. 1962. Lobotomy in Western Pennsylvania: Looking backward over ten years. *Am. J. Psychiatry, 119,* 503–510.

Walker, A. E. 1972. Varieties of retribution. In R. Gerber and P. McAnany (Eds.), *Contemporary punishment.* North Bend, Ind.: University of Notre Dame Press.

————. 1973. Man and his temporal lobes. *Surgical Neurology, 1,* 69–79.

Walsh, K. W. 1977. Neuropsychological aspects of modified leucotomy. In W. H. Sweet, S. Obrador, and A. G. Martin-Rodriguez (Eds.), *Neurosurgical treatment in psychiatry, pain, and epilepsy.* Baltimore: University Park Press. Pp. 163–174.

————. 1978. *Neuropsychology: A clinical approach.* New York: Churchill Livingstone.

Waltz, J. R., and Inbau, F. E. 1971. *Medical jurisprudence.* New York: Macmillan.

Waltz, J. R., and Scheuneman, T. W. 1970. Informed consent to therapy. *Northwestern Univ. Law Rev., 64,* 628–650.

Watson, J. P., and Marks, I. M. 1971. Relevant and irrelevant fear in flooding—A crossover study of phobic patients. *Behavior Therapy, 2,* 275–293.

Waxman, S. G., and Geschwind, N. 1975. The interictal behavior syndrome of temporal lobe epilepsy. *Arch. Gen. Psychiatry, 32,* 1580–1586.

Wechsler, D. W. 1945. A standardized memory scale for clinical use. *J. Psychology, 19,* 87–95.

————. 1946. *Wechsler-Bellevue Intelligence Scale, Form II.* New York: Psychological Corp.

————. 1955. *Wechsler Adult Intelligence Scale.* New York: Psychological Corp.

Weisskopf, V. F. 1972. What is an elementary particle? Unpublished manuscript of talk given at the 50th Anniversary Session of the General Assembly of the International Union of Pure and Applied Physics, September.

Wender, P. H. 1971. *Minimal brain dysfunction in children.* New York: Wiley Interscience.

Wexler, D. 1975. Reflections on the legal regulation of behavior modification in institutional settings. *Ariz. Law Rev., 17,* 132–143.

White, J. C., and Sweet, W. H. 1955. *Pain: Its mechanisms and neurosurgical control.* Springfield, Ill.: Charles C Thomas.

Whitehead, D. 1938. Improvement and recovery rates in dementia praecox without insulin therapy. *Psychiatric Quarterly, 12,* 409–413.

Whitty, C. W. M.; Duffield, J. E.; Tow, P. M.; and Cairns, H. 1952. Anterior cingulectomy in the treatment of mental disease. *Lancet, 262,* 475–481.

Wiener, N. 1948. Time, communications and the nervous system. *N.Y. Academy of Sciences Annals, 50,* 197–220.

Willett, R. A. 1960. The effects of psychosurgical procedure on behaviour. In H. J. Eysenck (Ed.), *Handbook of abnormal psychology.* London: Pitman. Pp. 566–610.

Williams, R. J. 1956. *Biochemical individuality: The basis for the genetotrophic concept.* New York: Wiley.

Williamson, F. 1975. Leucotomy for the relief of an obsessional neurosis. *Nursing Times, 71,* 812–815.

Wilson, D. H., and Chang, A. E. 1974. Bilateral anterior cingulectomy for the relief of intractable pain: Report of 23 patients. *Confinia Neurologica, 36,* 61–68.

Wilson, I., and Warland, E. H. 1947. Prefrontal leucotomy in a thousand cases. Report written for Great Britain Board of Control. London: Her Majesty's Stationery Office.

Winter, A. 1972. Depression and intractable pain treated by modified prefrontal lobotomy. *J. Medical Society, 69,* 757–759.

Wolpe, J. 1958. *Psychotherapy by reciprocal inhibition.* Stanford, Calif.: Stanford University Press.

Wonnenberger, M.; Henkel, D.; Arentewicz, G.; and Hasse, A. 1975. Studie zu einem Selbsthilfe-program für zwangneurotische Patienten. *Zeitschrift für Klinische Psychologie, 4,* 124–136.

Woodruff, R. A.; Goodwin, D. W.; and Guze, S. B. 1974. *Psychiatric diagnosis.* New York: Oxford University Press.

Wootton, B. 1963. *Crime and the criminal law: Reflections of a magistrate and social scientist.* London: Stevens & Sons.

Wynne, L. 1968. Methodologic and conceptual issues in the study of schizophrenics and their families. In D. Rosenthal and S. Kety (Eds.), *The transmission of schizophrenia.* New York: Pergamon. Pp. 185–199.

Yin, R. K. 1970. Face recognition by brain-injured patients: A dissociable disability? *Neuropsychologia, 8,* 395–402.

Zaidel, D., and Sperry, R. W. 1974. Memory impairment after commissurotomy in man. *Brain, 97,* 263–272.

Zigler, E., and Phillips, L. 1961. Psychiatric diagnosis: A critique. *J. Abnormal and Soc. Psychology, 63,* 607–618.

Zubin, J. 1967. Classification of the behavior disorders. In P. R. Farnsworth, O. McNemar and Q. McNemar (Eds.), *Annual Review of Psychology,* Vol. 18. Palo Alto, Calif.: Annual Reviews. Pp. 373–406.

Index of Names

Aarons, L., 50, 487, 521
Abrams, R., 404
Adams, J. E., 134
Akiskal, H. S., 287
Allen, F. A., 526
Alpers, B. J., 133
Andenaes, J., 523, 524, 525
Andersen, R., 458, 460, 491
Andy, O. J., 130, 155, 487
Annas, G. J., 386, 392, 393, 394, 398,
    493, 495, 496, 504
Arieti, S., 282, 284
Arjona, V., 161
Arnot, R., 490
Astrachan, M., 485

Bailey, H. R., 92, 155
Balasubramaniam, V., 48, 57, 83, 94,
    99, 153, 162, 199, 336, 491
Ballantine, H. T., Jr., 28, 64, 78, 106,
    109, 148, 153, 162, 165, 166, 167,
    539, 541
Bandura, A., 272, 304, 305
Barchas, J. D., 196
Bard, P., 57
Baretto, A. C., 27
Barlow, D. H., 304
Barnhart, B. A., 409
Barrera, M., Jr., 310
Barrett, C. L., 313
Bartlett, J. R., 63, 69, 96
Bateson, G., 319
Beall, J. G., Jr., 490
Bear, D. M., 48, 135, 136, 311, 540

Bechtereva, N. P., 61, 85
Beecher, H. K., 152, 325
Bell, C., 423
Bellack, A. S., 310
Benn, S., 525
Bentham, J., 523
Berg, E. A., 185
Berger, P. A., 196
Bergman, P., 316
Bernard, C., 349, 350
Bernstein, I., 114
Berry, R., 403
Bettis, D. B., 71, 98, 161, 162
Bingley, T., 151
Bird, D., 488
Birley, J., 117, 123
Bivens, L. W., 130
Blachly, P. H., 542
Blanchard, E. G., 305
Blaney, P. H., 290
Bluglass, R., 543
Blumer, D. P., 136
Boersma, K., 127
Bogen, J. E., 188
Bohm, D., 345, 346
Bond, E. D., 200
Bondartchuk, A. N., 85
Bosch, H., 15
Boulougournis, J., 127
Braceland, F. J., 200
Braginsky, B. M., 321
Braginsky, D. D., 321
Brakel, S. J., 409
Breggin, P. L., 487

583

Index of Topics